Functional
Neuroimaging

Functional
Neuroimaging
TECHNICAL FOUNDATIONS

Edited by

Robert W. Thatcher
M. Hallett
T. Zeffiro
E. Roy John
Michael Huerta*

Medical Neurology Branch
Clinical Neuroscience Division
National Institute of Neurological Disorders & Stroke
National Institutes of Health
Bethesda, Maryland

* Division of Neuroscience & Behavioral Science
National Institute of Mental Health
National Institutes of Health
Rockville, Maryland

Academic Press
San Diego   New York   Boston   London   Sydney   Tokyo   Toronto

Cover photograph: Combined surface and volume rendering of
reconstructed human brain. See Plate 33.

This book is printed on acid-free paper. ∞

Academic Press, Inc.
A Division of Harcourt Brace & Company
525 B Street, Suite 1900, San Diego, California 92101-4495

United Kingdom Edition published by
Academic Press Limited
24-28 Oval Road, London NW1 7DX

Library of Congress Cataloging-in-Publication Data

Functional neuroimaging : technical foundations / edited by Robert W.
    Thatcher ,,, [et al.].
        p.   cm.
        Includes bibliographical references and index.
        ISBN 0-12-685845-4
        1. Brain--Imaging.   2. Brain mapping.   3. Neural networks
    (Neurobiology)   I. Thatcher, Robert W.
    QP376.F773   1994
    612.8'2--dc20   93-37671

PRINTED IN THE UNITED STATES OF AMERICA
94   95   96   97   98   99   QW   9   8   7   6   5   4   3   2   1

Contents

I

RELATING STRUCTURE TO FUNCTION: LOCAL VERSUS SYSTEM PERSPECTIVES

1

Neural Models of Cortical Integration
Olaf Sporns, Giulio Tononi, and Gerald M. Edelman

2

Neural Modeling and Positron Emission Tomography
Barry Horwitz

3

Distribution-Free Statistical Analyses of Surface and Volumetric Maps
R. Clifford Blair and Walt Karniski

II

INTRASUBJECT ACTIVATION TECHNIQUES

4

Radiotracer Techniques for Functional Neuroimaging with Positron Emission Tomography
Peter Herscovitch

12

Three-Dimensional Surface-Based Spatial Normalization Using a Convex Hull

J. Hunter Downs III, Jack L. Lancaster, and Peter T. Fox

13

Statistical Probability Mapping of Brain Function and Structure

E. Roy John, Jian-Zhou Zhang, Jonathon D. Brodie, and Leslie S. Prichep

14

Three-Dimensional Correlative Imaging: Applications in Human Brain Mapping

A. C. Evans, D. L. Collins, P. Neelin, D. MacDonald, M. Kamber, and T. S. Marrett

15

Partial Volume Correction in Emission-Computed Tomography: Focus on Alzheimer Disease

Carolyn Cidis Meltzer and J. James Frost

16

Visualization and Warping of Multimodality Brain Imagery

Arthur W. Toga

17

Visualization Methods for Analysis of Multimodality Images

Richard A. Robb

18

Intersubject Comparison of PET Activation Data by MRI Matching

J. D. G. Watson

Contributors

Numbers in parentheses indicate the pages on which the authors' contributions begin.

R. Clifford Blair (19), Department of Epidemiology and Biostatistics and Department of Community and Family Health, College of Public Health, University of South Florida, Tampa, Florida 33612

Christian Bohm (121, 209), Department of Physics, University of Stockholm, S-10401 Stockholm, Sweden

Fred L. Bookstein (107), Center for Human Growth & Development, The University of Michigan, Ann Arbor, Michigan 48109

Mitchell Brigell (243), Department of Neurology, Loyola University Medical Center, Chicago, Illinois 60611

Jonathon D. Brodie (137), Department of Psychiatry, New York University Medical Center, New York, New York 10016

Raif Cakmur (243), Department of Neurology, Dokuz Eylul University, Izmir, Turkey

Verne S. Caviness, Jr. (201), Center for Morphometric Analysis, Department of Neurology, Massachusetts General Hospital, Harvard Medical School, Boston, Massachusetts 02214

Gastone Celesia (243), Department of Neurology, Loyola University Medical Center, Chicago, Illinois 60611

Chin-Tu Chen (233), Department of Radiology, The University of Chicago, Chicago, Illinois 60637

George T. Y. Chen (233), Department of Radiation and Cellular Oncology, The University of Chicago, Chicago, Illinois 60637

Simon R. Cherry (47), Department of Pharmacology, Imaging Sciences Division, Crump Institute for Biological Imaging, University of California, Los Angeles, School of Medicine, Los Angeles, California 90024

D. L. Collins (145), McConnell Brain Imaging Center, Montreal Neurological Institute, Montreal, Quebec, Canada H3A 2B4

Brian Cutillo (223), EEG Systems Laboratory & SAM Technology, San Francisco, California 94107

Gwendolyn Davis (95), The Research Imaging Center, University of Texas Health Science Center at San Antonio, San Antonio, Texas 78284

J. Hunter Downs III (131), Biomedical Image Analysis Division, Research Imaging Center, University of Texas Health Science Center at San Antonio, San Antonio, Texas 78284

Don DuRousseau (223), EEG Systems Laboratory & SAM Technology, San Francisco, California 94107

Gerald M. Edelman (1), The Neurosciences Institute, La Jolla, California 92037

Lars Eriksson (121, 209), Departments of Neuroradiology and Neurophysiology, Karolinska Institute/ Hospital, S-10401 Stockholm, Sweden

A. C. Evans (145), McConnell Brain Imaging Center, Montreal Neurological Institute, Montreal, Quebec, Canada H3A 2B4

Pauline A. Filipek (201), Center for Morphometric Analysis, Department of Neurology, Massachusetts General Hospital, Harvard Medical School, Boston, Massachusetts 02214

Peter T. Fox (95, 131), Biomedical Image Analysis Division, Research Imaging Center, University of Texas Health Science Center at San Antonio, San Antonio, Texas 78284

Karl J. Friston (79), The Neurosciences Institute, La Jolla, California 92037

J. James Frost (163), Department of Radiology, Division of Nuclear Medicine, The John Hopkins Medical Institution, Baltimore, Maryland 21287

Alan Gevins (223), EEG Systems Laboratory & SAM Technology, San Francisco, California 94107

Torgny Greitz (121, 209), Department of Neuroradiology, Karolinska Institute/Hospital, S-10401 Stockholm, Sweden

Ulf Grenander (217), Division of Applied Mathematics, Brown University, Providence, Rhode Island 02912

Robert Grzeszczuk (243), Department of Radiology, The University of Chicago, Chicago, Illinois 60637

Mark Hallett (251, 259, 269), Medical Neurology Branch, Clinical Neuroscience Program, National Institutes of Neurological Disorders and Stroke, National Institutes of Health, Bethesda, Maryland 20892

Peter Herscovitch (29), The Warren Grant Magnuson Clinical Center, National Institutes of Health, Bethesda, Maryland 20892

Hans Herzog (59), Institute of Medicine, Research Center Jülich, D-52425 Jülich, Germany

Barry Horwitz (9), Laboratory of Neurosciences, National Institute on Aging, National Institutes of Health, Bethesda, Maryland 20892

Martin Ingvar (121, 209), Department of Neurophysiology, Karolinska Institute/Hospital, S-10401 Stockholm, Sweden

Peter Jezzard (69), Laboratory of Cardiac Energetics, National Heart, Lung, and Blood Institute, National Institutes of Health, Bethesda, Maryland 20892

E. Roy John (137), Department of Psychiatry, New York University Medical Center, New York, New York 10016, and Nathan S. Kline Research Institute, Orangeburg, New York 10962

M. Kamber (145), McConnell Brain Imaging Center, Montreal Neurological Institute, Montreal, Quebec, Canada H3A 2B4

Walt Karniski (19), Department of Pediatrics, College of Medicine, University of South Florida, Tampa, Florida 33606

David N. Kennedy (201), Center for Morphometric Analysis, Departments of Neurology and Radiology, Massachusetts General Hospital, Harvard Medical School, Boston, Massachusetts 02214

Jack L. Lancaster (95, 131), Biomedical Image Analysis Division, Research Imaging Center, University of Texas Health Science Center at San Antonio, San Antonio, Texas 78284

Jian Le (223), EEG Systems Laboratory & SAM Technology, San Francisco, California 94107

Harrison Leong (223), EEG Systems Laboratory & SAM Technology, San Francisco, California 94107

David N. Levin (233, 243), Department of Radiology, The University of Chicago, Chicago, Illinois 60637

F. H. Lopes da Silva (279), Graduate School of Neurosciences, Institute of Neurobiology, Faculty of Biology, University of Amsterdam, 1098 SM Amsterdam, The Netherlands

D. MacDonald (145), McConnell Brain Imaging Center, Montreal Neurological Institute, Montreal, Quebec, Canada H3A 2B4

T. S. Marrett (145), McConnell Brain Imaging Center, Montreal Neurological Institute, Montreal, Quebec, Canada H3A 2B4

John C. Mazziotta (47), Departments of Neurology, Radiological Sciences, and Pharmacology, Division of Brain Mapping, University of California, Los Angeles, School of Medicine, Los Angeles, California 90024

Carolyn Cidis Meltzer (163), Department of Radiology, Division of Neuroradiology, The Johns Hopkins Medical Institutions, Baltimore, Maryland 21287

James W. Meyer (201), Center for Morphometric Analysis, Department of Neurology, Massachusetts General Hospital, Harvard Medical School, Boston, Massachusetts 02214

Shawn Mikiten (95), The Research Imaging Center, University of Texas Health Science Center at San Antonio, San Antonio, Texas 78284

Michael I. Miller (217), Department of Electrical Engineering, Electronic Signals and Systems Research Laboratory, Institute for Biomedical Computing, Washington University, St. Louis, Missouri 63110

P. Neelin (145), McConnell Brain Imaging Center, Montreal Neurological Institute, Montreal, Quebec, Canada H3A 2B4

Charles Pelizzari (233, 243), Department of Radiation and Cellular Oncology, The University of Chicago, Chicago, Illinois 60637

M. J. Peters (279), Department of Applied Physics, Low Temperature Division, University of Twente, Enschede, The Netherlands

Mark E. Pflieger (269), Neuroscan, Inc., El Paso, Texas 79902

Leslie S. Prichep (137), Department of Psychiatry, New York University Medical Center, New York, New York 10016, and Nathan S. Kline Research Institute, Orangeburg, New York 10962

Richard A. Robb (181), Biomedical Imaging Resource, Mayo Foundation, Rochester, Minnesota 55905

Robert L. Rogers (289), Neuromagnetism Laboratory, Epilepsy and Brain Mapping Center, Hospital of the Good Samaritan, Los Angeles, California 90017

Michael Smith (223), EEG Systems Laboratory & SAM Technology, San Francisco, California 94107

Jean-Paul Spire (243), Department of Neurology, The University of Chicago, Chicago, Illinois 60637

Olaf Sporns (1), The Neurosciences Institute, La Jolla, California 92037

Jeffrey A. Steck (243), Department of Neurology, The University of Chicago, Chicago, Illinois 60637

Robert W. Thatcher[1] (251, 259, 269), Medical Neurology Branch, Clinical Neuroscience Program, National Institutes of Neurological Disorders and Stroke, National Institutes of Health, Bethesda, Maryland 20892

Lennart Thurfjell (121, 209), Center for Image Analysis, Uppsala University, S-75237 Uppsala, Sweden

Arthur W. Toga (171), Laboratory of Neuro Imaging, Department of Neurology, University of California, Los Angeles, School of Medicine, Los Angeles, California 90024

Giulio Tononi (1), The Neurosciences Institute, La Jolla, California 92037

Camilo Toro (251, 259, 269), Medical Neurology Branch, Clinical Neuroscience Program, National Institutes of Neurological Disorders and Stroke, National Institutes of Health, Bethesda, Maryland 20892

Vernon L. Towle (243), Department of Neurology, The University of Chicago, Chicago, Illinois 60637

Robert Turner (69), Laboratory of Cardiac Energetics, National Heart, Lung, and Blood Institute, National Institutes of Health, Bethesda, Maryland 20892

Michael W. Vannier (217), Mallinckrodt Institute of Radiology, Washington University School of Medicine, St. Louis, Missouri 63110

Binseng Wang (251, 259), Biomedical Engineering and Instrumentation Program, National Center for Research Resources, and Human Motor Control Section, Medical Neurology Branch, National Institutes of Neurological Disorders and Stroke, National Institutes of Health, Bethesda, Maryland 20892

Eric M. Wassermann (251), Biomedical Engineering and Instrumentation Program, National Center for Research Resources, and Human Motor Control Section, Medical Neurology Branch, National Institute of Neurological Disorders and Stroke, National Institutes of Health, Bethesda, Maryland 20892

J. D. G. Watson[2] (191), Department of Anatomy, University College London, London WC1E 6BT, United Kingdom, and MRC Cyclotron Unit, Hammersmith Hospital, London W12 0HS, United Kingdom

H. J. Wieringa (279), Department of Applied Physics, Low Temperature Division, University of Twente, Enschede, The Netherlands

Roger P. Woods (47), Department of Neurology, Division of Brain Mapping, University of California, Los Angeles, School of Medicine, Los Angeles, California 90024

Thomas Zeffiro (251, 259), Biomedical Engineering and Instrumentation Program, National Center for Research Resources, and Human Motor Control Section, Medical Neurology Branch, National Institute of Neurological Disorders and Stroke, National Institutes of Health, Bethesda, Maryland 20892

Jian-Zhou Zhang (137), Department of Psychiatry, New York University Medical Center, New York, New York 10016, and Nathan S. Kline Research Institute, Orangeburg, New York 10962

[1] Present address: Veterans Affairs Medical Center, Neurology Service-151, Bay Pines, Florida 33504

[2] Present address: Department of Medicine, The University of Sydney, New South Wales, Australia 2006

Foreword

As part of the Human Brain Project, the National Institute of Mental Health (NIMH) encourages and supports advances in technology that facilitate the integration of all types of neuroscience information. Over the past decade, the NIMH has played an important role in encouraging and supporting the neuroimaging community to integrate structural and functional brain data. Neuroimaging represents a vast new frontier of methodology allowing us to visualize both structural and functional changes in the brains of intact functioning individuals. Because of its potential to greatly advance our understanding of normal and abnormal behavior, it is critical to the NIMH that these new methodologies be supported, and that information about their use and accuracy be disseminated quickly and widely.

The disciplines contributing to neuroscience include physics, biomathematics, and computer science, as well as neuropsychology, neurophysiology, and neuroanatomy. With so many varied groups of research scientists, areas of study, and modalities of research, integrating information has been difficult. By necessity, most researchers take a reductionist approach to their problems and work on a highly restricted aspect of brain function or even just one type of cell or brain nucleus. For this researcher, even maintaining an up-to-date knowledge base of colleagues' results in a restricted research area is difficult. This problem is now being addressed by a major federal initiative known as the Human Brain Project. This global effort will facilitate the integration of all knowledge on brain structure and function, making neuroscience more efficient and hastening our understanding of brain function and dysfunction. Of all fields comprising neuroscience, neuroimaging may be in the best position to take advantage of the Human Brain Project.

Around 1984 John Mazziotta and I had a number of discussions about the importance of the "new" imaging technologies and their associated problems.

As a scientist at NIMH, I felt that the capability to visually monitor the activity of the brain and visualize its structure would serve no field better than the research aimed at understanding mental disorders.

A major problem identified by researchers in this area is in integrating functional and structural information. One general solution to this problem lies in the combination and spatial alignment of data obtained by different modalities, such as magnetic resonance imaging (MRI) and positron emission tomography, using any of a variety of methods. This book discusses in detail the methods available to integrate this information across different modalities or, by the use of a single modality, MRI, to obtain both types of data. Other chapters focus on results from magnetoencephalography (MEG), which allows for the detection of electrical activity in the intact functioning human, below the level of the cortex, in a noninvasive manner. This approach to research has been pursued extensively by many groups of researchers throughout the world with success. Due to the enormous cost of this approach many groups are being forced to abandon MEG, perhaps prematurely.

The technological advances that will allow for greater and more in-depth study of the brain lie in front of us in an unpredictable time frame. We need new technologies to image structural and functional changes more precisely in functioning humans, both well and ill. New technologies are also needed to allow the study of the sites of therapeutic drug action in the brain; endogenous levels of neurotransmitters, their precursors, and metabolic products; states of activity of different receptor systems, as well as voltage-gated and transmitter-gated ion channels; and electrical activity of deep structures within the brain which when summated and measured from the skull provide the electrophysiology.

During the Decade of the Brain, neuroscientists will be afforded many new opportunities. These novel technologies will open new vistas toward understanding brain disorders. A major threat to this entire community is not the new knowledge afforded by these new technologies, but rather our inability to fully utilize this knowledge to understand brain structure and function. Even at this juncture we have a certain embarrassment of riches. Due to multiple "revolutions" in neuroscience and biology—neuroimaging, molecular and cellular biology, peptide and protein chemistry, pharmaceutical development, etc.—the amount of data available to any one researcher is overwhelming. This is reflected by the fact that there are more than 200 journals devoted to neuroscience and behavioral research, and that 40,000–50,000 neuroscientists are actively pursuing research worldwide.

The long-term objective of the Human Brain Project is to develop neuroscience databases and network systems that will be accessible to scientists around the world. Ultimately, these databases will allow neuroscience researchers, as well as clinicians, teachers, and students, to access the full range of information regarding current knowledge of the nervous system. The databases will contain information ranging from raw data, to data deposited as a supplement to published articles, to data highly synthesized from multiple sources, to directories of scientists and their areas of expertise. The network component

will ultimately allow global access to the databases and will permit scientists to share their data with each other in confidence, or in formats that are available to the public. The network will promote collaboration and cooperation across disciplinary and geographic borders. The development of this network is currently underway at the NIMH, the National Institute on Drug Abuse (NIDA), the National Science Foundation (NSF), the National Institute of Child Health and Human Development (NICHD), the National Institute on Aging (NIA), the National Institute on Deafness and Other Communication Disorders (NIDCD), the National Center for Research Resources (NCRR), the National Library of Medicine (NLM), the Office of Naval Research (ONR), and the National Aeronautics and Space Administration (NASA).

This book serves as a source of valuable information to neuroscientists today, and identifies technological breakthroughs and fresh insights in the uses of functional brain imaging. It is fitting that this book is published during the Decade of the Brain, since the discovery and demonstration of our capability to visually monitor both functionally and structurally the intact human brain is one of the events that led to the Presidential proclamation in 1990 making this the Decade of the Brain.

Stephen Koslow

Preface

Medical neuroimaging has evolved at an explosive rate in the past few years. High-resolution, three-dimensional anatomical information can now be obtained in a routine manner with magnetic resonance imaging (MRI) and computer-aided tomography (CT). Three-dimensional functional imaging of blood flow and metabolic information can be obtained from positron emission tomography (PET) images, and functional four-dimensional electrophysiology (EEG) and evoked potential information can be obtained using high-speed computers. Many laboratories throughout the world have successively superimposed various combinations of three-dimensional images to give enhanced anatomical and functional resolution. The three- and four-dimensional registration of different modalities of neuroimaging will require researchers and physicians to learn new techniques and to extract and combine the best features of each modality in order to better diagnose and plan for patient treatment. This explosion of new techniques also emphasizes the need to integrate and focus the efforts of scientists and clinicians to facilitate communication, establish standards, and develop training programs. The past five decades of growth of the science of the brain have witnessed an enormous differentiation of subdisciplines each with their own language and technologies, which is a further drive to integrate and find common ground within and between the subdisciplines. Although complete integration is impossible, it is in our power to integrate within families of subdisciplines. We believed that a sufficient number of scientific publications concerning the basic techniques of functional neuroimaging, as well as their clinical applications, warranted the creation of an edited volume with the goal of publishing in one place some of the most recent advancements in this field. It is principally these ideas and background which gave rise to this book.

Among the new subdisciplines of neuroscience is the field of functional neuroimaging in which both neural structure and function can be placed in registration. This subdiscipline principally encompasses EEG, magnetoencephalography (MEG), functional magnetic resonance imaging (FMRI), and PET with new technologies such as optical imaging and optical dyes still under development. This book is organized around the basic foundations of neural systems theory and image analysis and builds, in a stepwise manner, to the registration of different functional neuroimages.

The demand for integration and complementation is the engine that drives the effort to compile in one book the various neuroimaging technologies, such as MRI, PET, and EEG. A spectrum of structural and functional integration can occur through the synergism of these different imaging technologies, rendering new perspectives to each of the technologies. We recognized that a book was needed to encompass the outgrowth of fresh perspectives in functional neuroimaging, especially as they relate to clinical neuroscience. For purposes of clinical diagnosis and treatment there is a growing need to visualize the structural location of functional abnormalities of the brain. With the increasing image resolution of the MRI comes the opportunity to obtain a three-dimensional anatomical map upon which the functional images from FMRI, PET, EEG, and evoked potentials may be superimposed. Once adequate structural images are obtained, then registration of different functional images can create a spectrum of multimodal neuroimages from which more accurate diagnoses and a deeper understanding of brain abnormalities may emerge.

This book addresses the technical problems involved in the registration of MRI and PET, MRI and EEG/EP, and PET and EEG/EP, as well as critical conceptual issues regarding the registration of these modalities. Finally, it addresses research and clinical guidelines for future developments. The general goals are to discuss the technical problems of image registration, to present different approaches to intersubject and intrasubject analyses, to explore the synergistic advantages of multimodal integration, and to establish conceptual and practical guidelines for future developments. In the latter category, the issues of "normative" databases, intercampus exchange of information and the synergistic use of multivariate and univariate statistics to discriminate clinical populations will be addressed.

This book is organized into four sections: (I) Relating Structure to Function: Local versus System Perspectives; (II) Intrasubject Activation Techniques, (III) Intersubject Comparison Techniques (i.e., creation of normative databases and intercampus exchange of information), and (IV) Multimodal Registration Techniques. These sections are designed to build upon the theoretical foundations and mathematical techniques that are necessary for the understanding and maximal utilization of functional neuroimages. For example, Section I addresses issues such as the use of neural network modeling in functional neuroimaging (Sporns *et al.*, Chapter 1), how to relate spatial and temporal mappings (Horwitz, Chapter 2), and the general application of multivariate statistics and covariance analyses to functional neuroimaging (Blair and Karniski, Chapter 3). Section II addresses technical issues involved in activation techniques, such as blood flow versus metabolism (Herscovitch, Chapter 4). This chapter is especially important since it addresses the fundamental issues concerning the relationships between neuronal activity and blood flow. Section II also addresses advances in methods of intrasubject activation from PET (Woods *et al.*, Chapter 5 and Herzog, Chapter 6) to the functional MRI (Turner and Jezzard, Chapter 7). Section III is an extension and elaboration of Section II with special emphasis on the problems of intersubject comparisons and data-

base management. The problems of intersubject registration are further separated into probability mapping and registration to a brain atlas in Chapters 8 to 13 (Friston to John *et al.*) and registration to the MRI in Chapters 14 to 19 (Evans *et al.* to Kennedy *et al.*). Finally, Section IV addresses recent advances in multimodal registration in which various combinations of functional images are placed into registration. It begins with fundamental multimodal registration techniques in Chapters 20 to 22 (Ingvar *et al.* to Gevins *et al.*) and then extends the registration of three-dimensional spatial images to include the fourth dimension of time through the additional registration of EEG/ MEG dipoles in Chapters 23 to 29 (Pelizzari *et al.* to Rogers). The concept of four-dimensional tomographic EEG is explicitly introduced in Chapter 26 (Toro *et al.*) and Chapter 27 (Thatcher *et al.*) in which the temporal details of neural network switching are presented through PET and MRI registration and validation of EEG dipole sources followed by the computation of dipole coherence and phase.

The audience most interested in this volume will be neuroscientists in general, graduate students, psychologists, neuropsychologists, neurologists, neurosurgeons, radiologists, psychiatrists, and general practitioners interested in the use of EEG, MRI, and PET. A growing number of people are being trained to enter into the fields of functional neuroimaging, and the field is enjoying an increase in private and government funding. This increase in interest and funding is expected to continue into the foreseeable future and should result in new and exciting advances in both basic science and clinical applications. We hope that this book will aid in this effort by presenting cutting edge issues in a direct and readable manner.

Robert W. Thatcher

List of Color Plates

1

Neural Models of Cortical Integration

Olaf Sporns, Giulio Tononi, and Gerald M. Edelman

The Neurosciences Institute, La Jolla, California 92037

I. The Problem of Integration

In this chapter we review several computer models of the cerebral cortex that are rigorously based on anatomical and physiological data. They all focus on a key problem of brain function, the problem of *cortical integration*. The problem is posed because many studies have shown that the mammalian cerebral cortex is partitioned into numerous distinct areas, each specialized to carry out a relatively specific function (Zeki, 1978, 1990). In view of this degree of functional segregation the question of how neural activity in the various areas is integrated to form a unified percept of the world and to allow coherent behavioral responses arises.

A central aim of neuroscience since its very beginnings has been to identify the nature of neural integration (e.g., Sherrington, 1947), and the problem has recently received renewed attention (Damasio, 1989; Edelman, 1987, 1989; Engel *et al.*, 1992; Finkel and Edelman, 1989; Tononi *et al.*, 1992a, 1992b; Zeki, 1990). Most earlier attempts to explain integration have started from the notion that the visual cortex is organized hierarchically with a progressive increase in the specificity of its neurons from the sensory periphery to more central areas. According to one version of the model, perceptual integration is achieved by the confluence of diverse processing streams at a very high hierarchical level, or "master area." However, whereas there are areas of the brain that receive convergent inputs from multiple modalities or submodalities (Damasio, 1989), no single area has been identified that receives a sufficiently rich set of afferents to allow it to carry out a *universal* integrative function [for a contrasting view, see Young (1992)].

An alternative view of integration takes into account the cooperative interactions between different areas of the brain. This view is consistent with a characteristic anatomic feature of cortical organization: the abundance of reciprocal pathways linking functionally segregated areas. In the visual system, such reciprocal pathways exist between areas at the same or different hierarchical levels (Felleman and Van Essen, 1991). In addition neurons within each area are often densely and reciprocally interconnected [see, for example, Kisvarday and Eysel (1992)]. Some return projections are anatomically diffuse (Zeki and Shipp, 1988) and may serve a modulatory function, others can directly drive neurons in lower areas (Mignard and Malpeli, 1991). Edelman (1978) proposed that reciprocal pathways form the substrate of cortical integration by allowing the dynamic, bidirectional exchange of neural signals between areas in a process called *reentry*. Reentry can be defined as the "ongoing parallel signaling between separate maps along ordered anatomical connections" (Edelman, 1989). Modeling studies and experiments have shown that reentrant projections can directly influence the re-

FUNCTIONAL NEUROIMAGING

sponse properties of neurons (*constructive* function) and that reentry can give rise to patterns of temporal correlations (*correlative* function).

Recently, microelectrode recordings in the cat visual cortex have provided new evidence for the correlative function of reentry by revealing stimulus-dependent patterns of correlated neural activity. Gray and Singer (1989) reported that orientation-selective neurons show oscillatory discharges at around 40 Hz when presented with an optimally oriented stimulus. These oscillations can be observed in single cells (Jagadeesh *et al.*, 1992), as well as local populations of cells. Such populations, characterized by shared receptive field properties and temporally correlated discharge patterns, have been called *neuronal groups* (Edelman, 1978). Cortical oscillations have also been reported in motor cortex (Murthy and Fetz, 1992), inferotemporal cortex (Nakamura *et al.*, 1992), and visual cortex of the monkey (Kreiter and Singer, 1992).

Further experiments revealed widespread patterns of correlations in the cat visual system and provided support for the notion that these patterns depend on reentrant connectivity. When a single long light bar is moved across the receptive fields of spatially separated neurons with similar orientation specificity, cross-correlations reveal that their oscillatory responses are synchronized (Eckhorn *et al.*, 1988; Gray *et al.*, 1989). The synchronization becomes weaker if a gap is inserted into the stimulus contour and it disappears completely if two parts of the contour are moved separately and in opposite directions. Synchrony is established rapidly, often within 100 ms, and single episodes of coherency last for 50 to 500 ms. Frequency and phase of the oscillations vary within the range of 40–60 Hz and +/− 3 ms, respectively (Gray *et al.*, 1992). Synchronized neural activity was observed between cortical areas V1 and V2 (Eckhorn *et al.*, 1988; Nelson *et al.*, 1992) and between striate and extrastriate cortical areas (Engel *et al.*, 1991). Engel *et al.* (1991) have shown stimulus-dependent correlations between neurons located in the two hemispheres of cat visual cortex in response to two simultaneously presented stimuli, one on each side of the visual midline. These correlations disappear when the corpus callosum is transected, an indication that reentrant signaling is responsible for their generation. After transection, the hemispheres continue to show neuronal activity at normal levels; this supports the view that mean activity rates alone are an insufficient indicator of neural integration and that the temporal characteristics of neuronal firing play an important role in this process.

II. Neural Models of Integration

First, we will show how local populations of neurons may interact to produce locally correlated neuronal discharges. Then, we will address a specific and fundamental problem in visual perception, that of perceptual grouping and figure–ground segregation. We will see how temporal correlations might serve as the neural basis for these perceptual phenomena. We will also consider the effect of temporal correlations on behavior. Finally, we will briefly describe some key results obtained with a detailed model of the primate visual system.

A. Integration within Single Neuronal Groups

Experiments as well as modeling studies have suggested that individual cortical neurons are sensitive to temporal correlations in their inputs (Abeles, 1991; Bernander *et al.*, 1991). The discharge characteristics of a neuronal group are largely determined by cooperative interactions, and, typically, the correlated population activity is statistically more reliable than that of its constituent neurons. We have modeled neuronal groups in several computer simulations (Sporns *et al.*, 1989, 1991a, 1991b) (Fig. 1). We assumed that, within each group, cells are connected relatively sparsely and at random; for example, a given excitatory cell connects to 10% of all other excitatory cells within the group. Generally, intragroup connections are stronger relative to those between groups. In the simulations locally correlated oscillatory activity is generated by the interactions between excitatory cells and inhibitory cells within a group. The oscillation frequency depends critically on the temporal delay introduced by the recurrent inhibitory connections. In accordance with experimental results (Gray *et al.*, 1992), the instantaneous frequency of the oscillations varies significantly. This is due to the fact that each neuronal group acts as a population oscillator, composed of many sparsely connected and partly independent neurons. The coherent activity of such neuronal groups is statistically more reliable than the activity of each of its constituent neurons. Thus, neuronal groups represent a first, elementary step for establishing functionally significant correlations.

B. Figure–Ground Segregation

Temporal correlations as established by reentrant signaling may provide a key to the solution of a classi-

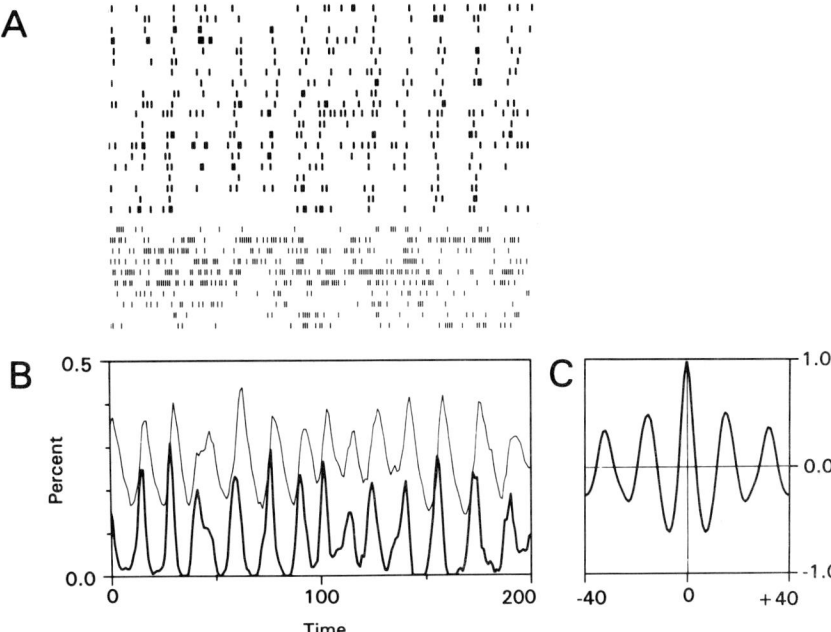

Figure 1 Rhythmic discharges in a simulated neuronal group. The group responds to an optimally oriented moving light bar and contains 160 excitatory and 80 inhibitory cells (Sporns *et al.*, 1989). (A) Firing patterns of 20 randomly selected excitatory (top) and 10 randomly selected inhibitory (bottom) cells for a time period of 200 ms. Excitatory cells discharge apparently irregularly, although a bursting pattern is occasionally observed. In the model, inhibitory neurons have a higher spontaneous firing rate that further obscures their oscillatory discharge pattern. (B) Population activity (analogous to a local field potential) of the same neuronal group recorded simultaneously with the single neurons shown in A. The rhythmic firing pattern of both the excitatory and inhibitory populations (thick and thin traces, respectively) is immediately apparent. The inhibitory population trails the excitatory one by several milliseconds. Note that the frequency shows considerable variations. (C) Autocorrelation of the excitatory cell population for the same time period shown in B.

cal problem in visual perception, that of perceptual grouping and figure–ground segregation. These two processes, both of fundamental importance in perceptual organization (Kanizsa, 1979), refer to the ability to group together elementary features into discrete objects and to segregate these objects from each other and from the background. At the beginning of this century, Gestalt psychologists thoroughly investigated the factors influencing grouping and the distinction between figure and ground. They described a number of perceptual laws, such as those of similarity, continuity, proximity, and common motion.

We have investigated the potential role of temporal correlations in perceptual grouping and figure–ground segregation in a model (Sporns *et al.*, 1991a) that consisted of an array of orientation- and direction-selective neuronal groups forming a map of visual space. These groups are linked by a pattern of reentrant connections similar to that existing in visual cortex. An important feature of the model is that synaptic efficacies of reentrant connections can change on a short time scale (within tens of milliseconds). In general, the efficacy among correlated groups increases (with the effect of rapidly amplifying and stabilizing the correlations) and that among uncorrelated groups decreases. These changes are transient; in the absence of activity, the efficacy rapidly (within 100–200 ms) returns to its resting value. Evidence for voltage-dependent, short-term increases in the efficacy of horizontal connections has been found in cat visual cortex (Gilbert, 1992; Hirsch and Gilbert, 1991). Fast modulation of synaptic efficacy has also been observed in other parts of the nervous system (e.g., Aertsen *et al.*, 1989, 1991; Ahissar *et al.*, 1992; Gochin *et al.*, 1991).

Figure 2 shows an example of the responses of the model. The groups responding to the bars that composed the object are rapidly linked by coherent oscillations (within 60–100 ms after stimulus onset) and are segregated from those groups responding to elements of the background. We found that the ability

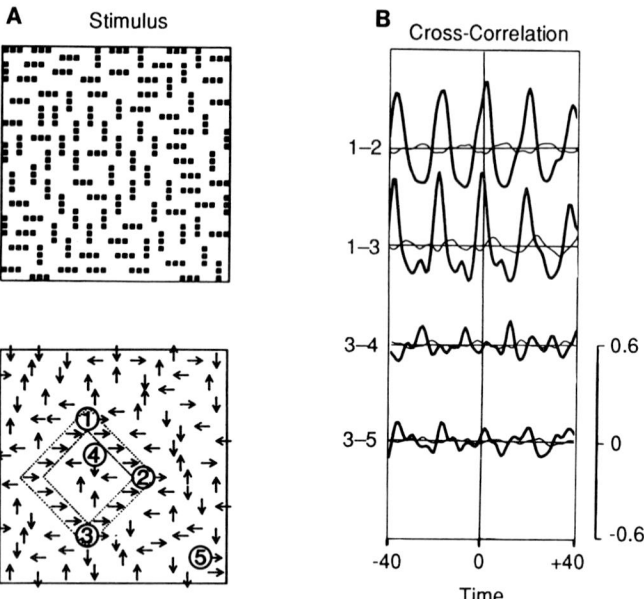

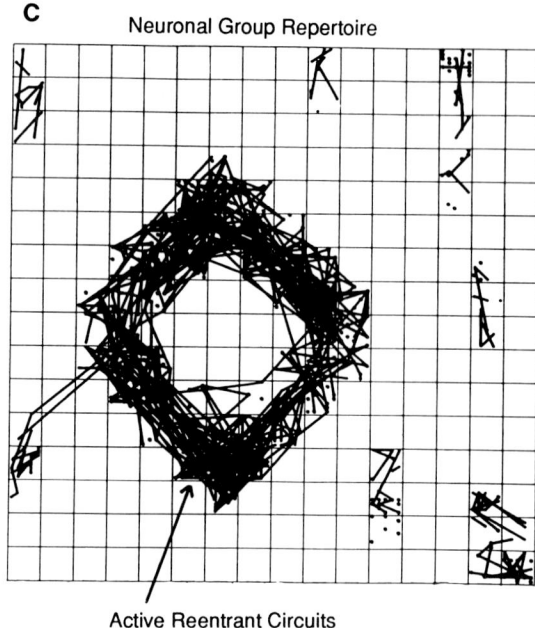

Active Reentrant Circuits

Figure 2 An example of grouping and segmentation in the model of Sporns *et al.* (1991a). (A) Stimulus presented to the model, consisting of a diamond-shaped figure, composed of vertically oriented bars, and a set of randomly oriented bars forming a background. In the top panel the bars are shown at their starting positions; the bottom panel shows their corresponding directions of movement indicated by arrows. Encircled numbers with arrows in the bottom panel refer to the locations of recorded neuronal activity; corresponding cross-correlations are displayed in B. "Electrodes" 1 and 2 recorded from neurons responding to Fig. 1; electrodes 3 and 4 recorded from neurons responding to Fig. 2. (B) Cross-correlograms of neuronal responses to the stimulus shown in A. Cross-correlograms are computed over a 100-ms sample period and subsequently averaged over 10 trials. Numbers refer to the locations of neuronal groups within the direction-selective repertoires (see A). Four correlograms are shown, computed between 201 and 300 ms after stimulus onset. The correlograms are scaled, and shift predictors (thin lines, averaged over nine shifts) are displayed for comparison. (C) Establishment of active (i.e., enhanced) reentrant connections among neuronal groups selective for vertically oriented bars moving to the right, 250 ms after the onset of the stimulus shown in A. Black lines indicate strongly enhanced functional connections. Reproduced with permission from Sporns *et al.* (1991a).

to establish specific linking (grouping) is directly related to the ability of achieving segmentation. Accordingly, there is no coherency among groups responding to elements of the figure and others responding to elements of the background; the latter include elements moving in the same direction as the figure, but placed some distance away. In the model, synchronization after stimulus onset is rapid and—in accordance with perceptual data—occurs usually within 100–200 ms. Multiple coherent episodes of varying length may occur at different times in different trials. Furthermore, synchrony is transient (between 100 and 500 ms), and its offset is fast, as would be clearly required by the fact that the visual scene continuously changes due to eye movements. In the model, episodes of correlated activity coincide with transient enhancement of reentrant connectivity due to short-term changes in synaptic efficacy. This would suggest that the perceptual time scale of several hundred milliseconds is in part determined by voltage-dependent effects at cortical synapses.

This computer model shows that, at least in principle, the neural basis for the integration and segregation of elementary features into objects and background might be represented by the pattern of temporal correlations among neuronal groups mediated by reentry. In addition, because the resulting grouping and segregation are consistent with the Gestalt laws of continuity, proximity, similarity, common orientation, and common motion, it suggests that the neural basis for these laws is to be found implicitly in the specific pattern of reentrant connectivity incorporated into the architecture.

Neurons are sensitive to temporal correlations in their inputs; thus, the timing of activity in one set of neurons can have a well-defined effect on the activity of other neurons and can ultimately influence behavior. In order to demonstrate this point (Tononi *et al.*, 1992a), we modified our grouping and segmentation model by adding a single group, called the effector, which is connected uniformly to all groups within the direction-selective network. The effector is sensitive to temporal correlations in its inputs and is able to trigger a behavioral response (pressing of a lever). After training with a number of stimuli the model responds selectively to a coherent square moving in a particular direction. It does not respond to squares moving in other directions, or to moving disconnected edges. The correct behavior depends on the presence of the individual attributes of the square as well as their "connectedness" or "Gestalt" reflected in the pattern of temporal correlations. Thus, the model shows in an elementary way how cooperative interactions leading to short-term correlations among neuronal groups may be used to integrate the relevant characteristics of the stimulus and to elicit an appropriate behavioral response. Supporting this notion are experimental results obtained from awake monkeys (Vaadia et al., 1991) that indicate that prefrontal neurons show correlated activity for short periods of time (250 ms) when a behavior occurs.

C. Cooperative Interactions among Multiple Cortical Areas

So far, we have dealt with integration at the level of neuronal groups and within a single cortical area. In order to explain the unity of visual perception across submodalities, we generalized these results and simultaneously tested both the constructive and correlative functions of reentry in a model of multiple areas of the visual system (Tononi et al., 1992b). We introduced a computational scheme that deals explicitly and efficiently with short-term temporal correlations among large numbers of units. The model receives visual input from a color camera and contains nine functionally segregated areas divided into three parallel anatomical streams for form, color, and motion; the areas are connected by reciprocal pathways (Plate 1). Altogether, 10,000 units are linked by about 1,000,000 connections between areas at different levels (forward and backward), between areas at the same level (lateral), and within an area (intrinsic). A precise description of the model is given in Tononi et al. (1992b).

We studied two psychophysical phenomena (the perception of form from motion and motion capture) that, respectively, illustrate the constructive and correlative functions of reentry. We showed that the reentrant interactions between the motion and the form streams can be used to construct responses to oriented lines from moving random dot fields (form from motion). In the model, the activity of a "higher" area of the motion stream (V5) is reentered into a "lower" area of the form stream (V1) and modifies its responses to an incoming stimulus. Motion capture in-

volves the illusory attribution of motion signals from a moving object to another object (defined by chromatic or color boundaries) that is actually stationary. Based on the model, we propose that the basis for the perceptual effect of motion capture is the emergence of short-term correlations between units in the motion and those in the color streams as a result of reentrant connections linking these streams.

The correlative properties of the model are explored further in simulations involving all three streams. When presented with a single object, the model solves the so-called "binding problem" and displays coherent unit activity both within and between different areas, including a nontopographic one. Two or more objects can be simultaneously differentiated. We show that coherent unit activity depends on the presence of reentrant pathways giving rise to widespread cooperative interactions among areas. In order to efficiently evaluate patterns of correlations we simultaneously display short-term correlations in a correlation matrix. Consecutive displays of the correlation matrix reflect the functional connectivity (Chapter 8) (Friston et al., 1993) of areas and units within areas over time.

A key characteristic of this model is that successful integration is linked to an observable output, a simulated foveation response. This eliminates the problem of deducing potential outputs by interpreting specific patterns of neural activity and correlations from the point of view of a privileged observer; it also shows that temporal correlations are not merely epiphenomena of neural activity. The foveation response is also used as a basis for conditioning. Reward for a correct discrimination response is mediated by activation of a saliency system that resembles diffuse projection systems in the brain, such as the monoaminergic and cholinergic systems. The simulated diffuse release of a modulatory substance from the saliency system regulates synaptic changes in multiple cortical pathways. After conditioning, the model performs a behavioral discrimination of objects that requires the integration through reentry of distributed information regarding shape, color, and location. This behavior depends critically upon the presence of short-term temporal correlations brought about by reentry and the fact that this does not require integration by a hierarchically superordinate area.

III. Summary and Conclusion

The purpose of this chapter was to show that the design of synthetic neural models of visual cortex can provide new insight into a fundamental problem of cortical function, the problem of neural integration.

Central to the solution of this problem are the patterns of temporal correlations that result from the cooperative reentrant interactions of multiple brain areas. The models discussed in this chapter

- are consistent with neuroanatomy and neurophysiology;
- illustrate cortical integration at multiple levels of organization (within local neuronal groups and within and between cortical areas);
- meet important constraints on the time scale of integration, which is in the range of hundreds of milliseconds; and
- show that patterns of correlations can have an effect on other neurons or directly on behavior.

We conclude that in addition to mechanisms of integration based on the confluence of signals in multimodal areas of the brain, reentrant signaling and the establishment of short-term correlations can serve to integrate distributed neural activity.

Acknowledgments

The author's research was carried out as part of the theoretical neurobiology research program at The Neurosciences Institute, which is supported through the Neurosciences Research Foundation. The Foundation receives major support for this research from the John D. and Catherine T. MacArthur Foundation and the Lucille P. Markey Charitable Trust. Olaf Sporns is a W. M. Keck Foundation Fellow.

References

Abeles, M. (1991). "Corticonics." Cambridge: Cambridge University Press.

Aertsen, A. M. H. J., Gerstein, G. L., Habib, M. K., and Palm, G. (1989). Dynamics of neuronal firing correlations: Modulation of "effective connectivity." *J. Neurophysiol.* **61**, 900–917.

Aertsen, A., Vaadia, E., Abeles, M., Ahissar, E., Bergman, H., Karmon, B., Lavner, Y., Margalit, E., Nelken, I., and Rotter, S. (1991). Neural interactions in the frontal cortex of a behaving monkey: Signs of dependence on stimulus context and behavioral state. *J. Hirnforsch.* **32**, 735–743.

Ahissar, M., Ahissar, E., Bergman, H., and Vaadia, E. (1992). Encoding of sound-source location and movement: Activity of single neurons and interactions between adjacent neurons in the monkey auditory cortex. *J. Neurophysiol.* **67**, 203–215.

Bernander, O., Douglas, R. J., Martin, K. A. C., and Koch, C. (1991). Synaptic background activity influences spatiotemporal integration in single pyramidal cells. *Proc. Nat. Acad. Sci. USA* **88**, 11,569–11,573.

Damasio, A. R. (1989). The brain binds entities and events by multiregional activation from convergence zones. *Neural Comput.* **1**, 123–132.

Eckhorn, R., Bauer, R., Jordan, W., Brosch, M., Kruse, W., Munk, M., and Reitboeck, H. J. (1988). Coherent oscillations: A mechanism of feature linking in the visual cortex? Multiple electrode and correlation analyses in the cat. *Biol. Cybernetics* **60**, 121–130.

Edelman, G. M. (1978). Group selection and phasic re-entrant signalling: A theory of higher brain function. *In* "The Mindful Brain" (G. M. Edelman and V. B. Mountcastle, Eds.), pp. 51–100. Cambridge, MA: MIT Press.

Edelman, G. M. (1987). "Neural Darwinism." New York: Basic Books.

Edelman, G. M. (1989). "The Remembered Present." New York: Basic Books.

Engel, A. K., König, P., Kreiter, A. K., and Singer, W. (1991). Interhemispheric synchronization of oscillatory neuronal responses in cat visual cortex. *Science* **252**, 1177–1179.

Engel, A. K., Kreiter, A. K., König, P., and Singer, W. (1991). Synchronization of oscillatory neuronal responses between striate and extrastriate visual cortical areas of the cat. *Proc. Nat. Acad. Sci. USA* **88**, 6048–6052.

Engel, A. K., König, P., Kreiter, A. K., Schillen, T. B., and Singer, W. (1992). Temporal coding in the visual cortex: New vistas on integration in the nervous system. *Trends Neurosci.* **15**, 218–226.

Felleman, D. J., and Van Essen, D. C. (1991). Distributed hierarchical processing in the primate cerebral cortex. *Cereb. Cortex* **1**, 1–47.

Finkel, L. H., and Edelman, G. M. (1989). The integration of distributed cortical systems by reentry: A computer simulation of interactive functionally segregated visual areas. *J. Neurosci.* **9**, 3188–3208.

Friston, K. J., Frith, C. D., Liddle, P. F., and Frackowiak, R. S. J. (1993). Functional connectivity: The principal component analysis of large (PET) data sets. *J. Cereb. Blood Flow Metab.* **13**, 5–14.

Gilbert, C. D. (1992). Horizontal integration and cortical dynamics. *Neuron* **9**, 1–13.

Gochin, P. M., Miller, E. K., Gross, C. G., and Gerstein, G. L. (1991). Functional interactions among neurons in inferior temporal cortex of the awake macaque. *Exp. Brain Res.* **84**, 505–516.

Gray, C. M., and Singer, W. (1989). Stimulus-specific neuronal oscillations in orientation columns of cat visual cortex. *Proc. Nat. Acad. Sci. USA* **86**, 1698–1702.

Gray, C. M., König, P., Engel, A. K., and Singer, W. (1989). Oscillatory responses in cat visual cortex exhibit inter-columnar synchronization which reflects global stimulus properties. *Nature* **338**, 334–337.

Gray, C. M., Engel, A. K., König, P., and Singer, W. (1992). Synchronization of oscillatory neuronal responses in cat striate cortex: Temporal properties. *Vis. Neurosci.* **8**, 337–347.

Hirsch, J. A., and Gilbert, C. D. (1991). Synaptic physiology of horizontal connections in the cat's visual cortex. *J. Neurosci.* **11**, 1800–1809.

Jagadeesh, B., Gray, C. M., and Ferster, D. (1992). Visually evoked oscillations of membrane potential in cells of cat visual cortex. *Science* **257**, 552–554.

Kanizsa, G. (1979). "Organization in Vision: Essays on Gestalt Perception." New York: Praeger.

Kisvarday, Z. F., and Eysel, U. T. (1992). Cellular organization of reciprocal patchy networks in layer III of cat visual cortex (Area 17). *Neuroscience* **46**, 275–286.

Kreiter, A. K., and Singer, W. (1992). Oscillatory neuronal responses in the visual cortex of the awake macaque monkey. *Eur. J. Neurosci.* **4**, 369–375.

Mignard, M., and Malpeli, J. G. (1991). Paths of information flow through visual cortex. *Science* **251**, 1249–1251.

Murthy, V. N., and Fetz, E. E. (1992). Coherent 25- to 35-Hz oscillations in the sensorimotor cortex of awake behaving monkeys. *Proc. Nat. Acad. Sci. USA* **89**, 5670–5674.

Nakamura, K., Mikami, A., and Kubota, K. (1992). Oscillatory neuronal activity related to visual short-term memory in monkey temporal pole. *NeuroReport* **3**, 117–120.

Nelson, J. I., Salin, P. A., Munk, M. H.-J., Arzi, M., and Bullier, J. (1992). Spatial and temporal coherence in cortico–cortical connections: A cross-correlation study in areas 17 and 18 in the cat. *Vis. Neurosci.* **9**, 21–37.

Sherrington, C. (1947). "The Integrative Action of the Nervous System." New Haven: Yale University Press.

Sporns, O., Gally, J. A., Reeke, G. N., Jr., and Edelman, G. M. (1989). Reentrant signaling among simulated neuronal groups leads to coherency in their oscillatory activity. *Proc. Nat. Acad. Sci. USA* **86**, 7265–7269.

Sporns, O., Tononi, G., and Edelman, G. M. (1991a). Modeling perceptual grouping and figure–ground segregation by means of active reentrant connections. *Proc. Nat. Acad. Sci. USA* **88**, 129–133.

Sporns, O., Tononi, G., and Edelman, G. M. (1991b). Dynamic interactions of neuronal groups and the problem of cortical integration. *In* "Nonlinear Dynamics and Neural Networks" (H. G. Schuster, Ed.), pp. 205–240. Weinheim, Germany: Verlag Chemie.

Tononi, G., Sporns, O., and Edelman, G. M. (1992a). The problem of neural integration: Induced rhythms and short-term correlations. *In* "Induced Rhythms in the Brain" (E. Basar and T. H. Bullock, Eds.), pp. 367–395. Boston: Birkhäuser.

Tononi, G., Sporns, O., and Edelman, G. M. (1992b). Reentry and the problem of integrating multiple cortical areas: Simulation of dynamic integration in the visual system. *Cereb. Cortex* **2**, 310–335.

Vaadia, E., Ahissar, E., Bergman, H., and Lavner, Y. (1991). Correlated activity of neurons: a neural code for higher brain functions? *In* "Neuronal Cooperativity" (J. Krüger, Ed.), pp. 249–279. Berlin: Springer.

Young, M. P. (1992). Objective analysis of the topological organization of the primate cortical visual system. *Nature* **358**, 152–154.

Zeki, S. (1978). Functional specialization in the visual cortex of the rhesus monkey. *Nature* **274**, 423–428.

Zeki, S., and Shipp, S. (1988). The functional logic of cortical connections. *Nature* **335**, 311–317.

Zeki, S. (1990). Parallelism and functional specialization in human visual cortex. *Cold Spring Harbor Symp. Quant. Biol.* **55**, 651–661.

2

Neural Modeling and Positron Emission Tomography

Barry Horwitz

Laboratory of Neurosciences, National Institute on Aging, National Institutes of Health, Bethesda, Maryland 20892

I. Introduction

The ability to assess how the brain and its component parts behave during normal cognitive, sensory, and motor performance, as well as in various brain diseases, has been greatly enhanced by the use of functional imaging techniques. Imaging techniques differ from one another in the particular aspect of neuronal activity that is chosen to represent functional activity. Electrical activity can be assessed employing electroencephalography (EEG) and magnetoencephalography (MEG). The use of cerebral blood flow or metabolism (henceforth called metabolic functional imaging) as a measure of brain functional activity originated with the work of Roy and Sherrington (1890). As brain cells function, they utilize energy [mainly for ion pumping (Mata *et al.*, 1980)], thus requiring cerebral glucose metabolism to reestablish energy stores. Cerebral blood flow is increased to supply the glucose and oxygen needed for energy metabolism. Metabolic functional brain activity in humans can be imaged using a variety of techniques, including the nontomographic xenon-133 method, and tomographic techniques such as single photon emission computed tomography (SPECT) and positron emission tomography (PET). The nontomographic method and SPECT use regional cerebral blood flow (rCBF) as their measure of functional activity, whereas PET can image rCBF as well as the local rate of glucose utilization (rCMRglc) or the regional rate of oxygen metabolism.

The advantages and disadvantages of each of these metabolic mapping technique for human studies were discussed in Haxby *et al.* (1991). Recently, magnetic resonance imaging (MRI) has been used to image brain functional activity (Kwong *et al.*, 1992; Ogawa *et al.*, 1992) employing techniques that are sensitive to blood flow and blood oxygenation. The discussion in this chapter will be devoted to metabolic imaging of functional activity, primarily with PET, unless indicated otherwise.

Brain metabolic mapping methods provide time-integrated measures of brain functional activity, but the time interval over which the integration occurs differs markedly for each method, from a low of about 5–10 s for MRI flow imaging, to about 1 min for [^{15}O]water rCBF/PET studies, to a high of about 20–30 min for rCMRglc/PET studies. Consequently, each imaging technique is best used with behavioral studies specifically designed for the appropriate time interval.

In a typical analysis of metabolic functional imaging data, values for specific regions of interest (ROIs) are determined, averaged across subjects, and group differences evaluated using some statistical procedure such as a *t* test. For multiple run PET/rCBF studies, within-subject differences can be determined using techniques such as pixel-by-pixel subtraction (Fox *et al.*, 1984), and, following intersubject averaging, areas of activation or deactivation can be found by a variety of statistical techniques, including outlier detection (Fox *et al.*, 1988; Mintun *et al.*, 1989). A more general procedure is statistical parametric mapping (SPM) (Friston *et al.*, 1991a), which allows for weighted comparisons among the different runs followed by the generation of pixel-based statistical maps.

Conventional analyses use the numbers obtained only as input to statistical analyses to ascertain group or task differences in particular brain regions. However, it is apparent that the brain consists of networks of interacting regions, as opposed to a number of independently acting regions, and that behaviors are mediated through the functioning of these networks (Luria, 1973; Horwitz, 1989; Damasio, 1989; Mesulam, 1990; Felleman and Van Essen, 1991; Kosslyn and Intriligator, 1992). Quantitative data obtained simultaneously from multiple brain areas are the kind of data that can be used in network analyses of brain function. Because the relationships among the activities of interacting network elements can become complicated, one needs to use a mathematical or computer model to grasp and articulate the interrelationships. Therefore, the complexity of network analysis implies that computational modeling of network behavior is necessary in order to use effectively functional neuroimaging data. What seems rather surprising is how little effort has gone into developing such models for metabolic functional neuroimaging data. In this chapter, I shall discuss our laboratory's work in this area. Recently, other researcher groups have begun modeling efforts, and I shall briefly mention their work as well.

II. A PET Study of Human Visual Processing

I first shall present some experimental PET data from our laboratory in order to have a concrete example with which to discuss modeling. The study (Haxby *et al.*, 1991a; Horwitz *et al.*, 1992a) was an investigation of the visual pathways involved in object identification and spatial localization. Studies in nonhuman primates have demonstrated the presence of many brain regions in posterior neocortex that respond to visual input (Desimone and Ungerleider, 1989; Felleman and Van Essen, 1991; Macko and Mishkin, 1985; Van Essen, 1985), which can be organized into two processing streams (Mishkin *et al.*, 1983; Ungerleider and Mishkin, 1982). The first passes from occipital cortex into inferior temporal cortex and is associated with object identification (Desimone and Ungerleider, 1989). The other goes from occipital cortex into parietal cortex and is involved with processing information about the spatial location of objects (Goldberg and Colby, 1989; Ungerleider and Mishkin, 1982). A number of studies, mostly of lesion effects in clinical cases, suggest that these two visual pathways also exist in

humans (Damasio *et al.*, 1989; Newcombe and Ratcliff, 1989).

Our PET study (Haxby *et al.*, 1991a) examined young men during performance of both a face matching task (object vision task) and a dot-location matching task (spatial vision task) in the same scanning session. Sample stimuli for both tasks are shown in Fig. 1. For all tasks, the subject indicated his choice by pressing a button with his left or right thumb (choices were counterbalanced). Scanning was performed using a Scanditronix PC1024-7B tomograph. To determine specific brain areas of activation, images of rCBF obtained during a sensorimotor control task (three empty squares) were subtracted pixel-by-pixel from images obtained during each of the two visual processing tasks. Figure 2 shows brain areas of significant activation for each task. During both tasks, there was bilateral activation of an area of ventral occipital cortex that may correspond to area V4 in the macaque monkey (Haxby *et al.*, 1991b). The face matching task also resulted in bilateral activation of an area of ventral occipitotemporal cortex that may correspond to area TEO in the macaque (Bonin and Bailey, 1947). During the dot-location matching task, there was bilateral activations of an area of occipitoparietal cortex and of superior parietal cortex. The latter may represent the human homologue of the macaque's area PG (Bonin and Bailey, 1947).

III. Covariance Analysis of Functional Neuroimaging Data

In a network one has elements or nodes that are interconnected with one another. One characterizes the state of a network in terms of the activity of each element, and the strength of the connection between each pair of elements. For a systems level network of brain regions, functional neuroimaging data can provide the values for the activity of each network component. In order to investigate the functional relations among network elements, some type of covariance analysis is required. The use of covariance analysis for determining functional interrelationships has been used for all measures of functional activity and for neural networks at both the systems level and the cellular level. For example, there have been covariance studies employing multiunit microelectrode-obtained data (Gerstein *et al.*, 1978), data from scalp-recorded electrical activity (Gevins *et al.*, 1985), data from optical recordings of brain activity (Shoham *et al.*, 1991), and cerebral metabolic measures of functional activity (Clark *et al.*, 1984; Friston and Frackowiak, 1991; Horwitz *et al.*, 1984, 1992a; McIntosh and Gonzalez-Lima,

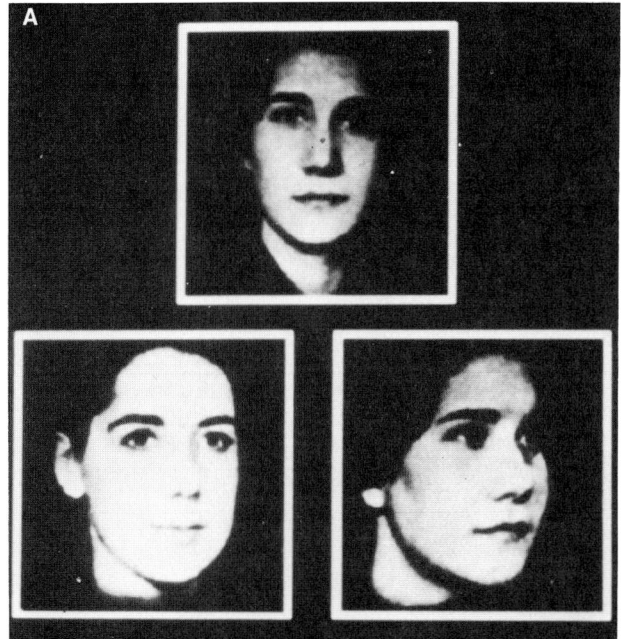
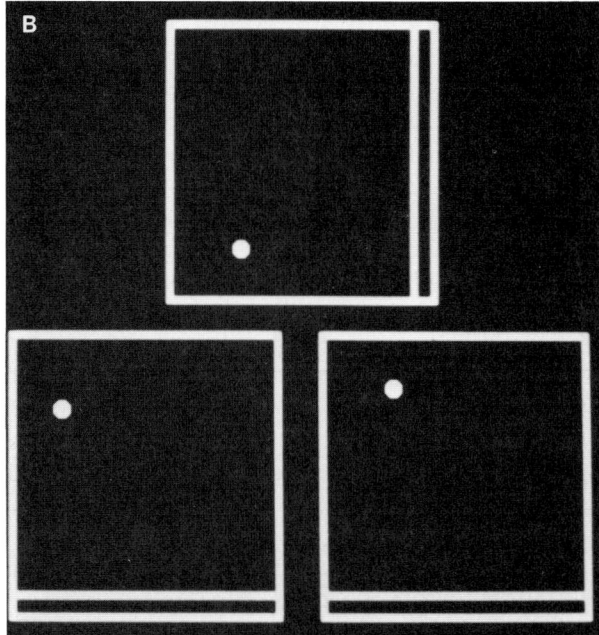

Figure 1 Items from the face matching (A) and dot-location matching (B) tasks. Faces are from the Benton Facial Recognition Test (Benton, 1974). Reprinted from Haxby *et al.* (1991a).

1991; Metter *et al.*, 1984). The fundamental assumption that all these approaches have in common is that neural units that function together have correlated activities.

One important reason for performing a covariance analysis is because a conventional analysis of a meta-bolic map does not always indicate all the elements that constitute the networks associated with a specific behavioral task. Compared to some control task, for example, a particular brain region may not demonstrate a change in blood flow or metabolism during a specific behavior. Such a region may have been part

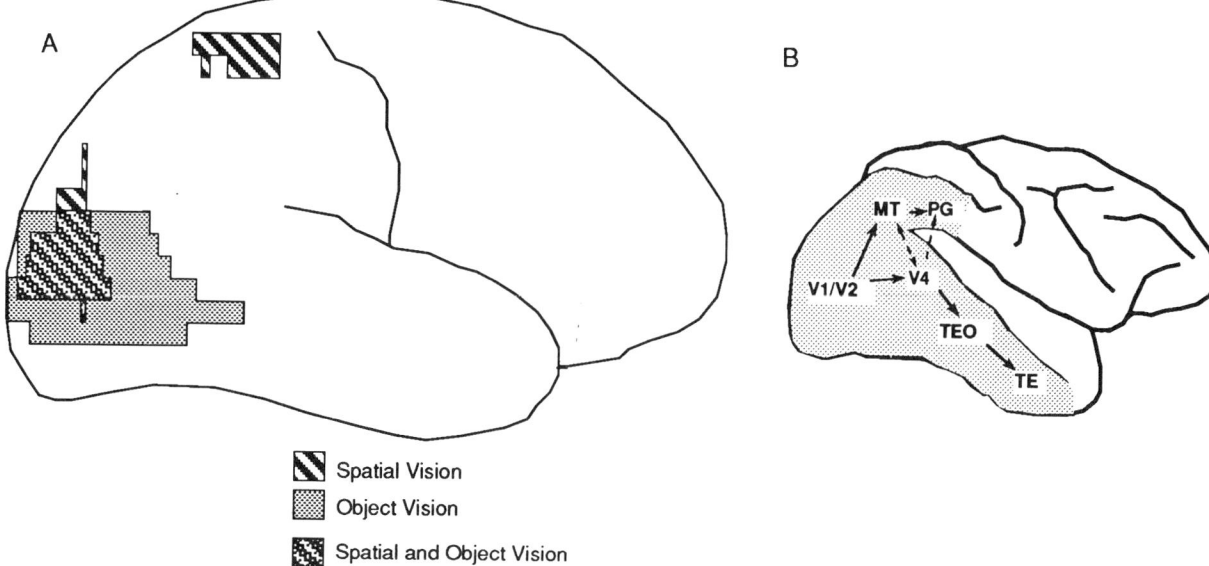

Figure 2 (A) Areas of significant increases in normalized rCBF during object vision (face matching) and spatial vision (dot-location matching). Activations, which were bilateral, are relative to the sensorimotor control task. (B) Map of major visual areas in macaque visual cortex, and their interconnections. Reprinted from Haxby *et al.* (1991a).

of one activated network during the control task, and a member of a second during the behavior under study. What have changed are the functional relations between this and other brain regions, not its net blood flow or metabolism. Covariance analysis is required to investigate such functional relations.

Our laboratory has investigated the functional relations among brain regions in humans using either rCMRglc or rCBF data obtained by PET (Horwitz *et al.*, 1984, 1987, 1992a). For a multirun rCBF study, correlations between pairs of regional normalized rCBF are determined for each run separately (data from each regional pair for one subject constitute one entry into the calculation of the correlation). A large correlation coefficient between two regions may indicate that the two are functionally associated during the task (Horwitz *et al.*, 1992a).

We use the rCBF data for the visual processing tasks discussed above to illustrate this procedure. The results of Haxby *et al.* (1991a) suggest that during face matching, the neural pathway between ventral occipital and occipitotemporal cortex is functionally activated, whereas during dot-location matching, the functionally activated neural pathway leads from occipital cortex into superior parietal cortex. These hypotheses were examined using correlations between normalized rCBF values for these areas (Horwitz *et al.*, 1992a). Data came from 17 healthy men aged 19–34 years. Correlations were performed on normalized (regional/global) rCBF values (not on subtracted data) for each task separately.

The normalized rCBF correlations among these regions are shown in Table 1. During face matching, significant ($p < 0.05$) correlations were found between normalized rCBF for the occipitotemporal and ventral occipital association areas ($r = 0.54$), as well as between normalized rCBF for the ventral occipital and occipitoparietal areas ($r = 0.52$) in the right hemisphere. During dot-location matching, significant correlations were found between the ventral association and the occipitoparietal areas ($r = 0.53$) and between the occipitoparietal area and the superior parietal region ($r = 0.60$) in the right hemisphere. However, the correlation between the last two regions in the right hemisphere was not significant ($r = -0.07$) during face matching, nor was the correlation between the ventral occipital association region and the occipitotemporal region in the right hemisphere during dot-location matching ($r = 0.26$). Most importantly, significant correlations among these regions were found only in the right hemisphere. None of the corresponding correlations between normalized rCBF among these regions in the left cerebral hemisphere achieved statistical significance.

Table 1 Correlations of Normalized rCBF between Extrastriate Regions for Visual Tasks

	Face matching task				Dot-location matching task			
	OAV	OT	OP	SP	OAV	OT	OP	SP
OAV	■	.54*	.52*	.33	■	.26	.53*	.37
OT	− .08	■	.41	− .06	.41	■	.48	− .19
OP	− .04	− .04	■	− .07	.29	.28	■	.60*
SP	.25	− .30	.04	■	− .04	.10	.40	■

Note. Correlations above and to the right of diagonal are for the right hemisphere, those below and to the left of the diagonal are for the left hemisphere. OAV, ventral occipital association cortex; OP, occipitoparietal cortex; OT, occipitotemporal cortex; SP, superior parietal cortex. From Horwitz *et al.* (1992a).

[a]Correlation significantly different from 0 ($p < 0.05$).

Recently, my collaborators and I have developed a way to perform this type of correlational analysis in conjunction with the SPM method of PET data analysis (Friston *et al.*, 1989, 1990, 1991a, 1991b). Individual PET data used for correlational analysis are stereotactically normalized and smoothed using part of the SPM system (Friston *et al.*, 1989, 1991b). For this procedure, each scan is rotated, resized, and reshaped to match a template PET scan that has the orientation and dimensions of the stereotactic brain atlas of Talairach and Tournoux (1988), which orients sagittal and horizontal sections parallel to the anterior commissure–posterior commisure (AC–PC) line. Brain coordinates in millimeters are expressed relative to an origin at the intersection between the AC–PC line and the midline. Stereotactically normalized images are then smoothed using a 2-cm (FWHM) Gaussian filter. Because of the smoothing, a pixel that shows the largest significant activation in normalized rCBF locally can be thought of as the center of a region of activation. To perform correlation analysis, a reference pixel is chosen, and all other pixels in the brain significantly correlated with the reference pixel are determined.

Comparing the face matching task to the baseline control task, a focus of activation in the right hemisphere was found whose Talairach coordinates are $x = 34$ mm, $y = -78$ mm, and $z = -12$ mm (J. V. Haxby, unpublished observations). This location is in the posterior fusiform gyrus (Brodmann area 18–19, as defined by the Talairach atlas). In the left hemisphere a homologous activation site was found ($x = -30$ mm, $y = -84$ mm, and $z = -12$ mm). These locations may represent a portion of the human analogue of V4. Each of these pixels was used as reference pixels for correlation analysis for data obtained during the face matching task. The top part of Plate 2 shows axial slices of all the pixels in the brain significantly correlated ($p < 0.01$) with the right hemisphere reference pixel, and the bottom part of Plate 2 shows the corresponding set of significant correlations when the reference pixel is in the left hemisphere. When the reference pixel is located in the right hemisphere, significant correlations in the right hemisphere include pixels in the midfusiform gyrus (Brodmann area 37), which is not the case when the reference pixel is in the left hemisphere. The midfusiform gyral location may represent part of the human analogue to TEO. This pixel-by-pixel correlational analysis substantiates the conclusions of the region-by-region correlation analysis presented above.

Thus, correlational analysis of normalized rCBF can detect functional interactions between components of brain networks associated with the performance of particular cognitive tasks. Specifically, both face matching and dot-location matching depend to a greater degree on functional interactions among posterior cortical areas in the right hemisphere than in the left, although the pixel-by-pixel subtraction method (Haxby *et al.*, 1991a) demonstrated bilateral activation of the specific areas described above. Other evidence suggests that in right-handed subjects the right hemisphere plays a dominant role in face matching as well as in various aspects of the dot-location matching task (Damasio *et al.*, 1990; Ditunno and Mann, 1990; Ellis, 1983; Newcombe and Ratcliff, 1989; Sergent, 1989).

One kind of analysis, therefore, leads to the conclusion of right hemisphere dominance for these tasks; the other, to bilateral involvement. A hypothesis that could reconcile the two findings is that the neurons mainly involved in the processing of information about faces and spatial relations are located in the right hemisphere, but have projections to the left hemisphere, and that the increased rCBF seen there results in part from transcallosal activation of the left hemisphere. Indeed, information about the stimuli must ultimately reach the left hemisphere, because 50% of the time a button in the right hand must be pressed to denote the correct choice. One implication of the above interpretation is that the pixel-by-pixel subtraction technique (or region-by-region analysis) may incorrectly indicate bilaterally symmetric regional involvement for a specific cognitive component.

The notion of "interregional functional relation" must be sharpened if it is to be used in a neural modeling environment. We do this using several definitions introduced previously (Horwitz, 1990). Two regions are *anatomically coupled* if there is an anatomical projection from one to the other. If that projection is activated to a significant degree, we say that the two

regions are *functionally coupled*. This will be the case under certain experimental conditions, and not others. This functional coupling may result in a large correlation between the functional activities of the two regions. It is also possible for two regions to demonstrate a strong covariance without being anatomically coupled (e.g., both may receive projections from a third region), which we call *functional association*.

In order to develop a systems-level neural model, we have to understand what aspects of regional activity lead to neurobiologically meaningful statements about functional relations between brain regions. Table 2 lists some of the possible reasons why two regions may have metabolic activities that strongly correlate [a fuller discussion of the neurobiological substrates of interregional correlations can be found in Horwitz *et al.* (1992b)]. Because correlations generally are performed using values normalized to global CBF, only those factors that affect regional covariation are included.

We think the first two entries are the most important factors. Large interregional correlations in normalized metabolic activities could be due to subject-to-subject differences in the time interval over which a given pair of regions are active during the performance of the task. For example, suppose for a specific part of a cognitive task, region A excites region B. In one subject, this activation occurs during 75% of the time interval, and in a second subject during 85% of the time interval. Assume that this 13% increase results in a 13% increase in measured rCBF in both regions. Changes of this sort would lead to a correlation in normalized rCBF between A and B. This factor could operate within-subject during repeated runs of the same task.

Likewise, suppose attention equally affects activity in two functionally coupled regions. As different subjects are scanned under the same conditions, attention may affect each subject to a different degree, again leading to correlated activity between the two regions. As before, this factor could operate within a subject during repeated runs of the same task. Other brain

Table 2 Sources of Covariance in Activities of Two Regions

a. Covariation in time spent on task during scan interval

b. Covariation in effect of other regions (e.g., attention)

c. Covariation in effect of stimulus parameters

d. Between-subject covariation in size and shape of an anatomical ROI

e. Between-subject differences in covariation of response due to packing density, etc.

Table 3 Neurobiological Factors That Can Alter
Functional Couplings if Stimulus Parameters
Are Changed

a. Number and distribution of activated synapses from the first
   to the second region may change.

b. Second region may be activated for a longer or shorter time
   interval.

c. Different attentional (or memory, etc.) requirements may lead
   to modulation of efficacy of synapses from the first to the second region.

d. Different subpopulations of neurons may be activated.

e. Drug effects could modulate the synapses from the first to
   the second region.

f. Disease may alter synapses between two regions.

systems also could behave in a similar fashion (e.g.,
memory).

We now want to consider the kind of experiment
where the stimulus set is altered during repeated runs
of the experiment (e.g., the stimuli are made progressively more difficult to discern). The functional coupling between two regions can either change or not
change as the stimulus set is varied. Table 3 lists within-subject factors that could lead to changes in the
functional coupling between two regions.

The functional coupling between two regions (A to
B, let us say) can change if the stimulus parameters
are modified. Even if small changes in the stimulus
set occur, the computational requirements on the
brain may lead to an altered relationship between two
regions. For example, suppose the task requires face
discrimination. If, during one run, the stimuli are
fairly easy to discriminate, the functional coupling
between two regions may have one value. If, during
another run, the emotional content of the faces plays
a greater role in the discrimination process, the functional coupling could have a different value. Drugs
or disease also could affect the functional coupling
between two regions.

The biological reasons for a quantitative change in
the functional coupling between two areas could be
one of the following. It may be that the number and
distribution of activated synaptic connections from
the first to the second region changes because of the
altered nature of the stimulus set. This could lead to
a relatively greater (or lesser) activation of the second
region following stimulus activation of the first. Alternatively, it could be that the calculational requirements for the new stimulus set results in activation
of the second region for a larger fraction of the scan
than was the case during the first run. Additionally,
a modification in the nature of the task could require

greater attention (or memory input, etc.). Inputs to
the second region from brain attentional circuits may
increase the efficacy of synapses from the first to the
second region, again leading to a change in the functional coupling between the two regions. Of course,
drugs and disease also could alter the synaptic relationship between two regions, either by directly
changing it, or by modulating it.

From the above considerations, it is apparent that
the correlations that are determined from experimental data are an indirect reflection of the functional
couplings. It is the functional couplings that provide
the link between regional metabolic measurements
and the underlying functional neurobiology. In the
next section of this chapter, we focus on the functional
couplings and how they are to be treated using computational neural modeling techniques.

IV. Simulation Modeling

Network models can be used in either a data-fitting
or a simulation mode. In the former, the model is
imposed on actual experimental data, and the values
of the model parameters that yield the closest fit between model and data are determined. In the latter,
predefined values of the parameters (along with randomly generated variability) are used to determine
how the model behaves. Presumably, if the model is
reasonable, the simulations provide a way to explore
brain activity under a variety of conditions, which
could aid in experimental design. In this section, we
discuss the simulation mode of network modeling,
whereas in the next, the data-fitting mode.

We have developed systems-level simulation network models for both rCMRglc data (Horwitz, 1990)
and PET/rCBF (Horwitz, 1991) that generate simulated rCBF or rCMRglc data for a number of "brain"
regions in a specified number of subjects. Activity
in each region is a sigmoidal function (used so that
simulated values in a region, like actual metabolic
data, have both upper and lower bounds) of the activities in some or all of the other regions. The quantity
that relates the activity in one region to that in a second
is called the functional coupling coefficient. Variability
in the simulated data is provided by the use of random
numbers. Correlation analysis is performed on these
simulated data, thus allowing us to relate patterns of
correlation coefficients to patterns of functional couplings.

In an rCBF simulation, we assume that there are
N subjects, n regions, and L separate scans during a
PET session on a single subject. The following equation
gives the activity (rCBF) in region i ($i = 1, 2, ..., n$)

of subject j (j = 1, …, N) during run k (k = 1, …, L):

$$rCBF_i^{(j)}(k)$$

$$= \frac{B_i^{(j)}(k)}{1 + K \exp\left[-\sum_{m=1}^{n} C_{im}^{(j)}(k)\, rCBF_m^{(j)}(k) - A_i^{(j)}(k) \right]}.$$

$$(1)$$

The maximum value $rCBF_i^{(j)}(k)$ can have is $B_i^{(j)}(k)$, whereas the minimum value is $B_i^{(j)}(k)/(1 + K)$. The functional coupling coefficient, $C_{im}^{(j)}(k)$, determines (in subject j during run k) how activity in region m affects activity in region i. The functional couplings will change as different experimental conditions (or subject groups) are simulated. The parameter $A_i^{(j)}(k)$ generates the activity that is inherent to region i, that is, the activity that would be present if all functional couplings equaled zero. This quantity represents activity local to region i and also activity in region i due to regions not explicitly in the model. Equation (1) constitutes a set of n nonlinear equations (for each subject during each run) that must be solved simultaneously.

The parameters $A_i^{(j)}(k)$ and $B_i^{(j)}(k)$ have components that vary randomly, allowing us to simulate data that possess within-subject, between-subject, and between-run variabilities seen in actual experimental data. The values of these parameters can be chosen so that simulated data emulate specific kinds of experimental data (e.g., human rCBF/PET data) [see Horwitz (1990) for details on how to find the values for the parameters]. A specific simulation is performed by specifying the values of the functional coupling coefficients for each run. Once the simulated data are generated, correlational analysis, as described above, can be performed on normalized values.

This simulation model has been used to address a number of issues. Because we "know the answer" (i.e., the explicit set of brain relationships), we can use simulations to partially validate conclusions suggested by actual experimental data. It was shown, for example, that a change in the functional coupling coefficient between two regions leads to a corresponding change in the correlation coefficient between the two regions (Horwitz, 1990, 1991; Horwitz *et al.*, 1992b).

Here, we use simulations to address the hypothesis mentioned earlier concerning the object and spatial vision data, i.e., that one could have bilateral activation (as seen using a pixel-by-pixel subtraction technique), along with large functional couplings only

within a single hemisphere. Figure 3 presents the results of a simulation to investigate this conjecture. Regions 1, 3, and 5 are in the right hemisphere, whereas regions 2, 4 and 6 are in the left. Regions 1 and 2 (e.g., striate and peristriate cortex) are functionally coupled to regions 3 and 4 (e.g., V4), each of which projects across the corpus callosum. However, only regions 3 and 5 (e.g., TEO) in the right hemisphere are functionally coupled, not regions 4 and 6. Region 5 does project across the corpus callosum to region 6. Two runs were simulated. The functional couplings between region 1 and region 3 and those between region 2 and region 4 were unchanged for the two runs, whereas the other functional couplings went from a value of zero during run 1 (baseline control task) to those specified in the figure during run 2 (cognitive task). Mean normalized rCBF in each region is shown in the figure, demonstrating significant increases for the extrastriate regions (3, 4, 5, and 6) in both hemispheres. If the analysis had ceased at this point, the conclusion would be that the cognitive task during run 2 was similarly performed by both hemispheres. However, the correlations demonstrate that the only significant within-hemisphere functional relation in extrastriate cortex was between region 3 and region 5, and not between region 4 and region 6. Thus, the correlational analysis adds the important insight that there is a marked hemispheric asymmetry in the functional relations among the regions, reflecting the marked asymmetry in the way in which the

Simulation Results: Hemispheric Asymmetries

REGION	RUN 1	RUN 2
1	0.99 ± .09	0.95 ± .11
2	0.97 ± .08	0.91 ± .15
3	1.32 ± .10	1.48 ± .13*
4	1.29 ± .08	1.47 ± .09*
5	0.89 ± .08	1.34 ± .07*
6	0.88 ± .07	1.09 ± .06*
r(3,5)	-0.24	0.61 *
r(4,6)	-0.22	0.16
c	0	.018
c'	.012	.012

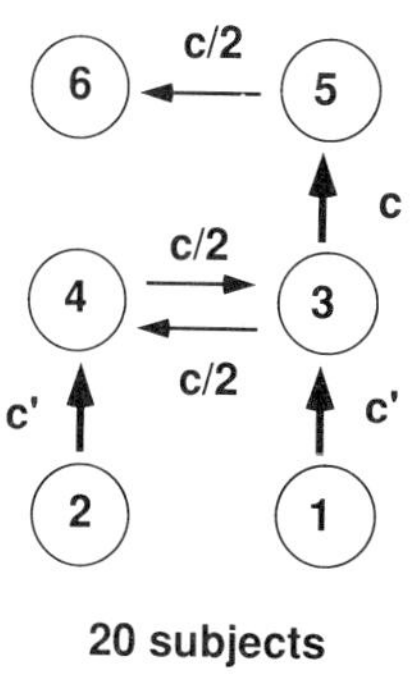

20 subjects

* p < .05

Figure 3 Simulation results corresponding to the configuration shown on the right. Regions 1, 3, and 5 are in the right hemisphere, whereas regions 2, 4, and 6 are in the left. The results from two runs are presented. The mean ± SD for normalized rCBF in each region is given, along with interregional correlation coefficients for region pairs 3–5 and 4–6. The table also gives the values of the functional coupling coefficients for each run. Modified from Horwitz *et al.* (1992b).

brain processes neural information. Of course, this simulation does not prove that this is the mechanism that occurs for the visual tasks whose rCBF data were discussed above. It does suggest that such a mechanism is not unreasonable.

V. Using Models to Fit Data

Simulations allow one to explore how changes in functional couplings result in alterations in network behavior. Finding the values of the functional couplings that actually correspond a particular cognitive, motor or sensory behavior requires adjusting the values of the functional coupling coefficients until good agreement is reached between actual experimental data and those generated by the model. If one is willing to use a linear model (rather than the sigmoidal model discussed above), a number of techniques exist for fitting data so that functional coupling coefficients can be determined. These approaches go under names such as path analysis or structural equation modeling (Joreskog and Sorbom, 1984; Loehlin, 1987). For data fitting, one selects a subset of regions whose interactions are of interest, and the functional coupling coefficients are determined. Requiring the functional coupling between two regions to be zero if no anatomical link between the two exits results in a reduction in the number of parameters that need to be fitted.

The first applications of this method to brain metabolic data were performed by McIntosh and Gonzalez-Lima (1991, 1992). In one study (McIntosh and Gonzalez-Lima, 1992), deoxyglucose (2DG) uptake was determined in the visual system of rats presented either with patterned light (square-wave gratings of various spatial frequencies) or darkness. The pattern of functional couplings for the two conditions between the most important rat visual areas are shown in Fig. 4. In darkness, the predominant positive couplings involved the tectocortical subsystem and the descending connections from secondary visual cortex, whereas, during patterned light, functional couplings were increased for the geniculocortical subsystem. The couplings in the tectocortical subsystem became smaller and reversed direction.

Recently, McIntosh et al. (1993) used structural equation modeling to determine the functional neural networks mediating the object and spatial vision tasks described above. The functional networks demonstrated differential involvement of the dorsal and ventral pathways. Interactions between the two pathways were important, as were interactions with regions in the frontal cortex. Network analysis permitted identification of the role played by specific regions in each

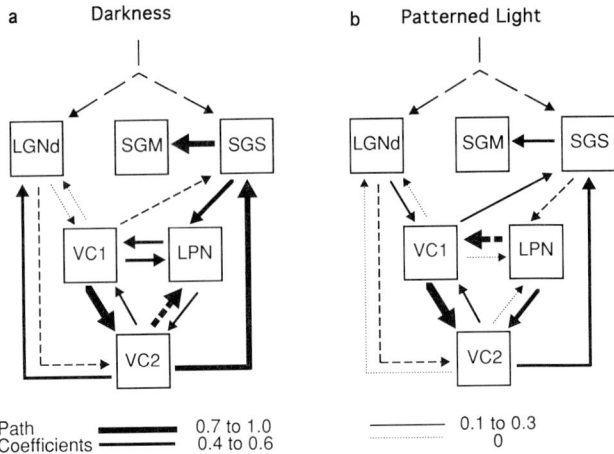

Figure 4 Structural equation modeling results for rats kept in darkness (a) and exposed to patterned light (b). The magnitude and directions of the functional coupling coefficients are shown. The magnitude is proportional to the line width. Positive coefficients are represented by solid arrows; negative coefficients are represented by dashed arrows. Dotted lines represent path coefficients of zero magnitude. LGNd: lateral geniculate n.; LPN: posterior thalamus; SGM and SGS: intermediate and superficial gray layers of superior colliculus; VC1 and VC2: primary and secondary visual cortex. Redrawn, with permission, from McIntosh et al. (1992).

task, which cannot be done by examining either the regional activations or the interregional correlations.

A different approach to data fitting was reported by Sun and Mazoyer (1991), who used a neural net procedure to demonstrate that mean rCMRglc values from a population of healthy normals form a stable, but nonunique, steady-state solution. Other approaches use principal component or factor analysis (Chapter 8) (Lagreze et al., 1991; Volkow et al., 1986). Starting with an interregional correlation matrix, one tries to find regional groupings that have strong correlations among themselves and weak correlations with other groupings. Each grouping is proposed to constitute a neural circuit. This method is more exploratory than the path analysis technique discussed above, but can be used as a starting point for path analysis.

VI. Network Modeling and Neurobiology

The neural network models described above are "macroscopic" or systems-level models, and the functional coupling coefficients are thus macroscopic or ensemble parameters, as are the quantitative values of rCBF or rCMRglc. The regional values and the functional couplings thus provide a description of the experimental paradigm. How these parameters vary as some independent variable in the experiment is modified (e.g., task difficulty, drug dose) become constraints on hypotheses purporting to explain how groups of neurons mediate the behavior under study.

As stated earlier, metabolic functional neuroimaging techniques (e.g., PET, functional MRI) provide time integrated values of regional functional activity. Given that the time scale for characterizing electrical activity in neural elements is on the order of a hundredth of a second, metabolic functional neuroimaging (even functional MRI, with its 5- to 10-s scale) represents time-integrated, rather than dynamic, neural activity. EEG and MEG, on the other hand, can provide measures of dynamic functional activity. As discussed by Toro (Chapter 26) and others, techniques like PET can be combined with EEG and MEG to provide constraints on finding the foci of electrical activity for specific tasks. These dynamic imaging techniques, however, are limited in their ability to determine values of functional activity at all spatial locations. In particular, noncortical sources generally cannot be interrogated.

A key role for systems-level neural modeling, therefore, will be to use metabolic functional neuroimaging data to generate the nodes of a network that would correspond to a specific cognitive, sensory or motor behavior, and the values of the functional couplings linking the nodes. EEG or MEG would provide measures of the dynamic temporal activity for some, but not necessarily all, of the nodes. Connecting these two different descriptions to one another will require neural models that relate the two kinds of functional activity to neuronal activity [i.e., what Churchland (1986) calls bridge theories]. Thus, it is through the different types of neural modeling that functional neuroimaging data can be best exploited and related to data obtained from other areas of neuroscience.

Acknowledgments

I thank Pamela Kirschner, Karl Friston, and Jose Maisog for help in developing some of the software associated with the studies described in this paper; James Haxby for the use of unpublished data; Stanley Rapoport for support; and A. Randy McIntosh for carefully reading the manuscript.

References

Benton, A. L. (1974). "The Revised Visual Retention Test: Clinical and Experimental Applications," Fourth ed. New York: Psychological Corp.

Bonin, G. v., and Bailey, P. (1947). "The Neocortex of Macaca Mulatta." Urbana, IL: University of Illinois Press.

Churchland, P. S. (1986). "Neurophilosophy: Toward a Unified Science of the Mind-Brain." Cambridge, MA: MIT Press.

Clark, C. M., Kessler, R., Buchsbaum, M. S., Margolin, R. A., and Holcomb, H. H. (1984). Correlational methods for determining regional coupling of cerebral glucose metabolism: A pilot study. *Biol. Psychiatry* **19**, 663–678.

Damasio, A. R. (1989). The brain binds entities and events by multiregional activation from convergence zones. *Neural Comput.* **1**, 123–132.

Damasio, A. R., Tranel, D., and Damasio, H. (1989). Disorders of visual recognition. *In* "Handbook of Neuropsychology" (H. Goodglass and A. R. Damasio, Eds.), pp. 317–332. Amsterdam: Elsevier.

Damasio, A. R., Tranel, D., and Damasio, H. (1990). Face agnosia and the neural substrates of memory. *Annu. Rev. Neurosci.* **13**, 89–109.

Desimone, R., and Ungerleider, L. G. (1989). Neural mechanisms of visual processing in monkeys. *In* "Handbook of Neuropsychology" (H. Goodglass and A. R. Damasio, Eds.), pp. 267–300. Amsterdam: Elsevier.

Ditunno, P. L., and Mann, V. A. (1990). Right hemisphere specialization for mental rotation in normals and brain damaged subjects. *Cortex* **26**, 177–188.

Ellis, H. D. (1983). The role of the right hemisphere in face perception. *In* "Functions of the Right Cerebral Hemisphere" (A. W. Young, Ed.), pp. 33–64. London: Academic Press.

Felleman, D. J., and Van Essen, D. C. (1991). Distributed hierarchical processing in primate cerebral cortex. *Cereb. Cortex* **1**, 1–47.

Fox, P. T., Mintun, M. A., Raichle, M. E., and Herscovitch, P. (1984). A noninvasive approach to quantitative functional brain mapping with H_2O^{15} and positron emission tomography. *J. Cereb. Blood Flow Metab.* **4**, 329–333.

Fox, P. T., Mintun, M. A., Reiman, E. M., and Raichle, M. E. (1988). Enhanced detection of focal brain responses using intersubject averaging and change-distribution analysis of subtracted PET images. *J. Cereb. Blood Flow Metab.* **8**, 642–653.

Friston, K. J., and Frackowiak, R. S. J. (1991). Imaging functional anatomy. *In* "Brain Work and Mental Activity (Alfred Benzon Symposium 31)" (N. A. Lassen, D. H. Ingvar, M. E. Raichle, and L. Friberg, Eds.), pp. 267–277. Copenhagen: Munksgaard.

Friston, K. J., Frith, C. D., Liddle, P. F., and Frackowiak, R. S. J. (1991a). Comparing functional (PET) images: The assessment of significant change. *J. Cereb. Blood Flow Metab.* **11**, 690–699.

Friston, K. J., Frith, C. D., Liddle, P. F., and Frackowiak, R. S. J. (1991b). Plastic transformation of PET images. *J. Comput. Assist. Tomogr.* **15**, 634–639.

Friston, K. J., Frith, C. D., Liddle, P. F., Lammertsma, A. A., Dolan, R. D., and Frackowiak, R. S. J. (1990). The relationship between local and global changes in PET scans. *J. Cereb. Blood Flow Metab.* **10**, 458–466.

Friston, K. J., Passingham, R. E., Nutt, J. G., Heather, J. D., Sawle, G. V., and Frackowiak, R. S. J. (1989). Localization in PET images: Direct fitting of the intercommissural (AC–PC) line. *J. Cereb. Blood Flow Metab.* **9**, 690–695.

Gerstein, G. L., Perkel, D. H., and Subramanian, K. N. (1978). Identification of functionally related neural assemblies. *Brain Res.* **140**, 43–62.

Gevins, A. S., Doyle, J. C., Cutillo, B. A., Schaffer, R. E., Tannehill, R. S., and Bressler, S. L. (1985). Neurocognitive pattern analysis of a visuospatial task: Rapidly-shifting foci of evoked correlations between electrodes. *Psychophysiology* **22**, 32–43.

Goldberg, M. E., and Colby, C. L. (1989). The neurophysiology of spatial vision. *In* "Handbook of Neuropsychology" (H. Goodglass and A. R. Damasio, Eds.), pp. 301–316. Amsterdam: Elsevier.

Haxby, J. V., Grady, C. L., Horwitz, B., Ungerleider, L. G., Mishkin, M., Carson, R. E., Herscovitch, P., Schapiro, M. B., and Rapoport, S. I. (1991a). Dissociation of object and spatial visual processing pathways in human extrastriate cortex. *Proc. Nat. Acad. Sci. USA* **88**, 1621–1625.

Haxby, J. V., Grady, C. L., Ungerleider, L. G., and Horwitz, B. (1991b). Mapping human functional neuroanatomy with brain work imaging. *Neuropsychologia* **29**, 539–555.

Horwitz, B. (1989). Functional neural systems analyzed by use of interregional correlations of glucose metabolism. *In* "Visuomotor Coordination" (J.-P. Ewert and M. A. Arbib, Eds.), pp. 873–892. New York: Plenum.

Horwitz, B. (1990). Simulating functional interactions in the brain: A model for examining correlations between regional cerebral metabolic rates. *Int. J. Biomed. Comput.* **26**, 149–170.

Horwitz, B. (1991). A network-simulation model for studying interregional correlations between regional rates of cerebral blood flow (rCBF). *Abstr. Soc. Neurosci.* **17**, 540.

Horwitz, B., Duara, R., and Rapoport, S. I. (1984). Intercorrelations of glucose metabolic rates between brain regions: Application to healthy males in a state of reduced sensory input. *J. Cereb. Blood Flow Metab.* **4**, 484–499.

Horwitz, B., Grady, C. L., Haxby, J. V., Ungerleider, L. G., Schapiro, M. B., Mishkin, M., and Rapoport, S. I. (1992a). Functional associations among human posterior extrastriate brain regions during object and spatial vision. *J. Cog. Neurosci.* **4**, 311–322.

Horwitz, B., Grady, C. L., Schlageter, N. L., Duara, R., and Rapoport, S. I. (1987). Intercorrelations of regional cerebral glucose metabolic rates in Alzheimer's disease. *Brain Res.* **407**, 294–306.

Horwitz, B., Soncrant, T. T., and Haxby, J. V. (1992b). Covariance analysis of functional interactions in the brain using metabolic and blood flow data. *In* "Advances in Metabolic Mapping Techniques for Brain Imaging of Behavioral and Learning Functions" (F. Gonzalez-Lima, T. Finkenstaedt, and H. Scheich, Eds.), pp. 189–217. Dordrecht, The Netherlands: Kluwer Academic Publishers.

Joreskog, K. G., and Sorbom, D. (1984). "LISREL VI: User's Guide," Third ed. Mooresville, IN: Scientific Software.

Kosslyn, S. M., and Intriligator, J. M. (1992). Is cognitive neuropsychology plausible? The perils of sitting on a one-legged stool. *J. Cog. Neurosci.* **4**, 96–106.

Kwong, K. K., Belliveau, J. W., Chesler, D. A., Goldberg, I. E., Weiskoff, R. M., Poncelet, B. P., Kennedy, D. N., Hoppel, B. E., Cohen, M. S., Turner, R., Cheng, H.-M., Brady, T. J., and Rosen, B. R. (1992). Dynamic magnetic resonance imaging of human brain activity during primary sensory stimulation. *Proc. Nat. Acad. Sci. USA* **89**, 5675–5679.

Lagreze, H. L., Hartmann, A., and Schaub, A. (1991). Factor imaging of cortical blood flow during behavioral activation: Interaction of neuronal networks in cognition. *J. Cereb. Blood Flow Metabol.* **11** (Suppl. 2), S369.

Loehlin, J. C. (1987). "Latent Variable Models: An Introduction to Factor, Path, and Structural Analysis." Hillsdale, NJ: Lawrence Erlbaum Associates.

Luria, A. R. (1973). "The Working Brain." New York: Basic Books.

Macko, K. A., and Mishkin, M. (1985). Metabolic mapping of higher-order visual areas in the monkey. *In* "Brain Imaging and Brain Function" (L. Sokoloff, Ed.), pp. 73–86. New York: Raven Press.

Mata, M., Fink, D. J., Gainer, H., Smith, C. B., Davidsen, L., Savaki, H., Schwartz, W. J., and Sokoloff, L. (1980). Activity-dependent energy metabolism in rat posterior pituitary primar-

ily reflects sodium pump activity. *J. Neurochem.* **34**, 213–215.

McIntosh, A. R., and Gonzalez-Lima, F. (1991). Structural modeling of functional neural pathways mapped with 2-deoxyglucose: Effect of acoustic startle habituation on the auditory system. *Brain Res.* **547**, 295–302.

McIntosh, A. R., and Gonzalez-Lima, F. (1992). Structural modeling of functional visual pathways mapped with 2-deoxyglucose: Effects of patterned light and footshock. *Brain Res.* **578**, 75–86.

McIntosh, A. R., Grady, C. L., Ungerleider, L. G., Haxby, J. V., Rapoport, S. I., and Horwitz, B. (1993). Network analysis of cortical visual pathways mapped with PET. *J. Neurosci.* (in press).

Mesulam, M.-M. (1990). Large-scale neurocognitive networks and distributed processing for attention, language, and memory. *Ann. Neurol.* **28**, 597–613.

Metter, E. J. Riege, W. H., Kuhl, D. E., and Phelps, M. E. (1984). Cerebral metabolic relationships for selected brain regions in healthy adults. *J. Cereb. Blood Flow Metab.* **4**, 1–7.

Mintun, M. A., Fox, P. T., and Raichle, M. E. (1989). A highly accurate method for localizing regions of neuronal activation in the human brain with positron emission tomography. *J. Cereb. Blood Flow Metab.* **9**, 96–103.

Mishkin, M., Ungerleider, L. G., and Macko, K. A. (1983). Object vision and spatial vision: Two cortical pathways. *Trends Neurosci.* **6**, 414–417.

Newcombe, F., and Ratcliff, G. (1989). Disorders of visuospatial analysis. *In* "Handbook of Neuropsychology" (H. Goodglass and A. R. Damasio, Eds.), pp. 333–356. Amsterdam: Elsevier.

Ogawa, S., Tank, D. W., Menon, R., Ellermann, J. M., Kim, S.-G., Merkle, H., and Ugurbil, K. (1992). Intrinsic signal changes accompanying sensory stimulation: Functional brain mapping with magnetic resonance imaging. *Proc. Nat. Acad. Sci. USA* **89**, 5951–5955.

Roy, C. S., and Sherrington, C. S. (1890). On the regulation of the blood supply of the brain. *J. Physiol.* (*London*) **11**, 85–105.

Sergent, J. (1989). Structural processing of faces. *In* "Handbook of Research on Face Processing" (A. W. Young and H. D. Ellis, Eds.), pp. 57–91. Amsterdam: North-Holland.

Shoham, D., Ullman, S., and Grinvald, A. (1991). Characterization of dynamic patterns of cortical activity by a small number of principal components. *Abstr. Soc. Neurosci.* **17**, 1089.

Sun, H., and Mazoyer, B. M. (1991). Simulations of a Hopfield neural network based on cerebral glucose metabolism regional correlations measured by positron tomography. *J. Cereb. Blood Flow Metab.* **11** (*Suppl. 2*), S371.

Talairach, J., and Tournoux, P. (1988). "Co-planar Stereotaxic Atlas of the Human Brain." New York: Thieme Medical Publishers.

Ungerleider, L. G., and Mishkin, M. (1982). Two cortical visual systems. *In* "Analysis of Visual Behavior" (D. J. Ingle, M. A. Goodale, and R. J. W. Mansfield, Eds.), pp. 549–586. Cambridge: MIT Press.

Van Essen, D. C. (1985). Functional organization of primate visual cortex. *In* "Cerebral Cortex" (A. Peters and E. G. Jones, Eds.), pp. 259–328. New York: Plenum Press.

Volkow, N. D., Brodie, J. D., Wolf, A. P., Gomez-Mont, F., Cancro, R., Van Gelder, P., Russell, J. A. G., and Overall, J. (1986). Brain organization in schizophrenia. *J. Cereb. Blood Flow Metab.* **6**, 441–446.

3

Distribution-Free Statistical Analyses of Surface and Volumetric Maps

R. Clifford Blair and Walt Karniski*

*Department of Epidemiology and Biostatistics and Department of Community and Family Health, College of Public Health, University of South Florida, Tampa, Florida 33612; and *Department of Pediatrics, College of Medicine, University of South Florida, Tampa, Florida 33606*

I. Introduction and Definition of the Problem

The statistical treatment of data collected in the course of PET, MRI, or EEG studies usually entails a number of problematic issues not adequately addressed by classical statistical methods. Of prime concern in this regard is the fact that such studies routinely generate tens, hundreds, or even thousands of data points for each subject evaluated. Thus, even in a simple research paradigm in which a single group of subjects is to be assessed under two treatment conditions, the investigator is likely to encounter difficulties in attempting to answer the routinely posed question of whether or not outcome variables (pixels, electrodes, etc.) were differentially impacted by the treatments.

A classical inferential approach to this problem would involve the application of Hotelling's one-sample T^2 test to the set of difference scores obtained by subtracting outcome values realized under one treatment from those produced by the second treatment. The null hypothesis to be tested is that all elements in the parameter vector of difference score means are equal to zero, whereas the alternative specifies that at least one of these elements is nonzero. But calculation of the T^2 test statistic requires that more subjects than variables be involved in the analysis—clearly an untenable condition in most studies of this sort. It should also be noted that even in instances in which

the number of subjects is only marginally greater than the number of variables, the power of the T^2 test may be so eroded as to render it incapable of detecting treatment induced effects of substantial proportions (Blair et al., 1992). Whereas various data reduction strategies (e.g., principal component analysis) may be employed to ameliorate this problem, it seems paradoxical that recent advances in spatial resolution should be analytically hampered by statistical tests that have failed to keep pace. We defer, for the moment, a discussion of the burdensome assumption of population multivariate normality that also underlies the T^2 test.

In the event that the omnibus question of whether or not treatments have differentially impacted outcomes can be answered in the affirmative, the researcher is likely to face a second, equally thorny, analytic difficulty. This difficulty stems from the need in most scientific inquiries of this type to identify individual elements (e.g., pixels or electrodes) that reflect treatment differences. Once again, the nature of PET, MRI, and EEG data renders classical methods of simultaneous inference, or multiple comparisons, inadequate for the task.

For example, the well known Bonferroni method controls experiment-wise error (EWE) by comparing each element level test result with a criterion probability obtained by dividing the desired level of EWE by the number of comparisons to be made. (We define

19

experimentwise error as the probability of rejecting one or more of the true element level null hypotheses.) Clearly, in the present context, such a strategy would tend to produce significance tests with little sensitivity to element level treatment differences. Part of the reason for this insensitivity can be found in the fact that the Bonferroni method fails to adjust critical values to reflect dependencies among comparisons. Thus, a dataset of low dimensionality would be treated in exactly the same manner as that used to treat a dataset of equal size with high dimmensionality. This shortcoming of the Bonferroni method is particularly important in studies in which spatially proximate data points are likely to be highly correlated. Whereas various modifications to the Bonferroni procedure have been made in order to increase its power (e.g., Holm, 1979; Hochberg, 1988), these modified tests are also unresponsive to the underlying data correlation structure, thereby producing unduly conservative results in many instances.

In the remainder of this chapter, we shall describe several simple, but effective, statistical tests that avoid various of the shortcomings discussed above. Specifically, we will describe and illustrate omnibus testing methods that (1) do not require an assumption of population multivariate normality for valid inference and (2) may be computed regardless of subject to variable ratios. In addition, we describe multiple testing procedures that are (1) exact, (2) distribution free, and (3) adaptive to underlying correlation patterns in the data. This last characteristic also implies that these tests will usually be more powerful than are unadaptive tests when they are used to assess correlated data. We now turn attention to these tests.

II. Omnibus Tests

The underlying theoretical justification for the tests to be discussed here is rooted in the well-known principles of permutation theory as developed by Pitman (1937) and Fisher (1966). For purposes of exposition, we confine our attention to the simple research design in which a single group of n subjects is to be observed under two treatment conditions. We also consider here the broad question of whether or not outcomes are differentially impacted by the two treatments. It must be emphasized, however, that the methods to be described here are quite general, thereby lending themselves to a broad range of research designs and questions. Further comments on this point will be made below.

In general, the sampling distribution of multivariate permutation statistics of the type considered here

is obtained by computing the desired test statistic on all possible permutations of the data vectors obtained on research subjects. Because all such permutations are equally likely when the null hypothesis of no treatment effect is true, a P value can then be obtained by counting the number of such statistics that exceed or equal the value of the test statistic computed on the data vectors as actually configured in the study and by dividing this count by the total number of permutations.

More formally, let $x_i = (x_{i1}, ..., x_{ip})$ and $y_i = (y_{i1}, ..., y_{ip})$ be p-dimensional vectors denoting observations taken on the ith subject under the first and second treatment conditions, respectively. Let $d_i = (x_{i1} - y_{i1}, ..., x_{ip} - y_{ip})$ denote the p-dimensional difference vector, which represents differences in responses to treatments. Let $-d_i$ denote the negative of the vector d_i. For instance, if $d_i = +d_i = (-1, 2, 4)$, then $-d_i = (1, -2, -4)$.

The significance level of a test statistic t, based on the permutation principle, is computed as follows. Let t_0 denote the value of the test statistic computed on the original data (i.e., all $+d_i$'s). For each of the 2^n possible assignments of $+$ and $-$ to the n vectors d_i, which are equally likely to occur under the null hypothesis of no difference in treatment effects, compute the value of the test statistic t. Count the number, $N(t_0)$, for which t is greater than or equal to t_0. The observed (one-sided) significance level of the test is then

$$P = \frac{N(t_0)}{2^n}.$$

Note that the number of permutations required for this testing method depends solely on n and not on p. This is an important characteristic of this test form because PET, MRI, and EEG studies routinely employ large numbers of data points associated with relatively few subjects. A second desirable quality of this method lies in the fact that it produces "exact" P values in the sense that t_0 is referenced to its true sampling distribution rather than one that has been approximated in some fashion. This in turn implies that no appeal must be made to a specific population form as is done, for example, with normal theory tests.

In the event that n is sufficiently large so as to make computation of all 2^n values of the test statistic impractical given available computer resources, an approximate form of the test can be employed (Edgington, 1969). The approximate version differs from the exact test in that, rather than computing all 2^n possible values of the test statistic, the approximate version uses a large (e.g., 10,000) random sample of such permutations. The associated P value is then computed as

$$P = \frac{N(t_0)}{M},$$

where M is the number of random permutations. The difference between the exact and the approximate tests is small when M is large.

One simple test statistic, useful for testing against broad classes of alternatives can be obtained as

$$t^2 = \sum_{j=1}^{p} t_j^2,$$

where t_j^2 denotes the square of the ordinary one-sample t statistic computed on the jth element of **d**. Figure 1 shows the results of a Monte Carlo study designed to estimate the power of t^2 for detecting differences between two dipoles located in an average adult sized skull with average conductivity of 3000 (ohm $\cdot$ cm^{-1}). In this study, voltages for 21 standard electrodes were generated using the homogeneous single sphere model described by Kavanagh *et al.* (1978), with additional components being added to simulate between and within subject variability. This method was used to produce data for two treatment conditions for each subject, with a different dipole location being asociated with each treatment. In order to obtain power estimates, this process was repeated 5000 times for each condition studied with t^2 being computed for each replication. The proportion of t^2 statistics falling in the 0.05 critical region was then used to estimate power.

As Fig. 1 shows, and as would be expected, the power of t^2 increases rapidly as the average distance between dipoles increases. Likewise, the power of t^2 is enhanced by increases in the number of subjects involved in the study. The Type I error validity of t^2 is attested to by the fact that a dipole separation of 0.0 (i.e., the null condition) produces a rejection rate of 5%, which is the intended level of significance for the test.

One of the most appealing properties of multivariate permutation tests lies in their adaptability to the research situation. Test statistics used in conjunction with classical parametric procedures must be expressed in forms that have known, or derivable, sampling distributions. This generally limits the domain of such statistics thereby excluding from consideration many otherwise attractive tests. For example, theory or previous research findings may suggest that treatments administered in a given research context are likely to differentially impact only a relatively small number of pixels or electrodes. In such a circumstance, a test that focuses on the largest element level difference rather than all element level differences as does t^2 can be quite sensitive to treatment differences. A statistic of this form, which we denote t_{max}, is defined as

$$t_{\text{max}} = t_j',$$

where t_j' is equal to the t_j that is greatest in absolute value.

As a final example of the flexibility of the permutation method, we define the statistic t_{sum} as

$$t_{\text{sum}} = \sum_{j=1}^{p} t_j.$$

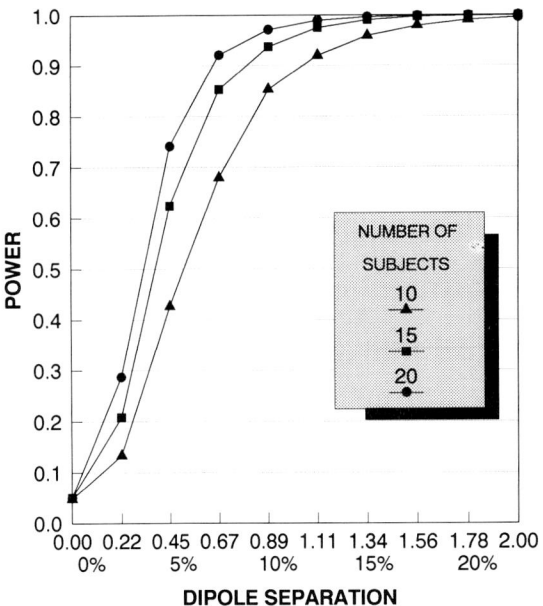

Figure 1 Power of the t^2 permutation as a function of dipole separation. This simulation was conducted on equivalent dipoles, generating voltage values at 21 electrodes when the number of subjects was always less than the number of variables (electrodes). When the dipoles were identical (true null condition), the power of the test was 5% at the 0.05 level, exactly as would be expected. As the dipoles moved apart, the t^2 permutation test identified the difference greater than 90% of the time for a dipole separation of 0.67 cm when only 20 subjects were present in the study.

This statistic has been shown to be quite powerful (Blair *et al.* 1992) in situations in which treatments induce element level changes that have the same algebraic sign as would occur, for example, with an increase in the magnitude of a dipole without an accompanying change in location. This statistic would not be appropriate in situations in which treatments caused increases at some element locations but decreases at others because the differently signed t_j would tend to sum toward zero.

Figure 2 shows the results of a Monte Carlo study that compared the power of t_{max}, t_{sum}, and a statistic denoted $t|sum|$ with that of Hotelling's T^2 test. $t|sum|$ is obtained by summing the absolute values of the t_j and generally has power similar to that of t^2. Unlike Hotelling's test, t_{max} and t_{sum} can be conducted as either one- or two-tailed tests. The suffix 1 or 2 is used in this figure to indicate one- and two-tailed versions, respectively. In this study multivariate normal data were generated with correlation between any two variables, j and j', given by

$$r_{jj'} = 1 - (j - j')\frac{1}{p} \quad j' = 1, ..., p; \quad j \geq j'.$$

As this figure shows, p took the values 4, 8, 16, 21, 32, and 48. A treatment effect was modeled by adding a value equal to 0.5σ to each variable, where σ represents the common standard deviation of the marginal distributions. For this simulation, all permutation tests were more powerful than Hotelling's T^2 test across all numbers of variables. Of particular interest is the fact that the power of T^2 declines sharply as the number of variables approaches the number of subjects, which was 10 in this case. When the number of variables reached 8, the power of T^2 was degraded to the point of being only slightly above α, thereby demonstrating an almost total lack of sensitivity to the treatment effect. Also important is the fact that, because $n = 10$, Hotelling's T^2 test could not be computed for those instances in which the number of variables was greater than 9. There is, of course, no such constraint on the permutation tests. In contrast to the pattern seen for T^2, the permutation tests show relatively stable power across all numbers of variables. (Results for $t_{sum}2$ and $t|sum|$ were sufficiently similar as to be virtually indistinguishable in this figure.) This stability is attributable to the constant effect size used to model the alternatives. Finally, as would be expected under this treatment model, one-sided permutation tests were more powerful than their two-sided counterparts.

It must be emphasized that the power of multivariate permutation tests will not always be greater than that of the T^2 test. In fact, in some instances the power of the parametric test can be substantially greater than that of the permutation tests. In general, the relative power of Hotelling's test and a given permutation test will depend upon (1) the permutation test chosen for the comparison, (2) the correlation structure of the data to be analyzed, (3) the form of the treatment effect, and (4) the number of subjects as compared with the number of variables in the study. Of course, the question of relative power becomes moot when the number of variables equals or exceeds the number

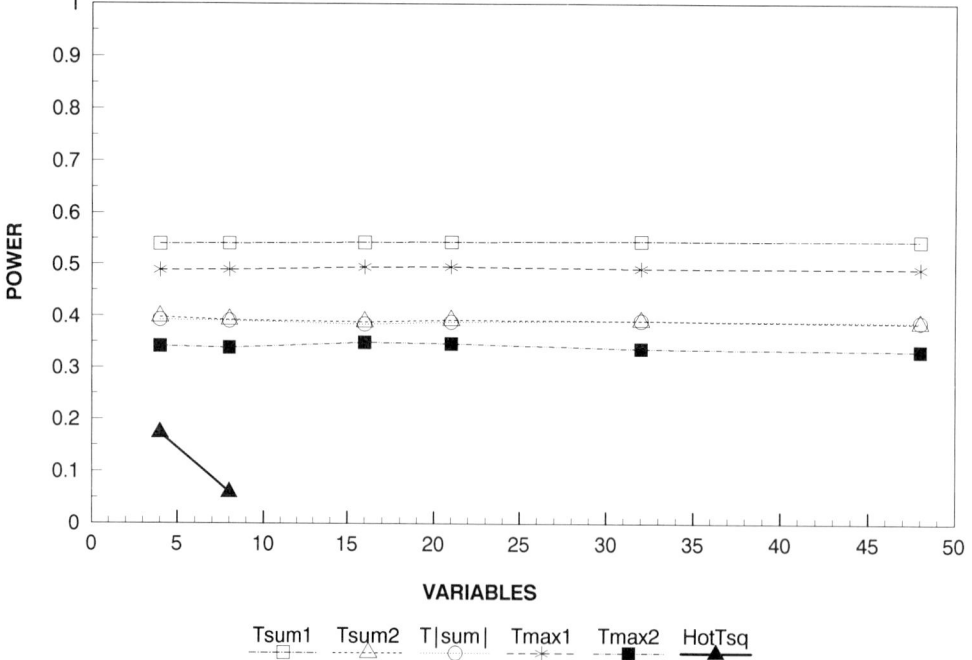

Figure 2 Power of Hotelling's T^2 and five different versions of the permutation test for a varying number of variables for 10 subjects. The power of the permutation tests remains stable as the number of variables (electrodes) increases and remains greater than Hotelling's T^2, whereas Hotelling's T^2 cannot be performed when the number of variables exceeds the number of subjects.

of subjects. The reader should also bear in mind that the T^2 test requires the assumption of population multivariate normality in order to assure Type I error validity, whereas no such assumption is needed for the permutation procedures.

III. Multiple Comparison Procedures

By their nature, the omnibus tests described above are restricted to dealing with broad-based questions concerning whether or not a difference in treatments has been realized in the course of a study. In most cases, however, not all elements (pixels, electrodes, etc.) will reflect treatment differences. It then may become vital for study purposes that elements that do show differences be identified. As applied to MRI or PET images, this is akin to the identification of the anatomic or functional locations. In the study design considered here, one might deal with this issue by conducting a paired-samples t test at each element, with significance being determined by reference to standard tables. This course will not be satisfactory if the researcher is concerned that the probability of one or more incorrect rejections not exceed some specified level. To this end, researchers often apply Bonferroni corrections to such tests, which consists of conducting each individual test at level α/m, where m is the number of such tests to be conducted and α is the desired experiment-wise error rate. As is well known, however, the Bonferroni method does not provide an exact test by setting EWE $= \alpha$, but rather guarantees only that EWE $\leq \alpha$. This, along with other factors, may result in a highly conservative test that lacks sensitivity to element-level treatment differences. This problem is likely to be particularly acute when data are highly correlated.

In this section we shall describe several multiple comparison procedures that provide more sensitivity for element-level testing than does the more familiar Bonferroni method. Some of these procedures have been previously described in the statistics literature, whereas others are appearing here for the first time. We begin with the previously described tests.

The Bonferroni method outlined above is sometime referred to as a "single-step" procedure in order to distinguish it from more recently developed "multistep" tests. One such procedure is the so called "step-down" test (Holm, 1979). Holm's test is conducted by ordering all of the P values obtained from element-level tests (p_i's) into $p_{(1)} \leq p_{(2)} \cdots \leq p_{(m)}$, so that $p_{(i)}$ is the ith smallest P value. The hypothesis corresponding to $p_{(i)}$ is denoted by $H_{(i)}$. According to this method, $H_{(i)}$ is rejected if and only if

$$p_{(j)} \leq \frac{\alpha}{m - j + 1} \quad \text{for all } j \leq i.$$

This means that the hypothesis $H_{(1)}$ is rejected when $p_{(1)}$, the smallest P value, is less than or equal to α/m, $H_{(2)}$ is rejected when $p_{(1)} \leq \alpha/m$ and $p_{(2)} \leq \alpha/(m - 1)$, and so on. Holm's modification of the Bonferroni test is superior to the traditional version in that it always produces the same EWE rate, as does the older method, but generally results in lower Type II errors for the element level tests. The advantage of this testing method is clearly seen in the fact that the size of the critical value used to determine significance is reduced as one steps down the testing sequence. This contrasts with the older single-step method, which employs a constant critical value.

While Holm's test provides important advantages over the older method, it still embodies a number of negative characteristics. For example, at the first step Holm's test employs the same critical value as does the Bonferroni method. Thus, if the first hypothesis cannot be rejected at the more stringent level, then the testing sequence is terminated and the advantages of the step-down procedure are not realized. Likewise, any nonsignificant result obtained on any but the last test leaves a subset of hypotheses untested. Also of concern is the fact that, like its older counterpart, Holm's test does not adjust critical values to account for correlations in the data. As a result, critical values may be larger than necessary, thereby resulting in an unduly conservative test.

A recently proposed test by Hochberg (1988) and Hochberg and Benjamini (1990) overcomes all but the last of the difficulties mentioned above in connection with Holm's method. Hochberg's test employs the same ordered P values, as does Holm's test, but proceeds in a "step-up" rather than step-down manner. This newer procedure begins by examining the largest P value, $p_{(m)}$. If $p_{(m)} \leq \alpha$, then $H_{(m)}$ and all other element-level hypotheses are rejected. In the event $H_{(m)}$ cannot be rejected, then this hypothesis is retained and $p_{(m-1)}$ is compared with $\alpha/2$. If the former is smaller, then $H_{(m-1)}$ and all other hypotheses with smaller P values are rejected. As described by Hochberg (1988), "Generally, one proceeds from highest to lowest P values, retaining $H_{(i)}$ if its P value satisfies $p_{(i)} > \alpha/(m - i + 1)$. One stops the procedure at the first ordered hypothesis when that inequality is reversed. This hypothesis is rejected and so are all hypotheses with lower or equal P values."

The testing sequence of Hochberg provides an advantage over that of Holm in that the former is not terminated by a nonsignificant result but continues until significance is attained or all hypotheses have been tested. This implies more powerful element level tests. Like Holm's test, however, Hochberg's procedure is unadaptive to data correlations and so may be conservative when these correlations are high. We now consider three tests that overcome, in a sense to be explained below, the conservative tendencies of the previously described procedures by using critical values that are adaptive to data correlations.

The sampling distribution discussed above in connection with the omnibus test denoted t_{max} can also be employed as the basis of a single-step multiple comparison procedure. It will be recalled that the sampling distribution for this statistic is constructed by forming the t statistics with greatest absolute value in each permutation into a reference distribution. An exact test is then carried out by comparing t_{max} with the critical values acquired from this distribution. A multiple comparison test that maintains EWE at level α is carried out by comparing each of the t statistics from the study sample with the t_{max} critical value. Hypotheses associated with any of the m statistics falling into this critical region would be rejected, whereas those associated with statistics not falling into this region would be retained. Control of EWE results from the fact that, by definition, all statistics in the study sample have an absolute value less than or equal to that of t_{max}. Therefore, rejection of any subset of t statistics in the study sample implies that t_{max} has also been rejected. Since the probability of rejecting t_{max} when all of the element-level hypotheses are true is α, it follows that the probability of one or more incorrect rejections is also equal to α. The situation where only a subset of element level hypotheses is true will be considered below. Figure 3 illustrates this multiple comparison method.

The upper panel of Fig. 3 depicts averaged frequent and rare waveforms obtained from 13 subjects during the course of a study of the temporal stability of auditory P3 derived from a standard oddball paradigm (Karniski and Blair, 1988). Each of these waveforms is made up of 500 time-point observations. The middle panel of this figure shows the average difference potential obtained by subtracting frequent from rare waveforms. The task at hand is to determine which of the 500 time points reflect rare–frequent differences. We wish to make this determination while not allowing the probability of EWE to exceed 0.05.

To this end, the lower panel of Fig. 3 shows a plot of the 500 t statistics computed at the individual time points. The sampling distribution of t_{max} yields two-tailed critical values of ± 4.468, which are shown as horizontal lines in this figure. Points falling above or below the horizontal lines can be declared statistically

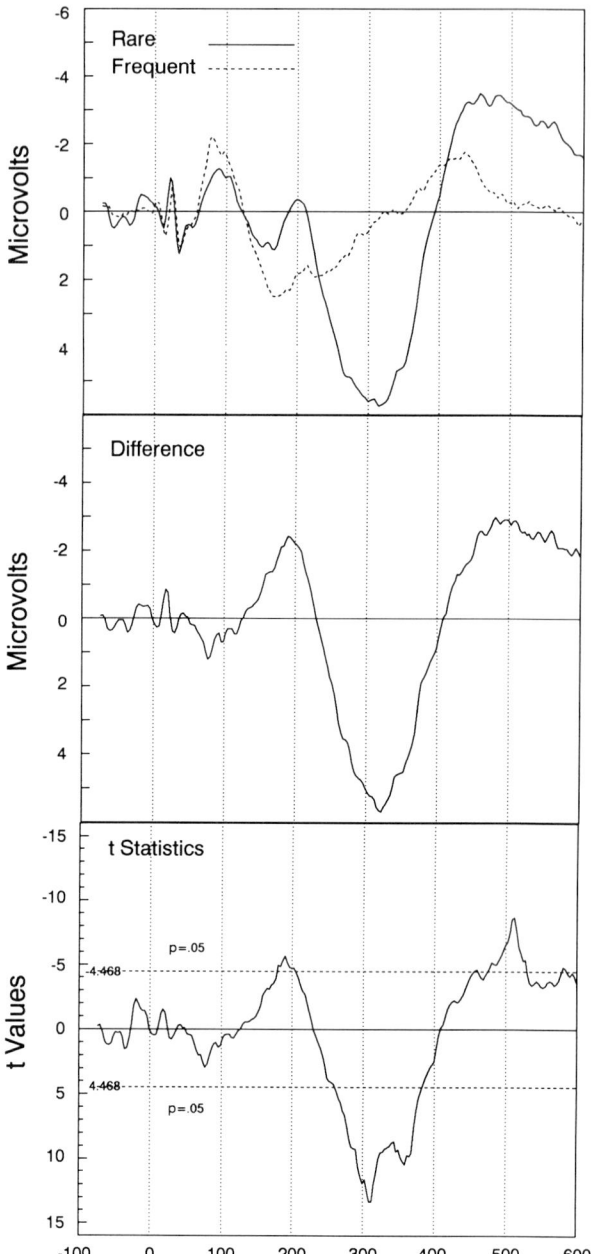

Figure 3 Averaged frequent and rare waveforms obtained from 13 subjects in a study of P300 (top); averaged difference potential waveform obtained by subtracting frequent from rare waveforms (middle); and plot of paired t statistics computed at each time point (bottom), with the horizontal dotted line representing the 0.05 critical value determined by the permutation test.

significant with assurance that EWE will not exceed 0.05.

It will be instructive to compare this single-step method of controlling Type I error with that afforded by Bonferroni adjustments. For the problem at hand, the Bonferroni method would be implemented by comparing each of the 500 test statistics with the critical value that cuts off $0.025/500 = 0.00005$ in each tail of a t distribution with 12 df. This critical value is 5.694, which is considerably larger than the 4.468 used with the permutation test. The difference in the critical values used by the two procedures is largely attributable to the fact that the data points that make up the waveform are correlated. Because the permutation method takes this dependency into account, whereas the Bonferroni method does not, the result is a less stringent critical value for the former procedure.

Permutation tests are conditioned on the data obtained in the research sample. This means that critical values reflect not only data shape as it exists in the sample, but also correlation patterns. An intuitive understanding of how the permutation method adjusts critical values to reflect correlations can be gained by considering the extreme case, in which all values obtained for a given subject are equal. In such a circumstance, all pairwise correlations would equal 1.0. It is obvious that no adjustment for multiple comparisons should be made in this case because all t statistics will have the same value meaning that, in reality, only a single test of hypothesis is being conducted. Because all t statistics in each permutation sample equal a common value, the resulting sampling distribution (of t_{max} for example) is exactly the same as that obtained if each subject were associated with but a single value. That is, the critical value in this case would be the same as that obtained for a univariate problem. If the correlations between variables are high but less than 1.0, the variability between t statistics in each permutation sample will be small and the value of the maximum statistic will tend to be only slightly larger (in absolute value) than that obtained for a univariate problem. As correlations between variables tend to zero, variability between t statistics in each permutation sample increase as will the variance of the sampling distribution. Thus, this method for performing multiple comparisons "automatically" adapts critical values to data dependencies without the necessity of estimating quantified representations of these dependencies. This has the important property of avoiding threats to test validity that often accompany such estimation procedures.

In the same sense that Holm's test is an improvement over the Bonferroni method, a step-down permutation test can be devised as an improvement over the single-step procedure discussed above. Such a test can be carried out by arranging the element-level t statistics from the study sample into descending order of absolute magnitude. The rules for the testing sequence are the same as those for Holm's test. That is,

one begins by comparing the t statistic with greatest absolute value with the critical value derived from its sampling distribution. If one wishes to maintain EWE at level α, then the appropriate critical value is the one that cuts off α in the tails (or tail in the case of a directional test) of the sampling distribution. Note that this first step uses the same critical value as does the single-step permutation test discussed above. If this first step is nonsignificant, then all null hypotheses are retained and testing is terminated. If not, $H_{(1)}$ is rejected and the second largest t statistic in absolute value is compared with the α level critical value derived from its sampling distribution. This process continues until either a nonsignificant result is obtained or all hypotheses have been rejected.

A key difference between the single-step and step-down tests resides in the fact that the single-step procedure uses the same sampling distribution for all comparisons, whereas the step-down test uses a different sampling distribution at each step of the testing sequence. The information in Table 1 will be used to help explain how the sampling distributions are constructed for the step-down test. In this table the 3×3 matrix under the heading "Permutation 1" is used to represent difference score observations obtained from each of three subjects (rows) on each of three variables (columns). For example, the values 2, 5, and -2 represent results obtained when observations taken on the second subject under one treatment condition are subtracted from those taken on the same subject under a different treatment condition, with such differences being taken on each of three variables. This matrix, along with the others shown in the table, represent all of the $2^3 = 8$ possible permutations of the data as described above. The t statistics computed on each of the variables is shown in parentheses beneath each data matrix. It must be remembered that Permutation 1 depicts the data as they were collected in the (fictitious) study.

At the first step, we test $t = 6.928$ for significance. The reference distribution for this test is formed by arranging the t statistics with the greatest absolute value in each data permutation in ascending order. The distribution thus obtained is -6.928, -3.972, -0.795, -0.758, 0.758, 0.795, 3.972, and 6.928. The obtained t value of 6.928 would be significant at the one-tailed $\alpha = 1/8$ or two-tailed $\alpha = 1/4$ level. Assuming significance, the t statistic that is second largest in absolute value (i.e., 1.732) is tested. Because the t statistic associated with the second variable has already been tested, the sampling distribution for the second step test must be formed solely from those t values that are associated with variables 1 or 3. That

Table 1   All Possible Permutations and Accompanying t Statistics for Data Used to Illustrate
Step-Up and Step-Down Permutation Tests

Permutation 1 (variables)			Permutation 2 (variables)			Permutation 3 (variables)			Permutation 4 (variables)		
1	2	3	1	2	3	1	2	3	1	2	3
1	3	-1	1	3	-1	1	3	-1	1	3	-1
2	5	-2	2	5	-2	-2	-5	2	-2	-5	2
0	4	1	0	-4	-1	0	4	1	0	-4	-1
(1.732: 6.928; -0.758)			(1.732; 0.487; -3.972)			(-0.374; 0.235; 0.758)			(-0.374; -0.795; 0.0)		

Permutation 5 (variables)			Permutation 6 (variables)			Permutation 7 (variables)			Permutation 8 (variables)		
1	2	3	1	2	3	1	2	3	1	2	3
-1	-3	1	-1	-3	1	-1	-3	1	-1	-3	1
2	5	-2	2	5	-2	-2	-5	2	-2	-5	2
0	4	1	0	-4	-1	0	4	1	0	-4	-1
(0.374: 0.795; 0.0)			(0.374; -0.235; -0.758)			(-1.732; -0.487; 3.972)			(-1.732; -6.928; 0.758)		

is, we once again take the t with greatest absolute value from each permutation but do so without regard to those values that were obtained on the second variable. This distribution is given by -3.972, -1.732, -0.758, -0.374, 0.374, 0.758, and 3.972. In this case the test value of 1.732 has an associated one-tailed P value of 1/4 and two-tailed P value of 1/2. The reference distribution for the third step test, if it were to be conducted, is created solely from values obtained from variable 3. This distribution is then -3.972, -0.758, -0.758, 0.0, 0.0, 0.758, 0.758, and 3.972. In general, and as illustrated here, the sampling distribution at each step is formed by ignoring values that are obtained from previously tested variables. As with the single-step test, the sampling distributions for this testing method are conditioned on the data correlations.

The reference distributions for the step-down tests described above can also serve as the basis for a step-up test. The advantages of such a test over the step-down version are essentially the same as those of Hochberg's test compared with Holm's test. The testing sequence of the step-up test would be the same as that of Hochberg. That is, after forming the reference distributions as described above, the t statistic with smallest absolute value is tested against its reference distribution. If significant, all hypotheses are rejected. If not, this hypothesis is retained and the next step-up test is performed. The sequence is continued as described above until either all hypotheses are retained or a rejection occurs.

In order to better understand the Type I error characteristics of these tests, it will be useful to distinguish

between two forms of EWE control. A test is said to maintian EWE level in a "weak" sense if this level is maintained only in the situation in which all tested null hypotheses are true. Fisher's (protected) LSD is a well-known test of this type. However, it is also highly desirable that a test maintain EWE level for a subset of true null hypotheses given that all other hypotheses are false. Tests that do this are said to maintain control in a "strong" sense.

Table 2 shows the results of a Monte Carlo study that examined Type I error characteristics of various tests discussed here. In this study, six multiple comparisons were carried out using moderately correlated data. Each EWE estimate was based on 100,000 repetitions of the assessed experimental condition. Estimates were obtained for situations in which all six hypotheses were true as well as the situation in which there were only three true hypotheses. Desired EWE was set to 0.05. As may be seen from this table, all

Table 2   Experimentwise Error Estimates for Selected
Multiple Comparison Procedures

	Number of True Null Hypotheses	
Statistic	6	3
Bonferroni	0.023	0.012
Holm	0.023	0.024
Hochberg	0.026	0.036
P(S-U)	0.050	0.050
P(S-U)	0.051	0.052

three parametric tests produced conservative results for all conditions studied. When all hypotheses were true, the step-down permutation test ($P(S\text{-}D)$) was exact, thereby maintaining level at the desired rate of 0.05. Whereas the step-up test ($P(S\text{-}U)$) generated a slightly liberal 0.051 level in this situation, this may be attributable to sampling error.

The step-down permutation test is not exact for the situation in which only a subset of hypotheses is true, but instead provides an upperbound for the desired level. The condition in which only three hypotheses were true was designed in such a manner as to test this upperbound. As can be seen, the step-down test produced a 0.05 upperbound, thereby maintaining the test level as desired. In contrast, the step-up test produced a 0.052 rate, which generates a 95% confidence interval that does not include 0.05. This suggests that a slight inflation might have taken place although the degree seems insignificant for practical purposes. In short, the step-down permutation test is exact when all null hypotheses are true and provides the appropriate upperbound when only a subset of hypotheses are true. There is evidence that the step-up test does not maintain exact levels in all situations, although results presented here (as well as extensive results not shown) suggest that the discrepancy is quite modest. By contrast, the older parametric tests were unduly conservative.

An example is presented in Plate 3 to demonstrate the relative sensitivity of the Bonferroni and multistep tests. To this end, a three-shell equivalent dipole model (Kavanagh *et al.*, 1978) was used to generate data at 100 electrodes for each of 20 subjects. For the first treatment condition, two mirror-image dipoles were simulated—one located in the left hemisphere of the head and the other in the right. The second condition was modeled by increasing the magnitude of the left dipole by 2% and decreasing the magnitude of the mirror-image dipole by the same amount. The grand average voltage maps produced by the two conditions are almost identical in appearance because, other than inter- and intrasubject variability, they differ only by a 2% magnitude change. The two condition maps were subtracted and scaled to produce the difference map. Paired-samples *t* tests performed at each electrode produced the map of *t* values with each of the electrodes that were found to be statistically significant by the permutation tests marked.

Of particular import is the fact that the Bonferroni method, using a constant critical value of 4.19, correctly identified seven of the electrodes as producing significant differences, whereas the Holm and Hochberg methods increased this number to eight. As can be seen, these latter tests rejected the hypothesis asso-

ciated with the eighth largest *t* statistic, using a critical value of 4.16. By contrast, the permutation tests correctly identified 10 electrodes, with a critical value of 3.84 being used to reject the hypothesis associated with the 10th largest *t* value.

In general, the relative power of the permutation and nonpermutation multistep tests will depend upon the degree of data correlation. We speculate that the Holm and Hochberg tests will be favored when correlations are small, whereas the permutation tests will excel when correlations are higher. Further study is needed to produce more definitive guidelines in this regard.

IV. Concluding Remarks

The inadequaticies of standard statistical methods such as Hotelling's T^2 and Bonferroni adjustments for analyzing data of the sort considered here seem apparent. Given the validity of this statement, it follows that other, more suitable methods should be identified or developed. To this end we have described, and examined some of the operating characteristics of, a number of such procedures. The foundation underlying some of these newer tests is the permutation method of significance assessment. This method provides a number of important advantages, among which are the following. (1) The permutation method of test construction has relatively deep historical roots, is well understood, and enjoys a great deal of respect in the statistics community. (2) Such tests are conditioned on the sample data implying, among other things, that they are distribution free and take into account the correlation structure as it exists in that data. This latter point means that no specific correlational form need be assumed nor is there any need to estimate some parameter that reflects this form. Thus, these tests avoid many of the sources of inference invalidity that hamper other methods. (3) Permutation methods are extremely flexible, thereby permitting the tailoring of test statistics for enhanced sensitivity to anticipated or important expressions of treatment impact. For example, changes in some specified area of a map may be considered more important than changes that may occur elsewhere. In such a situation, the researcher might differentially weigh the t_j^2 components of the omnibus t^2 statistic, with larger weights being assigned to the t_j^2 that are associated with the area of interest.

As a final comment on the flexibility of these methods, it should be noted that they are easily adapted to research designs other than those considered here. For example, by permuting data vectors between groups and appropriately transforming the data, multigroup repeated-measures designs can be analyzed, with tests for main effects, interactions, and multiple comparisons being carried out within a permutation framework. Such tests not only avoid normality assumptions but also the sphericity assumption that underlies the mixed model repeated measures approach. Under certain circumstances, even single-subject designs can be validly analyzed (Edgington, 1980).

One potential shortcoming of the methods discussed here lies in the discrete nature of the reference distributions. When samples are quite small (e.g., <5 or 6) the discreteness of the reference distribution may not permit the test to be conducted at a desired level, such as 0.05, but may instead force the researcher to choose a nontraditional level such as 0.03 or 0.07. This problem rapidly diminishes as sample size increases. One should also take into account the fact that parametric tests may fair even worse in this situation because they often lack robustness to departures from parametric assumptions when samples are small.

Historically, the principal shortcoming of permutation tests rests in the volume of calculations required for their application. The importance of this difficulty has waned in recent years with the development of high-speed, relatively inexpensive computers.

Historically, the principal shortcoming of permutation tests rests in the volume of calculations required for their application. The importance of this difficulty has waned in recent years with the development of high-speed, relatively inexpensive computers.

After considering the strengths and weaknesses of the permutation model, we conclude that this method offers significant potential for the development of more effective procedures for the analysis of neuroimaging data. We hope this chapter will serve to promote further development and research in this area.

References

Blair, R. C., Higgins, J. J., Karniski, W., and Kromrey, J. D. (1992). A study of multivariate permutation tests which may replace Hotelling's T^2 test in prescribed circumstances. *J. Multivar. Behav. Res.*, in press.

Edgington, E. S. (1969). Approximate randomization tests. *J. Psychol.* **72**, 143–149.

Edgington, E. S. (1980). Invited paper—Validity of randomization tests for one-subject experiments. *J. Educ. Stat.* **5**, 235–251.

Fisher, R. A. (1966). "The Design of Experiments," Eighth ed. New York: Hafner.

Hochberg, Y. (1988). A sharper Bonferroni procedure for multiple tests of significance. *Biometrika* **75**, 800–803.

Hochberg, Y., and Benjamini, Y. (1990). More powerful procedures for multiple significance testing. *Stat. Med.* **9**, 811–818.

Holm, S. (1979). A simple sequentially rejective multiple test procedure. *Scand. J. Stat.* **6**, 65–70.

Karniski, W., and Blair, R. C. (1988). Topographical and temporal stability of the P300. *Electroencephalogr. Clin. Neurophysiol.* **72**, 373–383.

Kavanagh, R. N., Darcey, T. M., Lehmann, D., and Fender, D. H. (1978). Evaluation of methods for three-dimensional localization of electrical sources in the human brain. *IEEE Trans. Biomed. Eng.* **25**, 421–429.

Pitman, E. J. G. (1937). Significance tests which may be applied to samples from any population I and II. *J. R. Stat. Soc.*, Suppl. 4, 119–130; 225–232.

4

Radiotracer Techniques for Functional Neuroimaging with Positron Emission Tomography

Peter Herscovitch

The Warren Grant Magnuson Clinical Center, National Institutes of Health, Bethesda, Maryland 20892

I. Introduction

This chapter attests to the importance of functional neuroimaging and to the increasing sophistication of the methods used to collect and analyze the images that are obtained. Although several methods are available for functional neuroimaging, positron emission tomography (PET) is currently the most widely used approach. PET is a nuclear medicine technique for performing regional physiologic measurements *in vivo*. The PET scanner provides tomographic images of the distribution of positron-emitting radioactive tracers in the body from which measurements such as blood flow and glucose metabolism can be obtained.

Conceptually, there are several components involved in performing measurements with PET. First, one requires tracer compounds of physiologic interest that are labeled with radioactive atoms that emit positrons. The positron-emitting radionuclides used most commonly to label PET radiotracers and their half-lives[1] are oxygen-15 (^{15}O; 2 min), nitrogen-13 (^{13}N; 10 min), carbon-11 (^{11}C; 20 min), and fluorine-18 (^{18}F; 110 min). A wide variety of positron-emitting radiopharmaceuticals has been synthesized to trace different physiologic processes. The second component, the

tomograph or scanner, consists of rings of radiation detectors arrayed around the body. It provides cross-sectional or tomographic images of the distribution of positron-emitting radioactivity in the body. Because of the special nature of the positron and the techniques used for image reconstruction, it is possible to obtain *absolute* radioactivity measurements from these images. Third, one requires a mathematical model that describes the *in vivo* behavior of the specific radiotracer used, that is the relationship over time between the amount of tracer presented to a brain region in its arterial input and the amount of tracer in the region. With an appropriate model, the physiologic process under study can be quantitated from measurements of radiotracer concentration in brain and blood. Finally, increasingly sophisticated methods have been developed to analyze PET images. These are used to provide anatomic localization in PET images and to detect areas of significant change in the physiologic measurements.

PET radiotracer techniques have been developed to study regional cerebral blood flow (rCBF) and blood volume; glucose, oxygen, and protein metabolism; neuroreceptor and transmitter systems; blood–brain barrier permeability; tissue pH; and tissue concentration of radiolabeled drugs. These techniques have been applied extensively to study both normal brain and neuropsychiatric disease (Grafton and Mazziotta, 1992; Mazière and Mazière, 1990). This chapter will describe the PET methods to measure local hemody-

---

[1] The half-life of a radioactive nuclide is the time taken for the radioactivity to decay to one-half of its original value. After six half-lives, less than 2% of the original amount of radioactivity remains.

namics and metabolism that are most commonly used to study functional brain activity. Experiments that have been performed to demonstrate the relationships between these measurements and local neuronal activity will also be reviewed. Techniques to analyze PET images of rCBF and metabolism and to correlate them with anatomic brain images are discussed elsewhere in this volume. The reader is referred to recent reviews for descriptions of PET instrumentation (Council on Scientific Affairs, 1988b; Evans *et al.*, 1991; Hoffman and Phelps, 1986; Karp *et al.*, 1991; Mazoyer *et al.*, 1991; Townsend *et al.*, 1991) and radiochemistry (Council on Scientific Affairs, 1988a; Fowler and Wolf, 1991; Kilbourn, 1990).

II. Glucose Metabolism

A. Deoxyglucose Method

The most widely used PET method is the measurement of regional cerebral glucose metabolism (rCMRGlu) with [18F]deoxyglucose (FDG). It is based on the deoxyglucose (DG) method that was developed to measure rCMRGlu in laboratory animals with 2-deoxy-D-[14C]glucose (Sokoloff, 1985; Sokoloff *et al.*,

1977). The DG method will be described in some detail because it is the basis of the FDG technique and because of the important role it has played in elucidating the relationship between local neuronal activity and metabolism.

DG is a glucose analogue that differs from glucose by the substitution of a hydrogen atom for the hydroxyl group on the second carbon atom. It is transported bidirectionally across the blood-brain barrier by the same transport system as glucose. In tissue, DG is phosphorylated by hexokinase as is glucose, to form [14C]deoxyglucose-6-phosphate (DG-6-P). Because of its anomalous structure, however, DG-6-P cannot be further metabolized. Also, there is little dephosphorylation of DG-6-P back to DG due to the low glucose-6-phosphatase activity in brain. As a result of this "metabolic trapping" of DG-6-P and its low membrane permeability, there is negligible loss of DG-6-P from tissue. This facilitates the calculation of rCMRGlu from measurements of local tissue radioactivity. Sokoloff developed a three-compartment mathematical model to describe DG behavior. The compartments consist of DG in plasma in brain capillaries, free DG in tissue, and DG-6-P in tissue (Fig. 1). Three rate constants describe the movement of tracer between these compartments. (The amount of

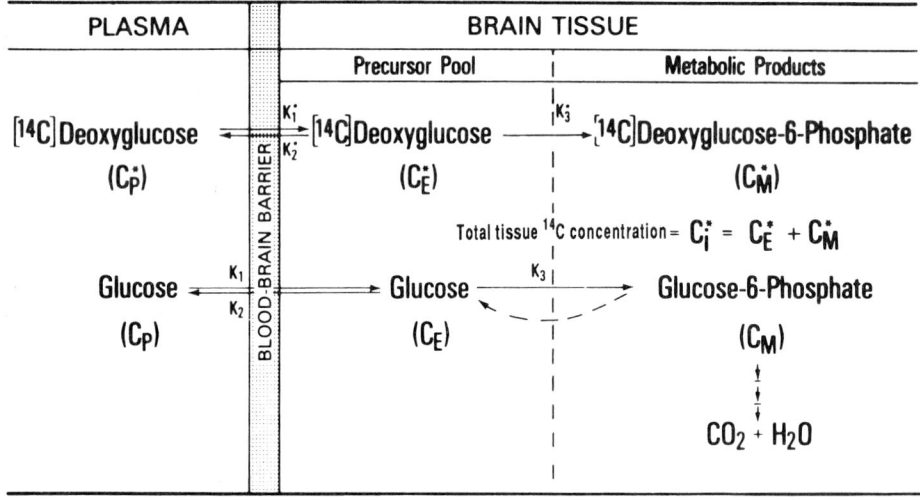

Figure 1 Sokoloff's three-compartment model to measure rCMRGlu with deoxyglucose (DG). The lower portion of the figure shows the metabolic fate of glucose in brain; the upper portion, that of DG. The three compartments consist of DG in plasma, DG in brain tissue, and DG-6-P in tissue. Rate constants describe the movement of DG between compartments: k_1^* and k_2^* for the bidirectional transport of DG across the blood-brain barrier and k_3^* for the phosphorylation of DG to DG-6-P. In the adaptation of this model to PET, 18F-labeled DG is used and a fourth rate constant, k_4^*, is added to account for dephosphorylation of FDG-6-P back to FDG. Recently however, the interpretation of k_4 as being required to account for the dephosphorylation of FDG-6-P has been questioned (Schmidt *et al.*, 1992). It has been suggested that the nonzero values of k_4 measured from PET data are observed because the radioactivity measurements are derived from heterogeneous tissue regions due to the limited spatial resolution of PET. From Sokoloff *et al.* (1977).

$$rCMRGlu = \frac{C_p}{LC} \cdot \frac{C(T) - k_1^* \exp[-(k_2^* + k_3^*)T] \int_0^T C_p^*(t) \exp[(k_2^* + k_3^*)t] \, dt}{\int_0^T C_p^*(t) \, dt - \exp[-(k_2^* + k_3^*)T] \int_0^T C_p^*(t) \exp[(k_2^* + k_3^*)t] \, dt}$$

$$= \frac{\text{Plasma glucose conc}}{\text{Lumped constant}} \cdot \frac{\text{Tissue radioactivity at time } T - \text{Free DG in tissue at time } T}{\text{Total amount of FDG entering tissue up to time } T}$$

Figure 2 Operational equation of the DG method to measure rCMRGlu. The equation is also expressed in words to aid in its understanding. $C(T)$ is the tissue radioactivity concentration measured at time T, typically 45 min after DG administration. The concentration of free DG in tissue at time T is calculated from the plasma glucose concentration of DG over time $[C_p^*(t)]$ and the rate constants. The difference between the two terms in the numerator equals the local DG-6-P that has been formed. The denominator represents the amount of DG delivered to tissue. Therefore, the ratio on the right-hand side equals the fractional rate of phosphorylation of DG. Multiplying this by C_p would give the rate of glucose phosphorylation if DG and glucose had the same behavior. Because this is not the case, the lumped constant (LC) is included to account for the difference. In the adaptation of the model to PET with FDG, a fourth rate constant (k_4^*) is included, and the operational equation is more complex.

tracer that leaves a compartment is proportional to the amount that is in the compartment; the rate constant is the constant of proportionality.)

An operational equation was derived to calculate rCMRGlu (Fig. 2). It contains terms readily measured in laboratory animals: the time course of DG concentration in plasma, the plasma glucose concentration, and the tissue radioactivity concentration at a single time point measured from autoradiographs. These are obtained by applying radioactive brain sections to photographic film. The equation also contains the three rate constants and a factor termed the lumped constant (LC), all of which must be specified. The LC corrects for the fact that a glucose analogue rather than glucose is used as the tracer. It accounts for the differences between glucose and DG in transport across the blood–brain barrier and in phosphorylation.

Neither the rate constants nor the LC can be routinely determined in each experimental animal. It was found to be possible, however, to use standard values for these terms that can be determined once in separate groups of animals. The rate constants are calculated from multiple measurements of tissue radioactivity obtained at different times after DG administration. Because their values were found to be uniform in gray and white matter, mean rate constants for gray matter and white matter can be used. The rate constants can vary in different experimental conditions, however. Therefore, a strategy was developed to minimize the error associated with using standard values (Mori *et al.*, 1990). The terms in the operational equation containing rate constants approach zero with increasing time. Therefore, a 45-min delay between DG injection and animal sacrifice was chosen to minimize error. A longer period was avoided to reduce loss of DG-6-P from tissue due to the small amount of glucose-6-phosphatase activity in brain and because of difficulty in maintaining a physiological steady state during long experimental periods. Theoretical arguments demonstrated that the LC is constant and uniform throughout brain under normal physiological conditions. A method was developed to measure the LC of whole brain from the ratio of the brain arterial-venous extraction fraction of DG to that of glucose. The whole-brain LC value, which is species dependent, is used.

The DG method has been widely applied in several species to study animal models of disease, brain development, pharmacologic interventions, and effects of functional activity in motor, visual, sensory, and other systems (Sokoloff, 1986). The power of the method was an obvious stimulus for its adaptation to PET.

B. PET FDG Technique

The method was adapted for PET by labeling DG with ^{18}F, a positron emitter with a 110-min half-life, to produce FDG (Huang *et al.*, 1980; Phelps *et al.*, 1979b; Reivich *et al.*, 1979). In tissue, FDG is phosphorylated to FDG-6-P, which is metabolically trapped in the same manner as DG. In order to obtain PET images from several brain levels with the early single-slice tomographs, it was necessary to scan well beyond the 45-min tracer uptake interval used in animals, and the potential for dephosphorylation of FDG-6-P, although small, was felt to be more important. To account for this, a fourth rate constant was added to the model. Average values for the four rate constants for both gray and white matter were calculated in a group of normal subjects from serial PET images obtained after FDG administration. Originally, a value for the LC was selected so that the average whole brain CMRGlu measured with FDG would equal that determined by earlier investigators with the more invasive Kety–Schmidt technique (Phelps et al., 1979b). The LC was subsequently measured in man from determinations of steady-state arterial and internal–jugular venous concentrations of FDG and glucose (Reivich et al., 1985). To implement the FDG technique, PET images are obtained starting 30–45 min after intravenous injection of 5–10 mCi of radiotracer (Kumar et al., 1992). Blood samples are collected to measure the concentrations of glucose and FDG in plasma as a function of time. Either peripheral arterial blood is obtained or venous sampling is performed from a hand heated to 44°C to "arterialize" venous blood (Phelps et al., 1979b). Scan duration is typically 5–10 min. The operational equation with standard values for the rate constants and LC is used to generate rCMRGlu images from the images of tissue counts and the blood measurements. Typical values of rCMRGlu in normal subjects with the measured value for the LC of 0.52 (Reivich et al., 1985) are 6–7 mg/(min-100 g) in gray matter and 2.5–3 mg/(min-100 g) in white matter (Azari et al., 1992; Camargo et al., 1992; Hatazawa et al., 1988; Sasaki et al., 1986; Tyler et al., 1988).[2]

C. Application of the DG Technique in Pathological Conditions

The accuracy of using standard values for the rate constants and LC has been the subject of considerable investigation (Baron et al., 1989; Cunningham and Cremer, 1985; Ingvar and Siesjö, 1985). The origina-

tors of the method noted that these parameters may change in abnormal conditions (Sokoloff, 1985; Sokoloff et al., 1977) and that use of incorrect values results in inaccurate calculation of rCMRGlu. Although the form of the operational equation lessens the impact of errors in the rate constants, incorrect rCMRGlu values can still be obtained in ischemia or tumor (Graham et al., 1989; Hawkins et al., 1986; Nakai et al., 1987; Wienhard et al., 1985). Several investigators suggested alternative formulations of the equation to decrease further its sensitivity to the rate constants and have also refined their calculation from sequential tomographic images (Brooks, 1982; Hutchins et al., 1984; Lammertsma et al., 1987; Wienhard et al., 1985). Experiments in both animals and humans have demonstrated that the LC also changes in certain pathological states. It increases in acute cerebral ischemia, postischemic tissue, and recent cerebral infarction (Nakai, 1987; Greenberg, 1992; Gjedde, 1985) as well as in hypoglycemia (Suda et al., 1990) and seizure (Ingvar and Siesjö, 1985), whereas in hyperglycemia it is decreased. The LC was also found to be increased in a brain tumor model in rats (Spence et al., 1990). Because calculated rCMRGlu is inversely proportional to the LC (see Fig. 2), the use of an incorrect value leads to a corresponding error in the calculation. Thus, it is necessary to redetermine both the LC and the rate constants to avoid such errors in pathological conditions in which there is a gross abnormality of tissue or an imbalance between glucose supply and demand.

These issues have become increasingly understood, and the PET FDG method has been a powerful tool in clinical research. It has been widely used to study resting rCMRGlu in normal subjects and in various conditions, including postnatal brain development, healthy aging, dementia, movement disorders, epilepsy, and psychiatric conditions such as schizophrenia and affective disorder (Grafton and Mazziotta, 1992; Volkow and Fowler, 1992).

An alternative approach to measuring rCMRGlu with PET uses ^{11}C-labeled glucose (Blomqvist et al., 1990). [^{11}C]Glucose is transported and metabolized in the same fashion and at the same rate as glucose. Therefore, a correction factor such as the LC is not required to account for differences between radiotracer and glucose. A disadvantage is that the labeled metabolites of glucose, such as $^{11}CO_2$, are not all trapped in tissue. Thus, tracer models must account for the formation and egress of labeled metabolites. The use of [^{11}C]glucose is at a relatively early stage, but with further work it may become more widely applied, especially in pathological conditions.

[2] Because of the limited spatial resolution of PET, it is not possible to obtain measurements from "pure" gray matter or white matter regions (Mazziotta et al., 1981). For example, measurements from gray matter structures receive a contribution from surrounding white matter and cerebrospinal fluid, whereas white matter measurements often receive a contribution from adjacent gray matter. As a result, PET measurements of rCBF and metabolism are generally underestimated in gray matter and overestimated in white matter. Measured values depend upon the resolution of the scanner used.

D. Relationship between rCMRGlu and Local Functional Activity

Several fundamental experiments elucidated the relationship between local neuronal activity and rCMRGlu and provided an important basis for the use of DG. An increase in neuronal firing frequency produced by electrical stimulation results in a frequency-dependent increase in local glucose consumption (Yarowsky et al., 1985; Yarowsky et al., 1983). In the visual system in rat, rCMRGlu increases with the flash stimulus rate in superior colliculus and lateral geniculate (Toga and Collins, 1981). Early PET experiments with FDG in humans demonstrated graded increases in rCMRGlu in visual cortex with increasing complexity of visual stimuli (Phelps et al., 1981). In the resting state, approximately 30% of the brain's energy metabolism supports synaptic transmission; 30%, residual ion fluxes and transport; and 40%, other processes, such as axoplasmic transport and macromolecular synthesis (Astrup et al., 1981). Most of the brain's additional glucose consumption during functional activation is required by the ATP-dependent Na^+–K^+ pump to maintain ionic gradients across cell membranes, which must be restored after depolarization (Mata et al., 1980; Yarowsky and Ingvar, 1981). The site of largest metabolic demand is not the neuronal cell body, but rather the neuropil, where axons terminate and synapse with dendrites (Kadekaro et al., 1987; Schwartz et al., 1979). This is where neurons have the greatest surface-area-to-volume ratio and therefore where ion pumping across cell membranes is the greatest. These observations are important for the interpretation of rCMRGlu measurements; a local increase in rCMRGlu may not be due to increased local neuronal firing, but may reflect increased activity in neurons projecting to the locus (Wooten and Collins, 1981). Postsynaptic elements do, however, show increased glucose consumption as well (Yarowsky et al.,1985). Furthermore, it has been shown that inhibitory activity of axon terminals also increases energy consumption (Ackerman et al., 1984), so that rCMRGlu may represent neuronal activity that is, at least in part, inhibitory.

E. Use of rCMRGlu Measurements for PET Activation Studies

In spite of these observations relating rCMRGlu to neuronal activity, the use of FDG for functional activation studies has been relatively limited, although this was one of its pioneering applications (Mazziotta et al., 1982; Phelps et al., 1981). This is because the 110-min half-life of ^{18}F complicates the performance of repeat scans in the same session. As a result, some investigators compared different activation states in different subjects (Kushner et al., 1988), whereas others scanned the same subjects in control and activation conditions on different days (Phelps et al., 1981). Reivich and colleagues (1982) proposed the use of DG labeled with ^{11}C rather than ^{18}F. Its shorter half-life (20 min) results in more rapid decay of the radioactive background so that a repeat scan can be performed approximately 2 h later. An alternative approach to performing repeat measurements in one scan session involves two sequential FDG injections and scans (Brooks et al., 1987; Chang et al., 1987; Duara et al., 1992). Scan data used to compute rCMRGlu during the second scan are corrected for the residual FDG radioactivity remaining from the first injection. With these approaches, two neurobehavioural states can be studied in one scan session.

Another limitation of the method for activation studies is that it assumes rCMRGlu is constant from the time of FDG administration to the end of scanning. It may be difficult to maintain a constant neurobehavioral state, however, and the physiological brain response may habituate. If rCMRGlu changes, the measured rCMRGlu is approximately a weighted average of the metabolic values during the experiment, with the weightings proportional to the plasma FDG concentration at the corresponding times (Huang et al., 1981). Because plasma FDG concentration gradually falls several minutes after administration, the measurement is influenced predominantly by rCMRGlu during the early part of the experiment. These limitations of DG lead to the widespread use of rCBF measurements for functional activation studies, because they can be performed much more rapidly and frequently.

III. Cerebral Blood Volume

Regional cerebral blood volume (rCBV) is measured using red cells labeled with [^{11}C] or [^{15}O]carbon monoxide (CO) administered in trace amounts by inhalation (Grubb et al., 1978; Martin et al., 1987). The labeled CO binds avidly to hemoglobin and is therefore confined to the intravascular space. rCBV measurement with ^{11}CO was one of the earliest PET techniques (Grubb et al., 1978; Phelps et al., 1979a). ^{11}CO was useful with the early single-slice tomographs because the 20-min ^{11}C half-life permitted images to be obtained at multiple scan levels by repositioning the subject. It has been supplanted by $C^{15}O$, however (Martin et al., 1987). The 2-min half-life of ^{15}O results in more rapid decay of the radioactive background, so that further PET measurements can be made with little delay. rCBV is often measured in conjunction with measurements of rCBF and regional cerebral oxygen metabolism (rCMRO$_2$) that require ^{15}O-labeled tracers; using C^{15}O avoids having to change the cyclotron target. Finally, the use of ^{15}O results in lower radiation exposure (Kearfott, 1982).

Scanning is begun at least 2 min after administration of labeled CO, to allow labeled carboxyhemoglobin to equilibrate in the blood pool (Martin *et al.*, 1987). The scan lasts for about 5 min with C^{15}O; a longer duration is possible with ^{11}CO. Blood samples are drawn, typically one per minute. Usually arterial blood is used, because rCBV is most often measured at the same time as rCBF and rCMRO$_2$, and these measurements require arterial samples. rCBV is calculated in units of milliliters of blood/100 g of tissue[3] from the ratio of the radioactivity in brain to that in peripheral whole blood. Due to the behavior of red cells in the microvasculature, the hematocrit is less in brain than in peripheral large vessels (Rosenbloom, 1972). This difference must be taken into account because the radiotracer is bound to red cells. The following equation was originally proposed to calculate rCBV from the tissue radiotracer concentration C_t (counts/s-g) during the scan and the average blood radiotracer concentration C_{bl} (counts/s-ml) (Grubb *et al.*, 1978):

$$rCBV = \frac{C_t}{C_{bl} \cdot R}. \qquad (1)$$

R is the ratio of cerebral hematocrit to peripheral hematocrit. Before Eq. (1) is applied, C_{bl} and C_t are corrected for physical decay that occurs during the scan. This assumes that decay-corrected radioactivity remains constant during the scan. There is, however, a slight decrease due to equilibration of the label with slowly exchanging compartments in the body (Lammertsma *et al.*, 1988; Phelps *et al.*, 1979a; Videen *et al.*, 1987). An alternative calculation without decay correction is preferable (Videen *et al.*, 1987):

$$rCBV = \frac{C}{R \int_{T_1}^{T_2} C_{bl}(t) \, dt}. \qquad (2)$$

---

[3] PET provides radioactivity measurements per cubic centimeter of tissue, but blood volume, blood flow, and metabolism are conventionally quoted per 100 g tissue. Therefore, it is necessary to divide radioactivity measurements by the density of brain, 1.05 g/cm^3. For clarity, neither this nor the multiplication by 100 to convert to units of 100 g of tissue is shown explicitly.

C is the number of counts per gram of tissue recorded over the scan duration T_1 to T_2, and $C_{bl}(t)$ is the blood time–activity curve, not corrected for decay. A value of 0.85 has been used for R, based on data from nontomographic animal and human studies (Grubb *et al.*, 1978; Phelps *et al.*, 1979a). Cerebral hematocrit values directly calculated from plasma and red cell volumes measured with PET or SPECT indicate, however, that R is 0.70–0.75 (Lammertsma *et al.*, 1984; Sakai *et al.*, 1985). A representative image of rCBV is shown in Plate 4. Normal values for rCBV measured with PET are approximately 4–6 ml/100 g in gray matter and 2–3 ml/100 g in white matter (Lammertsma *et al.*, 1983; Perlmutter *et al.*, 1987).

The measurement of rCBV is of interest in cerebrovascular disease because it reflects vasodilation in response to decreased perfusion pressure, as may occur distal to a narrowed internal carotid artery (Powers, 1991). The rCBV/rCBF ratio, which equals the mean transit time for red cells through the cerebral circulation, increases with decreased cerebral perfusion pressure, reflecting a slowing of the cerebral circulation. Changes in rCBV also reflect the local vasodilation that occurs in association with the rCBF response during functional activation of brain (Fox and Raichle, 1986). However, the rCBF response is greater and also can be measured more rapidly, so that it is the preferable physiologic indicator. Finally, the measurement of rCBV is a component of certain other PET techniques. rCBV data are used to correct PET measurements for radiotracer that remains in the intravascular space, so that one can determine the amount of radiotracer that actually entered brain tissue. This is necessary to measure rCMRO$_2$ (see Section V).

IV. Cerebral Blood Flow

A. Kety Tissue-Autoradiographic Method to Measure rCBF

All methods used to measure rCBF with PET are based on an approach developed by Kety to measure rCBF in animals with diffusible radiotracers and tissue autoradiography (Kety, 1951, 1960; Landau *et al.*, 1955). Kety developed a one-compartment model to describe the *in vivo* behavior of tracers that can diffuse freely between blood and tissue. This model has been extensively used to measure rCBF in laboratory animals, typically with [^{14}C]iodoantipyrine (Ginsberg, 1987; Sakurada *et al.*, 1978). Because of its importance to the understanding of PET rCBF methods, the method will be reviewed in some detail.

With Kety's approach, the radiotracer is infused

intravenously over a brief time period, typically 1 min, and the animal is then sacrificed. Frequent blood samples are obtained to determine the arterial time–radioactivity curve. The regional brain radioactivity present at the end of the experiment is measured by quantitative autoradiography. An equation was developed to calculate rCBF from these measurements, based on several assumptions, two of which have important implications for PET: (1) the blood–brain barrier is freely permeable to the tracer (i.e., there is instantaneous diffusion equilibration of tracer between tissue and blood in a single capillary transit) and (2) the tissue region in which flow is measured is a single compartment that is uniform in flow and other properties.

The rate of change of tracer concentration in any brain region equals the rate at which the tracer is transported to the tissue in the cerebral arterial circulation, minus the rate at which it is washed out into the venous drainage. This concept, known as the Fick principle, can be expressed as

$$\frac{dC_t}{dt} = f C_a - f C_v, \tag{3}$$

where f is the tissue blood flow (ml/min-100 g), C_t is the tissue radiotracer concentration (counts/s-g), and C_a and C_v are the time-varying radiotracer concentrations (counts/s-ml) in the arterial input and venous drainage, respectively. The time–activity curve measured from a peripheral artery can be used for C_a. It is not possible, however, to measure C_v regionally. Therefore, Kety introduced a substitution for C_v in terms of C_t and the brain–blood partition coefficient (λ). λ for a diffusible tracer is the ratio of the tissue to blood radiotracer concentrations at equilibrium, i.e., $\lambda = C_t/C_v$. It can be measured independently in experiments based on this definition by administering the tracer and waiting for it to equilibrate throughout the body of the animal (Sakurada et al., 1978). Because its value represents the relative solubility of the tracer in tissue and blood, λ can also be calculated as the ratio of the solubilities of the tracer in tissue and blood (Herscovitch and Raichle, 1985b; Kety, 1951). When there is no limitation to diffusion of the tracer across the blood-brain barrier, tracer entering a region in the capillary blood will reach equilibrium with the tissue by the time of its exit. Because tracer in the local venous drainage is in equilibrium with that in tissue, C_v in Eq. (3) can be replaced by C_t/λ:

$$\frac{dC_t}{dt} = f(C_a - C_t/\lambda). \tag{4}$$

This equation can be rearranged and integrated to give

$$C_t(T) = f \int_0^T C_a(t) \exp[-f/\lambda(T - t)] \, dt. \tag{5}$$

According to Eq. (5), the local brain radiotracer concentration $C_t(T)$ at time T after onset of tracer administration depends upon the flow f, the arterial time–activity curve $C_a(t)$, and λ. The unknown parameter, f, can be calculated numerically using this equation from measurements of $C_t(T)$ and $C_a(t)$. The tissue autoradiographic method to measure rCBF has been widely used in awake and anesthetized animals during physiologic and pharmacologic manipulations, and in experimental models of disease, including seizures and cerebral ischemia (Ginsberg, 1987).

B. Adaptation of the Kety Model to PET

Kety's model, embodied in Eqs. (4) and (5), is the basis for methods to measure rCBF with PET, although it has been modified to adapt to the unique aspects of PET data. Several different approaches have been implemented. They share many features, however, including the administration of a diffusible, positron-emitting radiotracer; blood sampling to determine the time–activity curve in arterial blood; and the application of a modification of Eqs. (4) and (5) to generate images of rCBF from PET images of radioactivity. The tracer most commonly used is [^{15}O]water ($H_2^{15}O$). It can be administered directly by intravenous injection, or, alternatively, scan subjects can inhale [^{15}O]carbon dioxide ($C^{15}O_2$). The catalytic action of carbonic anhydrase in red blood cells in the pulmonary vasculature results in rapid transfer of the ^{15}O label to water (Frackowiak et al., 1980). $H_2^{15}O$ has several useful characteristics as a flow tracer. Water is a biologically inert, chemically stable compound that has no undesirable physiologic effects. $H_2^{15}O$ and $C^{15}O_2$ are easily synthesized. Because of the short half-life of ^{15}O, relatively large amounts of radioactivity can be used to obtain satisfactory PET images over brief time periods with an acceptable radiation exposure to the subject. Rapid decay of the radioactive background permits another PET measurement to be performed within 12 min. A value of λ for $H_2^{15}O$ to use in the tracer kinetic equation can be calculated easily from the ratio of the water contents of brain and blood (Herscovitch and Raichle, 1985b). The average value for λ in human brain is 0.90 ml/g; values in white matter (0.82 ml/g) and gray matter (0.98 ml/g) differ because of their different water contents.

1. Steady-State rCBF Method

This was the earliest widely used method to measure rCBF with PET (Frackowiak et al., 1980; Subram-

anyam *et al.*, 1978). The subject inhales trace amounts
of $C^{15}O_2$ delivered continuously in air at a fixed rate.
$H_2^{15}O$ is generated in the lungs and circulates throughout the body. After approximately 10 min, a steady
state is reached in which the blood radioactivity concentration becomes constant and the radioactivity delivered to any brain region becomes equal to that leav-
ing the region by washout and radioactive decay. The
distribution of radioactivity in the brain remains constant, and, because the rate of change of regional radioactivity is zero, Eq. (4) may be reformulated as

$$\frac{dC_t}{dt} = f(C_a - C_t/\lambda) - \alpha C_t = 0, \qquad (6)$$

where α is the decay constant of ^{15}O (i.e. ln 2/half-
life or 0.34/min) and αC_t is the loss of radiotracer due
to physical decay.[4] Solving for flow gives:

$$f = \frac{\alpha}{C_a/C_t - 1/\lambda}. \qquad (7)$$

C_a, the arterial radiotracer concentration, is determined by blood sampling and C_t, the tissue radiotracer
concentration, is measured with PET. An average
whole-brain value is used for λ. Equation (7) is applied
on a pixel-by-pixel basis to convert the PET image of
radioactivity to a quantitative rCBF image in units of
ml/(min-100 g). The steady-state method is applicable
with all tomographs but is particularly suited to tomographs that operate best at low count rates; the rate
of radiotracer delivery is adjusted to the count rate
capability of the tomograph. With the early, single-
ring tomographs, multiple brain levels could be imaged by repositioning the subject during continued
$C^{15}O_2$ inhalation. Validation studies in animals
showed that measured rCBF changed appropriately
in response to variations in arterial pCO_2 (Rhodes
et al., 1981) and was similar to that obtained with
a reference microsphere technique (Steinling *et al.*,
1985).

Most of the limitations of this method arise from
the nonlinear relationship in Eq. (7) between rCBF
and tissue radiotracer concentration C_t (see Fig. 3)
(Herscovitch and Raichle, 1983; Jones *et al.*, 1982; Lammertsma *et al.*, 1981, 1982). At higher flow levels, a
large change in rCBF produces a relatively smaller
change in brain ^{15}O concentration. Thus, small errors
in measurement of C_t produce proportionally larger
errors in measured rCBF. Calculated flow values are

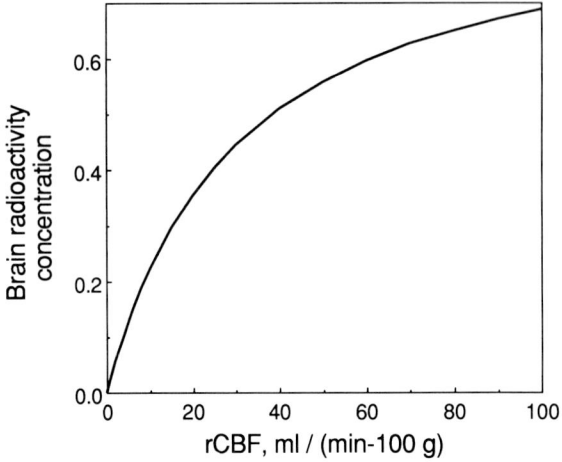

Figure 3 This graph illustrates the nonlinear relationship in Eq.
(7) between rCBF and tissue radioactivity concentration C_t (expressed as a fraction of arterial concentration C_a) for the steady-
state rCBF method. At higher flow levels, a large change in rCBF
produces a relatively smaller change in brain ^{15}O concentration.
Thus, an error in measurement of tissue radioactivity produces a
proportionately larger error in rCBF measurement.

also sensitive to measurement errors in C_a and to any
difference between the value of λ used in Eq. (7) and
its true value, which may vary if there are pathological
changes in brain water content. Another drawback
of the nonlinearity is the behavior of the method in
heterogeneous tissue regions. As noted above, the
basic model assumes that the measurement is made
in a uniform tissue region. Because of the limited
spatial resolution of PET (Mazziotta *et al.*, 1981), however, a regional radioactivity measurement usually
receives contributions from gray and white matter,
which have differing flow and λ values. The flow
measured in such a heterogeneous region underesti-
mates the true average flow by up to 20%. Because
of these limitations, as well as because of the cumber-
some method of tracer administration and the development of multislice scanners that can operate at high
count rates, the steady-state method has been largely
supplanted by methods that use bolus intravenous
injection of $H_2^{15}O$.

2. PET/Autoradiographic Method

An alternative approach is to measure rCBF after
bolus intravenous injection of $H_2^{15}O$ with a more direct adaptation of Kety's tissue autoradiographic
method. The method is not used in its original form
[Eq. (5)] because scanners cannot measure the instantaneous brain radiotracer concentration $C_t(T)$. A scan
must be performed over time to collect enough counts
to form a satisfactory PET image. Therefore, Eq. (5)
was modified by an integration over time of the count

---

[4] Note that the tissue autoradiographic method uses radiotracers
labeled with long-lived ^{14}C, so that the tracer equations [Eqs. (4)
and (5)] do not have to account for physical decay during the
experiment.

rate $C_t(T)$, from the scan start T_1 to the scan end T_2, to correspond to the summing process of tomographic data collection (Herscovitch *et al.*, 1983; Raichle *et al.*, 1983). In addition, rather than correcting the measurements of tissue and blood radioactivity for physical decay of ^{15}O, it is more convenient and accurate to incorporate the decay constant α explicitly (Videen *et al.*, 1987):

$$C = \int_{T_1}^{T_2} C_t(T) \, dT$$

$$= f \int_{T_1}^{T_2} \int_0^T C_a(t) \exp[-(f/\lambda + \alpha)(T - t)] \, dt \, dT. \quad (8)$$

Here, C is the local number of counts per gram of tissue recorded during the scan; neither C nor $C_a(t)$ are decay corrected. $H_2^{15}O$ is administered by bolus intravenous injection, and a brief scan, typically less than 1 min, is obtained after the radiotracer arrives in the head (Raichle *et al.*, 1983). The method has also been implemented using bolus inhalation of $C^{15}O_2$ (Kanno *et al.*, 1984). Blood is rapidly sampled through an arterial catheter to determine $C_a(t)$. Equation (8) can be solved numerically for flow by a variety of methods and is applied pixel-by-pixel to the image of tissue counts to obtain an rCBF image (Plate 5). CBF measurements obtained with this technique have been validated in the baboon by comparison to flow measured in the same animals by intracarotid injection of radiotracer and external residue detection (Raichle *et al.*, 1983).

The relationship between tissue counts and rCBF with the PET/autoradiographic method is almost linear; this has several advantages (Herscovitch *et al.*, 1983). Errors in measurement of tissue radioactivity result in approximately equivalent errors in rCBF; there is no amplification of error. Tissue heterogeneity results in only a small underestimation of flow and inaccuracy in the value of λ causes minimal error. Because the image of tissue counts closely reflects relative differences in regional flow, useful rCBF information can be obtained without an arterial time–activity curve (see Section IV.E). The PET/autoradiographic method does require a scanner that can operate at a high count rate; this is needed to give a statistically satisfactory image with a brief scan. Typically, 30–80 mCi are used, depending upon the performance characteristics of the scanner. Average values for rCBF in normal subjects obtained with either the steady-state method (Leenders *et al.*, 1990) or the PET/autoradiographic method (Herscovitch 1987; Perlmutter *et al.*, 1987) are in the range of 40–60 ml/(min-100 g) in gray matter and 20–30 ml/(min-100 g) in white matter.

3. Other Methods to Measure rCBF

Other approaches have been developed to measure rCBF, although they have been used less frequently in clinical research. They are also derived from the Kety model and use $H_2^{15}O$ or other diffusible flow tracers. The dynamic method involves collecting scan data over several minutes in the form of sequential, brief (e.g., 10–60 s) images after bolus administration of tracer. Equation (8) is used to describe the relationship between local tissue counts and flow for each scan frame:

$$C_i = f \int_{T_{i-1}}^{T_i} \int_0^T C_a(t) \exp[-(f/\lambda + \alpha)(T - t)] \, dt, \quad (9)$$

where the ith scan frame is obtained over the time interval T_{i-1} to T_i. A least-squares fitting method is used to estimate both rCBF and λ from the scan data (Holden *et al.*, 1981; Koeppe *et al.*, 1985). This method has also been implemented with dynamic scan data obtained from the start of a brief period of $C^{15}O_2$ inhalation (Lammertsma *et al.*, 1989).

Another approach uses scan data collected in two different forms after $H_2^{15}O$ injection (Alpert *et al.*, 1984; Huang *et al.*, 1982; Yokoi *et al.*, 1991). The terms in Eq. (4) or (5) are multiplied by two different, time-dependent weighting functions and the resultant two equations are solved explicitly for both rCBF and λ. Only two reconstructions, into which the weighting is incorporated, are necessary. Simple weighting functions corresponding to the use of decay- and nondecay-corrected scan data were originally used (Huang *et al.*, 1982). Their mathematical form can be optimized, however, to minimize the effect of image noise on calculated flow (Carson *et al.*, 1986). Data processing for the dynamic approach is more complex, but this is no longer a limitation with the use of powerful computers and efficient computational strategies (Koeppe *et al.*, 1985).

These methods have been less well studied and independent validation experiments have not been performed. Because λ for $H_2^{15}O$ is calculated, it is not necessary to specify its value. Measurement of λ may be of interest in pathological conditions affecting brain water, such as stroke and edema. However, the reported values of λ have not been consistent between methods (Lammertsma *et al.*, 1992), and further work is needed to validate these estimates.

4. Determination of the Arterial Time–Activity Curve

rCBF techniques using bolus administration of radiotracer require careful measurement of the arterial time–radioactivity curve. It is assumed that the curve measured from a peripheral artery, usually the radial, equals the arterial input to the brain. If this is not true, the rCBF calculation will be inaccurate. In fact, the radiotracer typically arrives at the radial artery several seconds later than in brain. In addition, there is dispersion or smearing of the curve as the tracer bolus traverses the arterial system; because the bolus travels farther to the peripheral artery, more dispersion occurs in the sampled curve. rCBF methods vary in their sensitivity to time delay and dispersion; the PET/autoradiographic method is most sensitive. Approaches have been developed to correct for these effects (Iida *et al.*, 1986, 1988; Lammertsma *et al.*, 1990; Meyer, 1989; Raichle *et al.*, 1983). Parameter estimation to determine delay, dispersion, and rCBF can be used, but because of statistical limitations, it is not possible to estimate all three for all image pixels. Instead, average brain values are used, obtained by fitting data from slice count rates or from brief sequential images of one or more brain slices. To simplify blood sampling, automated systems have been designed which continuously draw blood through tubing past a radiation detector (Eriksson and Kanno, 1991; Hutchins *et al.*, 1986). These produce a finely sampled blood curve and eliminate the radiation exposure to personnel that occurs during manual sampling.

C. Radiotracers for Flow Measurement with PET

rCBF methods that are based on the Kety model assume that the radiotracer is freely diffusible across the blood–brain barrier, so that, for a given arterial time–activity curve, the amount of tracer entering tissue depends only upon delivery to the region, that is, the local flow. Such a tracer is referred to as "flow limited." Unfortunately, $H_2^{15}O$ does not exhibit this ideal behavior. There is a limitation to diffusion across the blood–brain barrier, so that it does not freely equilibrate with brain tissue (Eichling *et al.*, 1974). With increasing CBF, there is a progressive decline in the extraction of $H_2^{15}O$ from blood by brain. This results in less tracer entering tissue than would be predicted by the flow model and an underestimation of rCBF, especially at higher flows. This has been demonstrated in baboon brain with the PET/autoradiographic method (Raichle *et al.*, 1983). There are, however, other PET flow tracers that are not diffusion limited, including radiolabeled butanol and fluoromethane. In a study that used the PET/autoradiographic method, $H_2^{15}O$ was found to underestimate rCBF by approximately 15% in comparison to [^{11}C]butanol (Herscovitch *et al.*, 1987). Although [^{11}C]butanol does provide more accurate rCBF estimates, its longer

half-life is inconvenient. Recently, a rapid synthesis of ^{15}O-labeled butanol has been developed (Berridge *et al.*, 1990, 1991). This tracer has several advantages, including absence of diffusion limitation, a short half-life, and intravenous method of administration, and may become increasingly popular. Another diffusible flow tracer is fluoromethane (CH_3F), an inert gas that can be labeled with either ^{11}C or ^{18}F (Herholz *et al.*, 1989; Holden *et al.*, 1981; Stone-Elander *et al.*, 1986). Its usefulness is limited, however, because of the less convenient inhalation mode of administration and the time (at least 30 min) required for its clearance from the body before another PET study can be performed.

D. Relationship between rCBF and Local Functional Activity

Several studies have demonstrated interrelationships among local flow, glucose metabolism, and functional activity. Sokoloff observed an increase in rCBF in visual pathways in the rat during photic stimulation, anticipating the use of rCBF measurements in man to map local brain responses during physiologic activation (Sokoloff, 1961). Other studies, using hydrogen clearance to monitor cortical flow in animals, demonstrated a flow response in somatosensory cortex during sensory stimulation; the response was related to both the stimulus frequency and the amplitude of the cortical-evoked potential (Leniger-Follert and Hossman, 1979). Coupling between cerebral blood flow and glucose metabolism has been demonstrated with the deoxyglucose and Kety rCBF methods. This has been done either using two matched groups of animals or with double-label techniques that permit both rCBF and rCMRGlu to be measured in the same animal. In the resting state, there is a tight correlation between local CBF and local glucose metabolism in both the awake and the anesthetized rat (Sokoloff, 1981). More recently, dynamic coupling of rCBF and rCMRGlu has been shown during somatosensory activation in the rat (Ginsberg *et al.*, 1987). In the human, coupling between rCBF and rCMRGlu measured with FDG has been demonstrated at rest (Baron *et al.*, 1984; Fox *et al.*, 1988) and in the occipital cortex during visual stimulation (Fox *et al.*, 1988). In addition, in the visual cortex, a linear relationship has been demonstrated between the rate of pattern-flash visual stimulus and the rCBF response (Fox and Raichle, 1984). These experiments, taken as a whole, provide a strong basis for the use of rCBF measurements to map local brain function. In fact, well before the introduction of PET, nontomographic methods were used to study rCBF in humans at rest and during functional activation. These methods used external radiation detectors to measure the clearance from different brain regions of freely diffusible radioactive gases, such as xenon-133, that were administered either by injection into the internal carotid artery or by inhalation (Lassen and Ingvar, 1963; Lassen et al., 1978; Obrist et al., 1967). In spite of the extensive literature relating to the use of rCBF to map local neuronal activity, however, it should be stressed that the physiologic mechanism responsible for the local flow response during neuronal activation remains to be elucidated (Lou et al., 1987).

E. Application of PET Measurements of rCBF

PET measurements of rCBF, mainly using $H_2{}^{15}O$, have been widely used to study normal brain and to assess rCBF abnormalities in a variety of neuropsychiatric diseases. The measurement of rCBF is also an integral component of PET techniques to measure $rCMRO_2$ with ^{15}O-oxygen (see Section V). Combined PET measurements of rCBV, rCBF, and $rCMRO_2$ have been extensively used to study the pathophysiology of cerebrovascular disease (Powers, 1988). The use of PET to map rCBF changes during functional brain mapping experiments has also become widespread. $H_2{}^{15}O$ is the most commonly used flow tracer for this application. Because of the short 2-min half-life of ^{15}O, multiple scans can be performed in each subject, separated by 10–12 min. Eight to ten flow measurements can be made during one scan session, allowing the subject to serve as his own control and to be studied under several different neurobehavioural conditions. In addition, these experiments can take advantage of the almost linear relationship between rCBF and tissue counts with a brief "autoradiographic" scan (Herscovitch et al., 1983). Because the $H_2{}^{15}O$ count image closely reflects differences in quantitative rCBF, relative changes in rCBF can be determined without arterial blood sampling and the application of a tracer model. This approach is now the most commonly used PET technique for functional brain mapping. Relative changes in rCBF during different tasks are determined by subtracting tissue count images that have been normalized for total brain radioactivity (Fox and Mintun, 1989).

V. Cerebral Oxygen Metabolism

A. Basic Principles of rCMRO_2 Measurement

$rCMRO_2$ is measured using scan data obtained with inhaled [^{15}O]oxygen ($^{15}O_2$). Two methods have been used in clinical research. One method was developed in conjunction with the steady-state rCBF technique and uses continuous inhalation of $^{15}O_2$ (Frackowiak et al., 1980; Jones et al., 1976; Subramanyam et al., 1978). The other uses a brief inhalation of $^{15}O_2$ and is a companion to the PET/autoradiographic rCBF technique (Mintun et al., 1984). The principles underlying these methods are similar. Only a fraction of the oxygen that is delivered to brain, approximately 0.40, is extracted by tissue and metabolized. Both methods measure this fraction, termed the oxygen extraction fraction (OEF). There essentially are no stores of oxygen in brain, and all extracted oxygen is metabolized. Therefore, $rCMRO_2$, in milliliters of O_2/(min-100 g), can be determined from the product of rOEF and the rate of oxygen delivered to brain, which equals rCBF multiplied by arterial oxygen content, that is,

$$rCMRO_2 = rOEF \cdot rCBF \cdot [O_2]. \qquad (10)$$

The basic assumptions describing the fate of the ^{15}O label are the same for both methods. The $^{15}O_2$ that enters tissue is metabolized to ^{15}O-labeled water of metabolism ($H_2{}^{15}O$), which washes out of brain. $H_2{}^{15}O$, produced not only by brain but also by the rest of the body, recirculates to brain and diffuses into and out of tissue, according to the kinetics described by the Kety model for diffusible tracers [Eqs. (5) and (8)]. Therefore, the tracer model must account for several sources that contribute to the measured ^{15}O activity: extracted $^{15}O_2$ that is metabolized to $H_2{}^{15}O$ and washed out of brain; recirculating $H_2{}^{15}O$; and unextracted $^{15}O_2$ in the brain's venous circulation. A large component of the measured radioactivity consists of intravascular, unextracted $^{15}O_2$. It is necessary to account for this component, so that it is not attributed to radioactivity in tissue from extracted $^{15}O_2$; otherwise, rOEF and $rCMRO_2$ would be overestimated. This requires an independent measurement of the intravascular volume, i.e., rCBV. Therefore, both the steady-state and the brief inhalation methods require three separate scans to measure rOEF and $rCMRO_2$: an rCBF scan, an rCBV scan, and a scan obtained with $^{15}O_2$. In addition, arterial blood samples are required to measure the components of radioactivity in blood: $^{15}O_2$ bound to hemoglobin, and [^{15}O]water of metabolism in plasma and red cells. To perform these measurements, it is necessary to centrifuge whole blood and count radioactivity in both plasma and whole blood.

B. PET Methods to Measure rCMRO_2

1. Steady-State Inhalation Method

Scanning is performed during continuous inhalation of $^{15}O_2$ mixed in air. rCBV is measured with continuous inhalation of $C^{15}O$ and rCBF with $C^{15}O_2$, as described in Sections III and IV.B.1. rOEF is computed with an equation that incorporates data from these three scans and from measurements of blood radioactivity (Frackowiak *et al.*, 1980; Lammertsma and Jones, 1983; Lammertsma *et al.*, 1983; Subramanyam *et al.*, 1978). As with the $C^{15}O_2$ rCBF technique, this method was particularly suited to the earlier tomographs that required low count rates or that had few slices. Blood sampling is relatively simple, because blood radiotracer concentrations remain constant during the procedure. Several error analyses of the method have been performed (Correia *et al.*, 1985; Herscovitch and Raichle, 1985a; Lammertsma *et al.*, 1981, 1982). Tissue heterogeneity has a small effect on rOEF calculation, but a large effect on calculated $rCMRO_2$ because the associated rCBF value is sensitive to heterogeneity. Measurement errors that may occur in rCBF, especially at higher flows, are also propagated in the $rCMRO_2$ calculation. During scanning, there may be a deviation from the steady-state requirement of constant arterial tracer concentration due to fluctuations in cyclotron delivery of ^{15}O-labeled gases or in the subject's respiratory pattern. The resulting inaccuracies in rCBF and $rCMRO_2$ calculation can be decreased by averaging data from several blood samples or by modifying the tracer equations (Lammertsma *et al.*, 1988; Meyer and Yamamoto, 1984; Senda *et al.*, 1988). Indirect validation experiments demonstrated that, with increasing arterial pCO_2, measured rCBF increased and rOEF decreased, whereas $rCMRO_2$ remained constant, as would be expected (Rhodes *et al.*, 1981). Validation studies in baboons in which rOEF was also directly determined from the cerebral arterial–venous oxygen difference demonstrated a 13% overestimation of rOEF (Baron *et al.*, 1981), most likely because the tracer model that was used at the time did not account for intravascular $^{15}O_2$ (Lammertsma and Jones, 1983).

2. Brief Inhalation Method

rOEF and $rCMRO_2$ can also be measured using a brief inhalation of $^{15}O_2$ in air (Herscovitch *et al.*, 1985; Mintun *et al.*, 1984; Videen *et al.*, 1987). A 40-s emission scan is obtained following $^{15}O_2$ inhalation, and arterial blood samples are collected for measurements of blood radioactivity. Rapid blood sampling and plasma separation must be performed. The method also involves measurement of rCBF with intravenous $H_2^{15}O$ and the PET/autoradiographic approach and of rCBV with inhaled $C^{15}O$. The equation used to calculate rOEF is shown in Fig. 4 and representative images of rOEF and $rCMRO_2$ are shown in Plate 6. As with the PET/autoradiographic technique for measuring rCBF,

this method requires a tomograph capable of operating at high count rates. Simulation studies have demonstrated that measurement errors in rCBV or rCBF cause approximately equivalent percentage errors in rOEF and $rCMRO_2$ values at high or normal levels of $rCMRO_2$, although errors are larger at low metabolic rates. Tissue heterogeneity has a small effect on $rCMRO_2$ values (Herscovitch and Raichle, 1985a). The method was validated in baboons against OEF measured by intracarotid injection of $^{15}O_2$ (Mintun *et al.*, 1984b). In these experiments, although rOEF was varied over a wide range by changing arterial pCO_2, $rCMRO_2$ varied little. Subsequent experiments validated the method for pathologic conditions of reduced $rCMRO_2$ (Altman *et al.*, 1991). This is important because the method is used to study cerebrovascular disease, in which reduced $rCMRO_2$ frequently occurs. Average values for $rCMRO_2$ in normal subjects obtained with the steady-state or the brief inhalation methods are typically in the range of 2.2–3.5 ml/(min-100 g) in gray-matter structures (Leenders *et al.*, 1990; Perlmutter *et al.*, 1987).

Both the steady-state and the brief inhalation methods require data from three scans obtained over the course of 30–60 min. It is assumed that rCBF, rCBV, and $rCMRO_2$ remain constant during this time. In addition, the subject's head must remain in the same position to maintain registration of the three images (Correia *et al.*, 1985). To overcome these difficulties, methods have been sought to estimate $rCMRO_2$ from a single scan obtained after $^{15}O_2$ administration. Although they give estimates of $rCMRO_2$ similar to those obtained with the brief inhalation method, direct validation studies have not been performed (Meyer *et al.*, 1987; Ohta *et al.*, 1992).

C. Application of PET Measurements of $rCMRO_2$

Although $rCMRO_2$ has been measured with PET in several neuropsychiatric diseases, the most frequent application has been to study the pathophysiology of cerebrovascular disease (Powers, 1988). In this case, information about the relationships among rCBV, rCBF, rOER, and $rCMRO_2$ is of interest, and the need to perform three scans is not a disadvantage. Of note, the accuracy of both methods in measuring $rCMRO_2$ is not substantially altered if there is focal pathology. In contrast, the FDG technique loses quantitative accuracy in cerebral ischemia, infarction, and tumor, as discussed in Section II.C.

In the resting state in humans, $rCMRO_2$ is closely coupled to both rCBF and rCMRGlu throughout the brain (Baron *et al.*,1984; Fox and Raichle, 1986). This

$$
\text{rOEF} = \frac{C - rCBF \int_{T_1}^{T_2} \int_0^T C_a^w(t) \exp[-k(T-t)]\, dt\, dT - rCBV \int_{T_1}^{T_2} C_a^o(t)\, dt}{rCBF \int_{T_1}^{T_2} \int_0^T C_a^o(t) \exp[-k(T-t)]\, dt\, dT - 0.835\, rCBV \int_{T_1}^{T_2} C_a^o(t)\, dt}
$$

$$
= \frac{\begin{array}{c}\text{Tissue radioactivity} \\ \text{measured with PET}\end{array} - \begin{array}{c}\text{Correction for recirculating} \\ \text{labeled water of metabolism}\end{array} - \begin{array}{c}\text{Correction for } {}^{15}O_2 \\ \text{intravascular radioactivity}\end{array}}{\begin{array}{c}\text{Theoretical tissue radioactivity} \\ \text{if oxygen extraction was 100\%}\end{array} - \begin{array}{c}\text{Correction for } {}^{15}O_2 \\ \text{intravascular radioactivity}\end{array}}
$$

where $\quad k = rCBF/(\text{partition coefficient of water}) + {}^{15}O$ decay constant

$\quad C_a^o(t) = $ measured arterial time-activity curve for ${}^{15}O_2$

$\quad C_a^w(t) = $ measured arterial time-activity curve for recirculating $H_2{}^{15}O$ of metabolism

Figure 4 Equation for the calculation of rOEF with the brief inhalation technique (Mintun *et al.*, 1984). rCBF and rCBV data are required for the calculation. The meaning of each term in the equation is given in word form. Note that the ratio of the first terms in the numerator and denominator would equal the rOEF, if no corrections for intravascular ${}^{15}O_2$ and recirculating $H_2{}^{15}O$ of metabolism were needed. Rather than correcting measurements of tissue and blood radioactivity for the physical decay of ${}^{15}O$ that occurs during the scan, it is more convenient and accurate to include decay explicitly in the equation (Videen *et al.*, 1987). $C_a^w(t)$, the arterial time–activity curve for recirculating of metabolism, is assumed to linearly increase from zero during the scan. It can therefore be determined from a single measurement of plasma radioactivity at the end of the scan (since all the ${}^{15}O_2$ activity is bound to red cells) and from the ratio of the fractional water contents of blood and plasma. $C_a^o(t)$, the arterial time–activity curve for ${}^{15}O_2$, is obtained by subtracting $C_a^w(t)$ from the whole blood radio activity curve. Although the equation is complex, an accurate simplification facilitates the calculation and the generation of rOEF images on a pixel-by-pixel basis (Herscovitch *et al.*, 1985). rCMRO$_2$ is then calculated as the product of rOEF, rCBF, and the arterial oxygen content.

is not the case during physiologic activation, however. When rCMRO$_2$ was measured during somatosensory activation, there was only a 5% increase in rCMRO$_2$, in spite of large increases in rCBF and rCMRGlu (Fox and Raichle, 1986; Fox *et al.*, 1988). This observation challenged the hypothesis that oxidative glucose metabolism or its products were directly involved in regulating the rCBF change that occurs during activation. In fact, there is considerable evidence that the classic metabolic candidates for coupling flow to metabolism, such as increased H$^+$ or decreased pO$_2$, may not be involved and that the rapid local vascular response precedes their appearance, if they are produced at all (Lou *et al.*, 1987). It has therefore been postulated that an intrinsic neural system may regulate acute flow changes (Lou *et al.*, 1987). Because of the poor CMRO$_2$ response during physiologic activation, the measurement of rCMRO$_2$ is of no practical value for activation experiments, even with a more convenient single scan approach. Measurement of rCBF with H$_2{}^{15}$O is the PET method of choice, in spite of the uncertainties about the mechanism underlying the flow response.

VI. Summary

This chapter has described the methods commonly used for functional neuroimaging with PET. In addition, important experiments demonstrating the relationships among cerebral blood flow, cerebral metabolism, and local neuronal activity have been reviewed.

Several approaches are available to measure cerebral blood flow and metabolism. Although their relative merits have been indicated, in general there is no "best" way to perform these measurements; a variety of tradeoffs are involved. This is especially true for rCBF methods, for which there are several computational strategies and radiopharmaceuticals. These methods differ in their formulation of the Kety model and in the manner of tracer admininstration and data collection. As a result, they have different sensitivities to sources of error such as tissue heterogeneity and inaccuracy in measurements of tissue and blood radioactivity (Baron *et al.*, 1989). In addition, practical issues relating to how and why a method is implemented must be taken into account (Alpert, 1991; Carson, 1991). The radiopharmaceutical, scanning protocol, and data processing requirements must be considered in relation to the resources available. The performance characteristics of the scanner used, such as sensitivity and ability to operate at high count rates, affect decisions about the amount of tracer administered and method of collecting scan data. For example, recent scanner designs permit removal of the lead septa between slices, resulting in true three-dimensional volume imaging and a substantial increase in scanner sensitivity (Townsend *et al.*, 1991). The reason a study is being performed also affects the choice of tracer method. Although both rCBF and rCMRGlu reflect changes in local neuronal activity, short scan duration and repeatability make rCBF methods preferable. Furthermore, because only relative flow differences are sought in functional brain mapping studies, a simple approach using single-frame scans without blood sampling is adequate. The diffusion limitation of $H_2^{15}O$ may result in underestimation of high flows, but this effect is well understood and has been accepted because of the tracer's convenience. In cerebral infarction, in which rCBF is decreased, diffusion limitation is less important.

Finally, it should be noted that radiotracer methods as well as PET instrumentation are constantly being refined. Current methods will be better understood and new approaches for measuring blood flow and metabolism will become available. In addition, further research should provide new insights into the relationship between cerebral blood flow and metabolism and functional brain activity.

References

Ackerman, R. F., Finch, D. M., Babb, T. L., and Engel, J. (1984). Increased glucose metabolism during long-duration recurrent inhibition of hippocampal pyramidal cells. *J. Neurosci.* **4**, 251–264.

Alpert, N. (1991). Optimization of regional cerebral blood flow measurements with PET. *J. Nucl. Med.* **32**, 1934–1936.

Alpert, N. M., Eriksson, L., Chang, J. Y., Bergstrom, M., Litton, J. E., Correia, J. A., Bohm, C., Ackerman, R. H., and Taveras, J. M. (1984). Strategy for the measurement of regional cerebral blood flow using short-lived tracers and emission tomography. *J. Cereb. Blood Flow Metab.* **4**, 28–34.

Altman, D. I., Lich, L. L., and Powers, W. J. (1991). Brief inhalation method to measure cerebral oxygen extraction with PET: Accuracy determination under pathologic conditions. *J. Nucl. Med.* **32**, 1738–1741.

Astrup, J., Sorensen, P. M., and Sorensen, H. R. (1981). Oxygen and glucose consumption related to Na^+–K^+ transport in canine brain. *Stroke* **12**, 726–730.

Azari, N. P., Rapoport, S. I., Salerno, J. A., Grady, C. L., Gonzalez-Aviles, A., Schapiro, M. B., and Horwitz, B. (1992). Interregional correlations of resting cerebral glucose metabolism in old and young women. *Brain Res.* **589**, 279–290.

Baron, J. C., Frackowiak, R. S. J., Herholz, K., Jones, T., Lammertsma, A. A., Mazoyer, B., and Weinhard, K. (1989). Use of PET methods for measurement of cerebral energy metabolism and hemodynamics in cerebrovascular disease. *J. Cereb. Blood Flow Metab.* **9**, 723–742.

Baron, J. C., Rougemont, D., Soussaline, F., Bustany, P., Crouzel, C., Bousser, M. G., and Comar, D. (1984). Local interrelationships of oxygen consumption and glucose utilization in normal subjects and in ischemic stroke patients: A positron emission tomographic study. *J. Cereb. Blood Flow Metab.* **4**, 140–149.

Baron, J. C., Steinling, M., Tanaka, T., Cavalheiro, E., Soussaline, F., and Collard, P. (1981). Quantitative measurement of CBF, oxygen extraction fraction (OEF) and $CMRO_2$ with the ^{15}O continuous inhalation technique and positron emission tomography (PET): Experimental evidence and normal values in man. *J. Cereb. Blood Flow Metab.* **1** (suppl. 1), S5–S6.

Berridge, M. S., Adler, L. P., Nelson, A. D., Cassidy, E. H., Muzic, R. F., Bednarczyk, E. M., and Miraldi, F. (1991). Measurement of human cerebral blood flow with [^{15}O]butanol and positron emission tomography. *J. Cereb. Blood Flow Metab.* **11**, 707–715.

Berridge, M. S., Cassidy, E. H., and Terris, A. H. (1990). A routine, automated synthesis of oxygen-15-labeled butanol for positron tomography. *J. Nucl. Med.* **31**, 1727–1731.

Blomqvist, G., Stone-Elander, S., Halldin, C., Roland, P. E., Widén, L., Lindqvist, M., Swahn, C.-G., Långström, B., and Wiesel, F. A. (1990). Positron emission tomographic measurements of cerebral glucose utilization using [1-^{11}C]D-glucose. *J. Cereb. Blood Flow Metab.* **11**, 467–483.

Brooks, R. A. (1982). Alternative formula for glucose utilization using labeled deoxyglucose. *J. Nucl. Med.* **23**, 538–539.

Brooks, R. A., Di Chiro, G., Zukerberg, B. W., Bairamian, D., and Larson, S. M. (1987). Test–retest studies of cerebral glucose metabolism using fluorine-18 deoxyglucose: Validation of method. *J. Nucl. Med.* **28**, 53–59.

Camargo, E. E., Szabo, Z., Links, J. M., Sostre, S., Dannals, R. F., and Wagner, H. N., Jr. (1992). The influence of biological and technical factors on the variability of global and regional brain metabolism of 2-[^{18}F]fluoro-2-deoxy-D-glucose. *J. Cereb. Blood Flow Metab.* **12**, 281–290.

Carson, R. E. (1991). The development and application of mathematical models in nuclear medicine. *J. Nucl. Med.* **32**, 2206–2208.

Carson, R. E., Huang, S.-C., and Green, M. V. (1986). Weighted integration method for local cerebral blood flow measurements with positron emission tomography. *J. Cereb. Blood Flow Metab.* **6**, 245–258.

Chang, J. Y., Duara, R., Barker, W., Apicella, A., and Finn, R. (1987). Two behavioral states studied in a single PET/FDG procedure: Theory, method, and preliminary results. *J. Nucl. Med.* **28**, 852–860.

Correia, J. A., Alpert, N. M., Buxton, R. B., and Ackerman, R. H. (1985). Analysis of some errors in the measurement of oxygen extraction and oxygen consumption by the equilibrium inhalation method. *J. Cereb. Blood Flow Metab.* **5**, 591–599.

Council on Scientific Affairs (1988a). Cyclotrons and radiopharmaceuticals in positron emission tomography. *JAMA* **259**, 1854–1860.

Council on Scientific Affairs (1988b). Instrumentation in positron emission tomography. *JAMA* **259**, 1351–1356.

Cunningham, V., and Cremer, J. E. (1985). Current assumptions behind the use of PET scanning for measuring glucose utilization in brain. *TINS* **8**, 96–99.

Duara, R., Barker, W. W., Chang, J., Yoshii, F., Loewenstein, D. A., and Pascal, S. (1992). Viability of neocortical function in behavioral activation state PET studies in Alzheimer disease. *J. Cereb. Blood Flow Metab.* **12**, 927–934.

Eichling, J. O., Raichle, M. E., Grubb, R. J., Jr., and Ter-Pogossian, M. M. (1974). Evidence of the limitations of water as a freely diffusible tracer in the brain of the rhesus monkey. *Circ. Res.* **35**, 358–364.

Eriksson, L., and Kanno, I. (1991). Blood sampling devices and measurements. *Med. Prog. Technol.* **17**, 249–257.

Evans, A. C., Thompson, C. J., Marrett, S., Meyer, E., and Mazza, M. (1991). Performance evaluation of the PC-2048: A new 15-slice encoded-crystal PET scanner for neurological studies. *IEEE Trans. Med. Imaging* **10**, 90–98.

Fowler, J. S., and Wolf, A. P. (1991). Recent advances in radiotracers for PET studies of the brain. *In* "Radiopharmaceuticals and Brain Pathology Studied with PET and SPECT" (M. Diksic and R. C. Reba, Eds.), pp. 11–34. Boca Raton: CRC Press.

Fox, P. T., and Mintun, M. A. (1989). Noninvasive functional brain mapping by change-distribution analysis of averaged PET images of H$_2$^{15}O tissue activity. *J. Nucl. Med.* **30**, 141–149.

Fox, P. T., and Raichle, M. E. (1984). Stimulus rate dependence of regional cerebral blood flow in human striate cortex, demonstrated by positron emission tomography. *J. Neurophysiol.* **51**, 1109–1120.

Fox, P. T., and Raichle, M. E. (1986). Focal physiological uncoupling of cerebral blood flow and oxidative metabolism somatosensory stimulation in human subjects. *Proc. Natl. Acad. Sci. USA* **83**, 1140–1144.

Fox, P. T., Raichle, M. E., Mintun, M. A., and Dence, C. (1988). Nonoxidative glucose consumption during focal physiologic neural activity. *Science* **241**, 462–464.

Frackowiak, R. S. J., Lenzi, G.-L., Jones, T., and Heather, J. D. (1980). Quantitative measurement of regional cerebral blood flow and oxygen metabolism in man using ^{15}O and positron emission tomography: Theory, procedure and normal values. *J. Comput. Assist. Tomogr.* **4**, 727–736.

Ginsberg, M. D. (1987). Autoradiographic measurement of local cerebral blood flow. *In* "Cerebral Blood Flow: Physiologic and Clinical Aspects" (J. H. Wood, Ed.), pp. 299–308. New York: McGraw–Hill.

Ginsberg, M. D., Dietrich, W. D., and Busto, R. (1987). Coupled forebrain increases of local cerebral glucose utilization and blood flow during physiologic stimulation of a somatosensory pathway in the rat: Demonstration by double-label autoradiography. *Neurology* **37**, 11–19.

Grafton, S. T., and Mazziotta, J. C. (1992). Cerebral pathophysiology evaluated with positron emission tomography. *In* "Diseases of the Nervous System: Clinical Neurobiology" (A. K. Asbury, G. M. McKhann, and W. I. McDonald, Eds.), pp. 1573–1588. Philadelphia: Saunders.

Graham, M. M., Spence, A. M., Muzi, M., and Abbott, G. L. (1989). Deoxyglucose kinetics in a rat brain tumor. *J. Cereb. Blood Flow Metab.* **9**, 315–322.

Grubb, R. L., Jr., Raichle, M. E., Higgins, C. S., and Eichling, J. O. (1978). Measurement of regional cerebral blood volume by emission tomography. *Ann. Neurol.* **4**, 322–328.

Hatazawa, J., Masatoshi, I., Matsuzawa, T., Ido, T., and Watanuki, S. (1988). Measurement of the ratio of cerebral oxygen consumption to glucose utilization by positron emission tomography: its consistency with the values determined by the Kety–Schmidt method in normal volunteers. *J. Cereb. Blood Flow Metab.* **8**, 426–432.

Hawkins, R. A., Phelps, M. E., and Huang, S.-C. (1986). Effects of temporal sampling, glucose metabolic rates, and disruptions of the blood-barrier on the FDG model with and without a vascular compartment: studies in human brain tumors with PET. *J. Cereb. Blood Flow Metab.* **6**, 170–183.

Herholz, K., Pietrzyk, U., Wienhard, K., Hebold, I., Pawlik, G., Wagner, R., Holthoff, V., Klinkhammer, P., and Heiss, W.-D. (1989). Regional cerebral blood flow measurement with intravenous [^{15}O]water bolus and [^{18}F]fluoromethane inhalation. *Stroke* **20**, 1174–1181.

Herscovitch, P., and Raichle, M. E. (1983). Effect of tissue heterogeneity on the measurement of cerebral blood flow with the equilibrium C^{15}O$_2$ inhalation technique. *J. Cereb. Blood Flow Metab.* **3**, 407–415.

Herscovitch, P., and Raichle, M. E. (1985a). Effect of tissue heterogeneity on the measurement of regional cerebral oxygen extraction and metabolic rate with positron emission tomography. *J. Cereb. Blood Flow Metab.* **5** (suppl. 1), S671–S672.

Herscovitch, P., and Raichle, M. E. (1985b). What is the correct value for the brain–blood partition coefficient of water? *J. Cereb. Blood Flow Metab.* **5**, 65–69.

Herscovitch, P., Markham, J., and Raichle, M. E. (1983). Brain blood flow measured with intravenous H$_2$^{15}O. I. Theory and error analysis. *J. Nucl. Med.* **24**, 782–789.

Herscovitch, P., Mintun, M. A., and Raichle, M. E. (1985). Brain oxygen utilization measured with oxygen-15 radiotracers and positron emission tomography: Generation of metabolic images. *J. Nucl. Med.* **26**, 416–417.

Herscovitch, P., Raichle, M. E., Kilbourn, M. R., and Welch, M. J. (1987). Positron emission tomographic measurements of cerebral blood flow and permeability-surface area product of water using [^{15}O]water and [^{11}C]butanol. *J. Cereb. Blood Flow Metab.* **7**, 527–542.

Hoffman, E. J., and Phelps, M. E. (1986). Positron emission tomography: Principles and quantitation. *In* "Positron Emission Tomography and Autoradiography" (M. E. Phelps, J. C. Mazziotta, and H. R. Schelbert, Eds.), pp. 237–286. New York: Raven Press.

Holden, J. E., Gatley, S. J., Hichwa, R. D., Ip, W. R., Shaughnessy, W. J., Nickles, R. J., and Polcyn, R. E. (1981). Cerebral blood flow using PET measurements of fluoromethane kinetics. *J. Nucl. Med.* **22**, 1084–1088.

Huang, S.-C., Carson, R. E., and Phelps, M. E. (1982). Measurement of local blood flow and distribution volume with short-lived isotopes: A general input technique. *J. Cereb. Blood Flow Metab.* **2**, 99–108.

Huang, S.-C., Phelps, M. E., Hoffman, E. J., and Kuhl, D. E. (1981). Error sensitivity of fluorodeoxyglucose method for measurement of cerebral metabolic rate of glucose. *J. Cereb. Blood Flow Metab.* **1**, 391–401.

Huang, S. C., Phelps, M. E., Hoffman, E. J., Sideris, K., Selin, C. J., and Kuhl, D. E. (1980). Noninvasive determination of local cerebral metabolic rate of glucose in man. *Am. J. Physiol.* **238**, E69–E82.

Hutchins, G. D., Hichwa, R. D., and Koeppe, R. A. (1986). A continuous flow input function detector for O-15 H$_2$O blood flow studies in positron emission tomography. *IEEE Trans. Nucl. Sci.* **33**, 546–549.

Hutchins, G. D., Holden, J. E., Koeppe, R. A., Halama, J. R., Gatley, S. J., and Nickles, R. J. (1984). Alternative approach to single-scan estimation of cerebral glucose metabolic rate using glucose analogs, with particular application to ischemia. *J. Cereb. Blood Flow Metab.* **4**, 35–40.

Iida, H., Kanno, I., Miura, S., Murakami, M., Takahashi, K., and Uemura, K. (1986). Error analysis of a quantitative cerebral blood flow measurement using $H_2^{15}O$ autoradiography and positron emission tomography, with respect to the dispersion of the input function. *J. Cereb. Blood Flow Metab.* **6**, 536–545.

Iida, H., Kanno, I., Miura, S., Murakami, M., Takahashi, K., and Uemura, K. (1988). Evaluation of regional differences of tracer appearance time in cerebral tissues using [^{15}O]water and dynamic positron emission tomography. *J. Cereb. Blood Flow Metab.* **8**, 285–288.

Ingvar, M., and Siesjö, B. K. (1985). Measurements of brain glucose utilization in pathological states: Problems and pitfalls. *In* "The Metabolism of the Human Brain Studied with Positron Emission Tomography" (T. Greitz, D. H. Ingvar, and L. Widén, Eds.), pp. 195–205. New York: Raven Press.

Jones, S. C., Greenberg, J. H., and Reivich, M. (1982). Error analysis for the determination of cerebral blood flow with the continuous inhalation of ^{15}O-labeled carbon dioxide and positron emission tomography. *J. Comput. Assist. Tomogr.* **6**, 116–124.

Jones, T., Chesler, D. A., and Ter-Pogossian, M. M. (1976). The continuous inhalation of oxygen-15 for assessing regional oxygen extraction in the brain of man. *Br. J. Radiol.* **49**, 339–343.

Kadekaro, M., Vance, W. H., Terrell, M. L., Gary, H., Jr., Eisenberg, H. M., and Sokoloff, L. (1987). Effects of antidromic stimulation of the ventral root on glucose utilization in the ventral horn of the spinal cord in the rate. *Proc. Natl. Acad. Sci. USA* **84**, 5492–5495.

Kanno, I., Lammertsma, A. A., Heather, J. D., Gibbs, J. M., Rhodes, C. G., Clark, J. C., and Jones, T. (1984). Measurement of cerebral blood flow using bolus inhalation of $C^{15}O_2$ and positron emission tomography: Description of the method and its comparison with the $C^{15}O_2$ continuous inhalation method. *J. Cereb. Blood Flow Metab.* **4**, 224–234.

Karp, J. S., Daube-Witherspoon, M. E., Hoffman, E. J., Lewellen, T. K., Links, J. M., Wong, W.-H., Hichwa, R. D., Casey, M. E., Colsher, J. G., Hitchens, R. E., Muehllehner, G., and Stoub, E. (1991). Performance standards in positron emission tomography. *J. Nucl. Med.* **32**, 2342–2350.

Kearfott, K. J. (1982). Absorbed dose estimates for positron emission tomography (PET): $C^{15}O$, ^{11}CO, and $CO^{15}O$. *J. Nucl. Med.* **23**, 1031–1037.

Kety, S. S. (1951). The theory and applications of the exchange of inert gas at the lungs and tissues. *Pharmacol. Rev.* **3**, 1–41.

Kety, S. S. (1960). Measurement of local blood flow by the exchange of an inert diffusible substance. *Methods Med. Res.* **8**, 228–236.

Kilbourn, M. R. (1990). "Fluorine-18 Labeling of Radiopharmaceuticals." Washington, DC: National Academy Press.

Koeppe, R. A., Holden, J. E., and Ip, W. R. (1985). Performance comparison of parameter estimation techniques for the quantitation of local cerebral blood flow by dynamic positron computed tomography. *J. Cereb. Blood Flow Metab.* **5**, 224–234.

Kumar, A., Braun, A., Schapiro, M., Grady, C., Carson, R., and Herscovitch, P. (1992). Cerebral glucose metabolic rates after 30 and 45 minute acquisitions: A comparative study. *J. Nucl. Med.* **33**, 2103–2105.

Kushner, M. J., Rosenquist, A., Alavi, A., Rosen, M., Dann, R., Frazekas, F., Bosley, T., Greenberg, J., and Reivich, M. (1988). Cerebral metabolism and patterned visual stimulation: A positron emission tomographic study of the human visual cortex. *Neurology* **38**, 89–95.

Lammertsma, A. A., and Jones, T. (1983). Correction for the presence of intravascular oxygen-15 in the steady state technique for measuring regional oxygen extraction ratio in the brain. 1. Description of the method. *J. Cereb. Blood Flow Metab.* **13**, 416–424.

Lammertsma, A. A., Brooks, D. J., Beaney, R. P., Turton, D. R., Kensett, M. J., Heather, J. D., Marshall, J., and Jones, T. (1984). *In vivo* measurement of regional cerebral haematocrit using positron emission tomography. *J. Cereb. Blood Flow Metab.* **4**, 317–322.

Lammertsma, A. A., Brooks, D. J., Frackowiak, R. S. J., Beany, R. P., Herold, S., Heather, J. D., Palmer, A. J., and Jones, T. (1987). Measurement of glucose utilization with [^{18}F]2-fluoro-2-deoxy-D-glucose: A comparison of different analytical methods. *J. Cereb. Blood Flow Metab.* **7**, 161–172.

Lammertsma, A. A., Correia, J. A., and Jones, T. (1988). Stability of arterial concentrations during continuous inhalation of $C^{15}O_2$ and $^{15}O_2$ and the effects on computed values of CBF and $CMRO_2$. *J. Cereb. Blood Flow Metab.* **8**, 411–417.

Lammertsma, A. A., Cunningham, V. J., Deiber, M. P., Heather, J. D., Bloomfield, P. M., Nutt, J., Frackowiak, R. S. J., and Jones, T. (1990). Combination of dynamic and integral methods for generating reproducible functional CBF images. *J. Cereb. Blood Flow Metab.* **10**, 675–686.

Lammertsma, A. A., Frackowiak, S. J., Hoffman, J. M., Huang, S.-C., Weinberg, I. N., Dahlbom, M., MacDonald, N. S., Hoffman, E. J., Mazziotta, J. C., Heather, J. D., Forse, G. R., Phelps, M. E., and Jones, T. (1989). The $C^{15}O_2$ build-up technique to measure regional cerebral blood flow and volume of distribution of water. *J. Cereb. Blood Flow Metab.* **9**, 461–470.

Lammertsma, A. A., Heather, J. D., Jones, T., Frackowiak, R. S. J., and Lenzi, G.-L. (1982). A statistical study of the steady state technique for measuring regional cerebral blood flow and oxygen utilization using ^{15}O. *J. Comput. Assist. Tomogr.* **6**, 566–573.

Lammertsma, A. A., Jones, T., Frackowiak, R. S. J., and Lenzi, G.-L. (1981). A theoretical study of the steady-state model for measuring regional cerebral blood flow and oxygen utilization using oxygen-15. *J. Comput. Assist. Tomogr.* **5**, 544–550.

Lammertsma, A. A., Martin, A. J., Friston, K. J., and Jones, T. (1992). *In vivo* measurement of the volume of distribution of water in cerebral grey matter: Effects on the calculation of regional cerebral blood flow. *J. Cereb. Blood Flow Metab.* **12**, 291–295.

Lammertsma, A. A., Wise, R. J. S., Heather, J. D., Gibbs, J. M., Leenders, K. L., Frackowiak, R. S. J., Rhodes, C. G., and Jones, T. (1983). Correction for the presence of intravascular oxygen-15 in the steady-state technique for measuring regional oxygen extraction ratio in the brain. 2. Results in normal subjects and brain tumor and stroke patients. *J. Cereb. Blood Flow Metab.* **3**, 425–431.

Landau, W. M., Freygang, W. H., Jr., Rowland, L. P., Sokoloff, L., and Kety, S. (1955). The local circulation of the living brain: Values in the unanesthetized and anesthetized cat. *Trans. Am. Neurol. Assoc.* **80**, 125–129.

Lassen, N. A., and Ingvar, D. H. (1963). Regional cerebral blood flow measurement in man. *Arch. Neurol.* **9**, 615–622.

Lassen, N. A., Ingvar, D. H., and Skinhoj, E. (1978). Brain function and blood flow. *Sci. Am.* **239**, 62–71.

Leenders, K. L., Perani, D., Lammertsma, A. A., Heather, J. D., Buckingham, P., Healy, M. J. R., Gibbs, J. M., Wise, R. J. S.,

Hatazawa, J., Herold, S., Beaney, R. P., Brooks, D. J., Spinks, T., Rhodes, C., Frackowiak, R. S. J., and Jones, T. (1990). Cerebral blood flow, blood volume and oxygen utilization: Normal values and effect of age. *Brain* **113**, 27–47.

Leniger-Follert, E., and Hossman, K.-A. (1979). Simultaneous measurements of microflow and evoked potentials in the somatomotor cortex of rat brain during specific sensory activation. *Pflügers Arch.* **380**, 85–89.

Lou, H. C., Edvinsson, L., and MacKenzie, E. T. (1987). The concept of coupling blood flow to brain function: revision required? *Ann. Neurol.* **22**, 289–297.

Martin, W. R. W., Powers, W. J., and Raichle, M. E. (1987). Cerebral blood volume measured with inhaled C^{15}O and positron emission tomography. *J. Cereb. Blood Flow Metab.* **7**, 421–426.

Mata, M., Fink, D. J., Gainer, H., Smith, C. B., Davidsen, L., Savaki, H., Schwartz, W. J., and Sokoloff, L. (1980). Activity-dependent energy metabolism in rat posterior pituitary primarily reflects sodium pump activity. *J. Neurochem.* **34**, 213–215.

Mazière, B., and Mazière, M. (1990). Where have we got to with neuroreceptor mapping of the human brain? *Eur. J. Nucl. Med.* **16**, 817–835.

Mazoyer, B., Trebossen, R., Deutch, R., Casey, M., and Blohm, K. (1991). Physical characteristics of the ECAT 953B/31: A new high resolution brain positron tomograph. *IEEE Trans. Med. Imaging* **10**, 499–504.

Mazziotta, J. C., Phelps, M. E., Carson, R. E., and Kuhl, D. E. (1982). Tomographic mapping of human cerebral metabolism: Auditory stimulation. *Neurology* **32**, 921–37.

Mazziotta, J. C., Phelps, M. E., Plummer, D., and Kuhl, D. E. (1981). Quantitation in positron computed tomography. 5. Physical–anatomical effects. *J. Comput. Assist. Tomogr.* **5**, 734–743.

Meyer, E. (1989). Simultaneous correction for tracer arrival delay and dispersion in CBF measurements by the H$_2$^{15}O autoradiographic method and dynamic PET. *J. Nucl. Med.* **30**, 1069–1078.

Meyer, E., Tyler, J. L., Thompson, C. J., Redies, C., Diksic, M., and Hakim, A. M. (1987). Estimation of cerebral oxygen utilization rate by single-bolus ^{15}O$_2$ inhalation and dynamic positron emission tomography. *J. Cereb. Blood Flow Metab.* **7**, 403–414.

Meyer, E., and Yamamoto, Y. L. (1984). The requirement for constant arterial radioactivity in the C^{15}O$_2$ steady-state blood-flow model. *J. Nucl. Med.* **25**, 455–560.

Mintun, M. A., Raichle, M. E., Martin, W. R. W., and Herscovitch, P. (1984). Brain oxygen utilization measured with O-15 radiotracers and positron emission tomography. *J. Nucl. Med.* **25**, 177–187.

Mori, K., Schmidt, K., Jay, T., Palombo, E., Nelson, T., Lucignani, G., Pettigrew, K., Kennedy, C., and Sokoloff, L. (1990). Optimal duration of experimental period in measurement of local cerebral glucose utilization with the deoxyglucose method. *J. Neurochem.* **54**, 307–319.

Nakai, H., Yamamoto, Y. L., Diksic, M., Matsuda, H., Takara, E., Meyer, E., and Redies, C. (1987). Time-dependent changes of lumped and rate constants in the deoxyglucose method in experimental cerebral ischemia. *J. Cereb. Blood Flow Metab.* **7**, 640–648.

Obrist, W. D., Thompson, H. K., King, C. H., and Wang, H. S. (1967). Determination of regional cerebral blood flow by inhalation of xenon-133. *Circ. Res.* **20**, 124–135.

Ohta, S., Meyer, E., Thompson, C. J., and Gjedde, A. (1992). Oxygen consumption of the living human brain measured after a single inhalation of positron emitting oxygen. *J. Cereb. Blood Flow Metab.* **12**, 179–192.

Perlmutter, J. S., Powers, W. J., Herscovitch, P., Fox, P. T., and Raichle, M. E. (1987). Regional asymmetries of cerebral blood

flow, blood volume, oxygen utilization and extraction in normal subjects. *J. Cereb. Blood Flow Metab.* **7**, 64–67.

Phelps, M. E., Huang, S. C., Hoffman, E. J., and Kuhl, D. E. (1979a). Validation of tomographic measurement of cerebral blood volume with C-11-labeled carboxyhemoglobin. *J. Nucl. Med.* **20**, 328–334.

Phelps, M. E., Huang, S. C., Hoffman, E. J., Selin, C., Sokoloff, L., and Kuhl, D. E. (1979b). Tomographic measurement of local cerebral glucose metabolic rate in humans with (F-18) 2-fluoro-2-deoxy-D-glucose: Validation of method. *Ann. Neurol.* **6**, 371–388.

Phelps, M. E., Mazziotta, J. C., Kuhl, D. E., Nuwer, M., Packwood, J., Metter, J., and Engel, J., Jr. (1981). Tomographic mapping of human cerebral metabolism: Visual stimulation and deprivation. *Neurology* **31**, 517–529.

Powers, W. J. (1988). Positron emission tomography in the evaluation of cerebrovascular disease: Clinical applications? *In* "Clinical Neuroimaging" (W. H. Theodore, Ed.), pp. 49–74. New York: Alan R. Liss.

Powers, W. J. (1991). Cerebral hemodynamics in ischemic cerebrovascular disease. *Ann. Neurol.* **29**, 231–240.

Raichle, M. E., Martin, W. R. W., Herscovitch, P., Mintun, M. A., and Markham, J. (1983). Brain blood flow measured with intravenous H$_2$^{15}O. II. Implementation and validation. *J. Nucl. Med.* **24**, 790–798.

Reivich, M., Alavi, A., Wolf, A., Fowler, J., Russell, J., Arnett, C., MacGregor, R. R., Shiue, C. Y., Atkins, H., Anand, A., Dann, R., and Greenberg, J. H. (1985). Glucose metabolic rate kinetic model parameter determination in humans: The lumped constants and rate constants for [^{18}F]fluorodeoxyglucose and [^{11}C]deoxyglucose. *J. Cereb. Blood Flow Metab.* **5**, 179–192.

Reivich, M., Alavi, A., Wolf, A., Greenberg, J. H., Fowler, J., Christman, D., MacGregor, R., Jones, S. C., London, J., Shiue, C., and Yonekura, Y. (1982). Use of 2-deoxy-D[1-^{11}C]glucose for the determination of local cerebral glucose metabolism in humans: Variation within and between subjects. *J. Cereb. Blood Flow Metab.* **2**, 307–319.

Reivich, M., Kuhl, D., Wolf, A., Greenberg, J., Phelps, M., Ido, T., Casella, V., Fowler, J., Hoffman, E., Alavi, A., Som, P., and Sokoloff, L. (1979). The [^{18}F]fluorodeoxyglucose method for the measurement of local cerebral glucose utilization in man. *Circ. Res.* **44**, 127–137.

Rhodes, C. G., Lenzi, G. L., Frackowiak, R. S. J., Jones, T., and Pozzilli, C. (1981). Measurement of CBF and CMRO$_2$ using continuous inhalation of C^{15}O$_2$ and ^{15}O$_2$: Experimental validation using CO$_2$ reactivity in the anaesthetised dog. *J. Neurol. Sci.* **50**, 381–389.

Rosenbloom, W. I. (1972). Can plasma skimming or inconstancy of regional hematocrit introduce serious errors in regional cerebral blood flow measurements or their interpretation. *Stroke* **3**, 248–254.

Sakai, F., Nakazawa, K., Tazaki, Y., Ishii, K., Hino, H., Igarushi, H., and Kanda, T. (1985). Regional cerebral blood volume and hematocrit measured in normal numan volunteers by single-photon emission computed tomography. *J. Cereb. Blood Flow Metab.* **5**, 207–213.

Sakurada, O., Kennedy, C., Jehle, J., Brown, J. D., Carbon, G. L., and Sokoloff, L. (1978). Measurement of local cerebral blood flow with iodo[^{14}C]antipyrine. *Am. J. Physiol.* **234**, H59–H66.

Sasaki, H., Kanno, I., Murakami, M., Shishido, F., and Uemera, K. (1986). Tomographic mapping of kinetic rate constants in the fluorodeoxyglucose model using dynamic positron emission tomography. *J. Cereb. Blood Flow Metab.* **6**, 447–454.

Schmidt, K., Lucignani, G., Moresco, R. M., Rizzo, G., Gilardi, M. C., Messa, C., Colombo, F., Fazio, F., and Sokoloff, L. (1992). Errors introduced by tissue heterogeneity in estimation of local cerebral glucose utilization with current kinetic models of the [18F]fluorodeoxyglucose method. *J. Cereb. Blood Flow Metab.* **12**, 823–834.

Schwartz, W. J., Smith, C. B., Davidsen, L., Savaki, H., Sokoloff, L., Mata, M., Fink, D. J., and Gainer, H. (1979). Metabolic mapping of functional activity in the hypothalamoneurohypo-physial system of the rat. *Science* **205**, 723–725.

Senda, M., Buxton, R. B., Alpert, N. M., Correia, J. A., Mackay, B. C., Weise, S. B., and Ackerman, R. H. (1988). The 15O steady-state method: Correction for variation in arterial concentration. *J. Cereb. Blood Flow Metab.* **8**, 681–690.

Sokoloff, L. (1961). Local cerebral circulation at rest and during altered cerebral activity induced by anesthesia or visual stimulation. *In* "Regional Neurochemistry" (S. S. Kety and J. Elkes, Eds.), pp. 107–117. New York: Pergamon.

Sokoloff, L. (1981). Relationships among local functional activity, energy metabolism, and blood flow in the central nervous system. *Fed. Proc.* **40**, 2311–2316.

Sokoloff, L. (1985). Basic principles in imaging of cerebral metabolic rates. *In* "Brain Imaging and Brain Function" (L. Sokoloff, Ed.), pp. 21–49. New York: Raven Press.

Sokoloff, L. (1986). Cerebral circulation, energy metabolism and protein synthesis: general characteristics and principles of measurement. *In* "Positron Emission Tomography and Autoradiography" (M. E. Phelps, J. C. Mazziotta, and H. R. Schelbert, Eds.), pp. 1–71. New York: Raven Press.

Sokoloff, L., Reivich, M., Kennedy, C., Des Rosiers, M. H., Patlak, C. S., Pettigrew, K. D., Sakurada, O., and Shinohara, M. (1977). The [14C]deoxyglucose method for the measurement of local cerebral glucose utilization: Theory, procedure, and normal values in the conscious and anesthetized albino rat. *J. Neurochem.* **28**, 897–916.

Spence, A. M., Graham, M. M., Muzi, M., Abbott, G. L., Krohn, K. A., Kapoor, R., and Woods, S. D. (1990). Deoxyglucose lumped constant estimated in a transplanted rat astrocytic glioma by the hexose utilization index. *J. Cereb. Blood Flow Metab.* **10**, 190–198.

Steinling, M., Baron, J. C., Maziere, B., Lasjaunias, P., Loc'h, C., Cabanis, E. A., and Guillon, B. (1985). Tomographic measurement of cerebral blood flow by the 68Ga-labelled-microsphere and continuous-C15O2-inhalation methods. *Eur. J. Nucl. Med.* **11**, 29–32.

Stone-Elander, S., Roland, P., Eriksson, L., Litton, J.-E., and Johnstrom, P. (1986). The preparation of 11C-labelled fluoromethane for the study of regional cerebral blood flow using positron emission tomography. *Eur. J. Nucl. Med.* **12**, 236–239.

Subramanyam, R., Alpert, N. M., Hoop, B., Jr., Brownell, G. L., and Taveras, J. M. (1978). A model for regional cerebral oxygen distribution during continuous inhalation of 15O2, C15O, and C15O2. *J. Nucl. Med.* **19**, 13–53.

Suda, S., Shinohara, M., Miyaoka, M., Lucignani, G., Kennedy, C., and Sokoloff, L. (1990). The lumped constant of the deoxyglucose method in hypoglycemia: Effects of moderate hypoglycemia on local cerebral glucose utilization in the rat. *J. Cereb. Blood Flow Metab.* **10**, 499–509.

Ter-Pogossian, M. M., Ficke, D. C., Hood, J. T., Sr., Yamamoto, M., and Mullani, N. A. (1982). PETT VI: A positron emission tomograph utilizing cesium fluoride scintillation detectors. *J. Comput. Assist. Tomogr.* **6**, 125–133.

Toga, A. W., and Collins, R. C. (1981). Metabolic response of optic centers to visual stimuli in the albino rat: anatomical and physiological considerations. *J. Comp. Neurol.* **199**, 443–464.

Townsend, D. W., Geissbuhler, A., Defrise, M., Hoffman, E. J., Spinks, T., Bailey, D. L., Gilardi, M.-C., and Jones, T. (1991). Fully three-dimensional reconstruction for a PET camera with retractable septa. *IEEE Trans. Med. Imaging* **10**, 505–512.

Tyler, J. L., Strother, S. C., Zatorre, R. J., Alivisatos, B., Worsley, K. J., Diksic, M., and Yamamoto, Y. L. (1988). Stability of regional cerebral glucose metabolism in the normal brain measured by positron emission tomography. *J. Nucl. Med.* **29**, 631–642.

Videen, T. O., Perlmutter, J. S., Herscovitch, P., and Raichle, M. E. (1987). Brain blood volume, flow, and oxygen utilization measured with 15O radiotracers and positron emisison tomography: revised metabolic computations. *J. Cereb. Blood Flow Metab.* **7**, 513–516.

Volkow, N., and Fowler, J. S. (1992). Neuropsychiatric disorders: investigation of schizophrenia and substance abuse. *Sem. Nuc. Med.* **22**, 254–267.

Wienhard, K., Pawlik, G., Herholz, K., Wagner, R., and Heiss, W.-D. (1985). Estimation of local cerebral glucose utilization by positron emission tomography of [18F]2-fluoro-2-deoxy-D-glucose: A critical appraisal of optimization procedures. *J. Cereb. Blood Flow Metab.* **5**, 115–125.

Wooten, G. F., and Collins, R. C. (1981). Metabolic effects of unilateral lesions of the substantia nigra. *J. Neurosci.* **1**, 285–291.

Yarowsky, P. J., and Ingvar, D. H. (1981). Neuronal activity and energy metabolism. *Fed. Proc.* **40**, 2353–2362.

Yarowsky, P., Crane, A., and Sokoloff, L. (1985). Metabolic activation of specific postsynaptic elements in superior cervical ganglion by antidromic stimulation of external carotid nerve. *Brain Res.* **334**, 330–334.

Yarowsky, P., Kadekaro, M., and Sokoloff, L. (1983). Frequency-dependent activation of glucose utilization in the superior cervical ganglion by electrical stimulation of cervical sympathetic trunk. *Proc. Natl. Acad. Sci. USA* **80**, 4179–4183.

Yokoi, T., Kanno, I., Iida, H., Miura, S., and Uemura, K. (1991). A new approach of weighted integration technique based on accumulated images using dynamic PET and H2 15O. *J. Cereb. Blood Flow Metab.* **11**, 492–501.

5

Optimizing Activation Methods: Tomographic Mapping of Functional Cerebral Activity

Roger P. Woods,* John C. Mazziotta,*† and Simon R. Cherry‡

Departments of Neurology,* Radiological Sciences,† and Pharmacology,† Division of Brain Mapping and Department of Pharmacology,‡ Imaging Sciences Division, Crump Institute for Biological Imaging, University of California, Los Angeles, School of Medicine, Los Angeles, California 90024

I. Optimizing Methods

The comprehensive understanding of human functional neuroanatomy will require the careful collection of data from a wide range of methodologies. The integration of these individual data sets will result in an ever-growing and a more comprehensive perspective of the functional organization of the human and non-human primate brain. Already, a vast array of methods exists for this process. The oldest and most time honored is that of the clinical–pathologic correlation of patients with cerebral injuries and the subsequent analysis of the individual's brain at postmortem. The ability to provide high-resolution structural brain images *in vivo* using X-ray computed tomography (CT) and magnetic resonance imaging (MRI) has allowed this process to continue at a macroscopic level during life. Functional data can be obtained from positron emission tomography (PET), single photon emission computed tomography (SPECT), electroencephalography (EEG), magnetoencephalography (MEG), magnetic resonance spectroscopy (MRS), diffusion and cerebral blood volume imaging with functional MRI (fMRI), and intraoperative stimulation and recording, as well as transcranial magnetic stimulation (TMS) (Mazziotta and Gilman, 1992). Thus, the inventory of available techniques to examine the structure and function of the human brain, not only at postmortem but also during life, is impressive and ever growing.

Likewise, the spatial and temporal resolution as well as the sampling capabilities of these techniques continue to improve and will, in the future, be augmented by methods currently not even imagined today.

This chapter will focus on the methods and approaches used to optimize data collected from these individual modalities as well as the current directions and speculation about future ways to integrate information within and between both subjects and methods. It is important to the investigator to understand both the method and the biological process under study. Detailed knowledge of both will provide the most accurate and appropriate as well as efficient means by which to use a technique to explore cerebral structure and function. By optimizing the accuracy and reproducibility of data from each technique and integrating across techniques in subjects, the most comprehensive view of brain function will emerge. The integration of data from all these methods and populations will provide a product that will be of greater value and use than the individual sum of the parts. Because of the authors' experience with PET, many of the following examples will be described in terms of their applicability to PET. Nevertheless, the approaches described herein should find general applicability for most, if not all, of the methods listed above. Important considerations in optimizing the acquisition of individual datasets and the integration of data between modalities can be well served by observing and understanding the following points:

47

Methodologic

1. The technique must be able to detect subtle signals superimposed on an extremely noisy background.
2. The technique must either prevent or compensate for any changes in the position of the subject's head with respect to the detector system during the course of the measurements.
3. The technique must be able to localize the neuroanatomic source of a signal.

Physiologic

1. A behavioral task must be shown to produce a consistent detectable change in a physiologic signal when compared with a control task.
2. Because behavioral tasks generally involve integration of multiple functional components, it is usually necessary to perform further validation experiments to determine which functional feature of the task is actually responsible for the physiologic signal.

In order to be able to better address the physiologic problems described above, we have systematically investigated new solutions to the three methodologic problems. One of our primary criteria in developing these new methods is that they should not require pooling of data from multiple subjects. While developed for and discussed with relation to PET, many of the solutions are applicable to other brain mapping methods as well. This article describes the background for these new solutions, the theory behind their implementation, and some of the experiments performed to validate the methods. In addition, some specific examples will be provided to illustrate practical applications of these methods to answer questions using analysis of data from single subjects.

II. Maximize Signal to Noise in Data Acquisition

PET $H_2^{15}O$ images are intrinsically noisy. One of the major factors that has impeded the use of $H_2^{15}O$ techniques in individual subjects is the fact that the dose that can be administered to a normal subject is limited by the amount of radiation exposure. Current guidelines at UCLA restrict the dose of $H_2^{15}O$ that can be administered to a normal subject to 300 mCi per year. Standard imaging techniques generally use 50 mCi of $H_2^{15}O$ per trial, allowing for a total of six trials per subject to be distributed among stimulation and control states. Consequently, it has not been possible to improve signal-to-noise levels by simply averaging

together a large number of studies of the same individual. The standard solution to this problem has been to pool data from multiple subjects to improve signal-to-noise ratios in the subject population as a whole (Fox *et al.*, 1988). If all brains were identical functionally and anatomically and if images from different subjects could all be precisely aligned with one another, pooling of data from six trials across 10 subjects would improve signal-to-noise ratios as much as performing 60 trials in a single subject. However, functional and anatomic variability and misregistration will result in less satisfactory results and could potentially even be worse than simply analyzing each subject individually.

Given that the maximal dose of radiation is fixed, the only alternative to intersubject data pooling is to try to improve the amount of signal that is actually detected by the PET scanner. Careful consideration of the physics, instrumentation, and kinetics of $H_2^{15}O$ imaging show that there are three major ways that signal-to-noise levels might be improved:

1. Improving scanner detector geometry to increase the sensitivity of the instrument. This issue is addressed by a new acquisition method known as three-dimensional (3D) PET imaging (Townsend *et al.*, 1991; Cherry *et al.*, 1991).
2. Decreasing the number of decay events that go undetected due to scanner dead time by administering a greater number of trials using smaller injected doses. This method will be referred to as dose fractionation.
3. Modifying the stimulation and control paradigms to exploit the fact that high blood flow levels in a particular brain region during the initial phase of a scan results in deposition of large amounts of tracer in the region but that sustained high blood flow levels in later phases allow that tracer to be washed out again. This issue will be discussed under the heading of optimization of tracer kinetics.

A. Three-Dimensional Data Acquisition with Dose Fractionation

Positron emission tomography is based on the fact that positron annihilation generates two 511-keV gamma rays that travel away from the site of annihilation at an angle of 180° to each other. PET scanners are configured to test for the nearly simultaneous arrival of gamma rays at any two of hundreds of spatially distinct detectors. When such events are detected, they are assumed to result from a positron annihilation event somewhere along the line connecting the two detectors. In conventional two-dimensional (2D) scanning, only decay events that emit gamma rays along lines that are roughly parallel to the scanner's imaging planes can be detected. Decay events oriented more obliquely are deliberately excluded by collimators that prevent gamma rays traveling at such angles from ever reaching the detectors, and simultaneous events recorded on widely separated planes are not scored during conventional 2D scanning. Consequently, 2D scanning detects only a small fraction of the total number of decay events that could be utilized to reconstruct a PET image.

There are two major reasons that PET scanners have previously relied on 2D imaging techniques. The first reason is that reconstruction of images based on all coincidence events detectable in a PET scanner is mathematically far more complicated than standard 2D reconstruction methods. The mathematics of such reconstructions has been developed only recently (Townsend *et al.*, 1991; Cherry *et al.*, 1991) and 3D image reconstruction requires orders of magnitude more computation time than conventional 2D reconstruction. The second reason that 3D imaging has not been widely utilized is that removal of the collimating septa that separate the various planes also greatly increases the likelihood of detecting gamma ray pairs in which one of the gamma rays has been deflected from its original path as a result of physical interactions with intervening matter. Such interactions are referred to as scattering events and they result in incorrect localization of the positron annihilation event that generated the scattered photon pair. Fortunately, scattering events largely cancel out when images are subtracted from one another, so this process is of considerably less concern for activation studies than it is for reconstruction of images to be used for absolute quantitation.

Dead time, the refractory period during which a scanner detection cannot record data following an event, increases as the amount of radioactivity in the field increases. All other things being equal, dead time considerations suggest that multiple studies acquired with very small doses of $H_2^{15}O$ should provide better signal-to-noise ratios than the equivalent dose injected as a single bolus and acquired as a single study.

In addition to this physical argument in favor of dose fractionation, there is also a biological argument. By increasing the number of trials per condition, dose fractionation effectively increases the amount of time over which blood flow is being measured. Any temporal fluctuations in blood flow that are uncorrelated with the specific task being performed are more likely to be minimized by averaging over a greater time period. Consequently, dose fractionation should decrease biological noise as well as improving counting statistics.

Three-dimensional imaging and dose fractionation are complementary concepts in the sense that dead time considerations demand that the injected dose of $H_2^{15}O$ be decreased from the 50 mCi used for conventional studies when performing 3D studies. If the dose is not decreased, the increased sensitivity will result in an enormous increase in the fraction of decay events that are lost due to dead time. Results from phantom studies suggest that doses should not exceed 10 to 15 mCi of $H_2^{15}O$ per injection. This would then allow for 20 to 30 repeat studies of an individual without exceeding the 300 mCi limit for normal subjects (Fig. 1).

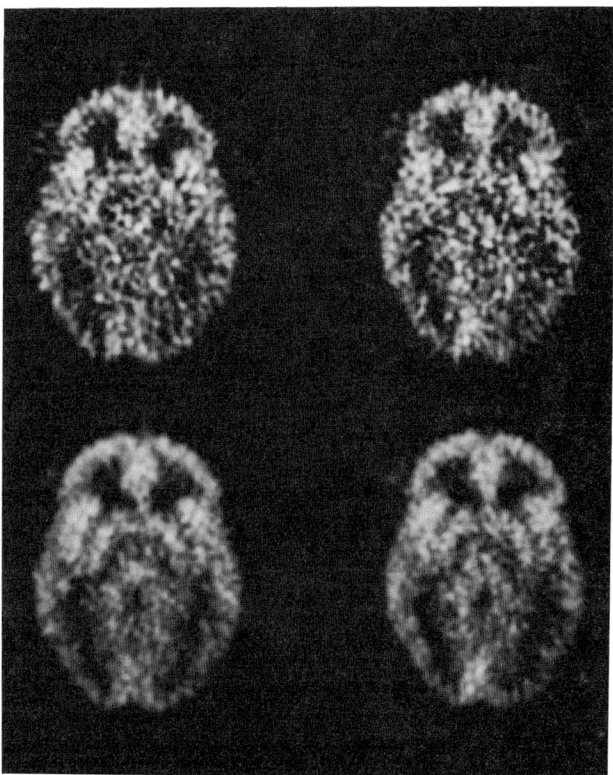

Figure 1 Direct comparison of conventional 2D and fractionated 3D imaging methods. All four images represent the same tomographic slice of a single subject, and all images were acquired during a single scanning session. The scans on the left were obtained with the subject at rest, and the scans on the right were obtained with the subject viewing an 8-Hz left-hemifield alternating checkerboard pattern. Each image in the figure represents data based on a total of 40 mCi of $H_2^{15}O$. The images on the top row are conventional 2D scans acquired after single 40-mCi injections. The images on the bottom row were acquired using 3D imaging, and each represents averaged values from four 10-mCi injections. The right occipital response (images are displayed with the right hemisphere on the left) to visual stimulation is readily apparent on the 3D images but is much more difficult to discern on the 2D images. Quantitative measurements demonstrated a twofold improvement in signal-to-noise ratios using the fractionated 3D acquisition method.

B. Optimization of Tracer Kinetics

Although the half-life of ^{15}O is 123 s, standard PET methods acquire images only for 45 to 90 s after the tracer reaches the brain (Mintun *et al.*, 1989; Kanno, *et al.*, 1991). Given the 123-s half-life, this means that the scanner is collecting data during only a small fraction of the available time and thus only a small fraction of the total decay events. Limited imaging times are based on the empirical observation that signal-to-noise levels actually decrease when longer data collection times are used (Mintun *et al.*, 1989; Kanno *et al.*, 1991; Volkow *et al.*, 1991). Although this seems paradoxical, the physical basis for this observation is now clear. When $H_2^{15}O$ is injected, it is initially distributed to the tissues in proportion to regional blood flow. This initial wash-in phase is largely a first-pass effect. After the first pass, the blood perfusing the tissue actually has a lower concentration of $H_2^{15}O$ than the tissue itself, so $H_2^{15}O$ is actually washed back out of the tissue as it becomes more evenly distributed within the intravascular compartment. The rate of wash-out is determined by regional blood flow, with more rapid wash-out in more highly perfused areas. If regional blood flow remains constant throughout the wash-in and wash-out periods, it is theoretically possible for the counts in well-perfused areas to drop below those in less-well-perfused areas as a result of continued wash-out. This progressive degradation and possible inversion of signal accounts for the deterioration in signal-to-noise ratios as scanning times are increased.

An understanding of the physical basis of the problem leads to some straightforward ways to exploit this understanding to improve signal-to-noise levels. The first step is to decrease the rate of wash-out in activated regions by stopping the stimulation task after which useful data can continue to be acquired (Volkow *et al.*, 1991). A second, less obvious alternative is to actually use the fact that wash-out occurs to further augment the difference between stimulation and control images. In this case, the stimulation state would consist of a stimulation task during wash-in phase and a control task during the wash-out phase, whereas the control state would consist of the control task during the wash-in phase and the stimulation task during the wash-out phase. Based on kinetic models, this approach should further extend the practical imaging time and lead to further improvements in signal-to-noise ratios of 15%, and we expect that even greater improvements may be seen by optimizing the exact timing of the changes between stimulations and control states.

III. Image Registration

The alignment and registration of datasets can be performed within and between modalities as well as within and between subjects. A large and ever-growing literature describes methods that have been applied to solve various aspects of this problem. The most simple situation is the alignment and registration of datasets from the same subject obtained using the same method or modality. An example would include serial MRI studies of a patient with a growing brain tumor or a battery of PET studies with the subject performing different tasks during different administrations of radiopharmaceuticals. These are examples of intrasubject, intramodality registration problems. Attempts to solve these experimental issues have included the use of rigid fixation devices for the head, fiducial markers, and other approaches. The optimal method should be independent of the particular modality employed, its spatial resolution, and the exact acquisition parameters for the subject. Additionally, it should be easy to perform, low cost, nonlabor intensive, and, if possible, totally automated.

A. Within Subject, within Modality

Subject movement is a problem even with the use of fairly restrictive head restraint devices (Mazziotta and Koslow, 1987). Once movement has occurred, there are two options for dealing with the problem. The first option is to discard the misregistered data. In the case of head movements that occur during a scan itself, this may be the only viable option. However, for head movements that occur between scans, throwing out misregistered data may result in eliminating half of all the trials due to a single movement midway through the study. Whereas it may be practical to discard some data or even to completely exclude all data from a given subject in experiments using pooled multisubject analysis, dose limitations do not allow more data to be collected to replace the discarded data in individual analysis cases.

The second option is to try to reregister the data. Methods for data registration will be discussed in more detail in the next section; many of these methods are poorly suited for registration of $H_2^{15}O$ images because of the difficulty in defining identifiable landmarks or surfaces in such images and because PET scanners generally cannot span the entire brain in the axial field of view. Computer algorithms that maximize some overall measure of goodness-of-fit provide a viable alternative in this setting (Woods *et al.*, 1992; Minoshima *et al.*, 1992).

Data registration is even more problematic when

subjects are scanned in repeat sessions on different days. Even with careful attention to external landmarks, it is difficult to reposition a subject accurately. In this situation, even perfect retrospective reorientation of the data may not prevent large quantitative errors due to partial volume and interpolation effects (Woods *et al.*, 1992). Repeat imaging sessions to follow the progression of a disease process or to evaluate the effects of some therapeutic intervention are likely to be an intrinsic part of the design of studies of individual patients, so some means of prospectively repositioning the patient correctly before the repeat study would be very beneficial.

We have developed a computer algorithm to perform automated image registration of PET data to compensate for interscan subject movement (Fig. 2). The algorithm iteratively seeks to minimize the standard deviation across all brain voxels of the ratio of one image to the other as a function of spatial orientation. The algorithm normalizes the standard deviation by dividing it by the mean ratio of one image to the other prior to minimization. In order to produce an unbiased result, two normalized standard deviations are calculated, one with a given study in the numerator of the ratio and the other with the study in the denominator. It is the average of these two values

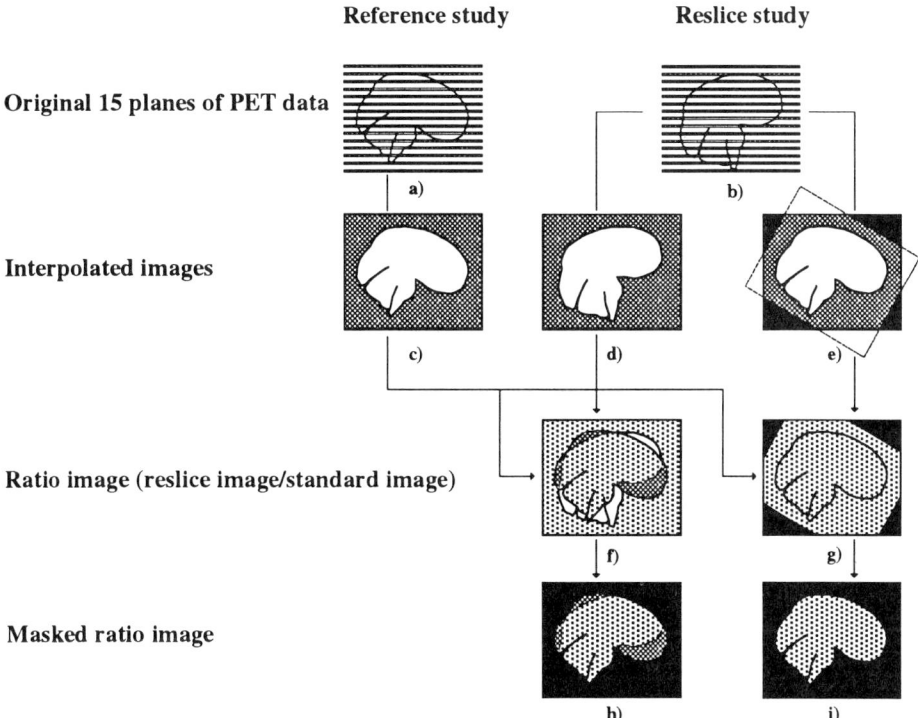

Figure 2 Rationale for the algorithm used to reorient PET images to correct for head movement relative to the scanner. One of the two scans is designated as the reference study (a) and the other, as the reslice study (b). The original tomographic images (15 planes) are interpolated to generate cubic voxels before the two images are compared (second row). In the case of the reference study, this interpolation is performed once and the results are stored to be assessed again with each iteration. Because the reslice study is reoriented with each iteration, the interpolation must be repeated each time to take the new orientation into account. Image d represents the first interpolation (no realignment), and e represents the final interpolation (optimal realignment). After interpolation, an image is formed that represents the ratio of the reslice study to the reference study on a voxel-by-voxel basis (third row). This image is masked to exclude any voxels that were outside the brain on the reference image (fourth row). The standard deviation of the remaining voxels is normalized by dividing it by the mean voxel value and is used as an index of how well the images are registered. When the reorientation parameters are poor, the masked ratio image has heterogeneous values and a large normalized standard deviation. When the reorientation parameters are optimized, the masked ratio image is maximally homogeneous and the normalized standard deviation is minimized. With each iteration, the algorithm computes the first and second derivatives of the normalized standard deviation with respect to each of the reorientation parameters and uses these values to move toward the minimum normalized standard deviation. The algorithm converges when all of the first derivatives are very close to zero. Reproduced with permission from Woods *et al.* (1992).

that is minimized. Further details about this algorithm have been reported (Woods *et al.*, 1992).

To validate the image registration algorithm, data were generated by imaging a realistic three-dimensional Lucite human brain phantom (Hoffman *et al.*, 1991) filled with an aqueous solution of [^{18}F]fluorodeoxyglucose (FDG). The internal cavity of this phantom conforms to brain gray matter structures and the resulting PET images are very similar to those obtained in real human H$_2$^{15}O or ^{18}FDG PET studies. Activation sites can be simulated in the phantom by inserting small balloons filled with a higher concentration of FDG.

By moving the scanner gantry and bed, the phantom was imaged (2D mode) at a variety of orientations. Because the gantry and bed are calibrated, it is possible to calculate the correct repositioning to align any two scans directly from their relative gantry and bed positions. The phantom imaging times and ^{18}FDG concentrations were adjusted to generate images with counting statistics similar to those seen in typical human H$_2$^{15}O studies, and one-half of the images were obtained with simulated cortical activation sites to test the sensitivity of the algorithm to focal activations. A total of 31 separate scans were performed with rotations of as much as 35° and translations of as much as 10 mm between different image pairs.

After reconstruction, the automated image registration algorithm was used to calculate the parameters needed to reorient the 930 pairwise permutations of images to compensate for the spatial misregistration induced by moving the gantry and bed between acquisitions. These registration parameters were then compared with the correct values known from the relative gantry and bed positions. Mean and maximal registration errors were calculated for each point in the brain to characterize the overall accuracy of the algorithm. The speed and accuracy of the algorithm was measured as a function of image resolution by applying postreconstruction smoothing of the data using a uniform smoothing filter.

As a means of minimizing misalignment across separate imaging sessions, a modified version of the automated image registration algorithm was developed for the purpose of online registration. Instead of providing parameters to reorient one image to fit the other, this algorithm generates new scanner gantry and bed positions so that images acquired in this new position will match the orientation of a previous scan as precisely as possible. In addition to quantitative validation using phantom emission data, this algorithm was also evaluated qualitatively using both emission and transmission data from human subjects.

Figure 3 shows the results of the 930 different comparisons of the Hoffman brain phantom imaged 31

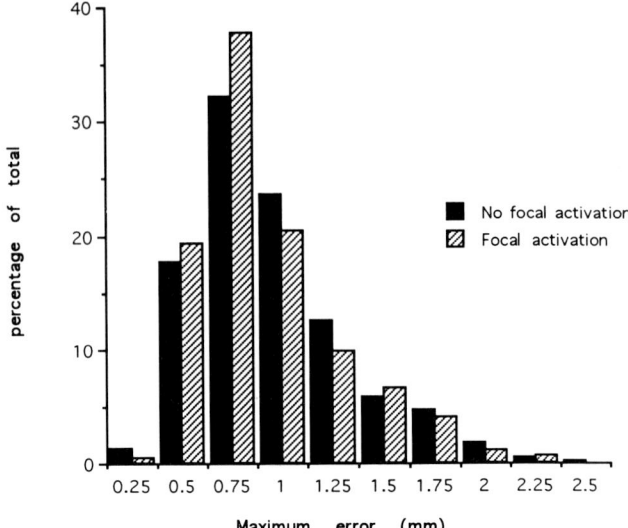

Figure 3 Accuracy of the intrasubject, intramodality alignment algorithm. The Hoffman brain phantom was imaged in a variety of different positions with angular displacements as large as 35° and linear translations up to 1 cm. The reorientation parameters derived by the registration algorithm were compared to the known values and the maximum three-dimensional error for any point in the brain was calculated for each image pair. Focal activation sites were simulated in some of the data sets using small balloons filled with a higher concentration of FDG than that that was used to fill the rest of the phantom. The maximum errors are displayed in histogram format. A total of 930 pairwise comparisons are represented. The results demonstrate that the approach is accurate to around 1.745 mm, which is the width of the voxels in the reconstructed images. Reproduced with permission from Woods *et al.* (1992).

different times in a variety of orientations with and without simulated focal activation sites. The maximal three-dimensional errors in registration were generally less than the width of a voxel in the reconstructed images (1.745 mm). The presence of simulated activation sites did not adversely affect the registration. The algorithm performance was quite fast with computation times of 3–6 min on a Sun SPARCstation 2.

We have used this algorithm on a routine basis for the past 18 months for registration of both normal and abnormal PET images and have not yet noted any failures to properly register the data. In addition, we have repeatedly used the algorithm prospectively to reposition the scanner gantry and bed on the basis of a transmission scan produced with an external germanium ring source and have found that this prospective repositioning is more accurate than we can achieve with careful manual repositioning.

B. Within Subject, between Modality

Methods to align and register datasets between modalities for an individual subject represent the next level of complexity to this overall problem. In this circumstance one might envision comparisons between functional data acquired with PET or EEG and structural information from MRI or CT. Approaches to this intrasubject, intermodality problem have employed fiducial markers, external head restraints, surface contour fitting, and purely statistical approaches. Optimal criteria for the solution of this problem are similar to those stated above the for intrasubject, intramodality case.

One of the strengths of PET studies is that they provide a three-dimensional map of brain function in the form of a series of two-dimensional images. With improving spatial resolution, PET blood flow images are capable of providing a great deal of information about the shape of the brain and about the location of many structures, particularly the well-delineated subcortical gray matter structures such as the thalamus, caudate, and putamen. Unfortunately, it is not currently possible to identify many cortical landmarks in PET studies. This lack of cortical landmarks makes it difficult to translate the three-dimensional map provided by the PET study into some more general frame of reference.

This localization problem is not unique to individual subject analysis. In fact, it is equally, if not more, important in pooled intersubject analyses because improvements in signal-to-noise ratios are dependent upon superimposition of analogous structures across subjects. The approach taken most commonly is to use a limited number of landmarks identifiable on the PET dataset to perform a stereotactic spatial transformation of the data into a common space. Modified versions of the stereotactic method of Talairach and Tournoux (1988) (Talairach *et al.*, 1967; Fox *et al.*, 1985) are used most commonly and involve identification of a line in the midsagittal plane (the anterior commissure–posterior commissure line or some approximation of it) and identification of extreme points on a coordinate system orthogonal to this line. Because both the extreme top and the extreme bottom points of the brain are rarely included simultaneously in the limited axial field of view of the PET scanner, these points must often be approximated by other means.

A fundamental assumption underlying the stereotactic method is that, even though cortical structures of any given individual may be matched poorly to the corresponding structures of some other individual (see Fig. 6), the average location of a particular

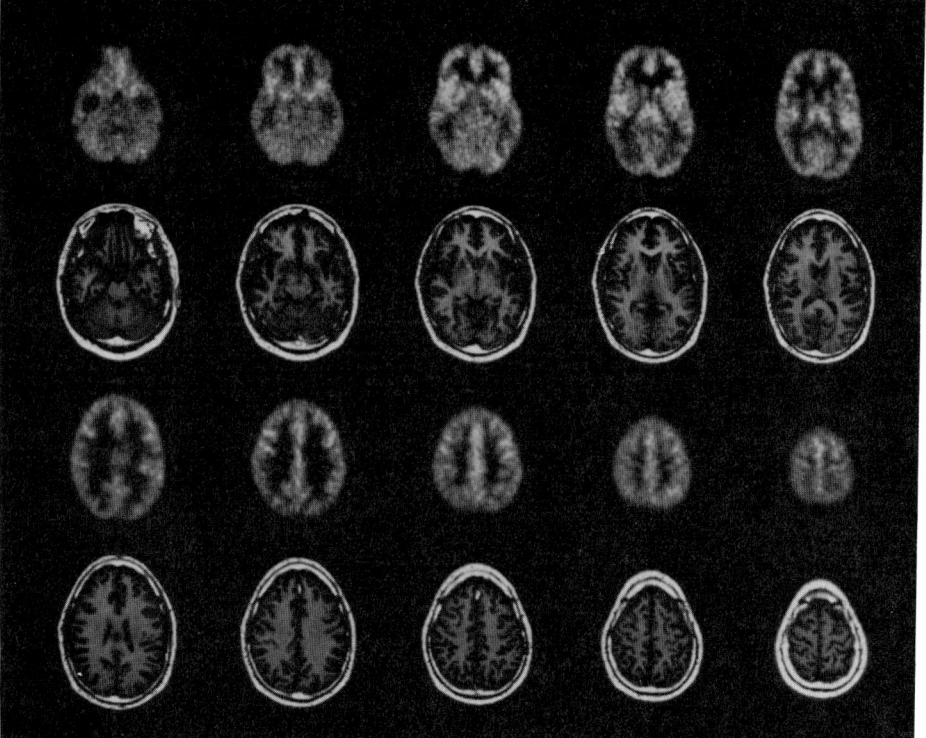

Figure 4   Registered $H_2^{15}O$ PET–MRI dataset chosen at random from 25 such datasets used for qualitative validation of the MRI–PET registration algorithm. The PET dataset represents the sum of six registered 2D $H_2^{15}O$ image sets from this subject. The accuracy of the registration can be judged by examining specific landmarks, including the gyrus rectus (1st image starting from the upper left), the heads of the caudate (3rd through 5th images), the location of the most anterior and most posterior boundaries of the corpus callosum (3rd through 6th images), the course of the parietooccipital sulcus (6th and 7th images), the location and shape of the central sulcus (9th and 10th images), and the location of numerous other landmarks around the cortical rim.

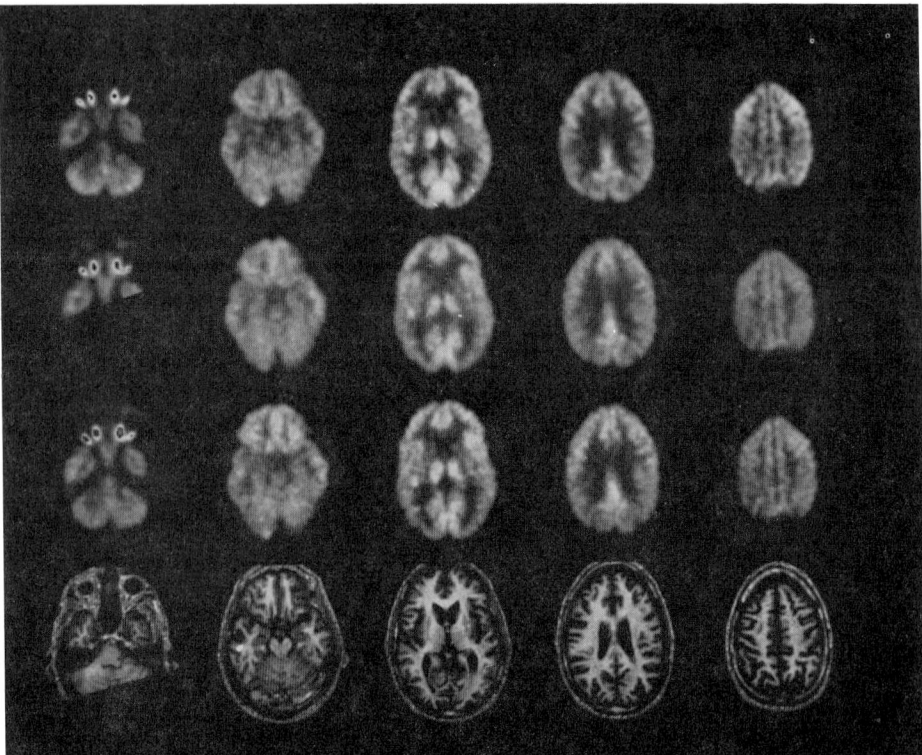

Figure 5 Use of the registration algorithms for longitudinal followup of a patient with Huntington's disease. This currently 40-year-old man with Huntington's disease had an initial FDG–PET study in 1989 (top row). A followup study was performed in 1990, and the PET–PET algorithm was used retrospectively to reslice the 1990 data to match those of the 1989 study. When the patient returned for a third study in 1991, a scout scan was performed near the end of the FDG uptake period, and the registration algorithm was used to reposition the scanner gantry and bed so that the imaging planes acquired after repositioning would match the imaging planes of the first study (row three) without the need for reslicing. Such prospective registration prior to acquisition minimizes errors due to partial volume effects and interpolation errors. An MRI scan obtained in 1991 was registered to match the PET studies using the MRI–PET algorithm. Note that the atrophied heads of the caudates can still be easily recognized on the MRI scan (third column) and that this anatomic information helps to confirm localization of the caudate on the sequential PET studies. Localization without registration of the data is likely to be less consistent across studies and less accurate anatomically.

structure in a random sample of subjects from a population will be fairly consistent across samples. Unfortunately, there is no published method for interconverting Talairach coordinates and gyral landmarks for any population (the atlas of Talairach and Tournoux is based on the brain of a single subject whose brain is not necessarily typical of any population), and it has not been demonstrated that such interconversions are independent of sex, handedness, ethnic origin, race, or other factors. Whereas the standard stereotactic method might be adequate for pooled data, Fig. 6 clearly demonstrates that it cannot be relied upon as the sole source of anatomic information for the purpose of individual subject analysis.

The main alternative to the stereotactic approach is to use MRI scanning to define the individual's gyral anatomy directly. This requires some means of performing cross modality registration of the MRI and PET datasets. Several different approaches have been developed for performing such registration:

1. The use of head holders or stereotactic frames with attached external fiducials that can be seen on MRI and PET images (Mazziotta and Koslow, 1987; Zhang *et al.*, 1990). This method is well suited to circumstances in which perfect registration is critical and the use of a stereotactic frame bolted to the subject's skull can be justified. However, for routine usage, less rigidly fixed head holders can allow movement of the brain relative to the fiducials resulting in misregistration. Such methods must be applied prospectively and require considerable time and effort.

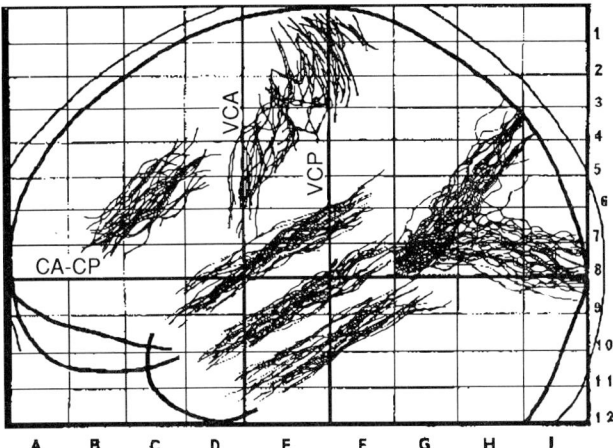

Figure 6 Demonstration of the anatomic variability that remains unaccounted for when different brains are mapped into Talairach space. The traced lines represent mapped projections of the inferior frontal sulcus; the superior, middle, and inferior temporal sulci; the central sulcus; the parietooccipital sulcus; and the calcarine sulcus onto the midsagittal plane. The first four landmarks were identified on 30 postmortem hemispheres and the central sulcus was identified in 20 postmortem hemispheres. The parietooccipital and calcarine sulci were identified on encephalograms of 30 patients. Intersubject variability on the order of 1 cm is readily evident from the figure. Note that this is an underestimate of true variability because variations orthogonal to the sagittal plane cannot be measured on a sagittal projection. The line labeled CA–CP passes through the anterior and posterior commissures by definition. Lines VCA and VCP pass through the anterior and posterior commissures, respectively, and are orthogonal to line CA–CP by definition. Modified from Talairach *et al.* (1967).

2. The use of internal anatomic landmarks for registration (Evans *et al.*, 1989). This method requires an expert user to directly identify common landmarks on the MRI and PET datasets. Precise identification of landmarks on PET datasets is made difficult by the comparatively poor resolution of the images. As discussed above, cortical landmarks are difficult to identify, so registration is mostly dependent on subcortical landmarks that tend to be clustered near the center of the brain. Whereas accuracy should increase with the number of common landmarks identified, the time required for an expert to locate a large number of such landmarks makes this method unattractive.

3. Determination of principal axes for registration (Alpert *et al.*, 1990). This method of registration has the advantage of being very fast and relatively free of user interaction. Unfortunately, it is sensitive to incomplete imaging of the brain. The limited axial field of view in PET images almost always leads to an incomplete dataset.

4. The use of a surface matching algorithm to register images (Pelizzari *et al.*, 1989). Because the skull cannot be seen on PET emission images and the sur-

face of the brain is difficult to identify precisely on emission images, this method uses the skull as identified on a transmission scan obtained using an external positron emitting ring source as a proxy for the emission images. Registration using this method assumes that the subject's head does not move relative to the scanner between the transmission and emission studies. If this assumption is met, the method works relatively well, although it does not exploit all of the anatomic information available in the images.

A modified version of the within-modality registration algorithm described above was generated to allow cross-modality registration of MRI and PET images (Figs. 4 and 5). The major difference between the two algorithms is that the cross-modality algorithm segments the MRI into 256 different partitions based on voxel value. This extensive partitioning increases the likelihood that each partition will represent a single homogeneous tissue type. Partitioning into different tissue types is necessary because the ratio of a PET voxel value to the corresponding MRI voxel value when the images are properly aligned will be different for different tissues. For example, gray matter will have a high pixel value on the PET study and a low pixel value on a T_1-weighted MRI study, whereas white matter values will be the reverse and CSF will appear dark on both types of studies. With such diverse ratios across tissues, it would be inappropriate to try to maximize the uniformity of the ratio of one image to the other across tissue types, but maximization within each tissue type is a reasonable approach. The algorithm computes the standard deviation of the PET voxel values corresponding to the MRI voxels in each partition, divides this value by the MRI voxel value for that partition, and computes a weighted average standard deviation across all partitions. This value is iteratively minimized as a function of spatial orientaion using a method analogous to the within-modality algorithm.

Qualitative validation of this algorithm was performed by direct inspection of identifiable landmarks on 25 consecutive 2D water studies and the registered MRI scans from the same subjects. Figure 4 shows data from 1 of these 25 MRI $H_2^{15}O$–PET pairs aligned using the MRI–PET registration algorithm. The excellent correspondence of landmarks seen in this figure is typical of the group. No evidence for misregistration was found in any of the 25 subjects.

The method was validated quantitatively using data obtained from candidates for epilepsy surgery who underwent clinically indicated MRI and ^{18}FDG studies with stereotactic frames attached to their skulls. Both image sets were collected on the same day without removal of the frame between scans. Fiducial plates attached to the stereotactic frame filled with copper sulfate during MRI scanning and with positron emitting germanium strips during PET scanning served as a standard for registering the images. Because the fiducials consisted of linear channels imbedded in the plates, a series of multivariate least-squares regressions of the fiducial positions was used to obtain the best estimate of the correct alignment parameters.

Alignment using the MRI–PET algorithm resulted in resliced image sets that were almost indistinguishable from those aligned using the fiducial markers, and the maximum discrepancy in any direction for any point in the brain for a typical subject was 2 mm. The mean and maximum discrepancies for six subjects with fiducial data demonstrate that the worst three-dimensional discrepancy for any subject was 2.7 mm, and the mean discrepancy was 1.3 mm for the group.

The algorithm converged very rapidly with the FDG data, requiring less than 10 min in all cases. Registration times for the $H_2^{15}O$ data were more variable and typically required 30 to 40 min.

C. Among Subjects

The most vexing registration problem is the rigorous comparison of structural and functional data among subjects in a population. The solution to this problem must address the wide range of structural and functional variability that exists among different individuals within a species. Proportionality schemes such as those proposed by Talairach and colleagues (Talairach *et al.*, 1967; Talairach and Tournoux, 1988) represent some of the most widely used and earliest attempts at solving this problem. The shortcomings of simple proportionality and scaling approaches are

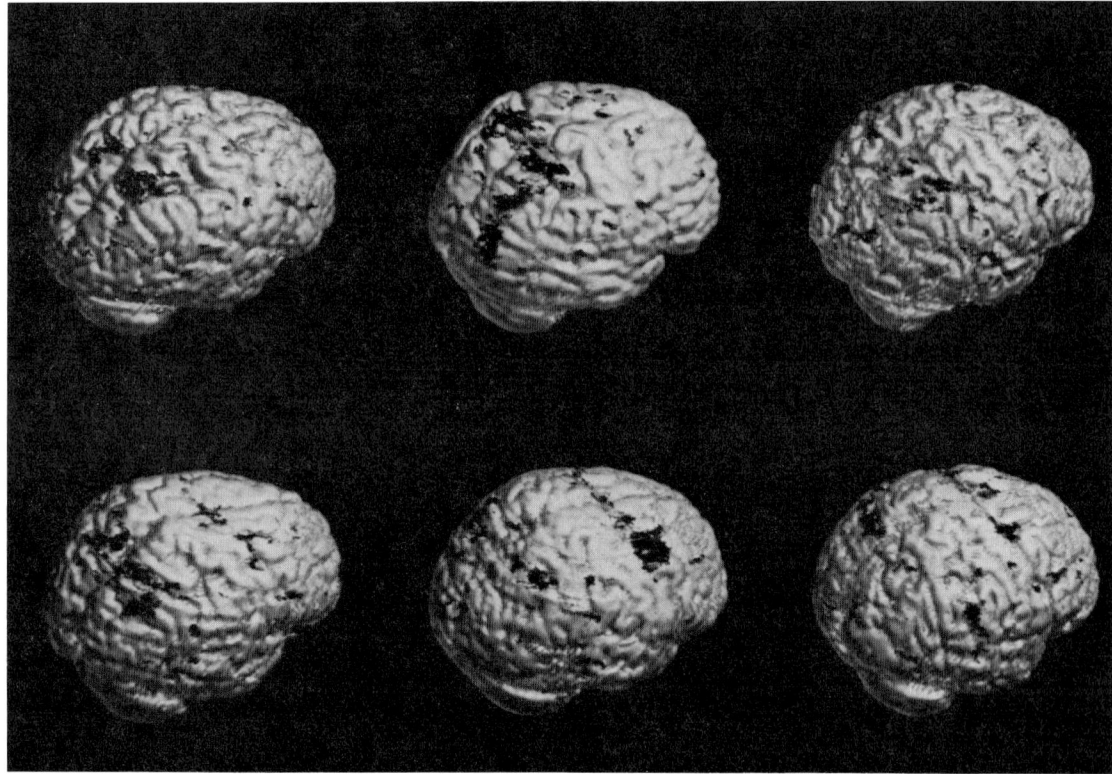

Figure 7 Anatomic localization and intersubject variability in normal subjects performing visually guided saccades. Six normal subjects were studied in 2D mode, and saccade tasks were compared with a control state consisting of visual fixation. The PET–PET registration algorithm was used to correct for head movements between scans, and the MRI–PET algorithm was used to align data from the two imaging modalities. In addition, the intersubject registration algorithm was used to orient and rescale each subject's data into a common orientation. Shaded areas demonstrated statistically significant increases in blood flow during the saccade tasks. The specific orientation used for surface rendering in this figure was chosen to optimize display the parietal activation site. Note the consistent activation bilaterally along the intraparietal sulcus. Activation in the premotor area (dorsal surface near the midline immediately anterior to the precentral gyrus) and the frontal eye fields (dorsolateral surface immediately anterior to the precentral gyrus) was more variable across subjects. Other areas show considerably greater variability. This study demonstrates the effectiveness of individual analysis for identification and localization of activation sites.

becoming more well known (Fig. 6). The intersubject registration problem is the most complex and least explored of the alignment and registration problems. In order to have clear insight into and a rigorous understanding of the commonalities and variabilities among subjects, in terms of brain structure and function, solutions to the intersubject issue must be achieved. Research currently in progress in our laboratory is directed toward facilitating intersubject comparison by extending the intrasubject, intramodality alignment algorithm described above (Fig. 7).

IV. Paradigm Development and Design

Of critical importance in the design of physiological and psychological paradigms for use in functional activation techniques is the concept that the fewest number of variables should change between states. That is, when comparing one behavioral or pharmacological condition with another, one should attempt to make the general behavioral condition of the subject as consistent as possible, while altering only one variable. Because it is impossible to have a "resting" condition for the human brain to serve as a control state, one attempts to maintain consistency between states and assumes that the subtraction of datasets acquired between control and "activation" states will cancel all but the activity associated with the altered variable. Obvious conditions to observe would include ambient room conditions such as sound, conversation, and visual stimuli. Less obvious, and often neglected, features might include time of day; ingestion of compounds with cerebral effects, such as nicotine and caffeine; circadian rhythm; and phase of the menstrual cycle. The more these and other variables within and between subjects can be made consistent, the more likely the experimentally induced change will result in a specific and clear signal in the subtracted datasets that can be rigorously interpreted.

V. Conclusion

The understanding of the functional organization of the human brain, even at a macroscopic level, represents one of the most challenging and daunting problems facing the scientific community today. The large and ever-growing number of methods that can be brought to bear on this issue are encouraging. The optimal use of each method and the integration of datasets acquired between methods provide the best hope for comprehensive insights into the structure and function of the human brain. This process will require the development of not only rigorous scientific methods but also common standards and communication links between investigators and laboratories in order to pool data for the best-integrated product. Such approaches, by their very definition, will require a degree of cooperation, as opposed to competition, that has not been part of the typical sociology of scientific endeavor. It is, however, only by such a collaborative and cooperative approach that an efficient means by which to address these issues can be obtained and the cost can be reduced to the point where such a project is feasible. If achieved, the results would be valuable and far reaching in their application to normal learning, development, aging, and cerebral disorders and their treatment.

Acknowledgments

The authors acknowledge Robert Knowlton, M.D., for participating in these studies; Ron Sumida and Larry Pang for technical assistance with scanning; and CTI, Inc., Knoxville, Tennessee, for the use of the Sun SPARCstation. This work was supported by Department of Energy Cooperative Agreement DE-FC03-87ER 60615, National Institutes of Mental Health Grant R01-MH37916, and NIH-NINDS Grant P01-NS15654.

References

Alpert, N. M., Bradshaw, J. F., Kennedy, D., and Correia, J. A. (1990). The principal axes transformation—A method for image registration. *J. Nucl. Med.* **31,** 1717–1722.

Cherry, S. R., Dahlblom, M., and Hoffman, E. J. (1991). 3D PET using conventional multislice tomograph without septa. *J. Comput. Assist. Tomogr.* **15,** 655–668.

Fox, P. T., Mintun, M. A., Reiman, E. M., and Raichle, M. E. (1988). Enhanced detection of focal brain responses using intersubject averaging and change-distribution analysis of subtracted PET images. *J. Cereb. Blood Flow Metab.* **8,** 642–653.

Fox, P. T., Perlmutter, J. S., and Raichle, M. E. (1985). A stereotactic method of anatomical localization for positron emission tomography. *J. Comput. Assist. Tomogr.* **9,** 141–153.

Evans, A. C., Marrett, S., Collins, L., and Peters, T. M. (1989). Anatomical-functional correlative analysis of the human brain using three dimensional imaging systems. *SPIE Med. Imaging III: Image Processing* **1092,** 264–274.

Hoffman, E. J., Cutler, P. D., Guerrero, T. M., Digby, W. M., and Mazziotta, J. C. (1991). Assessment of accuracy of PET utilizing a 3-D phantom to simulate the activity distribution of [18F]fluorodeoxyglucose uptake in the human brain. *J. Cereb. Blood Flow Metab.* **11,** A17–A25.

Kanno, I., Iida, H., Miura, S., and Murakami, M. (1991). Optimal scan time of oxygen-15-labeled water injection method for measurement of cerebral blood flow. *J. Nucl. Med.* **32,** 1931–1934.

Mazziotta, J. C., and Gilman, S. (1992). "Clinical Brain Imaging: Principles and Applications." Philadelphia: F. A. Davis.

Mazziotta, J. C., and Koslow, S. H. (1987). Assessment of goals and obstacles in data acquisition in analysis from emission tomography: Report of a series of international workshops. *J. Cereb. Blood Flow Metab.* **7,** S1–S31.

Minoshima, S., Berger, K. L., Lee, K. S., and Mintun, M. A. (1992). An automated method for rotational correction and centering of three-dimensional functional brain images. *J. Nucl. Med.* **33,** 1579–1589.

Mintun, M. A., Raichle, M. E., and Quarles, R. P. (1989). Length of PET data acquisition inversely affects ability to detect focal areas of brain activation [Abstr.] *J. Cereb. Blood Flow Metab.* **9**(Suppl. 1), S349.

Pelizzari, C. A., Chen, G. T., Spelbring, D. R., Weichselbaum, R. R., and Chen, C. T. (1989). Accurate three-dimensional registration of CT, PET, and/or MR images of the brain. *J. Comput. Assist Tomogr.* **13,** 20–26.

Talairach, J., Szikla, G., Tournoux, P., *et al.* (1967). "Atlas d'Anatomie Stereotaxique du Telecephale." Paris: Masson.

Talairach, J., and Tournoux, P. (1988). "Co-Planar Stereotaxic Atlas of the Human Brain: 3-Dimensional Proportional System: An Approach to Cerebral Imaging." New York: Thieme.

Townsend, D. W., Geissbuhler, A., Defrise, M., Hoffman, E. J., Spinks, T. J., Bailey, D. L., Gilardi, M. C., and Jones, T. (1991). Fully three-dimensional reconstruction for a PET camera with retractable septa. *IEEE Trans. Med. Imaging* **10,** 505–512.

Volkow, N. D., Mullani, N., Gould, L. K., Adler, S. S., and Gatley, S. J. (1991). Sensitivity of measurements of regional brain activation with oxygen-15-water and PET to time of stimulation and period of image reconstruction. *J. Nucl. Med.* **32,** 58–61.

Woods, R. P., Cherry, S. R., and Mazziotta, J. C. (1992). Rapid automated algorithm for aligning and reslicing PET images. *J. Comput. Assist. Tomogr.* **16,** 620–633.

Zhang, J., Levesque, M. F., Wilson, C. L., Harper, R. M., Engel, J., Jr., Lufkin, R., and Behnke, E. J. (1990). Multimodality imaging of brain structures for stereotactic surgery. *Radiology* **175,** 435–441.

6

Cortical Activation by Auditory Stimulation Studied with Positron Emission Tomography

Hans Herzog

Institute of Medicine, Research Center Jülich, D-52425 Jülich, Germany

I. Introduction

One of the major applications of positron emission tomography (PET) is in neurofunctional imaging. The assessment of regional cerebral functions in humans with radiotracers was first introduced by Lassen and co-workers (1978), who studied changes of regional cerebral blood flow (rCBF) in response to various stimuli. Employing the Kety–Schmidt technique and a freely diffusible, metabolically inert tracer such as ^{133}Xe, they used a battery of 254 scintillation detectors to measure increases of rCBF. With this technique they were able to demonstrate neuronal activation, especially in superficial cortical areas. The auditory cortex was one of the sensory systems investigated first (Roland *et al.*, 1981). These studies certified previous findings from animal research on the auditory system. The introduction of single photon emission computed tomography (SPECT) confirmed these early results with more precise regional definition. Nevertheless, this approach suffers from such disadvantages as low image resolution and the limited capability of regional quantitation.

The development of PET overcomes these shortcomings by providing several ways to assess neuronal activation. Blood flow and energy turnover, represented by oxygen and glucose consumption, are correlated with neuronal activation (Sokoloff, 1981; Yarowsky and Ingvar, 1981), so that PET measurements of

any of these three physiological parameters can be employed in functional imaging.

After a short description of the central auditory pathways, we will review PET examinations of cortical activation due to auditory stimulation. It is beyond the scope of this chapter to describe in detail the PET methods that are used in the different studies, but their main characteristics are mentioned.

II. The Central Auditory Pathways

The structures of the central auditory pathway are located in the brain stem, the midbrain, the posterior part of the internal capsule, and the temporal cortex. The first bipolar neuron of the auditory pathway leads from the hair cells of the cochlea, via the spiral ganglion, to the ventral and the dorsal part of the cochlear nucleus. From here most fibers cross to the contralateral side, partly as the second neuron and partly after being switched to the third neuron. The auditory pathway continues from the brain stem, past the lateral lemniscus with its dorsal nucleus—where some fibers cross—toward the inferior colliculus in the midbrain. Here the fifth neuron projects to the ipsilateral medial geniculate body inside the thalamus, whereas some fibers first cross to the opposite inferior colliculus. The medial geniculate nucleus with its dorsal, ventral, and medial parts is the origin of auditory radiation, which reaches the auditory cortex via the internal capsule. The auditory cortex is located in the superior transverse temporal gyri, which corresponds to Brodmann's areas 41 and 42. Whereas the distal parts of the auditory pathway are innervated exclusively by acoustic stimuli, only a small part of the primary auditory cortex is purely auditory. The rest receives other sensory stimuli as well. Neuroanatomic studies have shown that the primary cortex is connected to association areas in the same hemisphere, i.e., Wernicke's area (area 22, according to Brodmann) in the dorsal superior temporal gyrus, which is concerned with sensory speech processing, and Broca's area (areas 44 and 45 according to Brodmann) in the posterior inferior frontal lobe, which is considered to be responsible for motor speech processing. These secondary areas are related to many other structures in the brain. The primary auditory cortex is also linked to the contralateral cortex via the corpus callosum.

Three features of the auditory pathways are especially remarkable: the binaural innervation from the brain stem upward, the tonotopic representation of the cochlea in all parts of the auditory pathway, and, finally, the multisensory input in most parts of the primary auditory center.

III. Studies in Subjects with Normal Hearing

A. Activation by Simple Stimuli

Very few PET studies that examined the cortical activation caused by simple sounds or tones have been published. One of these studies tested if PET can confirm a tonotopic organization in the human primary auditory cortex as it is known in the primary cortex of animals. Lauter and co-workers (1985) investigated activation in the primary auditory cortex using the single-scan technique to measure rCBF.

Most PET techniques of measuring rCBF are based on ^{15}O-labeled tracers. The short, 2-min half-life of ^{15}O allows a sequence of several (e.g., six) scans, each 15–20 min apart. To quantify rCBF with ^{15}O-labeled tracers, two techniques were developed: the steady-state inhalation technique (Frackowiak et al., 1980), in which $C^{15}O_2$ gas is inhaled, and the single-scan technique (Herscovitch et al., 1983), which uses $H_2^{15}O$ injected as a bolus. The first technique has been applied mainly in the assessment of cerebrovascular diseases, whereas the single-scan technique has been used mainly for activation studies. Because this method requires a scan duration of less than 1 min, habituation plays no part during the time of stimulation. In contrast the steady-state inhalation method requires 10–15 min for a single study so that habitua-

tion must be taken into account. Although the single-scan technique allows an absolute quantitation of rCBF, it may be simplified for use in activation studies. Often only the *relative* change of rCBF due to a specific stimulus is of interest. Because the tissue uptake of $H_2^{15}O$ recorded by the single scan is nearly proportional to that of rCBF, at least in the range of normal rCBF values, some activation studies have utilized only the PET measurement itself without any blood data (Fox and Mintun, 1989).

Lauter and co-workers (1985) studied the tonotopic organization of the auditory cortex by presenting a pure tone with a frequency of 500 Hz, or 4 kHz monaurally (in only one ear), to normal-hearing, blindfolded volunteers. In each subject, four control scans, two before and two after the stimulation scans, were performed. The stimulation scans were also doubled, two for the 500-Hz tone and two for the 4-kHz tone. The results of the paired scans were averaged. Changes in rCBF were measured as percentage differences between control and stimulation scans. The results of this study confirmed the tonotopic organization of the human primary auditory cortex. The 500-Hz tone stimulation caused more activation in the lateral than in the medial part of the auditory cortex contralateral to the stimulated ear, whereas the medial part was more strongly activated by the higher tone of 4 kHz.

Cortical activation due to binaurally presented frequency modulated (FM) sound was studied by Griffiths and Brown (1991). rCBF was measured in six healthy right-handed male volunteers using inhaled $C^{15}O_2$ and a dynamic scanning technique (Lammertsma et al., 1989), which had been developed based on the steady-state inhalation technique. FM sound consisted of a 500-Hz tone modulated at 10 and 100 Hz. In addition, a pure 500-Hz tone was presented. Data analysis using statistical parametric images was performed as described by Friston and co-workers (1990). The parametric images were derived from data averaged over all examined subjects. The only significant activation was found in the left anterolateral occipital cortex at a modulation frequency of 100 HZ, but not at 10 Hz. Other possible activations, e.g., in the auditory cortex, were not reported. The authors speculated that the activated area, which is regarded as a visual association area, might process motion in the auditory space. Such motion is, of course, more pronounced for a modulation frequency of 100 Hz than for one of 10 Hz.

Recent studies directed in part toward the analysis of word processing, demonstrated that the frequency with which auditory stimuli are presented is closely related to the extent of activation of the primary cortex. When nouns were presented at different frequencies, i.e., from 10 to 90 words per minute, a linear relationship between the rate of stimulation and the increase in rCBF was found bilaterally in the pirmary auditory cortex and in middle regions of the superior temporal gyri, whereas in Wernicke's area on the left side an activation independent of the presentation rate was observed (Price *et al.*, 1992). In a study of word comprehension and retrieval, no increase in rCBF was measured in the primary auditory cortex when words were presented aurally at a frequency of 15 words per minute, whereas frequencies of more than 26 words per minute resulted in an elevated rCBF (Wise *et al.*, 1991).

B. Activation by Complex Stimuli

In the early 1980s, PET studies using complex auditory stimuli were reported by the groups at UCLA and the University of Pennsylvania. The main aims of these studies were to investigate cortical activation as a function of the side of the stimulated ear, the stimulus content, and the task strategy. In these studies, the regional metabolic rate of glucose consumption (rCMRGlc) was utilized as an indicator of neuronal activation. rCMRGlc was measured using the common single-scan technique after injection of [^{18}F]fluorodeoxyglucose (FDG) (Reivich *et al.*, 1979; Phelps *et al.*, 1979).

Mazziotta and co-workers (1984a) presented oral and nonoral stimuli to several groups of four to eight normal, right-handed volunteers. The data found in the stimulation studies were compared with the means of the results in a different group of normal, right-handed volunteers, who were studied at rest and under partial or total sensory (auditory, visual, or both) deprivation. The results of these control studies were communicated separately (Mazziotta and Phelps, 1984b). In right-handed individuals, the left cerebral hemisphere is regarded as dominant and responsible for the processing of language, whereas the right hemisphere is primarily dedicated to image and spatial processing. Therefore, it might be expected that the content and strategy of the processing of the stimuli are reflected by the site of activation. On the other hand, most fibers of the auditory pathway cross to the contralateral side, so that the main activation might be seen in the hemisphere opposite the stimulated ear. In order to answer this question, about half of each group was stimulated on the right side and the other half, on the left side. In spite of these monaural presentations, a common bilateral activation of the auditory cortex with an insignificant trend to a higher contralateral response was observed (Mazziotta and Phelps, 1984b). When an oral stimulus (a Sherlock Holmes story) was used, asymmetry was found, responses on the left being consistently greater than those on the right, in the frontal, lateral occipital, and posterior superior temporal cortices.

A second group of eight normal volunteers was stimulated (five on the right side; three on the left side) with tone sequences presented in pairs. Their task was to identify possible differences between the first and the second sequence. After a poststudy interview, the individuals were divided into two groups, one ($n = 5$) that did not use visual imagery to identify the single notes and a second ($n = 3$) that did. The first group showed consistently greater right hemisphere activation, whereas in all members of the second group there was an opposite asymmetry, with a higher rCMRGlc in the left hemisphere, especially in the posterior superior temporal cortex. A third test was performed in four musically unsophisticated subjects ($n = 2$ right-side stimulated; $n = 2$ left-side stimulated), who were asked to find differences between two single complex chords, which were presented as pairs. In this case, a general right-side metabolic asymmetry occurred in the frontal posterior temporal and temporooccipital cortices. Specific activations were found in the right superior posterior temporal and the temporoparietal regions of both sides.

Summarizing the results of this study, oral stimuli are preferentially processed by the left hemisphere, which is the dominant hemisphere in right-handed subjects. Nonoral stimuli caused a right-side asymmetry; i.e., they are processed primarily by the nondominant hemisphere. This finding was modified in those subjects who used their visual imagery to solve the task of tone identification. Here the dominant hemisphere was more active. Although the results in the single subgroups were consistent, only some of them were statistically significant. Therefore, Mazziotta and Phelps (1984b) concluded that a greater number of subjects would be needed to reach an acceptable level of significance.

In a later communication, Mazziotta *et al.* (1984c) reported a second evaluation of this study. Here the thalamus and the basal ganglia were specifically analyzed. In the group stimulated with the Sherlock Holmes story, the thalamus was activated bilaterally. This finding is consistent with the location of the medial geniculate body, which is part of the dorsal thalamus and the starting point of auditory radiation. On the other hand, no thalamic activation was found when nonoral stimuli were applied. Therefore, it might be concluded that the activation of the thalamus is dependent on the content of the stimulus.

Alavi and co-workers (1981) also studied the influence of the content of the stimulus on cortical glucose metabolism. They presented a factual story to one group ($n = 7$) and a meaningless story read in the Hungarian language to another group ($n = 7$). Each group was divided into right and left ear stimulation. Furthermore, a control group of eight men was studied without any specific stimulation. All subjects were normal, right-handed volunteers. In the control group, a minimum asymmetry was found. Those six members of the group listening to the factual story who paid attention throughout the scan showed a consistent activation of the right hemisphere, exceeding that in the region of the auditory cortex. The same result was observed in those subjects to whom the Hungarian story was presented. Thus, the ear of stimulation did not influence the outcomes. As all individuals were right-handed, this activation of the non-dominant hemisphere through the process of listening to language was surprising. In the discussion of their paper, the authors emphasized the importance of the additional task with which attention was assured: for the meaningful story the subjects had to recall the story after the scan, and for the Hungarian story a button had to been pressed when key stimuli embedded in the text were recognized. The authors speculated that the processing of these tasks might have activated the nondominant hemisphere more than the language processing activated the dominant hemisphere.

Contrary to the findings of Mazziotta et al. (1984a) and Alavi et al. (1981), Greenberg et al. (1981) found a consistent activation of the auditory cortex contralateral to the stimulated ear compared with their control group ($n = 6$), who had been examined with no aural or visual stimulation. This result was found in six normal-hearing, blindfolded volunteers to whom a factual story was presented monaurally (three right-sided, three left-sided). Here again the subjects were asked to recall the story after the PET scan. The relative difference of rCMRGlc between the contra- and the ipsilateral auditory cortex was $7 \pm 2.5\%$, whereas practically no asymmetry was found in the controls.

Using the single-scan technique to measure rCBF, Peterson and co-workers (1988) investigated 17 normal volunteers during binaural auditory stimulation by single words. This simple auditory stimulation was the first step in a hierarchic sequence of stimulation tasks to investigate single-word processing. The images taken of each subject during rest were subtracted from the images taken during the first stimulation, and these latter images were subtracted from the images of the second stimulation, etc. The results were averaged for the whole group, and the mean data were statistically analyzed to find the foci of activation (Fox et al., 1988). When single words were presented, cortical activation was found in the primary auditory

cortex and lateralized to the left in the temporoparietal, the anterior superior temporal, and the inferior anterior cingulate parts of the cortex. It was concluded that the activation in the temporoparietal and in the anterior superior temporal cortex is specific if words are used for stimuli. The temporoparietal region may play a role in phonological coding.

In a second test, the subjects had to repeat the spoken words. Here, cortical regions related to motor output became involved: the primary sensorimotor cortex, the supplementary motor area, the premotor area, and the inferior premotor sylvian area. The same areas were activated when visually rather than acoustically presented words had to be repeated aloud. When the subjects were tested for associations caused by the auditorily or visually presented words, additional foci besides those found during mere passive processing were revealed. These foci were mainly located in inferior prefrontal and cingulate regions and were similar for both kinds of stimulation.

The study of Peterson and co-workers (1988) clearly demonstrates how PET can aid in the investigation of the neuronal networks involved in speech processing when simple auditory stimuli are extended to sophisticated stimuli in combination with other sensory (e.g., visual) stimuli and associated tasks. Recently, further studies have been published on the same subject (Bartlett et al., 1987; Zatorre et al., 1991; Nenov et al., 1991; Wise et al., 1991; Howard et al., 1992).

IV. Studies in Patients with Hearing Deficits

All the papers discussed so far are based on inter-subject comparisons. In the early publications (Alavi et al., 1981; Mazziotta et al., 1984), separate groups of subjects were examined at rest and during stimulation. The individual single studies were evaluated by a region-of-interest technique, the results of each group, averaged; and the means, compared. More recent activation studies (Peterson et al., 1988; Seitz et al., 1990; Friston et al., 1990), especially those using ^{15}O-labeled tracers, utilized intrasubject controls, so that subtraction images between stimulation images and control images could be prepared. Subtraction images, however, are degraded by a high noise level, so that possible activations might be masked. Therefore, several groups have developed an intragroup averaging of the subtraction images. In order to take individual anatomic variations into account, the images are reoriented or scaled with the help of anatomical reference maps (Fox et al., 1985; Friston et al., 1989) or a standard brain atlas (Evans et al., 1988; Greitz et al., 1991) before averaging the images of the individual subjects. This method not only decreases the noise level but also enhances the signal found in activated areas. The disadvantage of this method is that standardization relative to a common reference system cannot correct for all intersubject variations. Whereas these variations may be neglected in the normal population, they have to be considered in patients. In the latter case, each subject must be evaluated by intrasubject comparison between control and stimulation, as was done in the next two studies discussed below.

In our own work, we emphasized the study of cortical activation in patients with hearing deficits. To the best of our knowledge, only the following few papers deal with auditory stimulation in patients with hearing deficits.

Normal-hearing persons have a bone conduction of up to 50 dB, so that a direct stimulation of the contralateral cochlea by attempted unilateral stimulation cannot be excluded. We studied one group of patients who were unilaterally deaf; the other group consisted of profoundly deaf patients with cochlear implants. In both groups of patients, a true one-sided auditory stimulation could be performed. Therefore, and because of the predominant crossover of the auditory pathway, one would expect a mainly contralateral cortical activation in these patients.

A. Studies in Unilaterally Deaf Patients

At the time we investigated the series of unilaterally deaf patients, only FDG was available as a tracer of brain function. In order to achieve a direct comparison between control and stimulation studies, a double-injection technique was used (Herzog *et al.*, 1988). Such a procedure has also been used by Chang *et al.* (1987). The direct short-term comparison was preferred to a pair of two single studies separated by one day, as the latter might be influenced by secondary, for example, psychological conditions, which cannot be controlled by the investigator. About 200 MBq of FDG were injected twice in four patients at an interval of 50 min. All patients were unilaterally deaf (two left-sided, two right-sided). Brain stem audiometry showed normal waves I–III and missing waves IV and V on the side of the deaf ear. Following the first injection (control, or baseline study), the patient was dynamically scanned at rest using the Scanditronix PET scanner PC4096-15WB with a resolution of 7 mm in reconstructed images (Rota Kops *et al.*, 1990). Following the second injection, another 50-min dynamic scan was acquired, during which rock music of 70 dB was presented as a stimulus. Parallel to both PET acquisitions, arterialized venous blood was withdrawn to monitor the plasma activity of FDG. Using

the dynamic PET data, a time–activity curve for the cortical tissue at the level of the auditory cortex was obtained. Image analysis was based on two images sets that were summed from 30 to 50 min after each injection. Due to the long half-life of ^{18}F, there was, in the second image, residual tracer activity, which originated from the control scan. In order to correct for this residual activity, the cortical time–activity curve was fitted to the interval of the control scan using the conventional three-compartment model of FDG kinetics (Phelps *et al.*, 1979) and extrapolated to the second scan period. This extrapolated curve represented the "background" curve of the residual tracer. Tracer uptake data from 30 to 50 min during the second scan were averaged first for the original measured uptake curve and then for the extrapolated curve of the residual tracer. The ratio of the resulting means was used to calculate a correction factor for the residual activity found in the second image. After the control image was multiplied by this factor, it was subtracted from the second image. The result was a modified image that showed cortical FDG uptake due only to the stimulation. After a corresponding correction of the plasma time–activity curve, two separate metabolic images of rCMRGlc (Plate 7) were calculated according to the formula suggested by Phelps *et al.* (1979). In the metabolic image during stimulation, areas of cortical activation were clearly displayed. These areas were the left and right auditory cortices, with a nearly symmetric activation. The mean ratio of rCMRGlc in the auditory cortex relative to the whole slice data was 1.13 on the ipsilateral and 1.12 on the contralateral side during control. These values increased to 1.41 and 1.40, respectively, due to stimulation.

B. Studies in Patients with Cochlear Implant

In another study, we investigated profoundly deaf patients who had received a cochlear implant, using ^{15}O-labeled water to measure changes in rCBF due to cortical activation. A similar study had been performed by our group some years before using the ECAT II PET camera and FDG scans during control and stimulation on separate days (Herzog *et al.*, 1986). Although the results of this study indicated the occurrence of cortical activation due to the cochlear implant, we were aware of problems caused by the long separation between the two studies and the limited image resolution of the ECAT II (about 15 mm).

Therefore, this investigation was repeated in different patients, after a high-resolution PET camera (Scanditronix PC4096-15WB) had been installed (Herzog *et al.*, 1991). Two of the patients were postlingually deaf;

i.e., complete hearing loss had occurred after they had learned to speak. The two other patients were prelingually deaf; i.e., they were bilaterally deaf from birth on. All four patients were right-handed and between 23 and 45 years old. The cochlear implant was connected to the cochlea with eight electrodes, in patients 1 and 2 on the left side and in patients 3 and 4 on the right. In each patient, six PET scans were acquired over 2 min, directly after the intravenous injection of 30–40 mCi $H_2^{15}O$ for each scan. The single injections were about 15 min apart. In this study a scan duration of 2 min was used instead of a duration of 40 s, which had been suggested by Herscovitch et al. (1983). The longer duration of 2 min equals the maximum duration of single scans of $H_2^{15}O$ as suggested by Kanno and colleagues (1987), who studied the effects of scan duration with its trade-off between the reduction of noise, on the one hand, and the nonlinearity between tissue activity and rCBF, on the other. The first and the fourth scan were acquired as control studies with the cochlear implant switched off. During other scans, the cochlear implant electronics were switched on, so that they transformed acoustic signals into electrical impulses that excited the auditory nerve directly. The acoustic signal consisted of white noise (WN) during the second and fifth scans and a sequence of words (WO) during the third and sixth scans. The sequence of words consisted of the Freiburger speech test (Weiland, 1954), which is used in the fitting of hearing aids and during the rehabilitation training following cochlear implant surgery. All subjects confirmed sensations of hearing when the cochlear implants were switched on. The scanner room was dimly lit and quiet, and the subjects kept their eyes open.

In this study, data analysis was based on images of cerebral $H_2^{15}O$ radioactivity rather than on rCBF images. The regional concentration of $H_2^{15}O$ is nearly linearly related to rCBF in the range of normal values when the single-scan technique is used. Therefore, relative changes of $H_2^{15}O$ radioactivity and rCBF or ratios of regional to global $H_2^{15}O$ radioactivity and rCBF are equivalent. This approach, for which no blood withdrawal is needed, has also been applied by other authors (Fox and Mintun, 1989). Regional tissue concentrations of $H_2^{15}O$ (c_T) were normalized to the mean c_T of the whole brain and expressed as c_R (relative tissue concentration). Thus, different amounts of injected activity were taken into account and intra- or interindividual comparisons became possible. In order to evaluate comparable PET images, 3 out of 15 acquired images were selected by comparing them with those brain slices in the anatomical reference atlas of Tailarach and Tournoux (1988), which include the primary and secondary auditory cortices. The ana-

tomical slices are parallel to the bicommissural line, whereas the PET images were aligned parallel to the canthomeatal line. However, both lines are parallel within narrow limits (Szikla et al., 1977). Plane 1 was selected at the level of the basal ganglia so that regions in Broca's area and the thalamus could be defined. Planes 2 and 3 were 6.5 and 13 mm higher, respectively, so that regions for the primary auditory cortex and Wernicke's area were found here.

In order to examine activations due to the cochlear implant, relative changes of c_R between control and stimulation were calculated in different ROIs. The fourth scan, which was performed as a second control scan, was not used after a preliminary evaluation. Acquired about 15 min after the WO scan, it obviously showed residual activity. Such a residual activation, persisting for 15 min after (visual) stimulation, was also found by Momose and co-workers (1991).

An elevation of rCBF in the auditory cortex was seen on the contralateral side in planes 2 and 3 and on the ipsilateral side in plane 2 for WN as well as for WO simulation. Using a matched pair sign test, the level of significance of these findings was $p = 0.06$. Thus, this study demonstrated that cochlear implant stimulation resulted in cortical activation not only in the postlingually, but also in the prelingually deaf patients (Plate 8). This finding was not anticipated, studies in the cat model having indicated atrophy of the auditory cortex in the case of prelingual deafness (Moore, 1985). Increases of c_R of more than 10% were also found for WN as well as for WO stimulation in the secondary auditory cortex (Wernicke's area). In plane 3, a significant level of $p = 0.06$ was reached by the activation in the contralateral Wernicke's area during WO stimulation. Whereas increases of c_R were observed in both hemispheres in the primary and secondary auditory cortices, contralateral activation was higher. In contrast to Wernicke's area, no indication of any activation could be found in Broca's area. This absence of activation in the auditory motor cortex is not surprising, as the patients remained silent during the investigation. ROIs defined over the thalamus, the location of the medial geniculate nucleus, gave variable results, so that no indication of activation could be defined, although here technical problems may have obscured any activation. Due to the small size of the medial geniculate nucleus, partial volume effects are unavoidable. Furthermore, image artifacts in the low-count images must be taken into account. However, studies with [^{14}C]deoxyglucose found activation in guinea pigs only in the inferior colliculus and not in the thalamus, when the cochlear nucleus was stimulated electrically (Evans et al., 1990).

The results found by our group are in agreement

with those of a case study performed by Ito and co-workers (1990). These authors examined one patient with a cochlear implant using measurements of the metabolic rates of glucose and oxygen. When the cochlear implant was not operative, metabolic rates in the auditory cortices were low compared with those of controls. When sound stimulation was presented via the cochlear implant, the metabolic rates returned to normal levels, demonstrating a bilateral activation of the auditory cortices by the cochlear implant.

V. Studies in Patients with Other Diseases

Auditory stimulation may also be helpful in the investigation of diseases that are caused by disorders other than those of the auditory pathway itself. Hagman and co-workers (1992) used an auditory version of the continuous performance test (CPT) to study cortical activation in dyslexic adults in comparison with a group of normal individuals. Several stop consonant–vowel syllables (a, da, ga, pa, ta) were presented binaurally and the syllable da was to be identified. rCMRglc was used as a parameter of neuronal activation. Whereas no effects were seen in the lateral parts of the different cortical lobes, a significant elevation of rCMRglc was found in the medial temporal lobe of both hemispheres. Thus, this part of the temporal lobe, which is close to the primary auditory cortex and to Wernicke's area, might be affected in dyslexia.

VI. Concluding Remarks

In this chapter, studies of neurofunctional imaging during auditory stimulation have been reviewed. Whereas most of these studies were performed in normal volunteers, only a few investigated patients with hearing deficits. Because the number of PET studies of auditory stimulation published up to now is relatively low and small groups were examined, only limited conclusions can be drawn. The most consistent finding is that *monaural stimulation causes a contralateral as well as an ipsilateral activation in the primary auditory cortex*. Although the contralateral activation was more intense than the ipsilateral, the ratio between them did not correspond to the predominant crossover of the auditory pathway. This finding was especially impressive in our studies with unilaterally and profoundly deaf patients, in whom a truly one-sided acoustic or electrically auditory stimulation could be performed. The results obtained by Mazziotta *et al.* (1982) and Alavi *et al.* (1981) suggest a depen-

dency of the ratio between contralateral and ipsilateral activation on the content of the stimulus. For these early studies, PET scanners with a low resolution of about 15 mm were used. Thus, there might be uncertainties about the precision of the activated areas. In order to verify these findings, it would be desirable to repeat these studies using a greater number of individuals and the high-resolution PET cameras now available. Other issues reported here, such as the cortical reaction to electrical auditory stimulation in patients with cochlear implants should be reexamined with respect to differences between post- and prelingually deaf patients. Given the demonstration of activation in the auditory cortex even in prelingually deaf patients, further studies could investigate if PET can be used as a tool to predict the benefit of implant surgery. As most neurologically caused hearing deficits involve parts of the auditory pathway distal from the primary auditory cortex, it would be advantageous to include the auditory centers in the midbrain and the brain stem in the study. The image resolution needed for such investigations is, however, not yet available, so that such work is hindered by partial volume problems.

It has already been emphasized above that, if activation studies are to be extended to patients, an interindividual averaging of subtraction images is no longer appropriate. On the other hand, it is often difficult to localize activated areas on the basis of PET images alone. Therefore, a method was developed by our co-workers at the Department of Neurology of the University Hospital at Düsseldorf that yields individual PET/MRI matching (Steinmetz *et al.*, 1992). Plate 9 gives an example of one of our most recent auditory studies using normal volunteers (manuscript to be published), in which the subtraction image, with zones activated during binaural word stimulation, is overlaid on the MRI image. With this superimposition, the activated zones can be anatomically localized in the individual subject. In order to exclude zones that represent noise, Knorr and co-workers (1993) developed a procedure to define a level of significance for each area found in the subtraction image. In our opinion, such procedures, which aim to achieve a reliable analysis of the individual patient, are absolutely necessary if activation studies with PET are to achieve clinical impact.

Acknowledgments

The author thanks Ms. D. Beaujean for her secretarial assistance. He is greatly indebted to Professor D. D. Patton, M.D. (Tucson, Arizona), and to Professor Altman, Ph.D., for their support in preparing the manuscript.

References

Alavi, A., Reivich, M., Greenberg, J., Hand, P., Rosenquist, A., Rintelmann, W., Christman, D., Fowler, J., Goldman, A., Mac-Gregor, R., and Wolf, A. (1981). Mapping of functional activity in brain with 18-fluoro-deoxyglucose. *Sem. Nucl. Med.* **9,** 24–31.

Bartlett, E. J., Brown, J. W., Wolf, A. P., and Brodie, J. D. (1987). Correlations between glucose metabolic rates in brain regions of healthy male adults at rest and during language stimulation. *Brain Language* **32,** 1–18.

Chang, J. Y., Duara, R., Barker, W. Apicella, A., Yoshii, F., Kelley, R. E., Ginsburg, M. D., and Boothe, T. E. (1987). Two behavioral states studied in a single PET/FDG procedure: Theory, method, and preliminary results. *J. Nucl. Med.* **28,** 852–860.

Evans, A. C., Beil, C., Marrett, S., Thompson, C. J., and Hakim, A. (1988). Anatomical–functional correlation using an adjustable MRI-based region of interest atlas with positron emission tomography. *J. Cereb. Blood Flow Metab.* **8,** 513–530.

Evans, D. A., Niparko, J. K., Altschuler, R. A., Frey, K. A., and Miller, J. M. (1990). Demonstration of prothetic activation of central auditory pathways using [^{14}C]-2-deoxyglucose. *Laryngoscope* **100,** 128–137.

Fox, P. T., Perlmutter, J. S., and Raichle, M. E. (1985). A stereotactic method of anatomical localization for positron emission tomography. *J. Comput. Assist. Tomogr.* **9,** 141–153.

Fox, P. T., Mintun, M. A., Reiman, E. M., and Raichle, M. E. (1988). Enhanced detection of focal brain responses using intersubject averaging and change-distribution analysis of subtracted PET images. *J. Cereb. Blood Flow Metab.* **8,** 642–653.

Fox, P. T., and Mintun, M. A. (1989). Noninvasive functional brain mapping by change-distribution analysis of averaged PET images of H$_2$^{15}O tissue activity. *J. Nucl. Med.* **24,** 790–798.

Frackowiak, R. S. J., Lenzi, G. L., Jones, T., and Heather, J. D. (1980). Quantitative measurement of regional cerebral blood flow and oxygen metabolism in man using ^{15}O and positron emission tomography: Theory, procedure and normal values. *J. Comput. Assist. Tomogr.* **4,** 727–736.

Friston, K. J., Passingham, R. E., Nutt, J. G., Heather, J. D., Sawle, G. V., and Frackowiak, R. S. J. (1989). Localization in PET images: Direct fitting of the intercommissural (AC–PC) line. *J. Cereb. Blood Flow Metab.* **9,** 690–695.

Friston, K. J., Frith, C. D., Liddle, P. F., Dolan, R. J., Lammertsma, A. A., and Frackowiak, R. S. J. (1990). The relationship between global and local changes in PET scans. *J. Cereb. Blood Flow Metab.* **10,** 458–466.

Friston, K. J., Frith, C. D., Liddle, P. F., and Frackowiak, R. S. J. (1991). Comparing functional (PET) images: The assessment of significant change. *J. Cereb. Blood Flow Metab.* **11,** 690–699.

Greenberg, J. H., Reivich, M., Alavi, A., Hand, P., Rosenquist, A., Rintelmann, W., Stein, A., Tusa, R., Dann, R., Christman, D., Fowler, J., MacGregor, B., and Wolf, A. (1981). Metabolic mapping of functional activity in human subjects with the (18-F) fluorodeoxyglucose technique. *Science* **212,** 678–680.

Greitz, T., Bohm, C., Holte, S., and Eriksson, L. (1991). A computerized brain atlas: Construction, anatomical content, and some applications. *J. Comput. Assist. Tomogr.* **15,** 26–38.

Griffiths, T. D., and Brown, W. D. (1991). XXII-13: Focal activation of human left area 19 during an auditory task. *J. Cereb. Blood Flow Metab.* **11**(Suppl. 2), S374.

Hagman, J. O., Wood, F., Buchsbaum, M. S., Tallal, P., Flowers, L., and Katz, W. (1992). Cerebral brain metabolism in adult dyslexic subjects assessed with positron emission tomography during performance of an auditory task. *Arch. Neurol.* **49,** 734–739.

Herscovitch, P., Markham, J., and Raichle, M. E. (1983). Brain blood flow measured with intravenous H$_2$^{15}O. I. Theory and error analysis. *J. Nucl. Med.* **24,** 782–789.

Herzog, H., Wieler, H., Morgenstern, C., Lipman, J., Langen, K.-J., Schmid, A., Rota, E., Patton, D., and Feinendegen, L. E. (1986). Demonstration of ipsilateral brain activation by noise in patients profoundly deaf with cochlear implant, or unilaterally deaf. *In* "Radioaktive Isotope in Klinik und Forschung" (W. Höfer and H. Bergmann, Eds.), Vol. 17, pp. 645–651. Wien: H. Egermann.

Herzog, H., Langen, K.-J., Kuwert, T., Rota Kops, E., Hennerici, M., Morgenstern, C., and Feinendegen, L. E. (1988). Cortical activation by motor and acoustic stimuli revealed by PET and repeated FDG-scans. *Eur. J. Nucl. Med.* **14,** 308. [Abstr.]

Herzog, H., Lamprecht, A., Kühn, A., Roden, W., Vosteen, K.-H., and Feinendegen, L. E. (1991). Cortical activation in profoundly deaf patients during cochlear implant stimulation demonstrated by H$_2$^{15}O PET. *J. Comput. Assist. Tomogr.* **15,** 369–375.

Howard, D., Patterson, K., Wise, R., Brown, W. D., Friston, K., Weiller, C., and Frackowiak, R. (1992). Distribution of cortical neural networks involved in word comprehension and word retrieval. *Brain,* **115,** 1769–1782.

Ito, J., Sakakibara, J., Honjo, I., Iwasaki, Y., and Yonekura, Y. (1990). Positron emission tomography study of auditory sensation in a patient with a cochlear implant. *Arch. Otolaryngol. Head Neck Surg.* **116,** 1437–1439.

Kanno, I., Iida, H., Miura, S., Murakami, M., Takahashi, K., Sasaki, H., Inugami, A., Shishido, F., and Uemura, K. (1987). A system for cerebral blood flow measurement using an H$_2$^{15}O autographic method and positron emission tomography. *J. Cereb. Blood Flow Metab.* **7,** 143–153.

Knorr, U., Weder, B., Kleinschmidt, A., Wirrwar, A., Huang, Y., Herzog, H., and Seitz, R. J. (1993). Identification of task-specific rCBF changes in individual subjects: Validation and application for PET. *J. Comput. Assist. Tomogr.* **17,** 517–528.

Lammertsma, A. A., Frackowiak, R. S. J., Hoffman, J. M., Huang, S. C., Weinberg, I. N., Dahlbom, M., MacDonald, N. S., Hoffman, E. J., Mazziotta, J. C., Heather, J. D., Forse, G. R., Phelps, M. E., and Jones, T. (1989) The C^{15}O$_2$ build-up technique to measure regional cerebral blood flow and volume of distribution of water. *J. Cereb. Blood Flow Metab.* **9,** 461–470.

Lassen, N. A., Ingvar, D. H., and Skinhoj, E. (1978). Brain function and blood flow. *Sci. Am.* **67,** 50–59.

Lauter, J. L., Herscovitch, P., Formby, C., and Raichle, M. E. (1985). Tonotopic organization in human auditory cortex revealed by positron emission tomography *Hear Res.* **20,** 199–205.

Mazziotta, J. C., Phelps, M. E., Carson, R. E., and Kuhl, D. E. (1984a). Tomographic mapping of human cerebral metabolism: Auditory stimulation. *Neurology* **32,** 921–937.

Mazziotta, J. C., and Phelps, M. E. (1984b). Human sensory stimulation and deprivation: Positron emission tomographic results and strategies. *Ann. Neurol.* **15**(Suppl.), 50–60.

Mazziotta, J. C., Phelps, M. E., and Carson, R. E. (1984c). Tomographic mapping of human cerebral metabolism: Subcortical responses to auditory and visual stimulation. *Neurology* **34,** 825–828.

Momose, T., Sasaki, Y., Nishikawa, J., Nakashima, Y., Watanabe, T., Sano, I., Katayama, S., and Nakajima, T. (1991). Residual effect of physiological stimulation on cerebral blood flow measured by H$_2$^{15}O bolus injection method and PET. *J. Cereb. Blood Flow Metab.* **11**(Suppl. 2), S853.

Moore, D. R. (1985). Postnatal development of the mammalian central auditory system and the neural consequences of auditory deprivation. *Acta Otolaryngol.* **421**(Suppl.) 19–30.

Nenov, V. I., Halgren, E., Smith, M. E., Badier, J. M., Ropchan, J., Blahd, W. H., and Mandelkern, M. (1991). Localized brain metabolic response correlated with potentials evoked by words. *Behav. Brain Res.* **44,** 101–104.

Petersen, S. E., Fox, P. T., Posner, M. I., Mintun, M. A., and Raichle, M. E. (1988). Positron emission tomography studies of the cortical anatomy of single-word processing. *Nature* **311,** 585–589.

Phelps, M. E., Huang, S. C., Hoffman, E. J., Selin, C., Sokoloff, L., and Kuhl, D. E. (1979). Tomographic measurement of local cerebral glucose metabolic rate in humans with (F-18) 2-deoxy-D-glucose: Validation of method. *Ann. Neurol.* **6,** 371–388.

Price, C., Wise, R., Ramsay, S., Friston, K., Howard, D., Patterson, K., and Frackowiak, R. (1992). Regional response differences within the human auditory cortex when listening to words. *Neurosci. Lett.* **146,** 179–182.

Raichle, M. E., Martin, W. R. W., Herscovitch, P., Mintun, M. A., and Markham, J. (1983). Brain blood flow measured with intravenous $H_2^{15}O$. II. Implementation and validation. *J. Nucl. Med.* **24,** 790–798.

Reivich, M., Kuhl, D. E., Wolf, A., Greenberg, J., Phelps, M. E., Ido, T., Casella, V., Fowler, J., Hoffman, E., Alavi, A., Som, P., and Sokoloff, L. (1979). The $[^{18}F]$-fluorodeoxyglucose-method for the measurement of local cerebral glucose utilization in man. *Circ. Res.* **44,** 127–137.

Roland, P. E., Skinhoj, E., and Lassen, N. A. (1981). Focal activation of human cerebral cortex during auditory discrimination. *J. Neurophysiol.* **45,** 1139–1151.

Rota Kops, E., Herzog, H., Schmid, A., Holte, S., and Feinendegen, L. E. (1990). Performance characteristics of an eight-ring whole-body PET scanner. *J. Comput. Assist. Tomogr.* **14,** 437–445.

Seitz, R. J., Bohm, C., Greitz, T., Roland, P. E., Eriksson, L., Blomqvist, G., Rosenqvist, G., and Nordell, B. (1990). Accuracy and precision of the computerized brain atlas programme for localization and quantification in positron emission tomography. *J. Cereb. Blood Flow Metab.* **10,** 443–457.

Steinmetz, H., Huang, Y., Seitz, R. J., Knorr, U., Schlaug, G., Herzog, H., Hackländer, T., and Freund, H.-J. (1992). Individual integration of positron emission tomography and high-resolution magnetic resonance imaging. *J. Cereb. Blood Flow Metab.* **12,** 912–926.

Sokoloff, L. (1981). Relationships among local functional activity, energy metabolism, and blood flow in the central nervous system. *Fed. Proc.* **40,** 2311–2316.

Szikla, G., Bouvier, G., Hori, T., and Petrov, V. (1977). "Atlas of Vascular and Cerebral Cortical Localization." Berlin: Springer.

Talairach, J., and Tournoux, P. (1988). "Co-Planar Stereotaxic Atlas of the Human Brain: 3-Dimensional Proportional System: An Approach to Cerebral Imaging." Stuttgart: Thieme.

Weiland, E. (1954). "Neue Wörterteste für Sprachaudiometrie und über damit angestellte Untersuchungen an 96 Normalhörenden." Ph.D. thesis, University of Freiburg i.Br., Germany.

Wise, R., Chollet, F., Hadar, U., Friston, K., and Frackowiak, R. (1991). Distribution of cortical neural networks involved in word comprehension and word retrieval. *Brain* **114,** 1803–1817.

Yarowsky, G. J., and Ingvar, D. H. (1981). Neuronal activity and energy metabolism. *Fed. Proc.* **40,** 2353–2363.

Zatorre, R. J., Evans, A. C., Meyer, E., and Gjedde, A. (1991). Lateralization of phonetic and pitch discrimination in speech processing. *Science* **256,** 846–849.

7

Magnetic Resonance Studies of Brain Functional Activation Using Echo-Planar Imaging

Robert Turner and Peter Jezzard

Laboratory of Cardiac Energetics, National Heart, Lung, and Blood Institute, National Institutes of Health, Bethesda, Maryland 20892

I. Introduction

Recent developments in magnetic resonance imaging (MRI) have demonstrated the possibility of non-invasive mapping of human brain functional activity with good spatial and temporal resolution. The early results are most encouraging, appearing to offer substantially better functional brain maps than other non-invasive methods.

However, many research groups reporting successful studies using MRI have found it necessary to use nonstandard equipment and also a special method for obtaining MR images very rapidly, known as echo-planar imaging (EPI). This chapter will describe the features of MRI that enable it to form maps of functional brain activity, and the particular characteristics of EPI, showing how it differs from conventional MRI.

The historical development of functional MRI will then be described, with critical analyses of the methods presently available. These comprise techniques for measuring relative blood volume, relative blood flow, and relative blood oxygenation. Finally, current research in those laboratories pursuing functional MRI will be surveyed.

II. Conventional MRI

Since the production of the first useful MR brain images 14 years ago (Editors, 1978) a number of re-searchers have speculated on the possibility of showing brain physiology as well as anatomy by this means. MRI is a technique that is highly sensitive to flow, as well as to differences in proton environment, and so this hope was not entirely without foundation, given that neuronal activity is normally accompanied by an increase in perfusion. However, until recently image changes due to flow could be reliably seen only in larger vessels, and the time resolution for observing changes in flow was extremely limited, to some tens of seconds at best. This combination of features was not suitable for functional brain imaging.

Magnetic resonance imaging obtains an image of a section of a subject by means of the phenomenon of nuclear magnetic resonance. This denotes the interaction between the spins of nuclei (usually the hydrogen nuclei, or protons, in water) and imposed magnetic fields. Because the protons possess a small magnetic moment, a steady magnetic field tends to align them in the field direction. By imposing a radio frequency (*rf*) magnetic field with precisely that frequency that corresponds to the energy difference between alignment parallel to and that antiparallel to the steady field, the spins can be "flipped" into an alignment that is no longer along the field direction. This final alignment depends on the duration of the *rf* pulse and is frequently made equal to 90° from the static field direction, at which angle the maximum output signal is observable. Following the *rf* pulse, the energy is reemitted by the nuclear spins, in the form of an *rf*

69

magnetic field decaying over some tens of milliseconds as the spin system returns to equilibrium. This field can be detected by a suitably configured tuned coil, to give a signal called the free induction decay (FID).

Frequently an additional rf pulse, giving a flip angle of 180°, is applied following the initial pulse. This so-called "refocusing pulse" has the effect of reversing the dephasing of the spins after it is applied, to create a "spin echo" at a time twice that between the two rf pulses. Such imaging sequences are much less sensitive to the effects of static magnetic field inhomogeneity than those without a refocusing pulse, known as "gradient echo" sequences.

Spatial information regarding the subject is obtained by imposing, after the rf excitation pulse, an additional set of magnetic fields possessing linear variations in space in one or more of the directions of the three coordinate axes (Wehrli, 1992). The frequency of the received FID from spins in any particular subregion of the subject depends on the magnetic field at that point, and hence a frequency analysis of the voltage output of the rf receiver gives a map of the density of protons at any point in space.

The primary source of contrast in the image is thus the density of protons in the tissue, and, because the protons are mostly found as the H_2 component of water, this is effectively tissue water content. However, the time dependence of the FID, and the recovery of the spin system to equilibrium following rf excitation, allow two more contrast parameters to be extracted. These are the "longitudinal relaxation time," T_1, and the "transverse relaxation time," T_2. T_1 is the time constant describing the recovery of the entire spin system to thermal equilibrium, and T_2 describes the development of phase incoherence of excited spins before they actually relax to equilibrium. These times, which can be made to affect image intensity by a variety of stratagems, each depend on different properties of the environment in which the protons find themselves and so are diagnostically useful in discriminating abnormal tissue.

However, neither of the relaxation times, nor the proton density, is affected directly by electrical activity of neurons in the brain, and the water signal itself shows no modulation by the metabolic processes associated with neuronal activity. For MRI to be used for imaging of brain physiology a different approach is needed.

The fresh approach—to be precise, approaches—relies on the close association, first postulated by Roy and Sherrington (1890) between neural activity and blood flow. The 2–4% by volume of blood in the brain is sufficient to modify the MRI signal, especially as

there are a number of tricks whereby its effect may be enhanced. These tricks, to which we shall return later, consist of labeling the blood in various ways so that it affects MRI signal from surrounding tissue. Before we consider these methods, however, it is useful to analyze the problem of functional brain mapping in more depth.

III. Temporal Resolution Issues in Functional MRI

The brain is an organ that is specifically adapted to deal with sensory inputs which may be rapidly varying in time. Many stimuli are habituative, and (for instance) large areas of the extrastriate visual cortex appear to be devoted to perception of motion in the visual field. Brain tasks are by definition time limited. Thus it is highly desirable to have a method for imaging brain activity that is fast enough that localization of the rapid bursts of activity most characteristic of brain function, lasting no more than some tens of seconds, can be achieved.

This gives MRI something of a problem. In the form in which it has been developed commercially on a large scale, imaging times for a single slice of the brain are typically minutes. Also, as we will see, the techniques to be described work best when imaging is performed fast enough to avoid any motion artifact arising from brain pulsations, or involuntary head motion. The pursuit of functional brain mapping by MRI became serious only when a much faster, unconventional method of obtaining images, termed EPI (Mansfield, 1977; Cohen and Weisskoff, 1991; Stehling *et al.*, 1991) was implemented on an MR system with relatively high magnetic field. This configuration, to be described in further detail below, allows an image signal-to-noise ratio (SNR) high enough for functional studies, together with a time resolution of 1 s or less, and an acquisition time per image of 50 ms, short enough to prevent any motion artifact.

Other forms of fast MRI have been devised (Frahm *et al.*, 1992). Using a "flip angle" of less than 90°, which excites a smaller proportion of the total spin magnetization available, the rf pulse repeat time can be reduced to 10 ms or so, resulting in an image acquisition time of 1 or 2 s. However, this is achieved at the cost of a serious loss in the SNR, because of the reduction in the magnetization interrogated at each rf pulse. Furthermore, motion of the subject, even normal brain pulsation with the cardiac cycle, can cause severe distributed artifacts on the image. Time averaging of the image data can do much to restore the image quality. If the inevitable loss of time resolution can be tolerated, the improved spatial resolution available with this conventional gradient echo technique is advantageous.

IV. Echo-Planar Imaging

To appreciate how EPI differs from conventional MRI, consider Fig. 1. Figures 1A and 1B show the relationship between image space and the space in which MRI data is sampled, generally known as k space. A Fourier transform of the raw data acquired in k space gives the NMR image. Conventional MRI, as shown in Fig. 1C, uses a series of N (typically 128) rf pulses to interrogate the k-space representation of the object, each pulse being followed by, say, 256 samples of data at equal time intervals, corresponding to equal intervals in k space. A period TR of 0.4–2 s then elapses, to allow the nuclear spins to recover

before the next rf excitation pulse, when the next line of k space is sampled. It is clear that a total time of $N \cdot$ TR is required to obtain all the information needed to construct an image, usually more than 60 s.

By contrast, EPI samples all of the k-space data required after only one rf pulse. This must be done in a short time span, less than 100 ms, because the NMR signal following the rf excitation pulse, which arises from protons on water molecules, decays in this time. Thus the sampling rate must be unusually high—up to 500 kilosamples/s—and the scanning of k space must be rapid. This scanning (Fig. 1D) is performed by means of applying rapidly alternating magnetic field gradients. To obtain fast enough switching of these field gradients, very low inductance gradient coils and very powerful current amplifiers must be used, which are not standard MRI equipment.

Only four or five MR systems in the world can provide good quality echo-planar images of the human brain. Because the data are gathered very quickly, and the rf receiver bandwidth is large, the SNR may be poorer than that with a conventional MRI technique, taking more than 15 s to acquire an image. However, SNR increases approximately proportional to the magnetic field used by the scanner, and at the widely used field of 1.5 T the SNR in echo-planar images is adequate for most purposes. What is more, because this technique is totally free from motion artifact, image stability is excellent.

EPI has certain limitations. Ultimately the speed of acquisition and spatial resolution are limited by the fact that peripheral nerves are excited by the rapid switching of sufficiently large magnetic fields. This stimulation, while barely detectable as a slight tapping feeling at threshold, becomes painful at field levels only 20–40% higher (Budinger *et al.*, 1991). The result is that it is not feasible to obtain EPI images with a 20-cm FOV and 256- × 256-pixel matrix in less than 100 ms.

Furthermore, compared with conventional MRI, the data are acquired for a relatively long time after each rf pulse, because all the data for a given image are collected then. This results in greater vulnerability to image distortion caused by inhomogeneities in the static magnetic field. Whereas field correction algorithms can reduce these considerably, the configuration of the object itself introduces some field variations that cannot be corrected, because the object generally has a magnetic susceptibility different from that of the surrounding air. Thus, for instance, the regions of the brain above the nasal sinuses and near the petrous bone are poorly shown in EPI images, especially at higher field strength, where the susceptibility differences become more manifest.

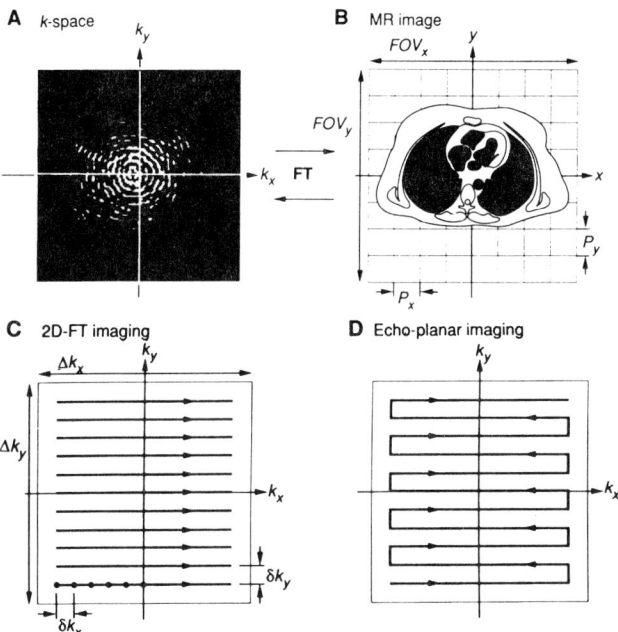

Figure 1 (A) MRI data displayed in k-space, the space defined by the time integral of the imaging magnetic field gradients, which corresponds to the time domain in which the MR data are sampled. (B) The MR image corresponding to these data, obtained by performing a Fourier transform. (C) In conventional 2D-FT MRI, the data in k-space are sampled in n consecutive acquisitions along lines parallel to the k_x axis, each line representing a digitally sampled gradient or spin echo. Nominal image resolution, or pixel size (P), is determined by the highest spatial frequencies sampled, $P_x = 2\pi/\Delta k_x$ and $P_y = 2\pi/\Delta k_y$. The field of view (FOV) is determined by $\text{FOV}_x = 2\pi/\delta k_x$ and $\text{FOV}_y = 2\pi/\delta k_y$. (D) In EPI, k-space is sampled in a single, continuous k-space trajectory within a fraction of a second. Reprinted with permission from Stehling *et al.* (1991): Copyright 1991 by the AAAS.

The problem is worsened when no *rf* refocussing pulse is used, because the spins have plenty of time to dephase. However, as we shall see, this phenomenon has unexpected advantages in regard to imaging of brain function.

V. The Use of Paramagnetic Tracers in Functional Brain MRI

A. Exogenous Contrast Agents

Using stable chelating compounds, a class of paramagnetic MR contrast agents of low toxicity has been developed in recent years, the best known of which is gadolinium diethylenetriaminepentaacetic acid (Gd-DTPA). Such agents do not cross the blood–brain barrier in healthy brain. By creating magnetic field gradients around the blood vessels, they produce a range of precession frequencies for the spins surrounding the vessels in a given voxel (Fig. 2). Hence, as a result of interference, there is a reduction of NMR signal, when gradient-echo imaging sequences are used, in which these field inhomogeneity effects are not canceled out by a second *rf* pulse. In this way, a small quantity of contrast agent (mean tissue concentration of 0.1 mmol/kg) can cause a decrease in image intensity in its passage through gray matter of perhaps 50%.

This change can be observed both in gradient-echo images and in spin-echo images. In this latter case the

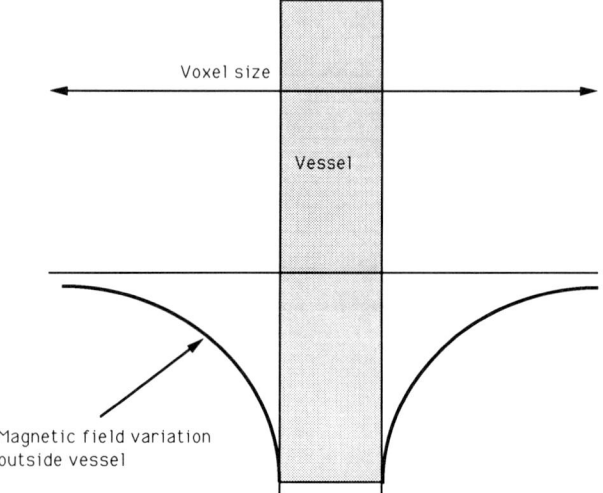

Figure 2 Diagram of the varying magnetic field in the tissue adjacent to a blood vessel containing a liquid (contrast agent or deoxygenated blood) that has a magnetic susceptibility different from that of tissue. Spins precess at a rate proportional to the magnetic field offset and thus lose their phase coherence in such magnetic field gradients.

change in signal results from the fact that during the time of the experiment the water molecules diffuse, by Brownian motion, through the regions of inhomogeneous magnetic field, creating a dispersion of the phase of the proton spins that the refocusing pulse cannot undo.

Thus the typical experiment is one in which a short bolus of contrast agent is intravenously injected, and successive MR images of the brain are obtained at short time intervals (1–2 s), while the concentration of contrast agent builds up and washes out. The total period over which this takes place is about 20 s. It is difficult to inject a bolus in less than about 4 s, and passage through the lungs increases the bolus width to 8 s or more.

B. Blood Volume and Flow Measurements

It is obvious that the change in image intensity while a bolus of contrast agent passes through tissue is closely related to blood flow. To extract a quantitative measure of blood flow, comparable to that obtained by tracer washout methods, or use of radioactive microspheres, is not easy, however. The important assumption is that the change in contrast, expressed as a change in relaxation rate, is proportional to the concentration of contrast agent in the tissue. Model calculations, for instance, by Fisel *et al.* (1991), show that this is approximately true over the range of concentrations typically used. Under these circumstances a measure of blood volume, V, can be obtained by integrating the logarithm of the signal change during the first pass of the contrast agent. Commonly, the first pass is discriminated from subsequent passages of the slowly excreted contrast agent by fitting the first peak in the curve to the gamma-variate function:

$$\Delta R_2 = c\, t^n e^{-t/b}, \tag{1}$$

where ΔR_2 is the change in relaxation rate (equal to the natural log of the attenuation of the signal from a given voxel), t is the time elapsed after the contrast agent enters the brain, and c, n, and b are adjustable parameters. Once this fit is made, a map of the integral of this curve may be made, which is roughly proportional to regional blood volume. The gray and white matter are distinguished purely by their different capillary density.

To derive a measure of blood flow requires in addition a measurement of the arterial input function of the contrast agent, and the use of the central volume theorem (Stewart, 1894). This is not a simple procedure and is not routinely done in MR studies of brain function.

C. Experimental Results

Striking results have been demonstrated showing functionally related changes in blood volume. The earliest of these studies was made by the group of Dr. Bruce Rosen at Massachusetts General Hospital, using a dog model (Belliveau *et al.*, 1990). Hypercapnia was used to induce changes in blood flow and blood volume from the normal resting state. EPI images were obtained at 1-s intervals, while a bolus of contrast agent passed through the brain. Calculated cerebral blood volume (CBV) was found to increase linearly with pCO_2, as expected.

Subsequent studies with human subjects have produced even more remarkable results (Belliveau *et al.*, 1991). The human visual cortex was investigated using photic stimulation, obtained with light-proof, patterned-flash stimulating goggles. For each subject, two intravenous injections of Gd-DTPA were made, with and without photic stimulation, each followed by 60 EPI images in the ensuing 45 s. The image slice, 8 or 10 mm in thickness, was aligned with the calcarine fissure, in order to maximize the volume of primary visual cortex within the field of view. In-plane resolution was as high as 1.5×1.5 mm. CBV maps were calculated for each condition, and difference maps were obtained.

In agreement with autoradiographically determined maps of visual cortex in animals, the difference maps show a well-demarcated activated region in the gray matter, not extending into white matter. The seven subjects tested all showed highly significant changes of blood volume in the activated region, up to 48%, and further work (Belliveau, 1992) has confirmed the robustness of the technique. Intersubject variation of the region activated (Belliveau *et al.*, 1991) may easily be observed, corresponding to anatomical variability in the positioning of the calcarine fissure and associated cortical tissue.

These experiments show that magnetic resonance imaging techniques can provide high-resolution functional maps of brain tissue involved in cognitive processing. There are limitations to the technique, however. The dose of contrast agent, which is excreted through the kidneys within a day, is sufficiently high that repeat studies cannot be made consecutively. A set of enough images to allow extraction of a CBV map cannot be obtained in less than 30 s, limiting temporal resolution. Finally, the method remains slightly invasive, although the toxicity of Gd-DTPA is low, and for more recently developed contrast agents it is still lower. These problems are circumvented in the next technique to be discussed, which also provides a measure of blood flow, but by creating an endogenous blood marker in the form of magnetically labeled spins.

VI. Magnetic Labeling of Perfusing Spins

The technique of using a preparatory *rf* pulse to invert or saturate the spins of protons in blood, before the imaging sequence proper has commenced, has been used for some time. MR angiography employs it to pick out spins in the larger blood vessels (Turner and Keller, 1991) by inverting the spins in a slice different from the imaging slice and observing their entry into the plane of the image. Flow velocity profiles in vessels may even be observed with this technique.

This suggested the following experiment (Williams *et al.*, 1992). A series of *rf* inversion pulses is provided to ensure continuous inversion of the water proton spins in the blood supply for a particular organ, in this case the brain. A bulk loss of signal is observed as these spins move into cells, canceling to a small extent the net spin of the intracellular protons. The effect depends directly on the tissue perfusion, and this quantity can be calculated from the loss of signal, together with a measure of the effective spin relaxation time when the inversion pulses are applied. A small correction must be applied, to allow for recovery of the normal spin magnetization while the inverted spins are in transit toward the tissue voxel under consideration. Maps of cerebral perfusion in absolute units are obtained, with reasonable SNR, given that the image intensity changes are only on the order of 5%. The technique has been validated using graded hypercapnia, as with the intravascular contrast agent method, and has also been used to show regional perfusion abnormalities in freeze-injured brain.

These initial results, using a conventional multipulse spin-echo imaging sequence, emphasized quantification of perfusion. If rapid observation of qualitative changes in regional perfusion is a priority, a simpler technique in which the spins in the imaging slice itself are inverted has merit. In this technique the recovery of signal in the imaging plane depends partly on how fast water proton spins are replaced by perfusion after the inversion pulse. The longitudinal relaxation time T_1 is changed (Williams *et al.*, 1992; Kwong *et al.*, 1992a, 1992b), such that

$$1/T_{1_{app}} = 1/T_1 + f/\lambda, \qquad (2)$$

where T_1 is the normal relaxation time without flow, $T_{1_{app}}$ is the relaxation time when blood flow effects are included, f is the blood flow in ml/g/s, and λ is the brain–blood partition coefficient (about 0.9 ml/g).

Thus a change in blood flow will cause a change in the observed $T_{1_{app}}$:

$$\Delta(1/T_{1_{app}}) = \Delta f/\lambda. \qquad (3)$$

A change in flow of 50 ml/100 g/min will thus cause a change of 2% in MR signal, when an inversion recovery sequence with the inversion time T_I is equal to the relaxation time T_1 (Kwong *et al.*, 1992a). Such a change is observable using an EPI inversion recovery sequence at a magnetic field at 1.5 T.

The group at Massachusetts General Hospital has used this effect, with human volunteers, to observe changes in CBF caused by photic stimulation (Kwong *et al.*, 1992a, 1992b). The experimental conditions were very similar to those described above for the contrast agent study, but this time no contrast agent was used. Image intensity changes corresponding to changes in perfusion showed excellent correlation with periods of photic stimulation, with an amplitide of about 1–2% of the baseline image intensity. The rise time of the perfusion increase on stimulation was observed to be about 9 s.

VII. Deoxygenation Contrast

A. Basic Principles

We turn now from flow to oxygen utilization. It has been known for a long time (Thulborn *et al.*, 1982; Brooks and Di Chiro, 1987) that the magnetic state of hemoglobin in red cells is strongly dependent on oxygen saturation. Deoxygenated blood is considerably more paramagnetic than oxygenated blood, the difference being about 0.2 ppm (Weisskoff and Kiihne, 1992). Ogawa *et al.* (1990) in a study of anesthetized rats, demonstrated at the high magnetic field of 4.7 T that this effect caused small blood vessels to appear larger on gradient echo images when blood oxygenation was lowered by using a particular anesthetic. Deoxygenated blood itself acts as an intravascular paramagnetic contrast agent, just as described earlier.

The effect was also noted by Turner *et al.* (1990), who used gradient-echo, echo-planar imaging to study cat brain before and within a few seconds after death. Experiments were performed on a 2-T animal scanner, using the gradient-echo EPI sequence, with a 40-ms echo time. With a field of view of 60 mm, an in-plane resolution of 1 mm was obtained. The observed image changes were not confined to the larger vessels, but caused an overall decrease in signal arising from brain tissue, primarily in the more highly perfused gray matter. Further experiments to observe

the time course of this effect (Turner *et al.*, 1991), using periods of 1–2 min of anoxia in cat brain, showed that the excellent time resolution of EPI allowed study of details such as a noticeable overshoot in cerebral blood oxygenation on recovery of normal breathing gases (Fig. 3). Images were collected at 3-s intervals. A detailed comparison of loss of signal in gray matter with arterial hemoglobin oxygen saturation sO_2 was made, showing a good linear correlation between change of relaxation rate and change of sO_2 (Turner *et al.*, 1992a) in the initial phase of the respiratory challenge. Further experiments were performed (Turner *et al.*, 1992a) in which the sO_2 in the cerebral vasculature itself was measured using a spectrophotometer coupled to an optical fiber monitoring the brain surface through a cranial window. The results were consistent with the hypothesis that the change of MR relaxation rate is proportional to the change in tissue deoxyhemoglobin concentration.

B. Human Brain Activation Studies

These results, demonstrating that the oxygen saturation of cerebral blood can be monitored by EPI with high temporal and spatial resolution, encouraged Kwong and co-workers (1992a, 1992b) at Massachusetts General Hospital to attempt the photic stimulation experiment described earlier, now using a simple gradient-echo EPI sequence for imaging. The echo time was 40 ms, and images were obtained with an in-plane spatial resolution of 1.5 mm and a slice thickness of 10 mm. This gave spectacular results. The hyperoxemia associated with brain functional activity (Frostig *et al.*, 1990) appears clearly in the primary visual cortex, as a signal increase of 2–3%.

At the higher field of 4 T, the effect on NMR signal caused by blood susceptibility changes has been found to be substantially greater, because the local magnetic field gradients are correspondingly larger. Turner *et al.* (1992b) and Ogawa *et al.* (1992) have demonstrated oxygenation changes associated with photic stimulation in human volunteers at this field. Typical changes in signal have been observed of up to 15% in visual cortex (Plate 10 and Fig. 4). Because the overall SNR at 4 T is considerably higher than that at the usual MRI field of 1.5 T, a gain in visibility of this effect of more than an order of magnitude has been obtained.

C. MR Technique Issues

It is worth making a comparison between EPI and conventional gradient-echo MRI. Whereas EPI's insensitivity to motion has its greatest value in cardiac

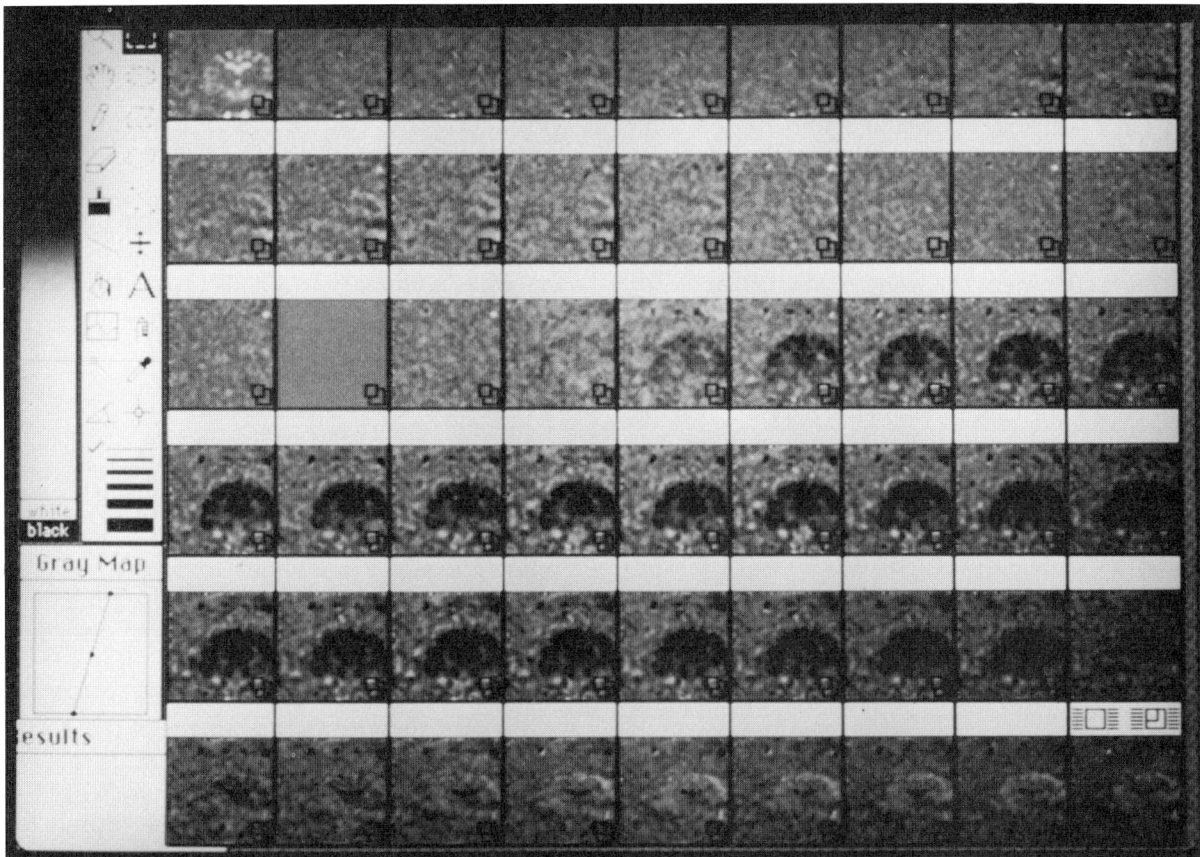

Figure 3 Sequential coronal difference images of a cat brain, at 3-s intervals, while the cat was subjected to respiratory anoxia (breathing pure N_2) from images 20 to 40. Image 20 was subtracted from each of the others to give this demonstration of contrast changes. The development of hypoxemia is well seen as a darkening primarily in gray matter, and the overshoot on recovery is also clearly visible. The first image shows enhancement of CSF due to the completely unsaturated condition of the spins at the outset of scanning. Images were obtained using a 2.0-T GE Omega 45-cm bore MR scanner, fitted with high performance Acustar gradient coils.

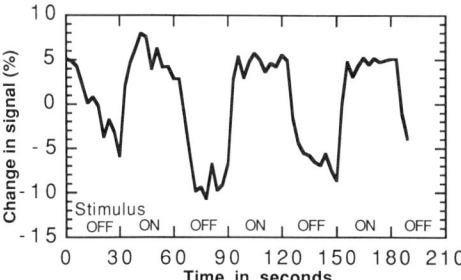

Figure 4 Variation of EPI image intensity for a 120-mm³ volume of cortical tissue beside the calcarine fissure in the brain of a normal volunteer experiencing photic stimulation. Sagittal images were obtained at a field of 4 T, and the photic stimulus was produced using light-tight goggles (Model S10VS, Grass Instruments) fitted with an array of LEDs that were activated at a frequency of 16 Hz for a period of 30 s in each minute. The change in signal is plotted as a percentage of the intensity in the fourth image.

imaging, it has proven to be highly beneficial in the brain. When conventional imaging is performed, the motion of the brain caused by arterial pulsation and involuntary head movements is often sufficient to cause a ghost in the phase encode direction amounting to a few percent of the image intensity. If time series of images are collected, the characteristically small image intensity variations associated with changes in regional CBF can be swamped by this ghosting. Averaging of successive images can reduce ghosting, but at the expense of further loss of time resolution.

It is fair to say that those few MR research laboratories that are equipped with EPI systems at fields of 1.0 T or higher have found it easy to observe the changes in gradient-echo EPI brain images due to functional activation, whereas considerable effort has been required to obtain images of sufficient quality and stability with conventional, low-flip-angle, fast imaging techniques to allow observation of the effect. To date, no successful studies have been reported employing conventional sequences to observe local changes in T_1 caused by variations in rCBF. The time resolution and SNR are poorer than with EPI, moreover, although the spatial resolution can be superior, and the images show less distortion and signal dropout caused by bulk field inhomogeneity.

Further experiments (Kwong et al., 1992a, 1992b; Bandettini et al., 1992a, 1992b) in which tactile hand stimulation was applied showed similar increases in blood oxygenation and flow in the region of the sensorimotor cortex corresponding to the hand representation. More recent results will be discussed in the next section.

D. Recent Studies

Credible reports, mostly presented at the 11th Annual Meeting of the Society of Magnetic Resonance in Medicine, 1992, of observation of changes in MR images during brain function have come from many laboratories (Turner et al., 1992b; Bandettini et al., 1992b; Sanders et al., 1992; Frahm et al., 1992; Blamire et al., 1992; Gore et al., 1992). Functional activation has been observed using oxygenation contrast MRI in the primary visual cortex (Plate 11), the extrastriate visual cortex, the hand (Plates 12 and 13), tongue and shoulder representations in the primary and associated motor and somatosensory cortices, and the left inferior frontal cortex (activated during word generation). Retinotopic mapping of the human visual cortex has been demonstrated (Schneider, 1992), using a standard gradient echo sequence. The following features are becoming apparent:

1. The regions of apparent activation (i.e., where the MR signal changes) are confined to gray matter, closely follow the borders of the sulci, and conform to appropriate functional areas of the brain, where these are known.

2. The changes seen come mainly from tissue surrounding smaller vessels; vessels of a diameter comparable to the voxel size do not dominate, although an increase of MR signal can clearly be seen in veins draining active brain regions.

3. The rise time to maximum of the effect is 5–10 s, reflecting the hemodynamic origin of the change of signal.

4. The signal rises above noise level within 1–3 s of the onset of stimulus.

5. The size of the effect depends on the intensity of the stimulus.

6. In theory, the change of signal can be affected by a change in blood arterial oxygenation, blood volume, blood flow, hematocrit, tissue oxygen uptake, and possibly blood velocity. Changes in blood flow apparently dominate, but the role of the other parameters awaits detailed modeling and experimental investigation.

7. The change in signal observable increases with the strength of the magnetic field used in the imaging system. Preliminary results (Turner et al., 1993) suggest that the dependence is greater than linear.

VIII. Discussion

The results described here, although very recent, are sufficiently robust and reproducible that they open up remarkable possibilities in functional brain imaging. The last two methods for observing brain activation are intrinsically different from previous brain mapping approaches. It is worthwhile to consider their advantages and disadvantages.

Perhaps the greatest advantage of these methods, which do not involve contrast agent, is that they are completely noninvasive. Repeated studies of the same subject in the same session are thus entirely feasible, allowing as much intrasubject data averaging as desired. Individual variations in the location and extent of activation for an endless variety of brain tasks are now open to exploration.

Second, the spatial resolution is considerably better than other relatively noninvasive techniques, such as positron emission tomography. MRI can give spatial resolution of 0.25 mm in plane over a human head, but this entails data acquisitions lasting many minutes to give adequate SNR. If a time resolution in brain functional studies of 1 or 2 s is required, the best spatial resolution likely to be attained is $1.25 \times 1.25 \times 5$ mm, which is still adequate to resolve details of the hand representation, for instance.

Third, for the spatial resolution mentioned, the temporal window now available allows mapping of brain activity at a time scale similar to that of changes in blood supply. The onset and cessation of hemodynamic response have been observed, for the first time in human brain (Kwong et al., 1992a, 1992b) to track the neural activation associated with performance of tasks.

The most serious disadvantage of these methods, albeit a temporary one, is that the effects in human brain have been best demonstrated on MR systems performing echo-planar imaging, and such systems, as mentioned previously, are few in number. Modifications to existing MR scanners to allow EPI are not simple, although several manufacturers are preparing suitable equipment upgrades.

There are, moreover, experimental concerns that need to be borne in mind. The first of these is that the observable changes are small, on the order of 4% of the total MR signal at the magnetic field of 1.5 T commonly used. Thus poor equipment stability, imperfect head immobilization, and involuntary motions such as brain pulsation caused by the cardiac or respiratory cycle may swamp the effect. Whereas a much larger effect is observable at 4 T, such magnets are expensive, and only three presently exist in clinical sites.

Second, it is the response in the blood that is being observed. This inevitably lags the neural response associated with brain activity and is somewhat less localized. In particular, the gradient-echo EPI technique, which detects blood oxygenation changes, is likely to be more sensitive to changes in larger venules than those in the smaller capillaries and thus may present a slightly distorted view of the region of activation. Further research is required to determine how severe a limitation this represents.

Moreover, the exquisite sensitivity obtainable by PET in study of particular neuroreceptors is unlikely to become available for MRI. The chemical multiplier effect, by which small changes in oxygen content of blood are amplified in the NMR signal from protons, cannot work for metabolites in concentrations in the micromolar range.

Nevertheless, it appears that a new era in functional brain imaging is beginning. The two latter methods mentioned here do not use contrast agents, are completely noninvasive, and permit unlimited within-subject functional studies, including studies of the effects of neuroactive drugs. Neuroscience institutions all over the world are gearing up for analysis of the enormous quantities of useful brain function data that are starting to pour out of MR laboratories. At least five such institutions have plans for installation of higher field MR systems dedicated to brain studies. Research into the functional organization of the brain; cerebral plasticity following trauma or amputation; learning; and mental illness will be accelerated by the relative ease, noninvasiveness and good spatial and temporal resolution of these techniques.

Acknowledgments

A substantial portion of this text is reprinted with permission from an article published in the *American Journal of Physiologic Imaging*. This survey would have been impossible without the continuing help and encouragement of Dr. Bruce Rosen, Dr. Ken Kwong, Dr. Mark Cohen, and Dr. Jack Belliveau, of the NMR Center, Massachusetts General Hospital; and of Dr. Alan Koretsky, of Carnegie Mellon University, Pittsburgh. Also I thank my collaborators at the *In Vivo* NMR Research Center at NIH, Dr. Denis Le Bihan, Dr. Robert Balaban, and Dr. Peter Jezzard; and in the National Institute for Neurological Disorders and Stroke, Dr. Tom Zeffiro, Dr. Leonardo Cohen, and Dr. Jordan Grafman.

References

Bandettini, P., *et al.* (1992a). Time course EPI of human brain function during task activation. *J. Magn. Reson. Imaging* **2P,** 76. [Abstr.]

Bandettini, P. A., *et al.* (1992b). Time course EPI of human brain function during task activation. *Magn. Reson. Med.* **25,** 390–397.

Belliveau, J. W., *et al.* (1990). Functional cerebral imaging by susceptibility-contrast NMR. *Magn. Reson. Med.* **14,** 538–546.

Belliveau, J. W., *et al.* (1991). Functional mapping of the human visual cortex by magnetic resonance imaging. *Science* **254,** 716–719.

Belliveau, J. W. (1992). Personal communication.

Blamire, A. M., *et al.* (1992). Echo-planar imaging of the activated human visual cortex shows a time delay between stimulus and activation. In "Proceedings of the 11th Annual Meeting of the Society of Magnetic Resonance in Medicine," p. 1823. [Abstr.]

Editors (1978). Britain's brains produce first NMR scan. *New Sci.* **80,** 588.

Brooks, R. A., and Di Chiro, G. (1987). Magnetic resonance imaging of stationary blood: A review. *Med. Phys.* **14,** 903–913.

Budinger, T. F., Fischer, H., Hentschel, D., Reinfeld, H. E., and Schmitt, F. (1991). Physiological effects of fast oscillating magnetic field gradients. *J. Comput. Assist. Tomogr.* **15,** 909–924.

Cohen, M. S., and Weisskoff, R. M. (1991). Ultra-fast imaging. *Magn. Reson. Imaging* **9,** 1–37.

Fisel, C. R., *et al.* (1991). MR contrast due to microscopically heterogenous magnetic susceptibility: Numerical simulations and applications to cerebral physiology. *Magn. Reson. Med.* **17,** 336.

Frahm, J., *et al.* (1992). Dynamic FLASH MRI of human brain oxygenation during photic stimulation. In "Proceedings of the 11th Annual Meeting of the Society of Magnetic Resonance in Medicine," p. 1820. [Abstr.]

Frahm, J., Gyngell, M. L., and Hänicke, W. (1992). Rapid scan techniques. In "Magnetic Resonance Imaging" (D. D. Stark and W. G. Bradley, Jr., Eds.), Vol. 1, p. 165. St. Louis: Mosby Year Book.

Frostig, R. D., Lieke, E. E., Ts'o, D. Y., and Grinvald, A. (1990). Cortical functional architecture and local coupling between neuronal activity and the microcirculation revealed by *in-vivo* high-resolution optical imaging of intrinsic signals. *Proc. Natl. Acad. Sci. USA* **87,** 6082–6086.

Gore, J. C., *et al.* (1992). Imaging regional brain activation at 1.5 T using conventional imaging techniques. In "Proceedings of the 11th Annual Meeting of the Society of Magnetic Resonance in Medicine," p. 1826. [Abstr.]

Kwong, K. K., *et al.* (1992a). Real time imaging of perfusion change and blood oxygenation change with EPI. In "Proceedings of the 10th Annual Meeting of the Society for Magnetic Resonance Imaging, New York, 1992," p. 301.

Kwong, K. K., *et al.* (1992b). Dynamic magnetic resonance imaging of human brain activity during primary sensory stimulation. *Proc. Natl. Acad. Sci. USA* **89,** 5675.

Mansfield, P. (1977). Multi-planar image formation using NMR spin echoes. *J. Phys. C* **10,** L55–L58.

Ogawa, S., *et al.* (1992). Intrinsic signal changes accompanying sensory stimulation—Functional brain mapping with magnetic resonance imaging. *Proc. Natl. Acad. Sci. USA* **89**, 5951–5955.

Ogawa, S., Lee, T.-M., Nayak, A. S., and Glynn, P. (1990). Oxygenation-sensitive contrast in magnetic resonance image of rodent brain at high magnetic fields. *Magn. Reson. Med.* **14**, 68–78.

Roy, C. S., and Sherrington, C. S. (1890). On the regulation of the blood-supply of the brain, *J. Physiol.* **11**, 85–108.

Sanders, J., *et al.* (1992). MR functional imaging without contrast on a clinical imager. *In* "Proceedings of the 11th Annual Meeting of the Society of Magnetic Resonance in Medicine," p. 1819. [Abstr.]

Schneider, W. (1992). Personal communication.

Stehling, M. K., Turner, R., and Mansfield, P. (1991). Echo-planar imaging: Magnetic resonance imaging in a fraction of a second. *Science* **254**, 43–50.

Stewart, G. N. (1894). Researches on the circulation time in organs and on the influences which affect it. *J. Physiol.* **15**, 1–89.

Thulborn, K. R., Waterton, J. C., Matthews, P. M., and Radda, G. K. (1982). Oxygenation dependence of the transverse relaxation time of water protons in whole blood at high field. *Biochim. Biophys. Acta* **714**, 265–270.

Turner, R., and Keller, P. (1991). Angiography and perfusion measurements by NMR. *Prog. NMR Spectrosc.* **23**, 93–133.

Turner, R., Le Bihan, D., Jezzard, P., Despres, D., and Taylor, J. (1992a). Time course imaging of blood deoxygenation in cat brain. *In* "Proceedings of the 11th Annual Meeting of the Society of Magnetic Resonance in Medicine," p. 918. [Abstr.]

Turner, R., *et al.* (1992b). Functional mapping of the human visual cortex at 4 tesla using deoxygenation contrast EPI. *In* "Proceedings of the 11th Annual Meeting of the Society of Magnetic Resonance in Medicine," p. 304. [Abstr.]

Turner, R., Jezzard, P., Wen, H., Kwong, K. K., Le Bihan, D., Zeffiro, T., and Balaban, R. S. (1993). Functional mapping of the human visual cortex at 4 tesla and 1.5 tesla using deoxygenation contrast EPI. *Magn. Reson. Med.,* **29**, 281–283.

Turner, R., Le Bihan, D., Maier, J., Vavrek, R., Hedges, L. K., and Pekar, J. (1990). Echo-planar imaging of intra-voxel incoherent motion. *Radiology* **177**, 407–414.

Turner, R., Le Bihan, D., Moonen, C. T. W., Despres, D., and Frank, J. (1991). Echo-planar time course MRI of cat brain deoxygenation changes. *Magn. Reson. Med.* **22**, 159–166.

Wehrli, F. W. (1992). Principles of magnetic resonance. *In* "Magnetic Resonance Imaging" (D. D. Stark and W. G. Bradley, Jr., Eds.), Vol. 1, p. 3. St. Louis: Mosby Year Book.

Weisskoff, R. M., and Kiihne, S. (1992). MRI susceptometry: Image-based measurement of absolute susceptibility of MR contrast agents and human blood. *Magn. Reson. Med.* **24**, 375–383.

Williams, D. S., Detre, J. A., Leigh, J. S., and Koretsky, A. P. (1992). Magnetic resonance imaging of perfusion using spin inversion of arterial water. *Proc. Natl. Acad. Sci. USA* **89**, 212–216.

8

Statistical Parametric Mapping

Karl J. Friston

The Neurosciences Institute, La Jolla, California 92037

I. Introduction

This chapter describes the ideas and techniques used in statistical parametric mapping. In one sense, statistics are the ultimate modality. They are dimensionless and allow information from different modalities to be compared or correlated. Statistical parametric maps (SPMs) are images with pixel values that are, under a null hypotheses, distributed according to a known (statistical) probability density function. SPMs are used to test specific null hypotheses, usually an equivalence or regional physiology or absence of correlation. SPMs are essentially images of change or correlational significance. Statistical parametric mapping involves a variety of analytical techniques. Those described here represent an internally consistent series of data transformations developed at the MRC Cyclotron Unit (Hammersmith Hospital, London). Each transformation appeals to a distinct and separate theory. The endpoint of these data transformations is the SPM.

Pixel values in the SPM are a statistical quotient, usually of the variance (differences) of interest and error variance (reliability) of the measurement. Increasing sensitivity means reducing of error variance. The remodeling and reduction of error variance is a constant theme found throughout the data analysis stream. The efficacy and nature of each data transformation are defined in terms of the error variance it

addresses. This is reflected in the descriptions below, which are structured around the source of error reduced and are presented in the order in which the transformations are performed. The most common experimental design, of repeated observations in different subjects, is the sensorimotor or cognitive activation paradigm. Consequently the analysis of activation studies will form the core of this chapter, namely the general case of k repeated measurements in n subjects.

The first half describes how SPMs are constructed. The second half provides empirical examples that show how SPMs can be used to assess (i) functional anatomy and specialization using activation studies, (ii) CNS plasticity with factorial designs, and (iii) functional connectivity using principal component analyses. The first half is a little dense and some readers may prefer to go straight to the second half and refer back for technical details.

II. Procedures

A. The Physiological Measurement

Neurophysiology is usually measured in terms of regional cerebral blood flow (rCBF), typically with a fast dynamic technique using ^{15}O radiolabeled water, administered intravenously or by $C^{15}O_2$ inhalation. Counts per pixel, per unit time, integrated over the acquisition period can be used as an index of rCBF or entered into a more complete analysis to generate images of actual rCBF using parameter estimation (Lammertsma et al., 1990). This parameterization removes variability due to technical idiosyncrasies but preserves rCBF changes of physiological significance. However, in any one brain the relative differences between integrated counts and estimated rCBF are so small, following global normalization, that parameter estimation is sometimes unnecessary. The justification for using integrated counts as a direct index holds given a strict condition; there is no *a priori* reason to expect a treatment effect on global measures. Treatment effects refer to those introduced by experimental design. It is unusual to find significant global differences in normal subjects during standard sensorimotor and cognitive activations. In our experience the only challenges that induce global differences are pharmacological. If the scope of the experimental question is limited to normal subjects, under physiological conditions, most investigators are comfortable using integrated counts per pixel as rCBF equivalents.

B. Stereotactic Differences

The coregister of homologous functional and anatomical loci from different subjects is the aim of stereotactic normalization. The simplifying assumption is that a correspondence exists between functional and structural anatomy. This assumption has been validated by the efficacy of stereotactic normalization in contributing to the detection of functional changes (Fox et al., 1988). Stereotactic normalization is a data transformation that reduces differences in brain position, size, and shape by mapping the image data into a standard stereotactic space. The space most widely used is defined by the atlas of Talairach and Tournoux (1988) and was first proposed by Fox et al. (1985). This space has now become the international standard for communicating PET results.

There are two sorts of stereotactic variance, positional and morphological. Morphological differences have linear (size) and nonlinear (shape) components. Stereotactic normalization deals with these differences by reducing a single nonlinear three-dimensional problem to a series of one-dimensional linear problems.

1. Positional Variance

Positional variance is removed by translation and reorientation of the volume image with reference to a standard line, the intercommissural line passing through the anterior commissure (AC) and posterior commissure (PC). This is alternatively known as the AC–PC line. The position of the AC–PC line can be estimated directly from morphological information in the primary (PET) image without reference to a mediating structural (e.g., MRI) scan. This estimation uses the functional contrast at gray–white matter boundaries. The feasibility of doing this was first demonstrated by using four landmarks that could be identified on coronal PET sections and that bear a constant relationship to the AC–PC line (Friston et al., 1989). The transverse level or height (z) of these landmarks was estimated for each of the coronal (y) levels. Linear regression was then used to estimate the AC–PC line. Construct validity was established with reference to the method described by Fox et al. (1985).

In order to increase reliability of the AC–PC line estimation the procedure has been automated; 15 coronal sections are sampled proportionally from the image. Each coronal section is matched, in a least-squares sense, to a standard template (average of many coronal sections following stereotactic normalization). This matching is in terms of z. The z displacement between the observed coronal section and the template defines the height of the AC–PC line. This procedure is repeated independently for all sections and the estimated AC–PC levels (z) regressed on the observed y. This regression is the AC–PC line estimate. Note that there is no explicit reference to the commissures or related structures. The functional profile over the entire brain volume contributes equally. In short, in contrast to earlier approaches, there are no morphometric landmarks because the procedure is correlative over the entire brain.

2. Brain Size

Brain size is defined by the bounding box in which it lies, the dimensions of which are simply determined by integrating the image over two dimensions to generate one-dimensional images. The lengths of these one-dimensional images are determined according to threshold criteria. Height is specified relative to the AC–PC line. The image is resliced parallel to the AC–PC line into 26 transverse sections that correspond to the drawings of the Talairach and Tournoux atlas (1988). These sections are linearly rescaled in x and y such that one pixel represents $2 \times 2 \times 4$ mm in the standard space.

3. Brain Shape

Each transverse section is mapped from Cartesian space to polar space. Each radius of the image in polar space is resampled according to the below theory: Let $g(x)$ be an observed continuous one-dimensional image (a radius of a polar image) and $\gamma(x)$ denote the desired image that approximates to a standard template $\tau(x)$. The transformation $g(x) - \gamma(x)$ is effected by resampling $g(x)$ according to distortion of the space (x) described by $\phi(x)$:

$$\gamma(x) = g[\phi(x)] = \tau(x) + \sigma(x). \qquad (1)$$

The difference between the observed image and the desired image is a slowly varying anatomical distortion in (of) space $[\phi(x)]$. The difference between the desired image and the template reflects a more rapidly varying difference due to functional changes $[\sigma(x)]$. All are continuous functions of x. The resampling function $\phi(x)$ is given by

$$\phi(x) \approx g^{-1}[\tau(x) + \sigma(x)], \qquad (2)$$

assuming $g^{-1}(\cdot)$ and $\tau(\cdot)$ are smooth monotonic functions (see below),

$$\phi(x) \approx g^{-1}[\tau(x)] + g^{-1}[\sigma(x)] = g^{-1}[\tau(x)] + \varepsilon(x), \qquad (3)$$

where $\varepsilon(x)$ is a high-frequency residual term. An estimate of $\phi(x)$ $[\phi'(x)]$ is obtained by applying the inverse image function to the template $g^{-1}[\tau(x)]$. The result is smoothed to reduce the effect of $\varepsilon(x)$ on the estimate $\phi'(x)$ [see Eq. (3)]. In practice, it is necessary to work with image integrals to ensure invertible, strictly increasing monotonic functions. For a fuller discussion, see Friston *et al.* (1991a). The key thing to note is that pixel values are not changed but moved according to the smooth resampling function. The smoothing affects the vectorial displacement of pixels $[\phi(x)]$, not the values themselves $[g(x)]$ (see Fig. 1).

This class of normalization has been validated by comparing linear and nonlinear sampling as described. In general cortical registration is significantly improved, whereas subcortical structures are less so. The approach is noniterative and noninteractive and therefore completely reliable.

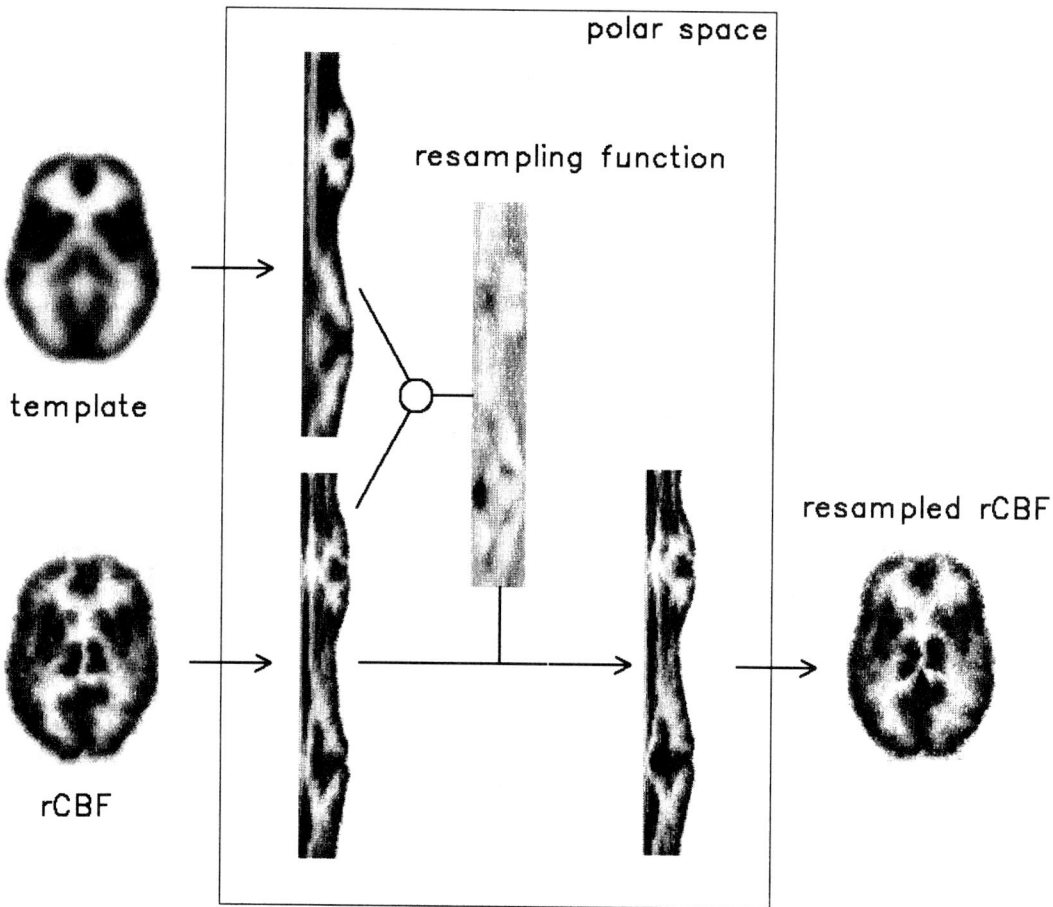

Figure 1 This schematic illustrates the nonlinear resampling of the Hoffman human brain phantom at 0 mm relative to the AC–PC line. Both observed $g(x)$ and template $\tau(x)$ sections are transformed from Cartesian to polar space and a resampling function $\phi(x)$ derived empirically for each radius (x) (row of the middle polar sections). The resampling function $\phi(x)$ is applied to the observed $g(x)$ polar section, which is then transformed back to Cartesian space. Brighter parts of the resampling function mean "resample the observed image from the left" (move to right) and darker parts mean "resample from the right." The derivation of $\phi(x)$ is described in the text.

C. Smoothing

1. Image Noise

This source of error variance can be reduced relative to signal by smoothing, or convolution. This is predicated on the observation that noise variance can be distributed in high spatial frequencies, whereas the signal cannot. The signal (differences in rCBF equivalents) must, by definition, have a spatial wavelength greater than the resolution of the acquisition system (because the signal must arise in resolvable structures). The highest spatial frequencies in noise are constrained only by the (Hanning) filter used in reconstruction (typically at 0.5 cycles per pixel).

2. Small-Scale Differences in Functional and Gyral Anatomy

There will always remain a spatial uncertainty about the position of a focal activation that remains after perfect stereotactic normalization. Functional specialization within a particular gyrus cannot be guaranteed from subject to subject and furthermore all subjects have slightly different gyral configurations. Convolution smooths a set of spatially dislocated activation foci into a center of common intersection. This intersection represents the cortical area evidencing a reliable increase in measured rCBF. Paradoxically the area of overlap can be smaller than the smoothing filter used, resulting in "hyperacute" spatial resolution.

Simulations and analytical solutions to maximizing this sort of signal recovery converge on surprisingly high degrees of smoothing. For typical resolutions of 8.5 mm (Spinks *et al.*, 1988), a Gaussian filter 20 mm in diameter is about optimal.

D. Global or Whole Brain Differences

A correction to rCBF estimates is usually required to account for the confounding effect of global CBF (gCBF) differences. This is achieved by covarying out the effect of gCBF using ANCOVA, a post hoc statistical adjustment with minimal assumptions. ANCOVA (Wildt and Ahtola, 1976; Friston *et al.*, 1990) is a generally accepted way of accounting for the effect of a nuisance variable or covariate (global activity for subject n under condition $k = G_{kn}$) on a dependent variable (observed rCBF $= C_{kn}$) to give an estimate of the subject independent, condition dependent variable (R_k) that would have been seen in the absence of covariate differences. The two linear models we have examined are defined by

$$C_{kn} = R_k + \beta(G_{kn} - E\{G_{kn}\}) \qquad (4)$$

$$C_{kn} = R_k + \beta_k(G_{kn} - E\{G_{kn}\}), \qquad (5)$$

where R_k is the adjusted regional index and $\beta_{[k]}$ is the regression slope (of C_{kn} on G_{kn}), reflecting the dependency of C_{kn} on G_{kn}. $E\{\cdot\}$ denotes expectation. Equation (4) contains only one term with a subscript k, and only k. This is the underlying regional effect that characterizes condition k. Because the regression slopes are parallel over all k conditions, the relative heights of the regression lines do not change with G_{kn}. For this reason, Eq. (4) is called the *independent model*. The activation effect from condition j to $i(R_i - R_j)$ does not depend on global activity. This can be remembered, somewhat metaphorically, by assuming that the physiological recruitment of cortical regions to perform a sensorimotor or cognitive operation does not depend on gCBF. Equation (5) is a more general case of Eq. (4) and allows for the regression slopes to change with condition $k(\beta_k)$. In this instance, the activation effect is two dimensional with an effect on R_k and an effect on β_k. Physiologically this is not easy to interpret. Because the activation component ($R_i - R_j$) depends on the level of global activity (i.e., convergent or divergent regression lines), this equation is called the *dependent model*. Note a special case of Eq. (5) (when $\beta_k = R_k/E\{G_{kn}\}$),

$$C_{kn} = R_k + R_k(G_{kn} - E\{G_{kn}\})/E\{G_{kn}\}$$

i.e.,

$$R_k = C_{kn}/(G_{kn}/E\{G_{kn}\}), \qquad (6)$$

is assumed in division by the whole brain mean. In this instance, the condition-specific, subject-independent factor (R_k) can be obtained by dividing the observed regional value (C_{kn}) by an estimate of the observed global index ($G_{kn}/E\{G_{kn}\}$). It is relatively straightforward to choose between Eqs. (4) and (5) by applying both to real data. Empirically it can be shown that applying the independent model [Eq. (4)] reveals a large number of pixels for which the null hypothesis that $R_i = R_j$ must be rejected. Conversely the dependent model [Eq. (5)] shows that the number of pixels for which β_k are different is less than chance expectation.

The rejection of the dependent model in favor of the independent model simplifies interpretation in that the activation effect is completely captured by an additive affect on R_k. See Fig. 2 for the regression analysis on real data implicit in the ANCOVA.

Marenco *et al.* (1991) find a substantial decrease in error variance and consequent increase in sensitivity with the ANCOVA model compared with division by global indices using SPECT and the Wisconsin Card Sort. Tempel *et al.* (1991) performed a regression anal-

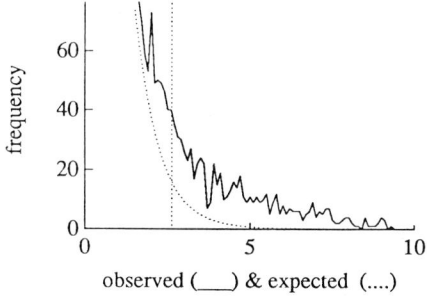
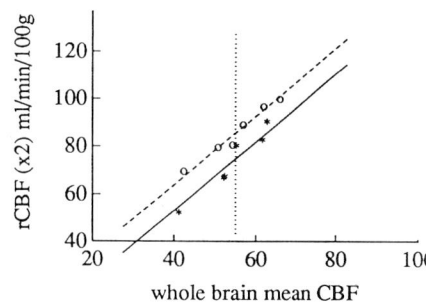

Figure 2 Right, the plotted regression analysis demonstrates graphically the effect of activation according to the *independent* ANCOVA model described in the text; namely, a vertical displacement in parallel regression lines of rCBF on gCBF. The solid line corresponds to a rest condition and the dotted line, a motor activation. Left, the distribution of the F ratio of variance attributable to treatment or condition and that due to error for all pixels in the slice from which the data in the regression were taken. Only the tail of the distribution is shown. The vertical line corresponds to $p < 0.05$. The solid line is the observed distribution and the dotted line, that expected under the null hypothesis.

ysis for several points during vibrotactile stimulation and rest and found only one example in which the B_k differed (at $p < 0.05$). Note that in the limiting case of $k = 1$ the ANCOVA adjustment reduces to a simple linear regression (see the study of schizophrenia below).

It is likely that the true relationship between relative regional and global indices is nonlinear, and therefore all linear models are invalid in a strict sense. The ANCOVA model with parallel regression slopes is probably the best, in that it allows for a linear approximation, over a small physiological range, to a generally nonlinear relationship.

E. Systematic Intersubject Differences

These are accounted for by using a completely randomized block design ANCOVA. The concept of a *block effect* accounts for the difference between a paired and an unpaired t test. The paired test is usually more sensitive because the variance not accounted for by the treatment is partitioned into true error variance and an intersubject (or block) variance. This refined modeling reduces the estimate of error variance and increases sensitivity. To generalize to k observations in n subjects, imagine an $n \times k$ data matrix with each subject along a row and conditions over columns. The means over columns and rows themselves have a variance. The variance of the means over rows represents error due to subject differences not under experimental control. This would normally contribute to error variance. It is this source of variance which is modeled and consequently removed by the block design. The variance in the k means over columns reflects diferences between the k conditions and has been introduced experimentally (treatment effect).

Typically the block effect is about *twice* the treatment effect.

By convention the grand mean ($E\{G_{nk}\}$) is set to 50 (Mintun *et al.*, 1989; Fox *et al.*, 1989), such that rCBF means can be interpreted as estimates adjusted to a mean of 50 ml/min/dl. Note that these estimates are actually expressed in arbitrary units, which is particularly relevant if the original data were integrated counts per pixel. Unless rCBF is estimated formally using parameter estimation, they are referred to as rCBF equivalents.

F. Constructing the SPM

The adjusted rCBFs are subject to the appropriate statistical test and the results assembled pixel by pixel into the SPM. The nature of the SPM is as diverse as any statistic one can imagine, from a simple t test to the factor loading following a principal component analysis (see below). In what follows we concentrate on the general case of k conditions in n subjects.

The significance of a particular profile of changes in the (k adjusted condition mean) rCBFs is tested with a weighted sum of the mean rCBFs at each pixel. The weights used are called a *contrast* and are chosen to reflect the changes that one is interested in. For example in an $A\ B\ C\ C\ B\ A$ design, an activation in conditions A, with respect to conditions C, would be tested with the contrast $1\ 0\ -1\ -1\ 0\ 1$. If the observed rCBF means are highly correlated with the contrast, then the sum will be large. The weighted sum is divided by (a function of) the adjusted error variance, estimated at each pixel. The resulting quotient has the t distribution under the null hypothesis that there is no correlation between the time-dependent rCBF changes and the contrast specified. It is important to note that the error variance used in constructing statistical parameteric maps is estimated for each brain region separately. This properly acknowledges that the underlying variablity in rCBF is not the same in different parts of the brain or under different experimental conditions. The use of contrasts preserves maximal flexibility by allowing pairwise, nonpairwise, orthogonal, nonorthogonal, and interaction comparisons. This flexibility takes comparison of condition means, and consequently experimental design, beyond a (cognitive) subtractive framework and into a more Boolean sphere. For example, conditions that are proposed to include a given cognitive component can be compared with all conditions that do not. This can be done even if no two brain states differ in, and only in, that component. Strictly speaking, a Boolean approach (e.g., what is in set A and is not in set B of conditions) should not become central, given that the contrast represents a linear sum of continuous variables.

This stage of analysis computes a t value for every pixel. Pixels at which the adjusted rCBF (equivalents) (mean over subjects and conditions) do not exceed 36 ml/min/dl are not analyzed further. Within the remaining (gray matter) brain regions a continuous smooth three-dimensional t image is created (SPM{t}). The object of further analysis is the interpretation of this direct test of the experimental hypothesis.

G. Assessing Significance

There are three approaches to interpreting the significance of SPMs (see Friston *et al.*, 1991b). Each is characterized by its own sort of null hypothesis (for computational and theoretical simplicity, the SPM{t} is actually transformed to the unit Gaussian distribution using a probability integral transform; this means changes are usually reported as Z scores).

1. Topographically Constrained Null Hypothesis

This is the simplest and states that there has been no change in rCBF at a single and specified brain location. This class of null hypothesis imposes a very selective interrogation of the data at, and only at, one brain region. Because of the smoothness inherent in the SPM{t} it is seldom necessary to specify the exact pixel *a priori*. This null hypothesis is rejected if the SPM{t} at the specified location exceeds, say, $p < 0.05$.

2. A Single Null Hypothesis Relating to the Profile of Activation

A profile of activation is defined as the *excursion set* of pixels above a threshold. There are as many

activation profiles as thresholds. For any arbitrary threshold, the null hypothesis states that this profile could have occurred by chance. The chance expectation of any profile can be assessed with the probability of getting the observed number of pixels (x) in the excursion set, or more, by chance. To estimate this probability one needs to know the distribution of x under the null hypothesis. This approach to testing the overall significance of activation profiles was first proposed in Friston *et al.* (1990) using a Poisson approximation for the probability distribution of x. This form of omnibus testing has no localizing power but represents a nonarbitrary test for outliers. It is nonarbitrary because the pixels subtending the "improbability" of chance occurrence are explicitly identified by the threshold chosen.

While the Poisson approximation is asymptotically correct in the limit of no smoothness, it is probably not appropriate for SPMs with substantial smoothness. The problem here is that although the expectation of x is known exactly (it is determined by the known univariate distribution of the statistic in question, the threshold, and the total number of pixels analyzed) the variance of x depends on smoothing. Although smoothness increases the probability of getting a large number of pixels in the excursion set by chance it *decreases* the chance probability of getting a large number of contiguous sets of pixels (regions). This is used to advantage in the third approach to assessing significance, which introduces a correction for the number of pixels analyzed.

If no correction for multiple comparisons is made (see below) then the threshold is usually set at some reasonably high level (e.g., $p < 0.001$). A level of $p < 0.001$ has been shown to protect from false positives using phantom activation simulations (Bailey *et al.*, 1991). In some comparisons (for example where the block effect cannot be removed in comparing two different cohorts) a very low threshold is used (e.g., $p < 0.05$). At this level, given about $3 \cdot 10^4$ pixels are analyzed, the expectation under the null hypothesis is 1500 (a sphere of about 7 pixels radius).

3. Multiple Null Hypotheses for Each Pixel

The final approach to interpretation treats the SPM{t} as many nonindependent univariate tests. There are as many null hypotheses as there are pixels. If the null hypothesis of no change is rejected for a specific location, then an independent activation can be localized to this site irrespective of changes elsewhere. This requires a threshold correction for multiple comparisons or the large number of null hypotheses being tested concurrently. This correction is not simple because the tests are not independent. Nonindependence is a consequence of smoothness.

For any given threshold the size of the excursion set will not depend on smoothness, but its spatial distribution will. A highly uncorrelated (rough) process will produce a large number of scattered regions subtending the excursion set. A very smooth process on the other hand is likely to have its entire excursion set in a single contiguous region. Although the univariate probability distribution of pixel values in the process is not a function of smoothness, the multivariate probability distribution of several neighboring pixels is. Account is taken of smoothing by defining the event of interest as the center of a contiguous subset of the excursion set (region). The probability (α) of this event (per pixel) is uniform over the image process and is a function of threshold (μ) and smoothness (s):

$$\alpha \approx (32 \cdot \pi \cdot s^2 \cdot \exp(\mu^2) \cdot p)^{-1}, \tag{7}$$

where p is equivalent probability in the absence of smoothing. s and FWHM are simply related:

$$\text{FWHM} = 2.3548 \cdot s. \tag{8}$$

An appropriate correction for multiple nonindependent univariate comparisons requires $\alpha = 0.05/N$, where N is the total number of pixels analyzed and $\alpha \cdot N$ is the expected number of regions. The above approximation is used to determine the threshold. This determination requires an estimate of s, obtained from the variance of the SPM field derivatives. These results were developed using the theory of stochastic processes (Cox and Miller, 1987) [see Friston et al. (1991b) for a full exposition].

Recent work by Worsley et al. (1992) has used the Euler characteristic of the excursion set as an estimate of the number of contiguous suprathreshold regions. This related approach gives almost identical results (in two dimensions).

Any or all of the three different hypotheses described above could be applied to the same data. The distinction between exploratory and confirmatory studies is often reiterated. This distinction is repeatedly acknowledged by my colleagues with a benevolent, if weary, air. Clearly, imaging studies can be treated as both exploratory and confirmatory depending on the nature of the hypothesis being tested.

SPMs are usually displayed in their entirety by viewing the brain space from orthogonal directions and displaying the highest valued pixel along any line of view (maximum intensity projection). These orthogonal projections can be thought of as statistical X rays highlighting statistically dense (significant) re-

gions. The data can be rendered onto drawings of the cortical surfaces to aid interpretation.

III. Applications

A. Functional Anatomy

1. An Activation Study

Consider this example from a six-subject study with three tasks presented twice (Frith et al., 1991) ($n = 6$, $k = 6$). The tasks were presented in balanced order to avoid monotonic time effects (this is standard practice in some units)—A B C C B A, where A is a word shadowing task, B is a semantic opposites task, and C is a paced verbal fluency task. All tasks were paced at one word per 2 s. Words in tasks A and B were high-frequency, concrete words. The design of this paradigm was predicated on cognitive subtraction (Petersen et al., 1989). The differences between A and B included semantic analysis, categorization, and retrieval. The key difference between A and C was the intentional aspect of word retrieval (intentional here means not specified by an extrinsic cue). This intensional component has been a major focus of our work using verbal fluency and memory challenges and reflects our interests in schizophrenia.

Figure 3 shows the comparison of tasks C and A (verbal fluency and word shadowing). The one-tailed SPM{t} were thresholded at $p = 0.001$ (no correction for multiple comparisons). The activation profile can be described as an extensive region in the left dorsolateral prefrontal cortex (DLPFC), including Broca's area (Brodmann's area, BA 44), and the anterior cingulate (bilaterally). There is a small region in the cerebellum that may or may not be significant. The decreases can be characterized as extensive bitemporal deactivations with a contribution from the posterior cingulate (bilateral). These are cursory but complete descriptions of the profiles. No one component of this profile is considered significant in its own right because a correction for multiple comparison was not made.

These results highlight a number of observations common to many cognitive activation profiles. First, if the cognitive differences between two tasks include an intentional component, the DLPFC is likely to be involved. Intentional tasks subsume (by definition) mnemonic tasks. Second, deactivations (rCBF decreases) characterize brain states with the same regional specificity and spatial extent typical of activations. Indeed one could look at the bitemporal deactivations as rCBF increases associated with extrinsically cued word generation (i.e., word shadowing

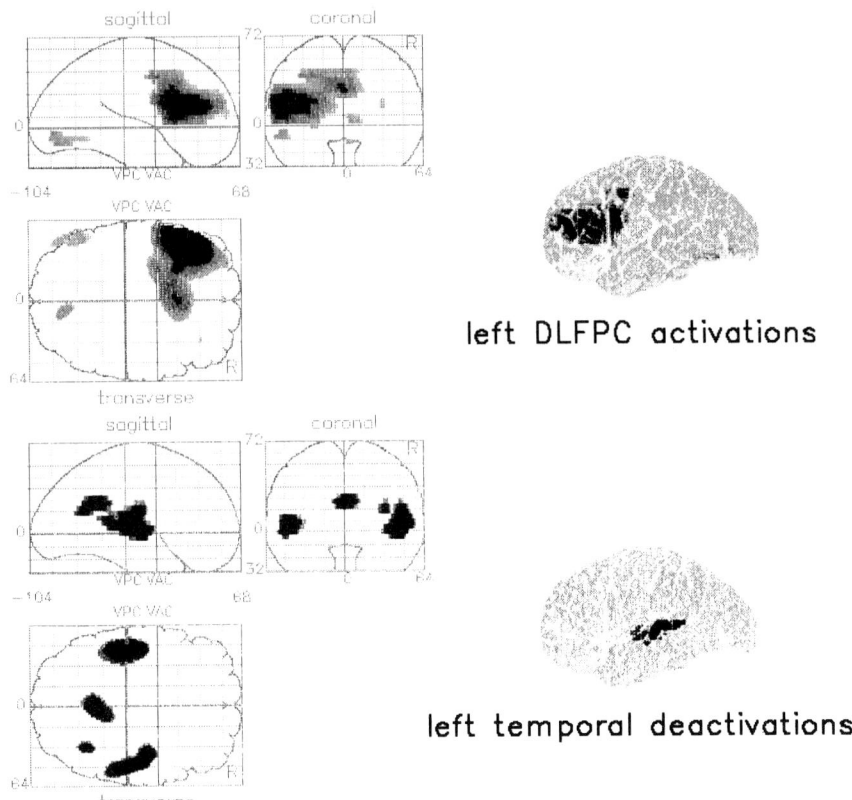

Figure 3 SPM{*t*} comparing two verbal fluency conditions with baseline (word shadowing conditions). The SPM has been thresholded at $p = 0.001$ with no correction for multiple comparisons. Because one-tailed levels were used, the increases (activations) and decreases (deactivations) are displayed separately. Each SPM{*t*} is displayed as a volume image from the back (top right), the side (top left), and top (bottom left) of the brain. The highest *t* value along any line of view is displayed. The standard stereotactic space is captured by the grid upon which the SPM{*t*} is superimposed (Talairach and Tournoux, 1988). The activation profile is described in the text but in summary shows a left DLPFC and bilateral anterior cingulate activation and bitemporal and posterior cingulate deactivations. The same excursion set of pixels has been divided into four sagittal blocks and the left lateral block, rendered onto a drawing of the cortical surface.

with verbal fluency as a control). Finally reciprocal changes in rCBF at remote sites is a common finding. Especially evident here are negatively correlated frontotemporal changes and a similar relationship between the anterior and the posterior parts of cingulate cortex. Both these correlations are seen in replication studies and other related (memory) paradigms.

2. Single Subjects and Single Conditions

The above is typical of the general $n \times k$ study. The SPM approach can be applied to many conditions in a single subject or indeed many subjects in the same state.

Figure 4 shows the rCBF increases attributed to morphine analgesia (see Jones *et al.*, 1991a). A 66-year-old man had had a well-differentiated squamous cell carcinoma of the left jaw, which was resected and

irradiated. Four days after completion of radiotherapy, he could tolerate left-sided jaw pain without diamorphine analgesia. The subject was scanned nine times every 15 min. After three scans he received an intravenous morphine infusion at 10 mg/h. The first three scans (in pain) were compared with the last five (subjectively rated pain free). The corresponding SPM{*t*} thresholded at $p < 0.001$ (no correction for multiple comparisons) is seen in Fig. 4 and highlights substantial increases in the right DLPFC (contralateral to the site of pain) and anterior cingulate. The later finding is particularly interesting given the finding of anterior cingulate responses to pain in normal subjects (Jones *et al.*, 1991b; Talbot *et al.*, 1991).

Figure 5 shows left parahippocampal correlates of symptomatic severity in 30 chronic schizophrenics. Thirty DSMIII-R (American Psychiatric Association,

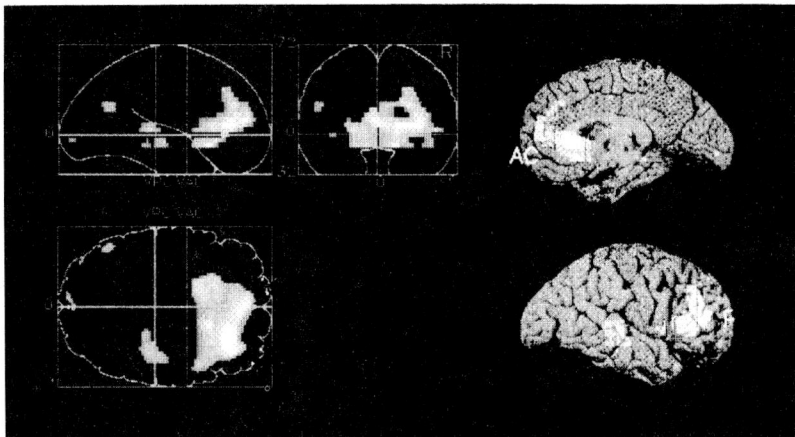

Figure 4 SPM{*t*} showing the significant increases ($p < 0.001$) in rCBF in a single subject repeatedly scanned during the induction of morphine analgesia.

1986) chronic schizophrenic patients all under the age of 55 were scanned under the same (rest) conditions. The selection criteria placed on emphasis on persistent and stable symptoms. Symptom ratings were made using CASH (Andreasen, 1987) and then subjected to factor analysis. This analysis revealed a three-dimensional structure to the behavioral data: psychomotor poverty, characterized by poverty of speech, movement, and feeling; a disorganization syndrome colored by inappropriate affect and incoherent speech with little informational content; and finally a dimension of positive experiential symptoms including delusions and hallucinations. The sum of these three factor scores provided an estimate of symptom severity that

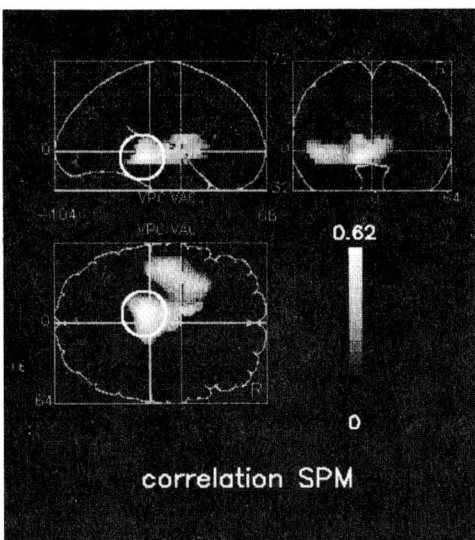

Figure 5 SPM{*ρ*} demonstrating marked positive correlations ($p < 0.05$) between symptom severity and adjusted rCBF in the left temporal region, mesencephalon, and basal ganglia (maximum correlation in the left parahippocampal gyrus-circled) in 30 DSMIII-R chronic schizophrenics.

received equal contributions from all (three) subsyndromes. This sum was correlated with adjusted rCBF at all pixels to generate a SPM{*ρ*}. Positive correlations thresholded at $p < 0.05$ (no correction for multiple comparisons) are displayed in Fig. 4. This statistic is equivalent to the partial correlation between overall symptom severity and rCBF, having accounted for the effect of global differences. The equivalent SPM{*ρ*} (not shown) for each of the separate subsyndromes revealed hypofrontality (Ingvar, 1974; DeLisi, 1985a, 1985b) for, and only for, the psychomotor poverty subsyndrome (see Liddle *et al.*, 1991; Friston *et al.*, 1992a).

Using the same analytical techniques and in particular the same standard stereotactic space allows the direct comparison of results on the functional anatomy of normal subjects and the physiological correlates of behavioral and cognitive deficits exhibited by patients. The relationship between stimulation experiments and disease or lesion studies has a long history in neuroscience. A landmark meeting, which took place on August 4th, 1881, to discuss localization of function in the cortex cerebri, addressed this issue. Goltz (1881), although accepting the results of electrical stimulation of the dog and monkey cortex (e.g., Ferrier, 1875), considered the excitation method inconclusive, in that movements elicited might have originated in related pathways or current could have spread to distant centers. "Ablation experiments were therefore essential to complement the results obtained by excitation" (Phillips *et al.*, 1984).

B. The Factorial Design—Cerebellar Plasticity

A natural extension of the SPM approach is the combination of two or more treatments in the same activation study. The appeal of this (*factorial*) design is that both the main effects and the interaction between treatments are measurable. An interaction is simply a difference in differences, in other words, the modulation of activation attributable to one treatment by a second. The first PET experiment in this class was perhaps the simplest imaginable and will serve as a concrete illustration of the idea.

Consider the synaptic changes that underlie motor learning. The cerebellum has long been thought to be implicated in motor learning (Marr, 1968; Albus, 1971; Ito *et al.*, 1974). Gilbert and Thach (1977) have demonstrated a reduction in the simple and complex spike activity of Purkinje cells in the cerebellum during motor learning in nonhuman primates. At a synaptic level, long-term depression (LTD) at synapses on apical dendrites of Purkinje cells, at the site of contact with parallel fibers, in neocerebellar cortex may be a key mechanism. Ito and colleagues (1989) have demonstrated LTD in synaptic efficacy following conjoint stimulation of parallel fibers and climbing fibers. If LTD in the neocerebellar cortex is associated with repeated practice of a novel motor task, it should be possible to image the neurophysiological correlates of these changes. It might be expected that physiological adaptation of the response to motor performance would be seen in the neocerebellum and the target area of Purkinje cell afferents (cerebellar nuclei) one synapse downstream. To test this hypothesis, subjects repeated *rest-finger opposition* task pairs three times. To ensure performance changes did not con-

found interpretation, finger opposition was entrained with a metronome. The two treatments in this example were *motor activation* and *time*. Motor activation had two levels (rest and practice) and time had three (first, second, and third trial pairs). The interaction term corresponds to physiological adaptation of the motor activation, namely an attenuation of the motor activation effect on rCBF over time (a difference in the differences). The results of this study (Friston *et al.*, 1992b, 1991c) were consistent with LTD in the cerebellum. Figure 6 shows two SPM{*t*}. The first represents the main effect of motor performance and is a typical motor activation profile (Deiber *et al.*, 1990). The second SPM{*t*} is the interaction term. This profile is strongest in the cerebellar cortex (ipsilateral to hand moved) and cerebellar nuclei. Additional components include the brain stem at the level of the inferior colliculi and a small portion of SMA (no data were obtained above this level). The contrasts (or weights) used to create the SPM{*t*} were:

	Condition (R, rest; A, practice)					
	R	A	R	A	R	A
Main effect of motor activation	−1	1	−1	1	−1	1
Interaction	−1	1	0	0	1	−1

There were no main effects of time at the threshold used ($p < 0.001$).

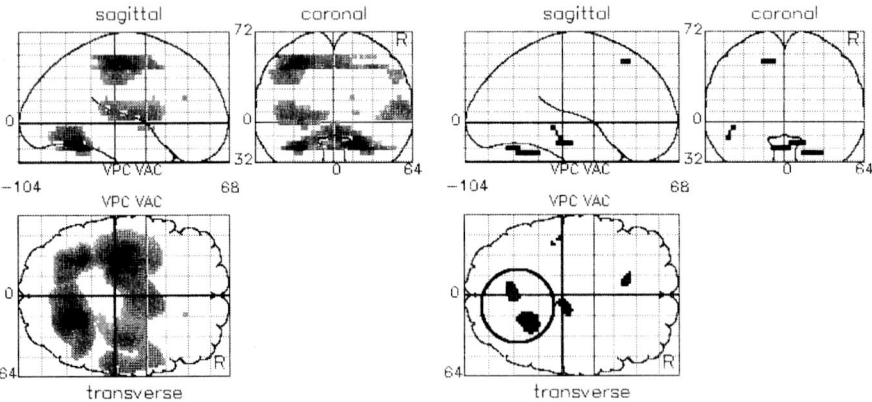

main effects of motor task   interaction SPM[t]

Figure 6 SPM{*t*}s depicting the main effect of motor activation and the interaction effect between motor activation and time (trial number). The one-tailed SPM{*t*}s are thresholded at $p = 0.001$ with no correction for multiple comparisons. The left SPM{*t*} shows increases and highlights the motor system from sensorimotor cortex to ipsilateral cerebellum. The interaction SPM{*t*} reflects adaptation of the activation effect. The components subtending this profile include the ipsilateral neocerebellum, the cerebellar midline at the level of the cerebellar nuclei, the brain stem, and a small portion of SMA at the edge of the field of view of the camera.

One clear application of the factorial design is to cross psychological and pharmacological treatments in a combined psychopharmacological paradigm. Indeed the study of neuromodulatory neurotransmitter systems requires a second treatment to elicit a physiological response that can be modulated (neuromodulation is here defined as an induced change in physiological response to an independent afferent input). This approach has been used with particular success by crossing subsupraspan memory tasks with the $5HT_{1A}$ partial agonist buspirone and the mixed dopamine agonist apomorphine (see Friston *et al.*, 1992c; Grasby *et al.*, 1992).

C. Functional and Effective Connectivity

In the past two decades the concept of *functional* or *effective connectivity* has been most thoroughly elaborated in the analysis of multiunit recordings of separable neuronal spike trains, recorded simultaneously from different brain areas (Gerstein and Perkel, 1969; Gerstein *et al.*, 1989). Temporal coherence among the activity of different neurones is commonly measured by cross-correlating their spike trains. The resulting correlograms are then interpreted as the signature of effective connectivity. In current approaches, effective connectivity is assessed as the joint probability of two neurones firing together as a function of time in an interstimulus interval (Aertsen and Preissl, 1991). There is a close relationship between the notion of effective connectivity and synaptic *efficacy*; "It is useful to describe the effective connectivity with a connectivity matrix of effective synaptic weights. Matrix elements would represent the effective influence by neurone *i* on neurone *j*" (Gerstein *et al.*, 1989). This definition is an essential and useful abstraction but lacks operational significance. In what follows, we reserve the term functional connectivity to mean *the observed temporal correlation between two electro/neurophysiological measurements from different parts of the brain*. Effective connectivity will refer to the underlying efficacy, which may or may not be measurable.

An exposition of functional connectivity based on PET physiological data can be reduced to an examination of its correlation structure. Correlation structure refers to the correlations observed over a time series in the same subject(s) (e.g., Friston *et al.*, 1991d; Lagreze *et al.*, 1991). This is very different from the analysis of correlations in cross-sectional data (acquired in different subjects in a single state). See Metter *et al.* (1984), Moeller *et al.* (1987), and Horwitz *et al.* (1984, 1990, 1991) for notable contributions to this related but separate field. Principal component analysis (PCA), as a first step, is most suited to the examination of correlations in a time series (Hope, 1968). PCA extracts

the important features of the correlation matrix in terms of principal components or eigenvectors. This approach is formally equivalent to the derivation of orthonormal spatial nodes from multiunit electrode recordings or multichannel EEGs [see the many chapters in Dvorak and Holden (1991)]. Spatial modes represent an elegant reorganization of a time series into a small number of distributed patterns. Within each mode, there are high correlations or high functional connectivity. Conversely, the temporal dynamics of different spatial modes are independent. Temporal dynamics refer to how much each mode contributes to activity over time.

The PCA of imaging data is not straightforward in the sense that the volume of data can be vast. This leads to computational memory problems when trying to find the principal components associated with the data covariance matrix. The simplest way to identify the principal components (eigenimages) is to use Singular Value Decomposition where:

$$[U\lambda V] = \text{SVD}\{M^T\}$$

and

$$M^T = U.\lambda V^T. \tag{9}$$

M is the data matrix with one column per pixel. U and V are unit matrices and λ is a diagonal matrix of singular values. Assuming M has been normalized to zero mean over columns, the eigenvector solution of the covariance matrix of $M (C\{M\})$ is simply U:

$$C\{M\} = M^T.M = U.\lambda^2.U^T$$

or

$$C\{M\}.U = U.\lambda^2. \tag{10}$$

An alternative approach was presented in Friston *et al.* (1993), which uses a recursive self calling algorithm. The advantage of recursive PCA over SVD is (a) that the entire data matrix does not have to be in working memory at any time and (b) recursive PCA lends itself to implementation on a parallel architecture. The disadvantages of recursive PCA are (a) it is more computationally expensive (requires more floating point operations) and (b) requires M to have a power of 2 columns.

1. Recursive PCA Analysis

The technique is modeled on "L" systems or string rewriting systems used in the construction of fractal and self-similar patterns. L systems were introduced by Lindenmayer in 1968 to model the growth of living organisms. In these systems, a pattern (primitive) that is composed of line segments is defined. According to (production) rules, each segment is replaced by the scaled pattern primitive. This primitive is constructed from line segments that are recursively replaced with smaller scaled primitives. No "drawing" actually occurs until the scale reaches a specified lower limit. See Voss (1988) for a full discussion. The charm of these systems is that the algorithm, which replaces each line segment of the primitive with smaller versions, calls itself recursively but implements pattern drawing only at the smallest scale. In a similar way, the PCA used here recursively calls itself until the size of the primitive data matrix reaches a lower limit. Let $\theta(M)$ denote the operation of the PCA operator $\theta\{\cdot\}$ on a data matrix (M), where M can be bisected $[M = (M_1 M_2)]$. The algorithm is defined by the following equivalence,

$$\theta\{M\} = \begin{pmatrix} \theta\{M_1\} & 0 \\ 0 & \theta\{M_2\} \end{pmatrix} \cdot \theta\{(M_1 \cdot \theta\{M_1\}M_2 \cdot \theta\{M_2\})\},$$

$$(11)$$

until the size of M reaches a lower limit ($S \geq 2.\text{rank}$ (M)). Then

$$\theta\{M\} = \varepsilon\{C\{M\}\} = Q_k, \qquad (12)$$

where Q_k are the largest $S/2$ eigenvectors of the covariance matrix of M ($= C\{M\}$). The operator $\theta\{\cdot\}$ recursively calls itself until the multiply bisected subpartitions reach a stopping criterion in terms of size (S) [see Friston *et al.* (1993) for a full description]. It should be noted that the key proposal here is that principal components or eigenimages are a powerful reorganization of the data and are directly related to the concept of functional connectivity. SVD and recursive PCA represent two computationally efficient ways of obtaining these eigenimages.

To pursue the functional connectivity implicated by intentional behavior, we repeated the word generation paradigm described above using word shadow-

First PC

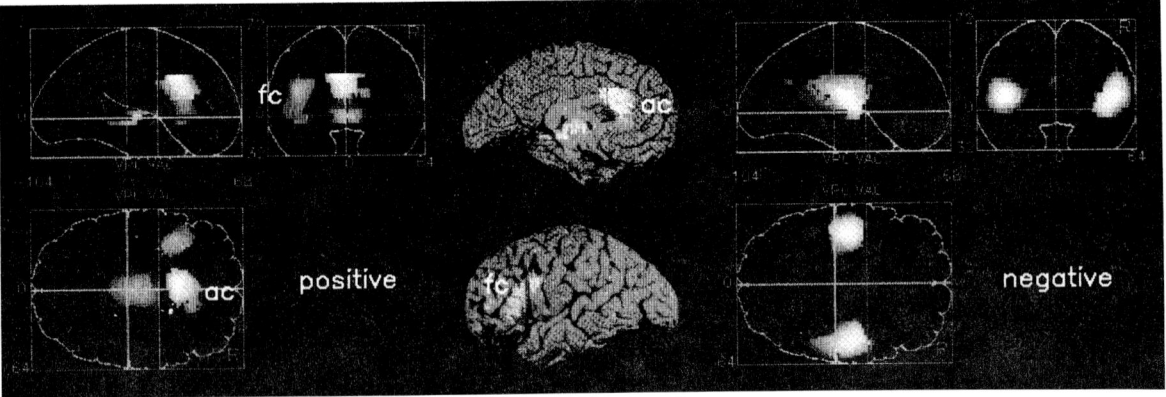

Second PC

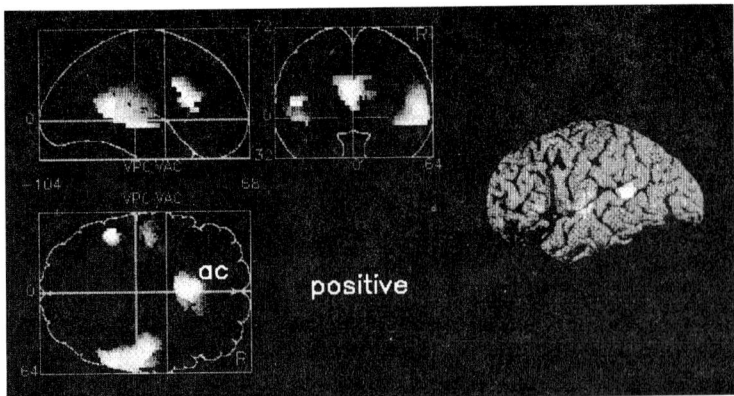

Figure 7 SPM{PC_1^+}, SPM{PC_1^-}, and SPM{PC_2^-}. First and second spatial modes for all voxels entered into the analysis (those with a nontrivial F: $p < 0.05$ following ANCOVA). Positive and negative loadings are shown for the first PC. Only positive loading are displayed for the second PC. ac, anterior cingulate; fc, left prefrontal cortex.

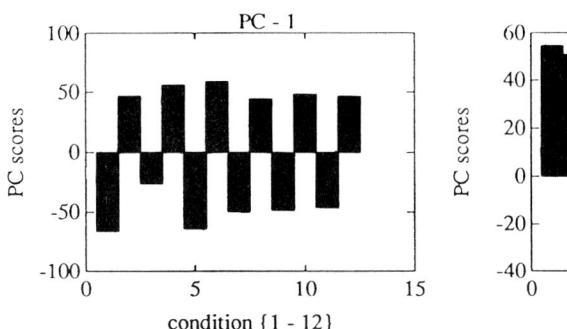
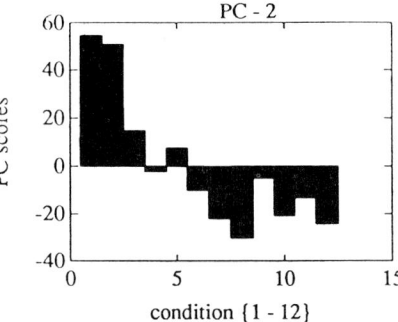

Figure 8 PC scores for the first two PCs or spatial modes. Conditions are baseline, fluency, baseline, ... These patterns suggest the first spatial mode is engaged by the task (i.e., variance introduced by experimental design). The second mode appears to reflect adaptation of absolute rCBF over the entire experiment.

ing and verbal fluency. Six subjects performed the two tasks alternately for 12 scans (order balanced across subjects). The mean adjusted rCBF equivalents for each of the $k = 12$ conditions were subject to recursive PCA analysis. The first two principal components, or spatial modes, accounted for almost all the variance observed (86%). The first mode accounted for 71% and the second, for 15% of variance. These are seen in Fig. 7. The third mode accounted for only 4%. The first spatial mode had positive loadings in the anterior cingulate (Brodmann's area, BA 24,32), the left dorsolateral prefrontal cortex (DLPFC BA 46) and Broca's area (BA 44), the thalamic nuclei, and the cerebellum. Negative loadings were seen bitemporally and in the posterior cingulate. This profile is a verbal fluency profile we discussed above (Fig. 3) (Frith *et al.*, 1991). We have not observed subcortical activation to be so reliable in previous data. The PC scores, reflecting the contribution of spatial modes to each condition (Fig. 8), testify to this interpretation. The first mode is very evident in the verbal fluency tasks, with correspondingly low scores on the baseline. Furthermore, these scores are largely invariant over time. The second principal component had its highest positive loading in the anterior cingulate and appears to correspond to a monotonic time effect with greatest prominence in the first three conditions (Fig. 8).

The two spatial modes may represent an *intentional* system critical for the intrinsic generation of words and a second *attentional* system whose physiology changes monotonically with time. This adaptation could reflect a decline in acquisition of perceptual set (Wise, 1989) as the tasks become familiar [see Posner *et al.* (1990) and Pardo *et al.* (1990) for evidence implicating the anterior cingulate in attention].

The functionally connected system corresponding to the first principal component accounted for 71% of the observable differences in adjusted mean rCBF from the 12 scans. This is a remarkable observation in that 71% of the variance in brain physiology was introduced by experimental design. This is a clear vindication of the PET technique in the investigation of functional anatomy and connectivity. Furthermore, the distributed system highlighted is in exact accord with that predicted from anatomical connectivity. All the components of this system (anterior cingulate, DLPFC, posterior cingulate, and superior temporal region) have dense and reciprocal connections (Pandta and Barnes, 1987; Goldman-Rakic, 1987, 1988).

IV. Conclusion

As the last section leaves us in a recursive frame of mind, the reader is referred to the introduction.

Acknowledgments

Thanks to colleagues at the MRC Cyclotron Unit for their contributions at both intellectual and technical levels. K.J.F. was funded by the Wellcome Trust during this work.

References

Aertsen, A., and Preissl, H. (1991). Dynamics of activity and connectivity in physiological neuronal networks. *In* "Non Linear Dynamics and Neuronal Networks" (Ed Schuster, Ed.), pp. 281–302. New York: HG VCH Publishers.

Albus, J. S. (1971). A theory of cerebellar function. *Math. Biosci.* **10**, 25–61.

American Psychiatric Association (1987). "Diagnostic and Statistical Manual of Mental Disorders," third ed. Washington, D.C.: American Psychiatric Press.

Andreasen, N. C. (1986). "Comprehensive Assessment of Symptoms and History." Iowa City, Iowa: University of Iowa, College of Medicine.

Bailey, D. L., Jones, T., Friston, K. J., Colebatch, J. G., and Frackowiak, R. S. J. (1991). Physical validation of statistical parameteric mapping. *J. Cereb. Blood Flow Metab.* **11**(Suppl. 2), S150.

Collings, S. N. (1977). "Mathematical Statistics: Its Setting and Scope," pp. 73–75. Milton Keynes, United Kingdom: The Open University Press.

Cox, D. R., and Miller, H. D. (1980). "The Theory of Stochastic Processes," pp. 272–336. New York: Chapman & Hall.

Deiber, N. P., Passingham, R. E., Colebatch, J. G., Friston, K. J., Nixon, P. D., and Frackowiak, R. S. J. (1991). Cortical areas and the selection of movement. *Exp. Brain Res.* **84**, 393–402.

Delisi, L. E., Holcomb, H., Cohen, R. M., *et al.* (1985a). Positron emission tomography in patients with and without neuroleptic medication. *J. Cereb. Blood Flow Metab.* **5**, 201–206.

Delisi, L. E., Buchsbaum, M. S., Holcomb, H., *et al.*, (1985b). Clinical correlates of decreased anteroposterior metabolic gradients in positron emission tomography (PET) of schizophrenic patients. *Am. J. Psych.* **142**, 78–81.

Dvorak, I., and Holden, A. V. (Eds.) (1991). "Mathematical Approaches to Brain Functioning Diagnostics," pp. 1–463. New York: Manchester University Press.

Ferrier, D. (1875). Experiments on the brain of monkeys. *Proc. R. Soc. London* **23**, 409–430.

Fox, P. T., Perlmutter, J. S., and Raichle, M. E. (1985). A stereotactic method of anatomical localization for positron emission tomography. *J. Comput. Assist. Tomogr.* **9**, 141–153.

Fox, P. T., Mintun, M. A., Reiman, E. M., and Raichle, M. E. (1988). Enhanced detection of focal brain responses using intersubject averaging and change distribution analysis of subtracted PET images. *J. Cereb. Blood Flow Metab.* **8**, 642–653.

Fox, P. T., and Mintun, M. A. (1989). Non-invasive functional brain mapping by change distribution analysis of averaged PET images of $H^{15}O_2$ tissue activity. *J. Nucl. Med.* **30**, 141–149.

Friston, K. J., Passingham, R. E., Nutt, J. G., Heather, J. D., Sawle, G. V., and Frackowiak, R. S. J. (1989). Localization in PET images: Direct fitting of the intercommissural (AC–PC) line. *J. Cereb. Blood Flow Metab.* **9**, 690–695.

Friston, K. J., Frith, C. D., Liddle, P. F., Lammertsma, A. A., Dolan, R. J., and Frackowiak, R. S. J. (1990). The relationship between local and global changes in PET scans. *J. Cereb. Blood Flow Metab.* **10**, 458–466.

Friston, K. J., Frith, C. D., Liddle, P. F., and Frackowiak, R. S. J. (1991a). Plastic transformation of PET images. *J. Comput. Assist. Tomogr.* **15**, 634–639.

Friston, K. J., Frith, C. D., Liddle, P. F., and Frackowiak, R. S. J. (1991b). Comparing functional (PET) images: The assessment of significant change. *J. Cereb. Blood Flow Metab.* **11**, 690–699.

Friston, K. J., Frith, C. D., Liddle, P. F., and Frackowiak, R. S. J. (1991c). The cerebellum in skill learning. *J. Cereb. Blood Flow Metab.* **11**(Suppl. 2), S440.

Friston, K. J., Frith, C. D., Liddle, P. F., and Frackowiak, R. S. J. (1991d). Investigating a network model of word generation with positron emission tomography. *Proc. R. Soc. London B* **244**, 101–106.

Friston, K. J., Liddle, P. F., Frith, C. D., Hirsch, S. R., and Frackowiak, R. S. J. (1992a). The left medial temporal lobe and schizophrenia: A PET study. *Brain* **115**, 367–382.

Friston, K. J., Frith, C. D., Liddle, P. F., and Frackowiak, R. S. J. (1992b). Motor practice and neurophysiological adaptation in the cerebellum: A positron emission study. *Proc. R. Soc. London B* **248**, 223–228.

Friston, K. J., Grasby, P., Bench, C., Frith, C. D., Cowen, P. J., Liddle, P. F., and Frackowiak, R. S. J. (1992c). Measuring the neuromodulatory effects of drugs in man with positron tomography. *Neurosci. Lett.* **141**, 106–110.

Friston, K. J., Frith, C. D., Liddle, P. F., and Frackowiak, R. S. J. (1993). Functional connectivity: The principal component analysis of large (PET) data sets. *J. Cereb. Blood Flow Metab.* **13**, 5–14.

Frith, C. D., Friston, K. J., Liddle, P. F., and Frackowiak, R. S. J. (1991). Willed action and the prefrontal cortex in man. *Proc. R. Soc. London B* **244**, 241–246.

Gerstein, G. L., and Perkel, D. H. (1969). Simultaneously recorded trains of action potentials: Analysis and functional interpretation. *Science* **164**, 828–830.

Gerstein, G. L., Bedenbaugh, P., and Aertsen, A. M. H. J. (1989). Neuronal assemblies. *IEEE Trans. Biomed. Eng.* **36**, 4–14.

Gilbert, P. F. C., and Thach, W. T. (1977). Purkinje cell activity during motor learning. *Brain Res.* **128**, 309–328.

Goldman-Rakic, P. S. (1987). Circuitry of primate frontal cortex and the regulation of behavior by representational memory. *In* "Handbook of Physiology: The Nervous System" (F. Plum and V. Mountcastle, Eds.), Vol. 5, pp. 373–417. Baltimore: Williams & Wilkins.

Goldman-Rakic, P. S. (1988). Topography of cognition: Parallel distributed networks in primate association cortex. *Annu. Rev. Neurosci.* **11**, 137–156.

Goltz, F. (1881). *In* "Transactions of the Seventh International Medical Congress" (W. J. W. MacCormac, Ed.), Vol. 1, pp. 218–228. London: Kolkmann.

Grasby, P. M., Friston, K. J., Bench, C., Cowen, P. J., Frith, C. D., Liddle, P. F., Frackowiak, R. S. J., and Dolan, R. J. (1992). The effects of the 5HT1A partial aginist buspirone on regional cerebral blood flow in man. *Psychopharmacology* **108**, 380–386.

Hope, K. (1968). "Methods of Multivariate Analysis," p. 64. London: University of London Press.

Horwitz, B., Duara, R., and Rappoport, S. I. (1984). Intercorrelations of glucose rates between brain regions: Application to healthy males in a reduced state of sensory input. *J. Cereb. Blood Flow Metab.* **4**, 484–499.

Horwitz, B. (1990). Simulating functional interactions in the brain: A model for examining correlations between regional cerebral metabolic rates. *Int. J. Biomed. Comput.* **26**, 149–170.

Horwitz, B., Grady, C., Haxby, J., Schapiro, M., Carson, R., Herscovitch, P., Ungerleider, L., Mishkin, M., and Rapoport, S. (1991). Object and spatial visual processing: Intercorrelations of regional cerebral blood flow among posterior brain regions. *J. Cereb. Blood Flow Metab.* **11**,(Suppl. 2), S380.

Ingvar, D. H., and Franzen, G. (1974). Abnormalities of cerebral blood flow distribution in patients with chronic schizophrenia. *Acta Psych. Scand.* **50**, 425–436.

Ito, M., Shida, T., Yagi, N., and Yamamoto, M. (1974). The cerebellar modification of rabbit's horizontal vestibulo-ocular reflex induced by sustained head rotation combined with visual stimulation. *Proc. Jpn. Acad. Sci.* **50**, 85–89.

Ito, M. (1989). Long term depression. *Annu. Rev. Neurosci.* **12**, 85–102.

Jones, A. K. P., Brown, W. D., Friston, K. J., Qi, L. Y., and Frackowiak, R. S. J. (1991a). Cortical and subcortical responses to pain in man using positron emission tomography. *Proc. R. Soc. London B* **244**, 39–44.

Jones, A. K. P., Friston, K. J., Qi, L. Y., Harris, M. Cunningham, V. J., Jones, T., Feinman, C., and Frackowiak, R. S. J. (1991b). Sites of action of morphine in the brain. *Lancet*, 338–825.

Liddle, P. F., Friston, K. J., Frith, C. D., Jones, T., Hirsch, S. R., and Frackowiak, R. S. J. (1992). Patterns of cerebral blood flow in schizophrenia. *Br. J. Psych.* **160,** 179–186.

Lagreze, H. L., Hartmann, A., and Shaub, L. (1991). A factor imaging of cortical blood flow during behavior activation: Interaction of neuronal networks in cognition. *J. Cereb. Blood Flow Metab.* **11,** S369.

Lammertsma, A. A., Cunningham, V. J., Deiber, M. P., Heather, J. D., Bloomfield, P. M., Nutt, J. G., Frackowiak, R. S. J., and Jones, T. (1990). Combination of dynamic and integral methods for generating reproducible functional CBF images. *J. Cereb. Blood Flow Metab.* **10,** 675–686.

Marenco, S., Coppola, R., Daniel, D. G., Zigun, J. R., Gorey, J. G., Jones, D. W., Berman, K. F., and Wienberger, D. R. (1991). rCBF activation with the Wisconsin card sort test in normal and schizophrenic subjects measured by SPECT. *J. Cereb. Blood Flow Metab.* **11**(Suppl. 2), S822.

Marr, D. (1969). A theory of cerebellar cortex. *J. Physiol.* **202,** 437–470.

Metter, E. J., Riege, W. H., Kuhl, D. E., and Phelps, M. E. (1984). Cerebral metabolic relationships for selected brain regions in healthy adults. *J. Cereb. Blood Flow Metab.* **4,** 1–7.

Mintun, M. A., Fox, P. T., and Raichle, M. E. (1989). A highly accurate method of localizing regions of neuronal activation in the human brain with positron emission tomography. *J. Cereb. Blood Flow Metab.* **9,** 96–103.

Moeller, J. R., Struther, S. C., Sidtis, J. J., and Rottenberg, D. A. (1987). Scaled subprofile model: A statistical approach to the analysis of functional patterns in positron emission tomographic data. *J. Cereb. Blood Flow Metab.* **7,** 649–658.

Pandya, D. N., and Barnes, C. L. (1987). Architecture and connections of the frontal lobes. *In* "The Frontal Lobes Revisited," pp. 41–71. The IRBN Press.

Pardo, J. V., Pardo, P. J., Janer, K. W., and Raichle, M. E. (1990). The anterior cingular cortex mediates processing selection in the Stroop attentional conflict paradigm. *Proc. Natl. Acad. Sci. USA* **87,** 256–259.

Petersen, S. E., Fox, P. T., Posner, M. I., Mintun, M., and Raichle, M. E. (1989). Positron emission tomographic studies of the processing of single words. *J. Cog. Neurosci.* **1,** 153–170.

Phillips, C. G., Zeki, S., and Barlow, H. B. (1984). Localization of function in the cerebral cortex: Past present and future. *Brain* **107,** 327–361.

Posner, M. L., Sandson, J., Dhawan, M., and Shulman, G. L. (1990). Is word recognition automatic? A cognitive–anatomical approach. *J. Cog. Neurosci.* **1,** 50–60.

Spinks, T. J., Jones, T., Gilardi, M. C., and Heather, J. D. (1988). Physical performance of the latest generation of commercial positron scanner. *IEEE Trans. Nucl. Sci.* **35,** 721–725.

Talairach, J., and Tournoux, P. (1988). "A Coplanar Stereotaxic Atlas of a Human Brain." Stuttgart: Thieme.

Talbot, J. D., Marrett, S., Evans, A. C., Meyer, E., Boshnell, and M. C., Duncan, G. H. (1991). Multiple representations of pain in human cerebral cortex. *Science* **251,** 1355–1358.

Tempel, L. W., Snyder, A. Z., and Raichle, M. E. (1991). PET measurement of regional and global cerebral blood flow at rest and with physiological activation. *J. Cereb. Blood Flow Metab.* **11**(Suppl. 2), S367.

Voss, R. F. (1988). Fractals in nature: From characterization to stimulation. *In* "The Science of Fractal Images" (H. Peitgen and D. Saupe, Eds.), pp. 21–69. New York: Springer-Verlag.

Wildt, A. R., and Ahtola, O. T. (1978). "Analysis of Covariance," p. 30. Beverly Hills/London: Sage Publications.

Wise, S. P. (1989). Frontal cortical activity and motor set. *In* "Neural Programming" (M. Ito, Ed.), p. 26. Tokyo: Japanese Scientific Societies Press.

Worsley, K. J., Evans, A. C., Marrett, S., and Neelin, P. (1992). A three-dimensional statistical analysis for rCBF activation studies in human brain. *J. Cereb. Blood Flow Metab.* **12,** 900–918.

9

BrainMap: A Database of Human Functional Brain Mapping

Peter T. Fox, Shawn Mikiten, Gwendolyn Davis, and Jack L. Lancaster

The Research Imaging Center, University of Texas Health Science Center at San Antonio,
San Antonio, Texas 78284

I. Introduction

The human functional brain-mapping community has a clear need for data visualization, data management, and data sharing. The computational and structural complexity of the human brain poses an unprecedented scientific challenge. As more and more laboratories accept this challenge, keeping abreast of the field has become difficult. Unwitting duplication of experiments on human subjects is wasteful preventable only through rapid dissemination of new findings. Electronic communication can provide a solution.

Human brain mapping is performed by several techniques. These include positron-emission tomography (PET), magnetoencephalography (MEG), electroencephalography (EEG), and functional magnetic resonance imaging (MRI). For localization of function, "PET has provided the best and most complete information on human functional brain organization" (Pechura and Martin, 1991). The reasons for this are several. Modern PET cameras have a field of view spanning the entire brain, with pixel sizes of 1–2 mm, slice widths of 3–6 mm, and spatial resolution of 4–6 mm. PET data are acquired in spatially precise two- or three-dimensional arrays. Activated neural populations can be localized to within a few millimeters (Fox *et al.*, 1986; Mintun *et al.*, 1989). Unlike MEG and EEG dipole localization by inverse solution, PET is equally precise for any number of focal activations. Because PET can scan the entire brain in as little as 40 s, study

a new behavioral condition every 10 min, and study numerous (8 to 10) behaviors in a single session, behaviorally sophisticated paradigms are widely used. PET's spatial precision, versatility, and paradigm sophistication have made PET the gold standard for functional brain mapping.

The PET brain-mapping literature is an obvious starting point for a database of human functional neuroanatomy. The field is sufficiently mature that methods for data analysis and a system for reporting of activated locations have become standardized (below). Application of these standards is almost universal (for functional activation studies), greatly facilitating database development. Although rich, the PET literature based on these standards is still of a manageable size, making this an opportune time for a database initiative. Finally, the technical evolution of other brain-mapping methods is quite rapid. The human brain-mapping literature will soon be in a phase of explosive growth. In developing a database for PET brain-mapping research, we will at least provide a model for database initiatives in other modalities. With sufficient forethought, BrainMap may even prove applicable to all modalities of human functional brain mapping, unifying these diverse communities.

II. Methodological Standards of the PET Brain-Mapping Community

In the PET brain-mapping community, standard methods for data analysis, data reduction, and data

FUNCTIONAL NEUROIMAGING

publication have evolved. Although methods are not identical among centers, differences are rather minor. These standards make communication among laboratories quite precise. Results from different laboratories can be compared and contrasted (i.e., meta-analyzed) quite meaningfully. These standards are the foundation upon which the BrainMap database has been erected.

A. The Bicommissural Coordinate Space

Bicommissural coordinates have become an international standard for reporting PET functional brain mapping. Virtually all PET brain-mapping laboratories now use bicommissural coordinates as their "least common denominator" for reporting locations of brain activation. The bicommissural coordinate space is defined by three orthogonal planes: the midsagittal plane, the plane through the anterior and posterior commissures and orthogonal to the midsagittal plane, and the plane through the anterior commissure and orthogonal to the prior two planes. Following alignment with these planes, a brain image is scaled along each axis to the dimensions of a standard brain (Fox *et al.*, 1985, 1988; Friston *et al.*, 1989; Talairach *et al.*, 1967; Talairach and Tournoux, 1988). After it is "warped" into the bicommissural space, each point in a brain image is labeled by an x–y–z address referable to the atlas brain.

Using coordinates to describe brain location is counterintuitive to many outside the field. Yet, the alternatives are limited. The most precise neuroanatomical methods are histological: cytoarchitectonics, myeloarchitectonics, connectivity, and histochemistry. With few exceptions—the stria of Genari can be seen on high-resolution MRI—histology is beyond the resolution limits of noninvasive imaging. Surface features (sulci and gyri) can be visualized by 3D rendering of anatomical images (MRI or X-ray computed tomography, CT). Cortical infoldings, however, vary among individuals in number, shape, and location. Although primary sensory and motor areas are typically localized to the bank of a primary sulcus, whether any consistent relationships exist between cortical folding patterns and higher-order cortical areas remains to be proved. Bicommissural coordinates ignore surface anatomy. Locations are described within a Cartesian space bounded by the overall shape of the brain. Intersubject variations in folding patterns and in the relation of functional areas to folding patterns introduce random noise, but do not systematically bias localization descriptions. Noise limits the ability to predict functional areas in individual sub-

jects, but does not prevent applying parametric statistics on groups of subjects. The effective use of bicommissural coordinates for intersubject averaging confirms that these variations are spatially random (Fox *et al.*, 1988; Lueck *et al.*, 1989).

The precision, objectivity, and wide use of bicommissural coordinates greatly simplify the task of developing a database of human brain mapping. Brain locations can be addressed without the ambiguities of conventional terminology (below). Voxel-based image analysis (below) complements the use of bicommissural coordinates. Together, these methods are highly suited to database use.

B. Voxel-Based Analytic Methods

The purpose of voxel-based image analysis is to determine the brain areas participating in a behavior in as precise and unbiased a manner as possible (Fox, 1991). Abandoning the traditional strategy of limited sampling (defining certain areas as being "of interest"), voxel-based methods analyze every volume element (voxel) within a dataset (50,000 values, or more). Although computationally intensive, these methods optimize the precision with which activated populations can be localized.

Image subtraction is the simplest voxel-based method. Pairs of images (task and control) are subtracted to create images of task-induced change. By registering images within the bicommissural coordinate space, multiple pairs of images (e.g., from several subjects) can be simultaneously analyzed, either as images of regional change or by computing "t" statistics, "z" scores, "p" values, or other statistical parameters images (Friston *et al.*, 1989). In images of regional change and related parameters, areas of neural activation appear as clusters of changed pixels (increased or decreased blood flow). The shape of an activated cluster approximates a 3D Gaussian, largely reflecting the spatial blurring of the image-reconstruction filter. Response locations are reported as the center of mass of these clusters.

Voxel-based analysis and center-of-mass localization are more precise than image resolution, so-called "hyperacuity" (Vernier acuity) (Fox *et al.*, 1986; Mintun *et al.*, 1989). For within-subject comparisons, even of averaged images, neural populations only a few millimeters apart can be separately localized with subtractive logic (Fox *et al.*, 1986). Comparisons of different groups of subjects are based on location coordinates, adding noise and increasing the variance (above). Among subjects, functional areas typically vary in location by less than a centimeter (Fox *et al.*,

1986, 1987). The combined use of voxel-based analysis and bicommissural coordinates provides efficient data reduction. An entire change-image array is reduced to a few hundred centers of mass. Each center is described by an x–y–z address and a magnitude expressed as percentage change, z score, or other statistical parameter.

C. Applicability of PET Methods to Other Human Brain-Mapping Techniques

PET brain-mapping standards promise to be surprisingly adaptable to other brain-mapping modalities. MRI brain mapping already uses voxel-based analyses, including image subtraction and imaging of statistical parameters. Using bicommissural coordinates poses no difficulty for MRI. Studies using this approach have already appeared (Belliveau *et al.,* 1991). EEG and MEG are more problematic, as these data types are not readily placed in tomographic or volumetric spatial arrays. Even within-subject coregistration to anatomical images (e.g., MRI and X-ray CT) does not fully resolve this problem. Increasing the number of channels (e.g., to 64 or 128) and applying accurate head models will be needed to create spatially precise data. After this is accomplished, transformation into bicommissural coordinates is quite simple.

III. Design Goals

The first step in building a database is to establish design goals. The purpose of the BrainMap database is to promote the user's ability to understand the functional anatomy of the human brain through rapid, exhaustive access to image-derived research on human functional neuroanatomy. Because "the organizing structure for information about the brain is neuroanatomy, which provides a construct for the functional expression of brain activity, ... it will be necessary to conjoin anatomy and function. ..." (Pechura and Martin, 1991). BrainMap's design is derived from the goal of relating function and location. Its design also reflects the standards and structure of PET brain-mapping data, as well as the needs and knowledge base of projected users.

A. A Searchable Atlas

"Neuroscience is an inherently visual science and, in this way, differs from other scientific fields" (Pechura and Martin, 1991). The complex spatial structure of the brain is best understood when the brain can be visualized. An efficient means of describing and depicting anatomy is the foundation of any neuroscience database. A key design goal, then, is that the user interface must include a digitized atlas of the human brain. This atlas should serve for visualizing the results of a query, and for initiating a query.

One approach to creating a searchable atlas is to segment the brain into regions (Evans *et al.,* 1988). Functional–anatomical associations are retrieved and analyzed on the basis of unique names for each region. Although it is superficially appealing, this approach has significant flaws. This strategy is best applied to medium-sized, well-demarcated structures. Very small structures are beneath the resolution of noninvasive images. Very large structures lack gross demarcations for functional boundaries. For example, the largest brain structure, the cerebral cortex, consists of an unknown but very large number of functional regions with no grossly apparent borders by which it can be subdivided. In fact, it is a goal of functional brain mapping to determine the functional parcellation of the cerebral cortex, in the absence of gross structural borders. Thus, no *a priori* subdivisions can be adequate. Further, the use of standard anatomical regions for database development would require that all laboratories use region-of-interest analysis for functional brain mapping. Brain-mapping laboratories, however, have largely abandoned region-of-interest analysis.

Bicommissural coordinates avoid the problems of *a priori* regional parcellation. Every location in the brain is assigned a unique coordinate. Activated locations are reported as the coordinate of the center of mass of the activated area, together with response magnitude and statistical significance. Any given structure, then, can be queried for reports of functional activation by identifying its center coordinate and a radius around that coordinate, rather than by a name or regional boundary. The logical appeal of the bicommissural coordinate system for data storage and retrieval, coupled with its widespread acceptance, mandates its central role in a database of human functional neuroanatomy.

B. Relating Psychology to Structure

In a database relating function to structure, the logic for storing and retrieving behavioral information must be no less robust than that for anatomy. This poses a problem. Just as the parcellations of the cerebral cortex are as not yet known, the elementary information-processing operations of the brain are as yet unknown. Consequently, the terminology of function is evolving, with no standards yet achieved. Nevertheless, the behavioral aspects of functional brain-mapping experiments must also be entered in the database.

Functional brain-mapping studies attempt to relate information-processing stages to brain locations (Posner *et al.*, 1988). Brain-mapping experiments are constructed as pairs of related behavioral conditions. Ideally, these pairs differ by a single cognitive component, whose location is revealed in the pixel-by-pixel comparison of the images from each condition. As the cognitive architecture of any task, however simple, is rarely known with certainty, an author's interpretation of the difference between two complex behaviors (and, therefore, of an area's function) is somewhat conjectural or hypothetical.

Brain-mapping experiments are based on behavioral conditions. A subject performs a task while the brain is imaged. Although the information-processing demands of a condition are hypothesized, the conditions themselves are a matter of observation. The instructions given to a subject, the stimuli presented, and the responses made all can be unequivocally described. However well-described, behavioral conditions do not ascribe functional properties to an area. They require interpretation.

In creating a database of human functional neuroanatomy, do we describe "functions" as bare descriptions of behavioral conditions or as information-processing interpretations? If we omit the author's functional interpretation, users may misinterpret the experiment. If we omit precise description of the behavioral conditions, users are prevented from entertaining alternative interpretations. Our design goal was to include both interpretation and observation. We hope that standards for description of behavior will emerge, possibly through BrainMap and similar projects.

C. Meta-analysis

Mapping the functional anatomy of the brain is not as clear-cut as mapping the amino-acid sequence of a gene. Placing a functional area "on the map" is only a first approximation. Defining the functional properties and functional interactions of an area is an ongoing process. Converging experiments bring deeper understanding and more detailed models, but not final answers. A database of functional neuroanatomy, then, should reflect the current state of knowledge and its ambiguities. The database should allow an overview without oversimplification. Enabling effi-

cient meta-analysis is a design goal that influences all aspects of database design and implementation.

The design goal of meta-analysis guides the selection of the forms of data to be included. Raw image data are bulky and require extensive postprocessing to be interpreted. On the other hand, reduced data are readily transported and compared among centers, if standards exist for postprocessing (above). Reduced data, however, must retain sufficient detail to allow alternative interpretations and analysis. Meta-analysis implies the ability to critique data quality. Methodological details such as the numbers of subjects used, the imaging modality and resolution, the response magnitude and level of statistical significance (preferably in terms of strength above background noise), and all pertinent behavioral measures must be included.

D. Broad Audience

Human brain mapping is a field at the crossroads of diverse disciplines. Interest in this field, then, is broad. A brain-mapping database should reflect this breadth and be designed to reach as wide an audience as possible. The data types and query structures must be relevant to scientists and clinicians across a wide range of disciplines. The interface must be intuitive to users widely variant in their knowledge of human neuroanatomy, psychology, brain imaging, and computer science. Finally, the larger environment within which the database is designed must be nonrestrictive; i.e., the hardware and software environment should be widely available, inexpensive, and readily learned.

E. What BrainMap Is Not

No tool can perform all functions. Design exclusions are as necessary as design goals. BrainMap was not designed as an archive of raw image data; rather it manages reduced data, ready for meta-analysis. BrainMap is not a "laboratory organizer," like the BrainBrowser (Bloom, 1991); rather, it is intended for meta-analysis of an entire field. BrainMap is not a teaching tool for neuroanatomy; rather, it is a tool for the functional brain-mapping research community. BrainMap is not a tool for postprocessing or analysis of raw data, like statistical parametric mapping (Friston *et al.*, 1989) or change-distribution analysis (Fox *et al.*, 1988); rather, the laboratory of origin reduces the data into a format amenable to meta-analysis. BrainMap is not an electronic bulletin board, like the Worm Community System (Schatz, 1991), or a citation index, like MedLine; *rather, BrainMap is an environment*

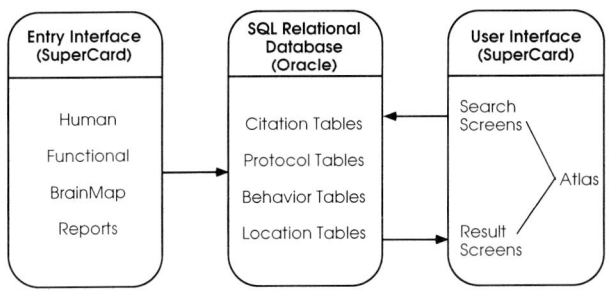

Figure 1 Database and interface interaction in BrainMap.

for in-depth exploration and interactive meta-analysis of the experimental literature of an expanding field.

IV. Implementation

BrainMap is implemented in three parts: a graphical user interface, a graphical entry interface, and a relational database (Fig. 1). The user queries the database through the user interface by search and report

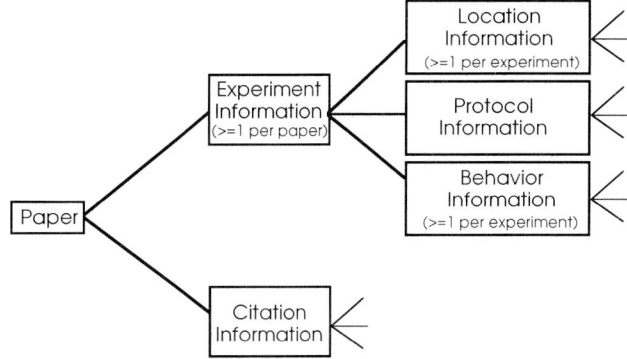

Figure 2 The database structure of BrainMap.

screens and a built-in, digitized brain atlas. The entry interface was initially designed for in-house use and will not be described here.

A. Database Design

BrainMap's database is constructed in a natural hierarchy (Fig. 2). The highest level is the *paper*. Each

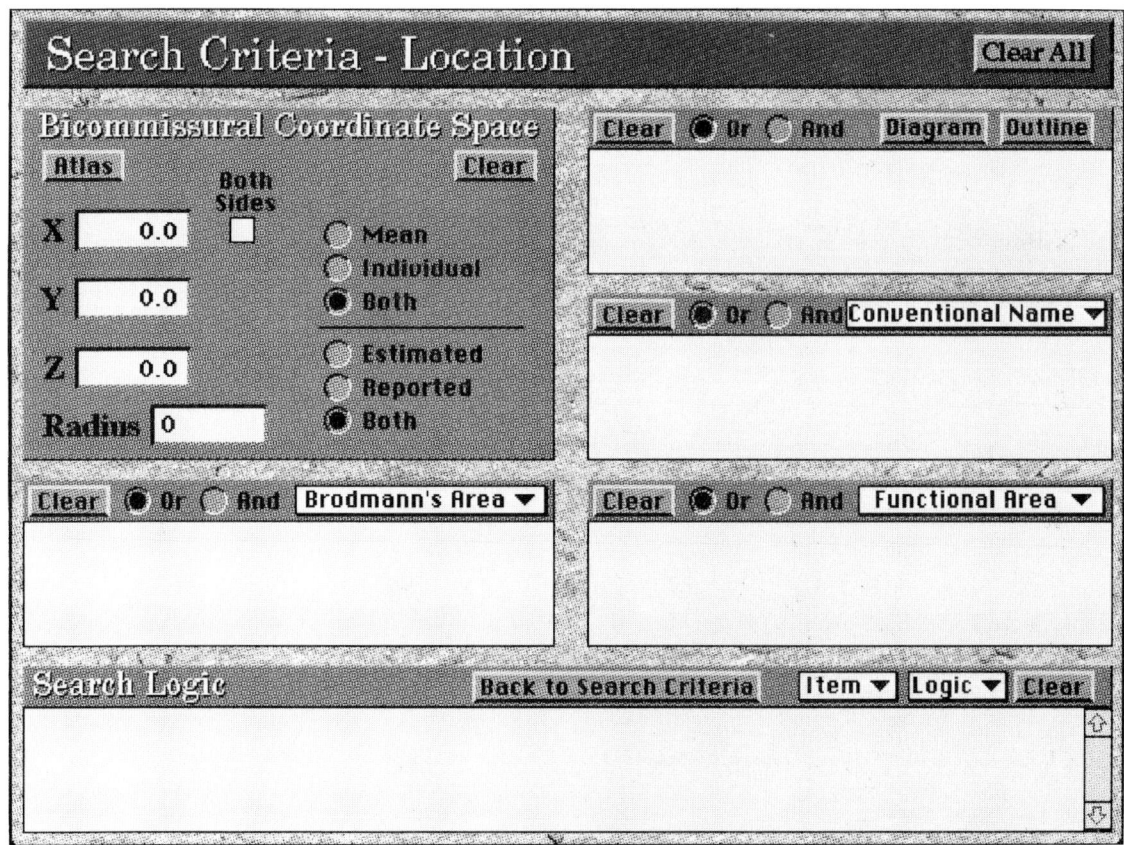

Figure 3 Location-based queries can be driven by stereotactic coordinates, lobar geometry, conventional anatomical names (e.g., putamen), Brodmann area, or functional names (e.g., area S1).

paper is divided into one or more *experiments*. An experiment is a grouping (typically a pairing) of behavioral conditions for which differentially activated locations are reported. *Behavioral conditions* are specified for each experiment. Methodological details are specified for each experiment, including imaging modality, tracer, patient population, etc. Each experiment reports one or more activated *locations*, the lowest level of the hierarchy. Each location (i.e., each $x–y–z$ coordinate) carries its links up the hierarchy, allowing information at the experiment and paper levels to be rapidly retrieved.

Queries follow four paths: location, behavior, reference, and protocol. A query can specify a single parameter in a single path or specify multiple parameters along multiple paths, with relations defined by Boolian logic.

1. Location Queries

Five anatomical schemes are used for data query (Fig. 3). The primary anatomical scheme is the bicommissural coordinate space (above). Brain locations are described as $x–y–z$ addresses. Findings published in bicommissural coordinates are flagged as "actual." When a mapping study does not publish coordinates but gives sufficent anatomical detail for an approximate coordinate to be entered, it is flagged as "estimated." "Clicking" on an atlas location automatically enters a coordinate for a search. A search can be broadened by specifying a range about that coordinate or by specifying several coordinates (Fig. 4). Search results are visualized by plotting the coordinates of activated locations into the digitized atlas. The digitized atlas is adapted from Talairach *et al.* (1967).

The second anatomical scheme is a geometrical parcellation of the cerebral cortex (Lobar geometry). The cortex is divided into three views: lateral, medial, and basal. Each view is divided into lobes along traditional boundaries: frontal, parietal, occipital, and temporal. Within each lobe, each axis is divided into three sections: anterior, middle, and posterior (Fig. 5).

The third anatomical search scheme, the conventional name, is the name applied to the activated location by the author. The conventional name is fairly powerful for structures with unequivocal boundaries and invariant names, such as subcortical nuclei. In

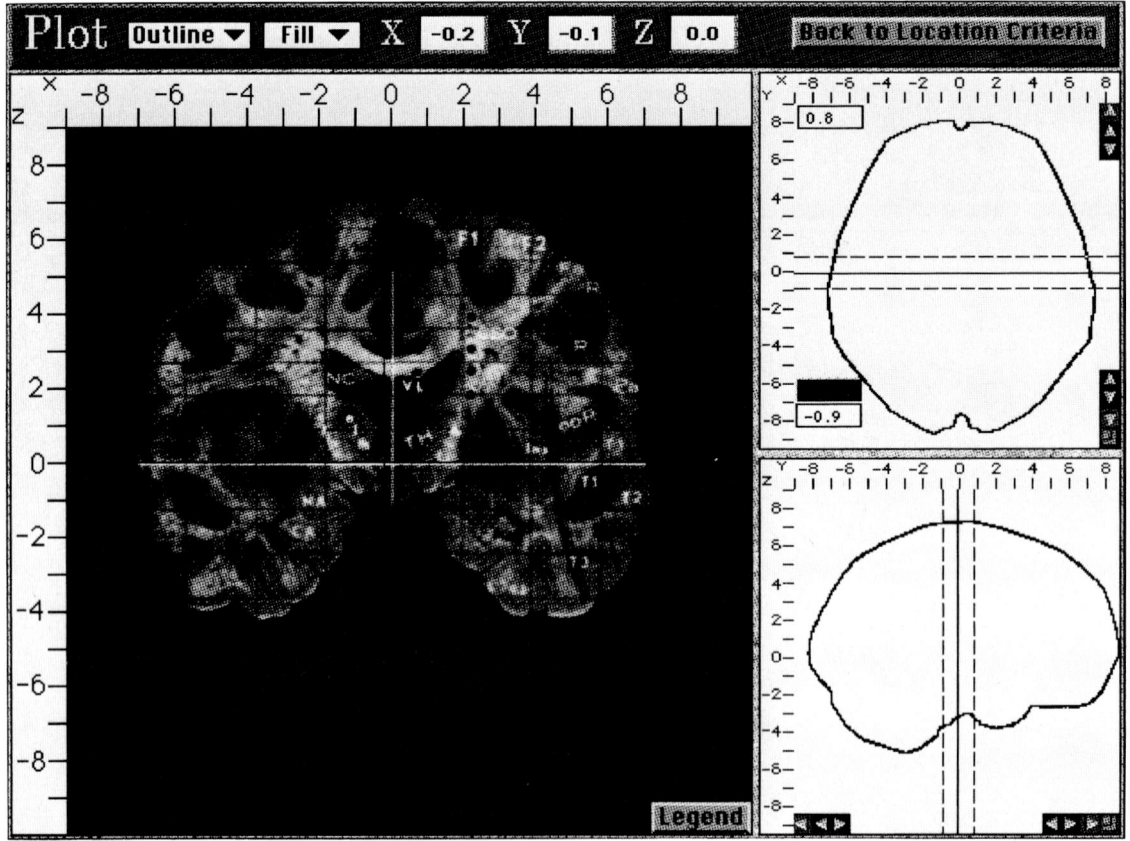

Figure 4   The digitized atlas can be used to initiate a location-based search, using stereotactic coordinates. "Clicking" on any location returns an $x–y–z$ address in the bicommissural coordinate space. The digitized brain atlas was adapted from plates published in Talairach *et al.* (1967).

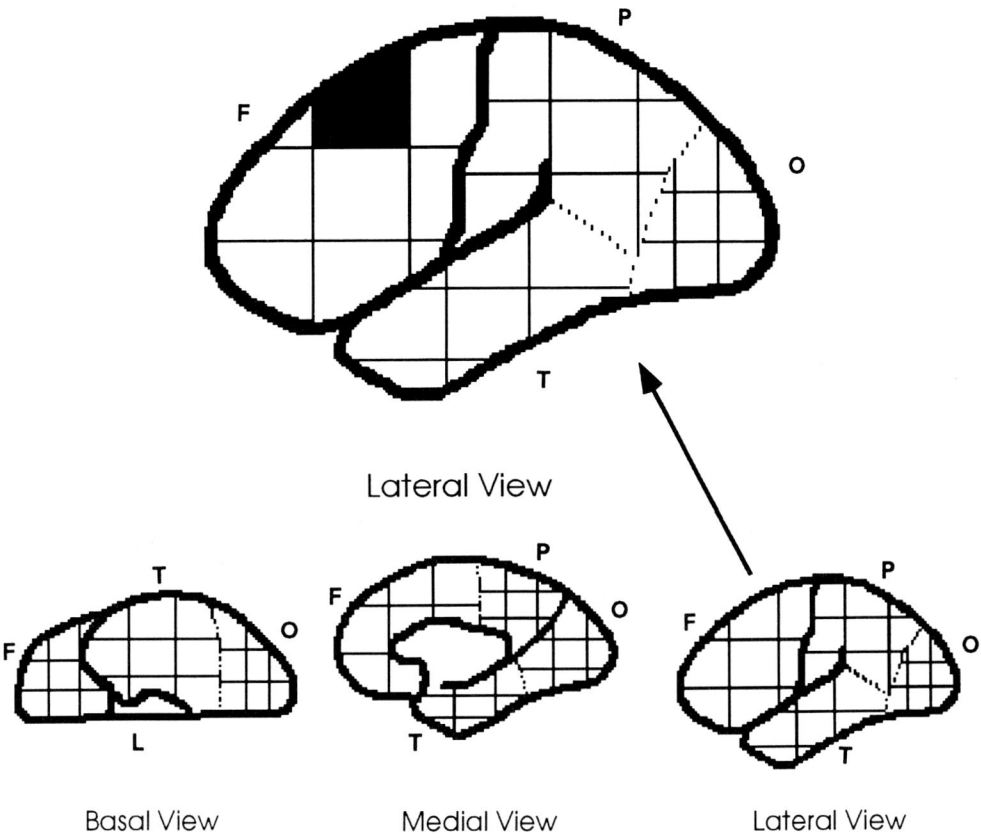

Figure 5 "Geometrical" anatomical searching. Brain locations are coded by surface (lateral, medial, and basal), by lobe (frontal, temporal, occipital, and parietal), and by sector.

the cerebral cortex, however, boundaries are vague and nomenclatures vary. Cortical locations may be named by gyral anatomy (e.g., the angular gyrus), Lobar geometry (e.g., dorsal lateral prefrontal cortex), and ill-defined quasi-anatomical names (e.g., Broca's area and supplementary motor area).

The fourth anatomical scheme is the Broadmann area. Brodmann areas apply only to the cerebral cortex. They are based solely on cytoarchitectonics, with no input from connectivity, histochemistry, or functional observations. For noninvasive imaging studies, this terminology is always presumed and never confirmed. Although Brodmann areas are by no means an ideal scheme for region naming, this nomenclature is widely used and does have some power for data storage and retrieval.

The fifth anatomical scheme, the functional area, names by the letter designations of functional areas, such as S1 for the primary somatosensory cortex or V1 for the primary visual cortex. This naming convention presumes interspecies homology, as these designations are derived from studies in other species using a variety of techniques including cytoarchitectonics,

myeloarchitectonics, histochemistry, and intracortical electrode recordings. Nevertheless, they are becoming popular in the human brain-mapping literature.

2. Behavioral Queries

Three schemes are used for encoding behavioral data (Fig. 6). The behavioral domain is a hierarchical categorization applicable to an entire experiment. The initial levels are perception, motion, cognition, and emotion. Perception is further subdivided by sensory modality (i.e., vision, audition, somesthesis, gustation, and olfaction). Each sensory modality is divided into submodalities. Vision is divided into color, shape, motion, depth, luminance, etc. Submodality categories are not comprehensive and will be expanded as needed. Behavioral domain classification should be accessible to users from virtually all backgrounds.

The second behavioral scheme is the task descriptor. Task descriptors are key words that classify experimental paradigms. Examples of task descriptors include "Stroop task," Wisconsin card sort," "continuous performance task," "Posner paradigm," and so forth. This query path is intended primarily for users

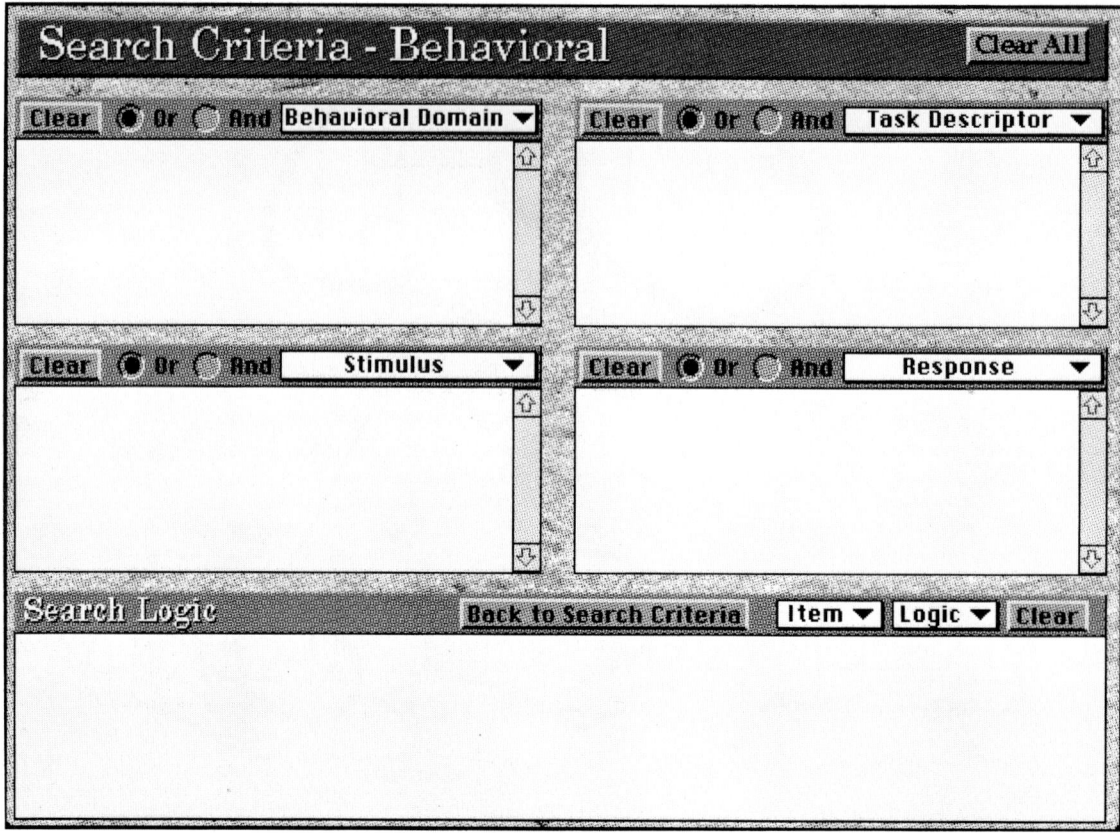

Figure 6 Behavioral queries can be developed with three distinct search axes. Behavioral domain is a general categorization of the entire experiment. Task descriptors are key words, often eponyms, that classify experimental paradigms used (e.g., Stroop task). Experimental specifications describe the behavioral conditions as stimulus, response, and instructions.

conversant in behavioral experimentation, although not necessarily in neurobehavioral imaging.

Experimental specification is the third behavioral scheme. This scheme specifies the stimulus, the response (i.e., physical movement), and the instructions given (i.e., the mental "set" established) for each behavioral condition. Entries are brief and hierarchical. Additional details about the experimental conditions are available as text fields excerpted from each manuscript, but cannot be used to initiate a query.

3. Reference (Citational) Queries

Each entry has complete location information: authors, title, year, journal, volume, page numbers, and key words. Each of these fields can be used to initiate a query. All current entries in each field are provided as a pop-up list of all available entries, allowing the user to restrict a search to possible values, even before a search is initiated.

4. Protocol (Methodological) Queries

This category searches the database for experiments with common methodological parameters such

as modality (PET, MEG, EEG, or MRI), tracer, subject population, statistical rigor, laboratory of origin, etc.

B. Graphical User Interface

The user interface is fully windowed and operates well in the multiwindowed environment of the Apple Macintosh II. The user moves through the search and display functions of the program through a series of special-purpose windows. Virtually all user actions are mouse driven. Functions are initiated by clicking soft buttons labeled with both text and icons. Search specifications are initially selected through buttons and further specified with pop-up lists of possible choices. Keyboard entries are allowed throughout, but are rarely advantageous.

The user interface includes a digitized atlas of the human brain (Fig. 7). High-resolution photographs from a bicommissural-coordinate-space atlas (Talairach, 1967) have been hand-detailed, creating outlines of cortical gray matter, white matter, ventricles, subcortical gray matter, and the cerebellum. The user has the option of viewing any plate as a gray-scale image,

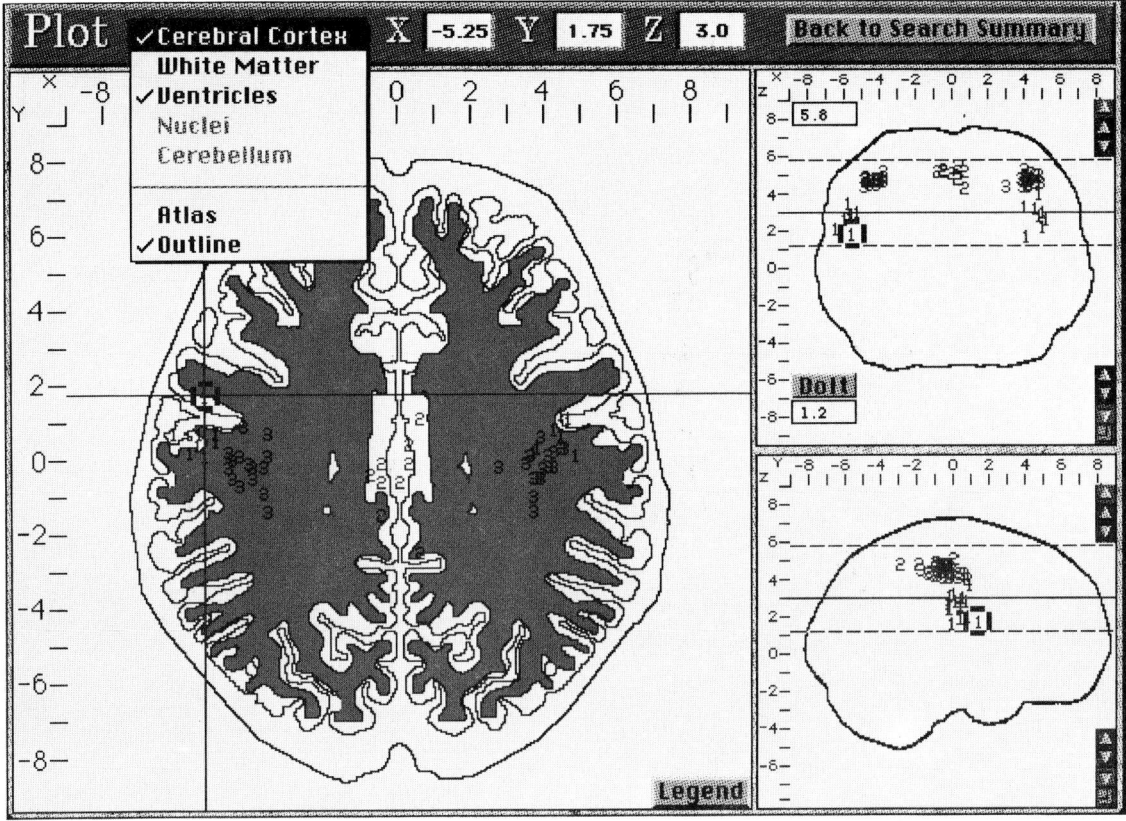

Figure 7 The user interface includes a digitized atlas of the human brain. High-resolution photographs from a bicommissural-coordinate-space atlas (Talairach *et al.*, 1967) have been hand-detailed, creating outlines of cortical gray matter, white matter, ventricles, subcortical gray matter, and the cerebellum.

region outlines, or filled regions in any combination. The plotting routines allow the locations associated with specific behaviors to be plotted onto brain sections or silhouettes in any of the three orthogonal views (Fig. 8). Points in the plot retain their relations to behavioral and citation data. Additionally, the plotting screen itself can initiate a search on anatomical criteria by selecting a location within the atlas. The user interface is distinct from the database. Thus, the current user interface could be modified or ported to other environments with no alteration in database design or function.

C. Environment

BrainMap has been developed in the Macintosh environment and operates on the Macintosh II series and *Quadra* series of computers. This environment choice reflected the low cost and wide availability of Macintosh computers, the sophistication of the Macintosh user interface and its fully windowed environment, the high quality of Macintosh graphics, and the sophistication of available prototype-development tools (i.e., SuperCard).

BrainMap's user interface was created in the SuperCard prototyping environment. Supercard is a set of tools for developing custom software on Macintosh computers. SuperCard combines two powerful metaphors for building software familiar to Macintosh users: windows and pulldown menus for navigating through a program, and cards and stacks of cards for storing information. Supercard is divided into an editing mode in which windows and related objects are defined, and an execute mode in which program scripts are attached to each object and the program is run. Supercard supports multiple windows, variable window sizes, 256 colors, and easy inclusion of external commands and functions. Finally, software developers can distribute standalone applications without licensing fees.

BrainMap's database is built in Oracle, a transact-SQL database management system. SQL is the industry standard for large-scale projects and has been called "the database of the 90's" (Gruber, 1990). In the Macintosh operating system, Oracle supports input and output using SuperCard or X-windows. Oracle-SQL code is embedded into BrainMap's user interface and entry interface. Through SuperCard, the

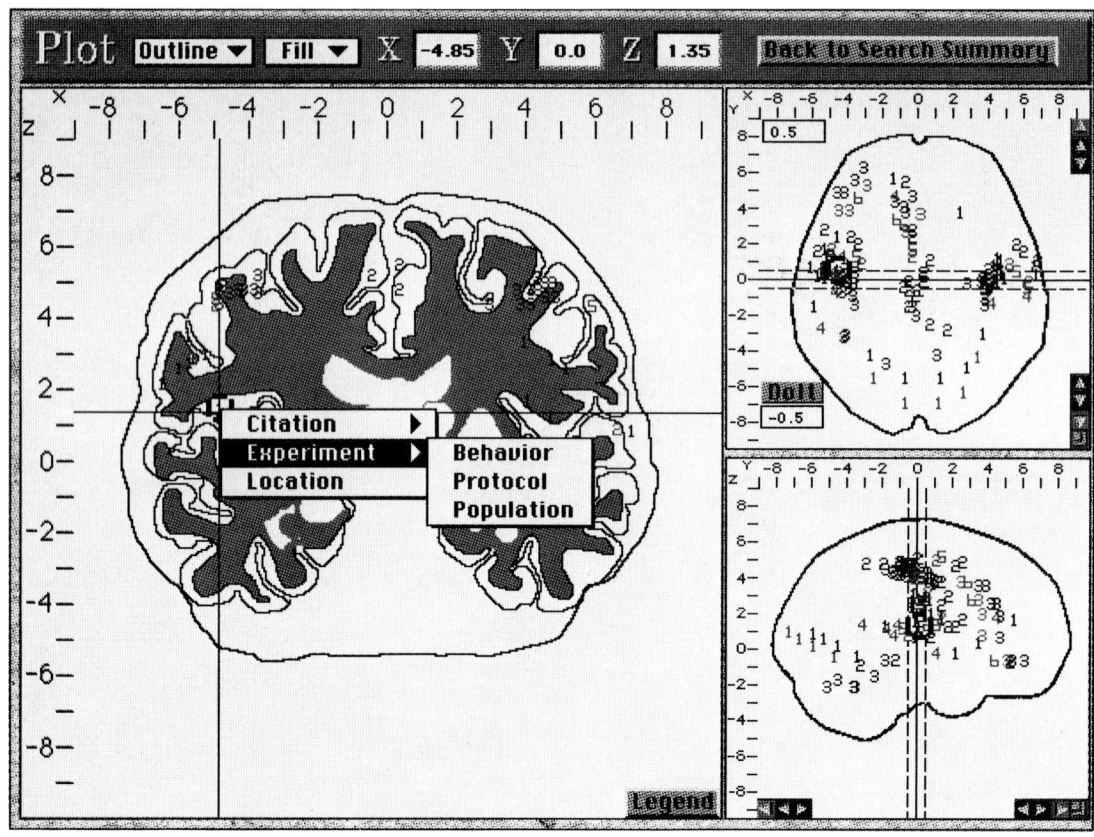

Figure 8 The digital atlas is used for displaying retrieved data. Locations reported as being significantly activated are plotted on the atlas.

BrainMap user interface issues SQL statements to drive query and entry. BrainMap operates both in a standalone mode and in a client/server mode. In standalone mode, a single Macintosh runs both the user interface and the database (in Oracle). In client/server mode, the user interface is run locally, but queries the database through a network link to the server. Because Oracle is highly portable, this software architecture will allow BrainMap's database to be served by a high-speed processor over Internet to multiple clients at remote sites.

V. Distribution and Further Development

A. Beta Testing

A beta version of BrainMap is complete. Refinement will incorporate input from brain-mapping laboratories. To this end, a BrainMap Advisory Group has been established. The Advisory Group includes representatives of the fields of PET, EEG, MEG, and MRI brain mapping, neuroscience database development, cognitive science, computational neurobiology,

and human and primate behavioral neuroscience. The Advisory Group began its interaction with the Brain-Map development team through a workshop (November 29 through December 1, 1992). The workshop provided a detailed critique of the BrainMap concept and sought consensus on its viability, prioritized future developments, and planned the means and scope of future distribution. Beta testing began at the end of Workshop I and will continue through Workshop III.

Data updates will be managed by the development site—the Research Imaging Center at the University of Texas Health Science Center at San Antonio. All brain-mapping laboratories using bicommissural coordinates are encouraged to submit preprints and high-quality copies of figures upon manuscript acceptance.

B. New Tools; New Environments

In the short term, development will be aimed at adding functions given highest priority at the initial workshop and in the early phases of beta testing. Tools for report generation will need to be designed. Tools for constructing and testing neural-systems models would be highly desirable (Friston *et al.*, 1991). Following beta testing, distribution will be expanded. The present strategy for expanded distribution is to port BrainMap's database (in Oracle) to a high-speed UNIX server; to serve the BrainMap database from a central location to clients running the user interface in client/server mode at remote sites through Internet, and to port the user interface to additional popular environments, such as Microsoft Windows for DOS and UNIX/X-windows/Motif.

Long-range goals of the Human BrainMap Database Project include incorporating datasets more inclusive than those in the published literature, developing the logic for inclusion of non-PET brain-mapping data (e.g., MRI, MEG, and EEG), building tools for local (in-house) comparisons of unpublished data (e.g., pilot data) with published data, and gaining community acceptance of BrainMap as an international, electronic registry for human brain-mapping data.

Acknowledgments

This research was supported by grants from the Low-Beer Foundation, the Office of Naval Research, the J. S. McDonnell Foundation, and IBM Academic Information Systems. We thank Richard Lucier and Steven Salzberg for an early critique of this project and, in particular, for expert advice on tools and strategies for prototyping databases.

References

Belliveau, J. W., Kennedy, D. N., McKinstry, R. C., Buchbinder, B. R., Weiskoff, R. M., Cohen, M. S., Vevea, J. M., Brady, T. J., and Rosen, B. R. (1991). Functional mapping of the human visual cortex by magnetic resonance imaging. *Science* **254**, 716–718.
Bloom, F. (1990). Databases of brain information. *In* "Three-Dimensional Neuroimaging" (A. Toga, Ed.). New York: Raven Press.
Evans, A. C., Beil, C., Marrett, S., Thompson, C. J., and Hakin, A. (1988). Anatocal–functional correlation using an adjustable MRI-based region of interest atlas with positron-emission tomography. *J. Cereb. Blood Flow Metab.* **8**, 513–530.
Fox, P. T. (1991). Physiological ROI definition by image subtraction. *J. Cereb. Blood Flow Metab.* **11**, A79–A82.
Fox, P. T., Burton, H., and Raichle, M. E. (1987). Mapping human somatosensory cortex with positron-emission tomography. *J. Neurosurg.* **63**, 34–43.
Fox, P. T., Mintun, M. E., Raichle, M. E., Miezin, F. M., Allman, J. M., and Van Essen, D. C. (1986). Mapping human visual cortex with positron-emission tomography. *Nature* **323**, 806–809.
Fox, P. T., Mintun, M. A., Reiman, E. M., and Raichle, M. E., (1988). Enhanced detection of focal brain responses using inter-subject averaging and change-distribution analysis of subtracted PET images. *J. Cereb. Blood Flow Metab.* **8**, 642–653.
Fox, P. T., Perlmuter, J. S., and Raichle, M. E. (1985). A stereotactic method of anatomical localization for positron emission tomography. *J. Comput. Assist. Tomogr.* **9**, 141–153.
Friston, K. J., Frith C. D., Liddle, P. F., and Frackowiak, R. S. J. (1991). Investigation of a network model of word generation with positron emission tomography. *Proc. R. Soc. London* **244**, 101–106.
Friston, K. J., Passingham, R. E., Nutt, J. G., Heather, J. D., Sawle, G. V., and Frackowiak, R. S. J. (1989). Localization in PET images: Direct fitting of the intercommissural (AC–PC) line. *J. Cereb. Blood Flow Metab.*, **9**, 690–695.
Gruber, M. (1990). "Understanding SQL." San Francisco. SYBEX, Inc.
Lueck, C., Zeki, S., Friston, K. J., Delber, M. P., Cope, P., Cunningham, V. J., Lammertsma, A. A., Kennard, C., and Frackowiak, R. S. J. (1989). A colour centre in the cerebral cortex of man. *Nature* **340**, 386–389.
Mintun, M. A., Fox, P. T., and Raichle, M. E. (1989). A highly accurate method of localizing regions of neuronal activity in the human brain with positron emission tomography. *J. Cereb. Blood Flow Metab.* **9**, 96–103.
Pechura, C. M., and Martin, J. B. (Eds.) (1991). "Mapping the Brain and Its Functions." Washington, D.C.: National Academy Press.
Posner, M. I., Petersen, S. E., Fox, P. T., and Raichle, M. E. (1988). Localization of cognitive functions in the human brain. *Science* **240**, 1627–1631.
Schatz, B. R. (1991). Building an electronic community system. *J. Management Inform. Syst.* **8**, 87–107.
Talairach, J., *et al.* (1967). "Atlas d'anatomie Stéréotaxique du Ttélencéphale." Paris: Masson.
Talairach, J., and Tournoux, P. (1988). "Co-Planar Stereotaxic Atlas of the Human Brain." New York: Thieme Medical Publishers.

10

Landmarks, Edges, Morphometrics, and the Brain Atlas Problem

Fred L. Bookstein

Center for Human Growth & Development, The University of Michigan, Ann Arbor, Michigan 48109

I. Introduction

Over the last decade, there have been major advances in *morphometrics,* the measurement of biological shape and shape change. Many innovations have woven together computational geometry, statistics, image analysis, and computer graphics into powerful new techniques that speak directly to the most important applied problems in medical image processing, such as the proposed collective neural structural–functional database that is the central concern of this volume. Underlying the scientific purposes of our initiative is a multifaceted problem of anatomical standardization: A methodology is wanting for coherently referring individual brains to the shared coordinate system of an "atlas." The standardization is required for diverse, overlapping scientific purposes, not only so that we can aggregate localized information over many specimens, but also so that we may correlate patterns in those distributed fields with patterns of anatomical variability (the problem of "endophrenology"). That is, we need not only to standardize images but also to represent the operations by which each was standardized in some analytically tractable way.

The power of the new morphometric methods derives from the fusion of these two purposes in a single joint algebraic/geometric formalism, the bald state-

ment of which seems at first almost unapproachably spare and technical. Let us define a *landmark* as a point with a biologically meaningful label, so that we can locate homologues for it in all the other forms of a dataset, and define an *edgel* as a landmark with a biologically meaningful orientation through it. Then the new formalism is as follows: We can construe arbitrary scenes of landmarks and edgels in two dimensions as deformations of a standard scene according to deformation functions, *thin-plate splines,* having formulas that are linear in the Cartesian coordinates of the landmarks and the edgels in the specimen; and similarly scenes of landmark points, edgels, and surfacels (normal directions through landmarks) in three dimensions. The standard scene may then be wholly replaced by a rigorous average of the specimen scenes after they have been unwarped, and the description of sample variation is reduced to ordinary variances and covariances of the deformations about the average, together with the variances and covariances of the pixels about their averages in this standardized coordinate system.

The new approach disentangles two sorts of geometry that apply to the selfsame medical image. One is a *horizontal* geometry of maps—locations of recognizable anatomical features. The other is a *vertical* geometry of surfaces—gray values or their multispectral extensions at each pixel of the image after it is standardized. Each geometry proffers its own descriptions of central tendencies ("averages") and variation, whereas horizontal and vertical are linked by a statisti-

---

The author retains the copyright to all figures in this chapter.

107

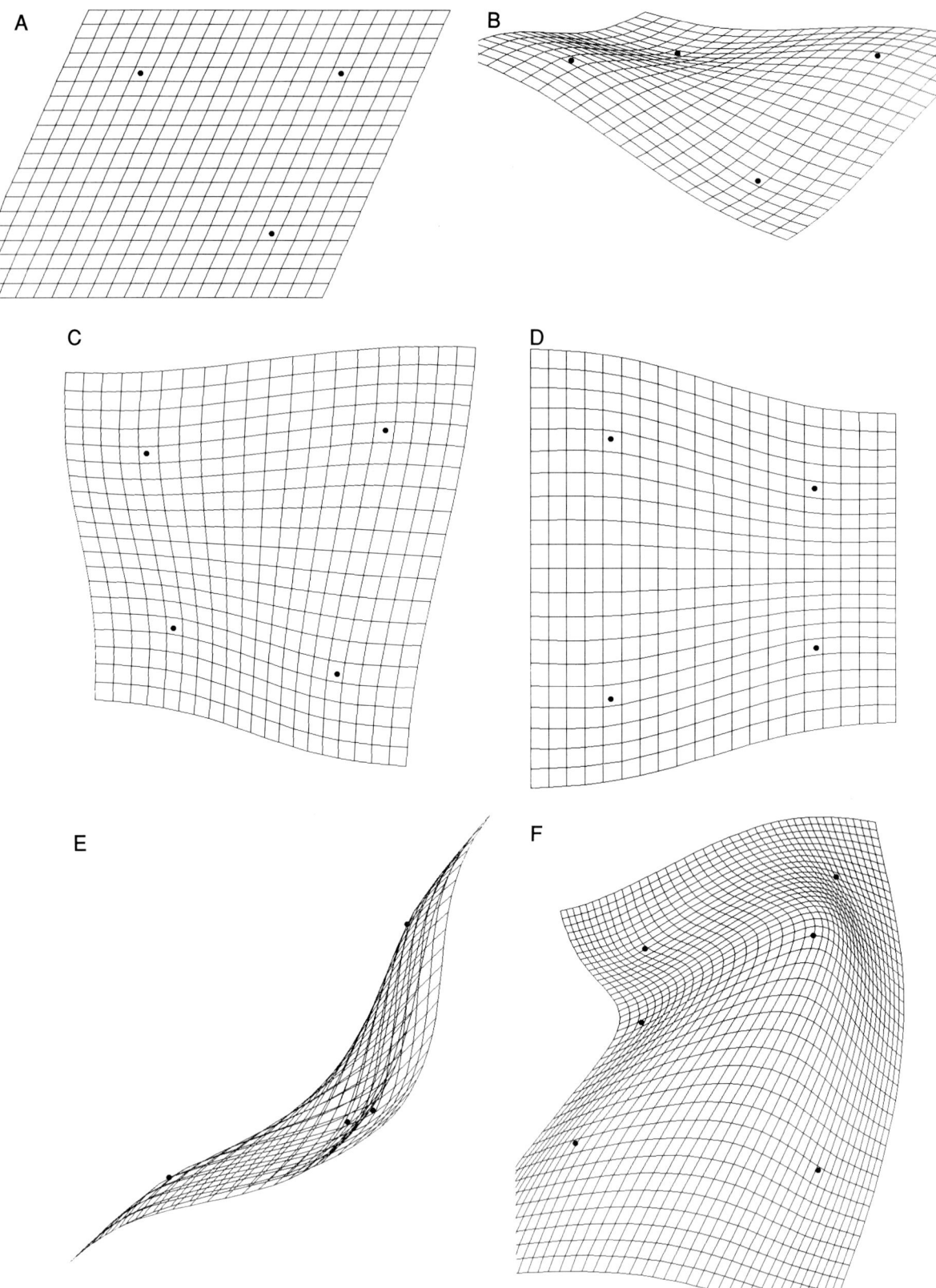

Figure 1 Thin-plate splines and deformations. (A) A simple shear can be imagined either as a deformation of a square grid or as a perspective view of a flat metal plate. (B) This particular plate is formed by raising the ends of one diagonal of a square of landmarks and lowering the ends of the other. (C and D) Viewed from different directions, and after arbitrary vertical rescaling, the plate represents deformations taking the square into any quadrilateral at all. (E) An extreme deformation of the square (side view of the original plate). (F) Surface or warp? The algebra of the thin-plate spline generates deformations of any number of landmarks that may be viewed as projections of plates (in general, one for the x coordinate and one for the y coordinate).

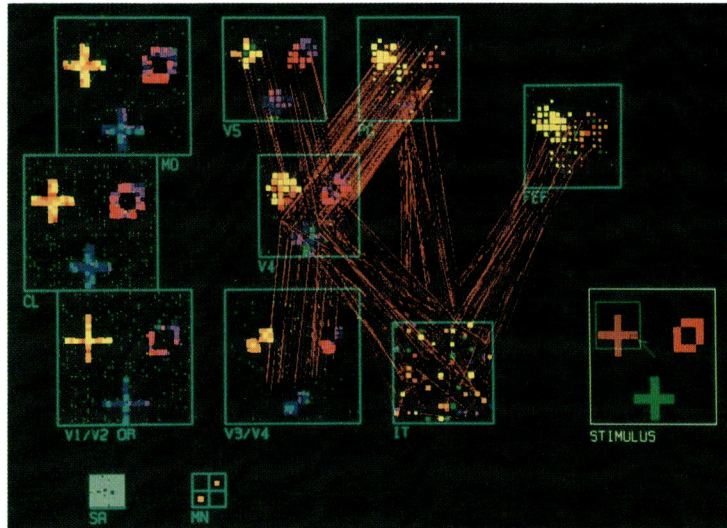

Plate 1 Responses of a model of primate visual cortex to various stimuli (final response pattern). Boxes stand for simulated visual areas and colored dots within the boxes, for neuronal groups. The size of each symbol codes for the activity level of the group, and color codes for the precise time of maximum discharge. Thus, units with identical or similar colors are correlated with zero time lag, and units with different colors are uncorrelated. Displayed are activity and correlation patterns after conditioning using a red cross as the reinforced object and during the presentation of three objects, a red cross, a red square, and a green cross. Units responding to the same object are correlated both within and between (topographic or nontopographic) areas. The three cohorts corresponding to the three different objects are segregated. This correlational structure depends critically on the presence and anatomical pattern of reentrant connections. About 5% of the connections that have been strengthened during conditioning are shown superimposed in shades of red. Note that strengthened connections appear among areas *V5, PG, FEF, V4, V3/V4,* and *IT* and that there is no preference for a particular position within the visual field. As a result of cooperative interactions along reentrant connectivity, the model produces a foveation response toward the red cross (the square window with white borders representing the center of the fovea has moved to the upper left; see arrow). Reproduced with permission from Tononi *et al.* (1992b).

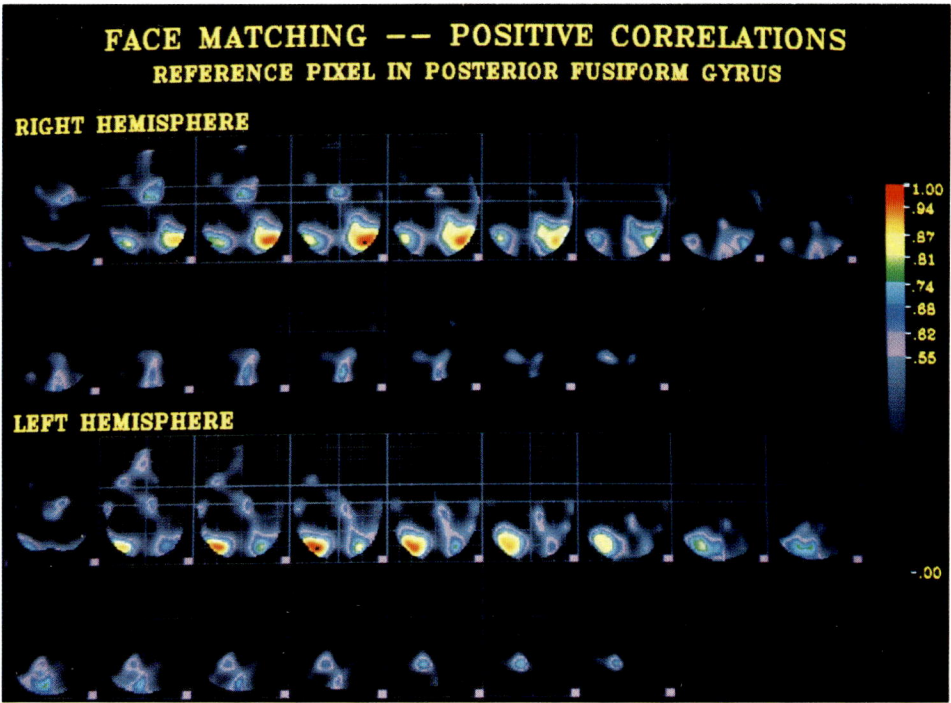

Plate 2 Axial PET slices showing all brain pixels whose normalized rCBF was significantly ($p<0.01$) and positively correlated with normalized rCBF of reference pixels in posterior fusiform gyrus (denoted by the black dots in the fourth slice from the left in the top line for each hemisphere) during face matching. Top, reference pixel in the right hemisphere with Talairach coordinates $x=34$ mm, $y=-78$ mm, and $z=-12$ mm; bottom, reference pixel in the left hemisphere with Talairach coordinates $x=-30$ mm, $y=-84$ mm, and $z=-12$ mm. The color scale represents the value of the correlation coefficient; the color of the square in the lower right corner of each slice indicates a significance level of $p<0.01$. In comparing corresponding slices when the reference pixels are in the right and left hemispheres, it is seen that the significant correlations extend more into anterior areas when the reference pixel is in the right hemisphere than when it is in the left.

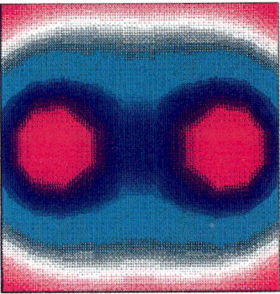

Condition 1

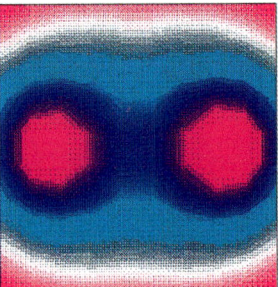

Condition 2

Plate 3 Multiple comparison permutation test. Example of the ability of the multiple comparison permutation test to identify which of the 100 electrodes differs between two conditions. Condition 1 is the voltage map generated by two mirror image dipoles in the left and right hemispheres (nose at top, left ear on left). Condition 2 was produced by increasing the magnitude of the left dipole 2% and decreasing the magnitude of the right dipole by the same amount. The maps are almost identical because of the small main effect. The difference map between the two conditions is shown in the middle, and paired *t* values are mapped on the right, with electrodes marked that were significantly different between the two conditions at the 0.05 level.

Magnitude Change 2%
Number Electrodes 100
Number Subjects   20

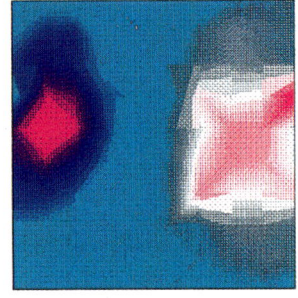 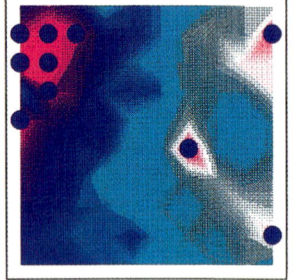

Difference   **T-values**

Global Tmax	T = 6.02, p < .0005
Bonferroni	T = 4.19, 7 elec
Holms/Hoch.	T = 4.16, 8 elec
Permutation,	T = 3.84, 10 elec

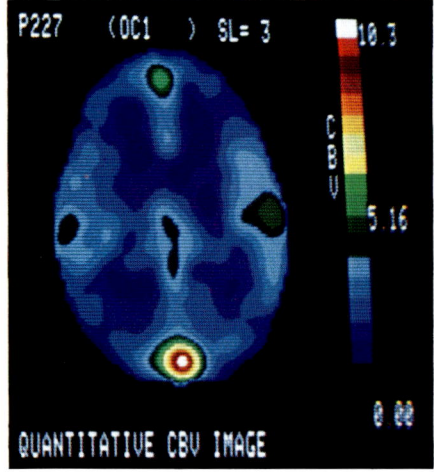

Plate 4 Quantitative image of rCBV measured with $C^{15}O$ administered by inhalation. The superior sagittal sinus is seen posteriorly, and differences in vascular density between gray and white matter are delineated. This image and those in subsequent figures were obtained with a PETT VI tomograph (Ter-Pogossian *et al.*, 1982) in a normal human subject. These are horizontal slices at the level of the thalamus, oriented such that anterior is up and left is to the reader's left.

Plate 5 Measurement of rCBF with bolus intravenous injection of $H_2^{15}O$ and the PET/autoradiographic method. The image on the left is of tissue counts (arbitrary units) accumulated during a 40-s scan following arrival of the tracer bolus in the head. The quantitative rCBF image on the right was obtained by applying Eq. (8) to the tissue count image. Because of the near linear relation between rCBF and tissue counts, the two images are very similar so that the image of tissue counts reflects regional differences in rCBF.

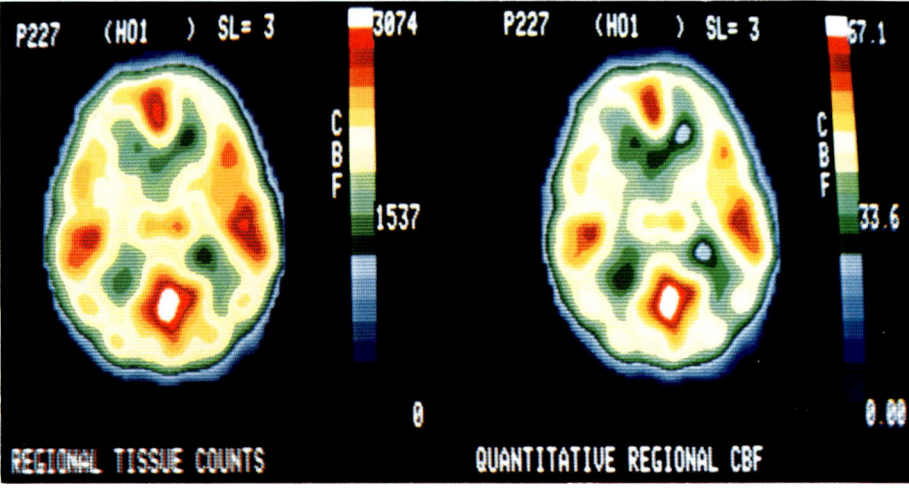

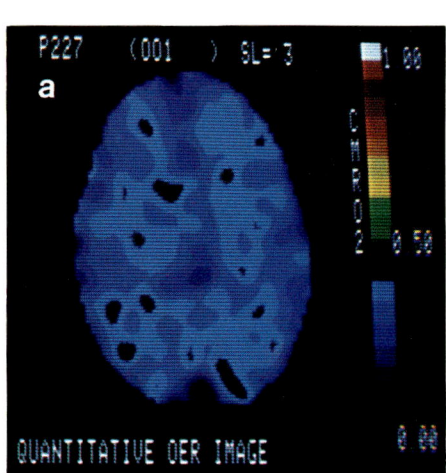
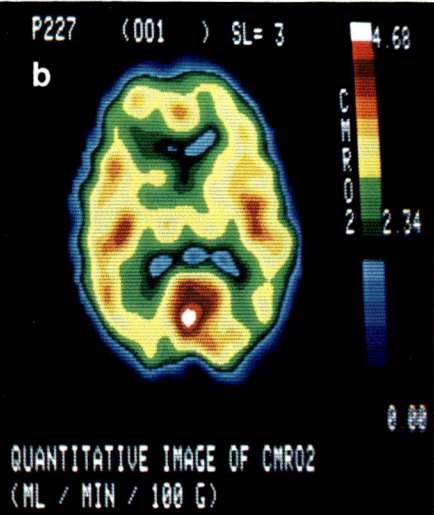

Plate 6 (a) Image of cerebral oxygen extraction fraction (rOEF) calculated from scan data obtained following the brief inhalation of $^{15}O_2$ as well as from the CBV and CBF images, according to the equation shown in Fig. 4. Note that the rOEF image is relatively uniform throughout the brain because oxygen metabolism and blood flow are matched throughout the brain in the resting state. (b) Image of the cerebral metabolic rate for oxygen (rCMRO$_2$). This is calculated from the product of OEF, CBF, and the arterial oxygen content.

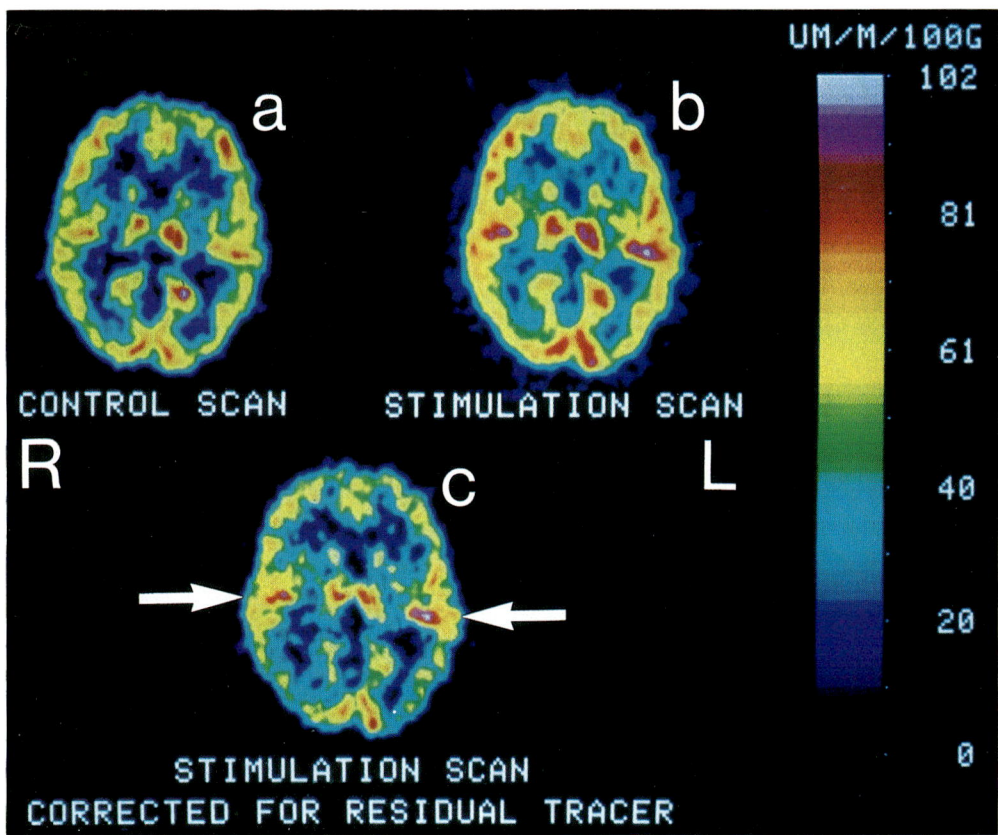

Plate 7 Symmetric activation in the primary auditory cortices (arrows) by monaural stimulation in a left-sided deaf patient. The bottom image (c) was obtained by subtracting the control image (a) times a constant factor from the image taken during the stimulation image (b).

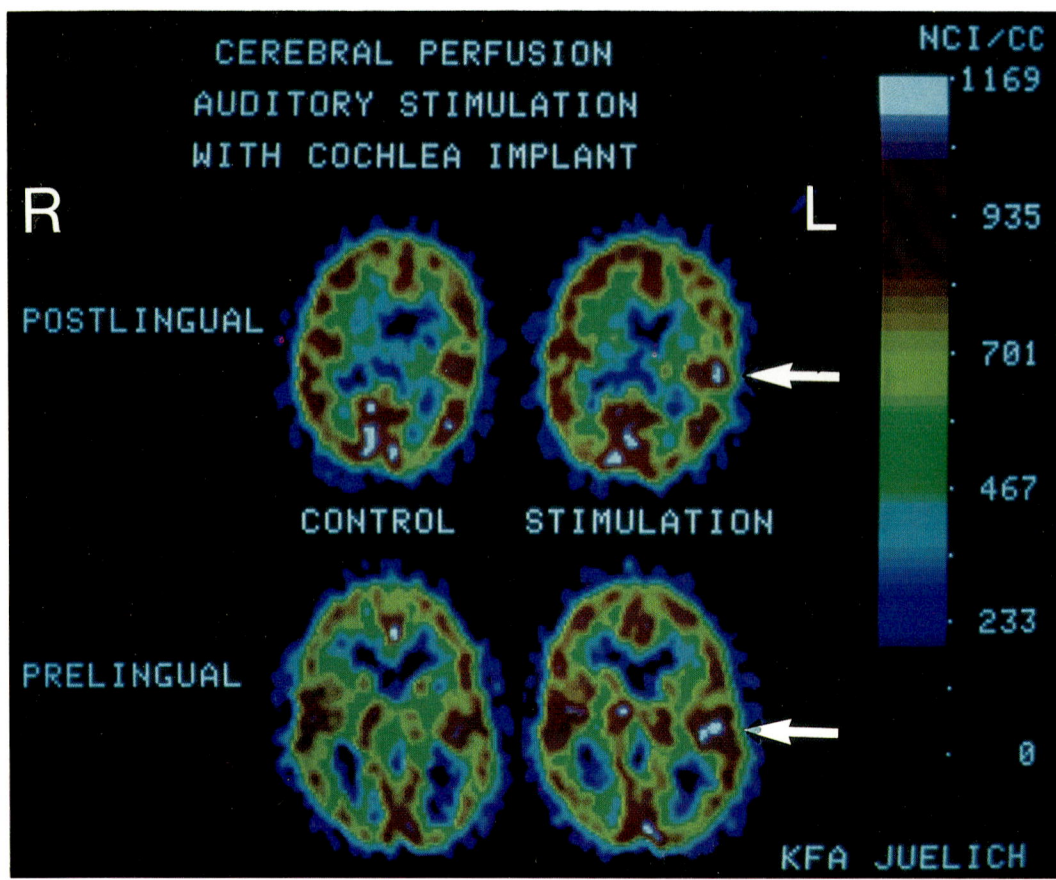

Plate 8 Using images of $H_2{}^{15}O$ activity, neuronal activation during cochlear implant stimulation is demonstrated in the auditory cortex (arrows) in a postlingually as well as in a prelingually deaf patient. In the postlingually deaf patient the implant was on the right side, and in the prelingually deaf patient it was on the left side.

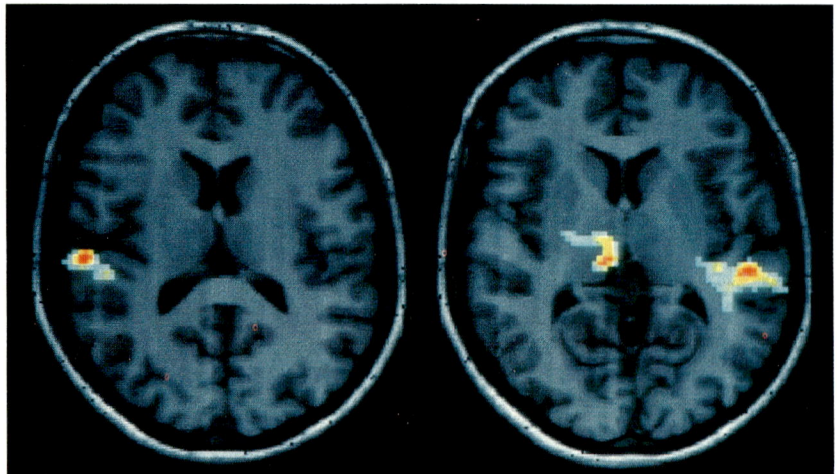

Plate 9 Integrated MRI/PET images with areas of high blood flow caused by binaural word stimulation in a normal volunteer. These areas located in the primary auditory cortex and the thalamus indicate significant neuronal activations as defined in a difference image between stimulation and rest.

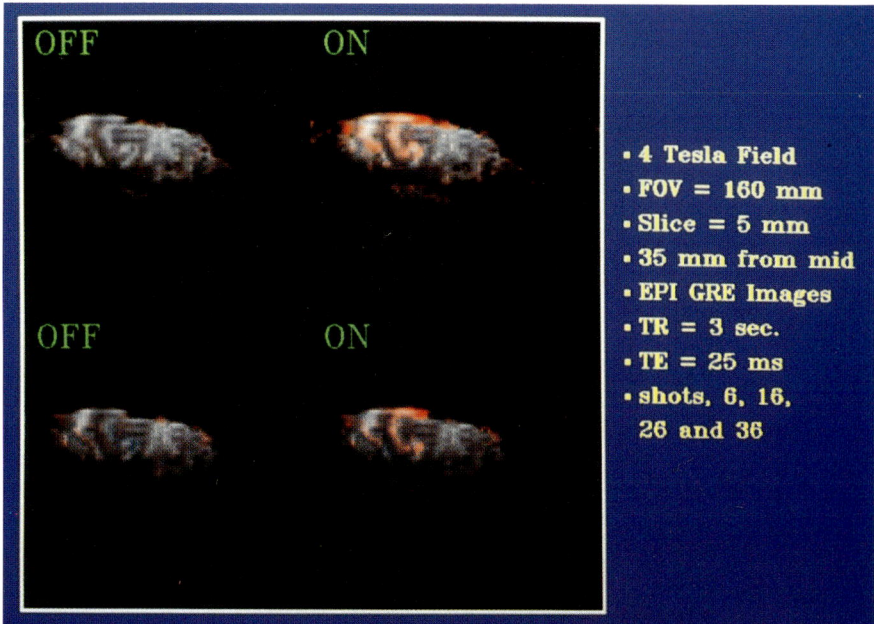

Plate 10 EPI parasagittal views at a magnetic field of 4 T of the hand representation areas around the central sulcus in a human volunteer. The posterior direction is to the left. Images were obtained using an rf surface coil to improve the signal-to-noise ratio and to restrict the field of view. The spatial resolution is 2. 5 mm in plane, the slice thickness is 5 mm, and each image was acquired in 45 ms. The volunteer was asked to tap each finger sequentially to the thumb as quickly as possible, for periods of 30 s alternating with 30-s rest periods. Sixty-four EPI images were obtained at 3-s intervals while this task was performed. For selected images, the image differences from the mean of rest images are shown superimposed in varying intensities of red on a rest image obtained at the beginning of the set. White matter appears dark and sulci appear bright with the image acquisition parameters used. Note the prominent central sulcus in the center of the image, which contains much of the hand representation motor cortex.

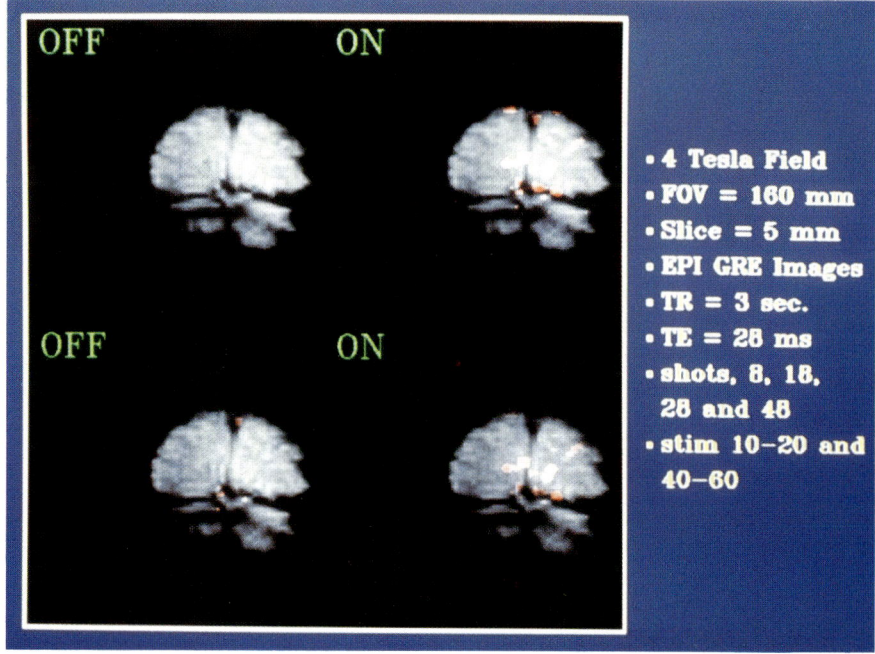

Plate 11 Coronal EPI images at 4 T through the occipital lobe of the brain of a normal volunteer. As in Plate 10, difference images have been overlaid in color on a gray scale rest image. Photic stimulation was produced as in Fig. 4 by means of binocular goggles fitted with LEDs. Note the large image changes in the primary V1 cortex in the calcarine sulcus, and the additional activation in a more superior lateral location.

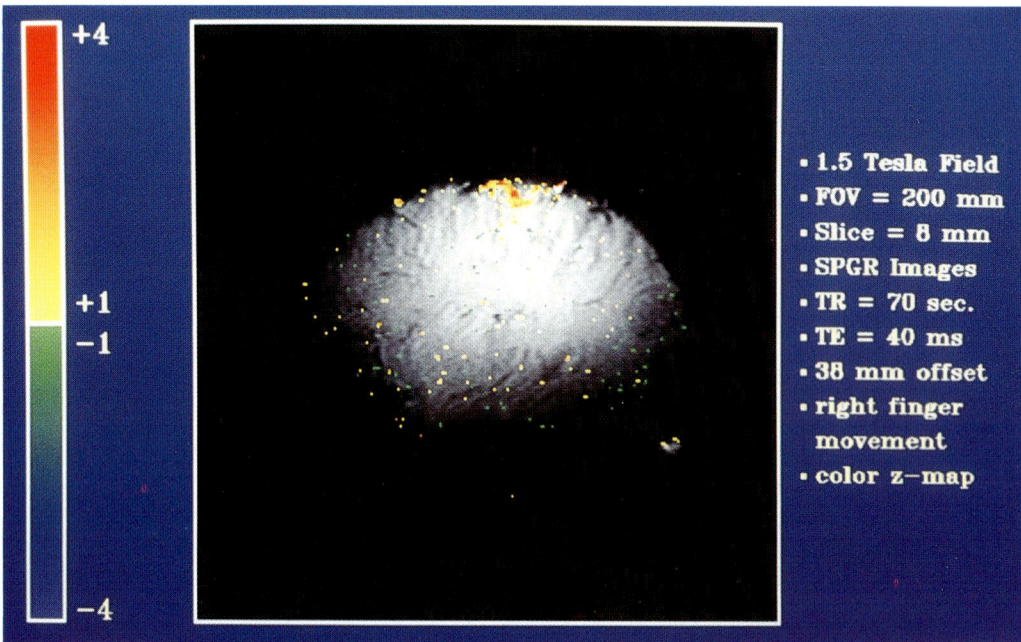

Plate 12 Spoiled grass (SPGR) imaging of response in the hand representation of a normal volunteer to the hand motor task described in the caption for Plate 10. Each of 40 parasagittal source images took 7 s to acquire, with an rf pulse repetition time TR of 70 ms. The color overlay in this figure shows the mean difference image, between the activated and rest states, plotted in units of the standard deviation in each pixel during the resting state, the "z-map." This map is overlaid on a gray-scale source image. The maximum departure of any pixel during activation from the rest state is about 5%. Images were obtained with a conventional MRI sequence on a standard 1.5-T GE Signa system. The echo time was 40 ms, in-plane resolution, 1.6 mm, and slice thickness, 8 mm.

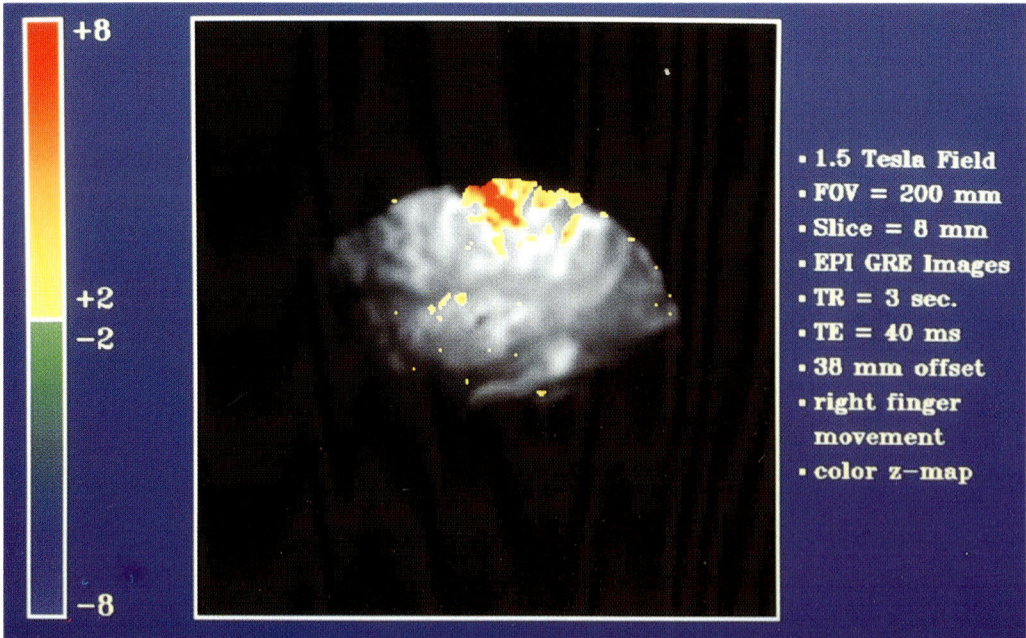

Plate 13 EPI imaging of the same subject performing the same task, during the same session, as that shown in Plate 12. The pixel resolution was 3.2 mm in plane, and the image acquisition time 80 ms, but the echo time, slice position, and slice thickness were identical to those of the previous figure. The mean difference image is again shown as a color overlay z-map. The improved SNR of the EPI data is manifested by the larger area of significant activation, and the higher values of z obtained at the focus of activation. Sixty-four images at 3-s intervals were obtained using a 1.5-T GE Signa MRI fitted with a special small gradient coil allowing acquisition of EPI images. The maximum image difference between activated and resting states was about 5%, as before.

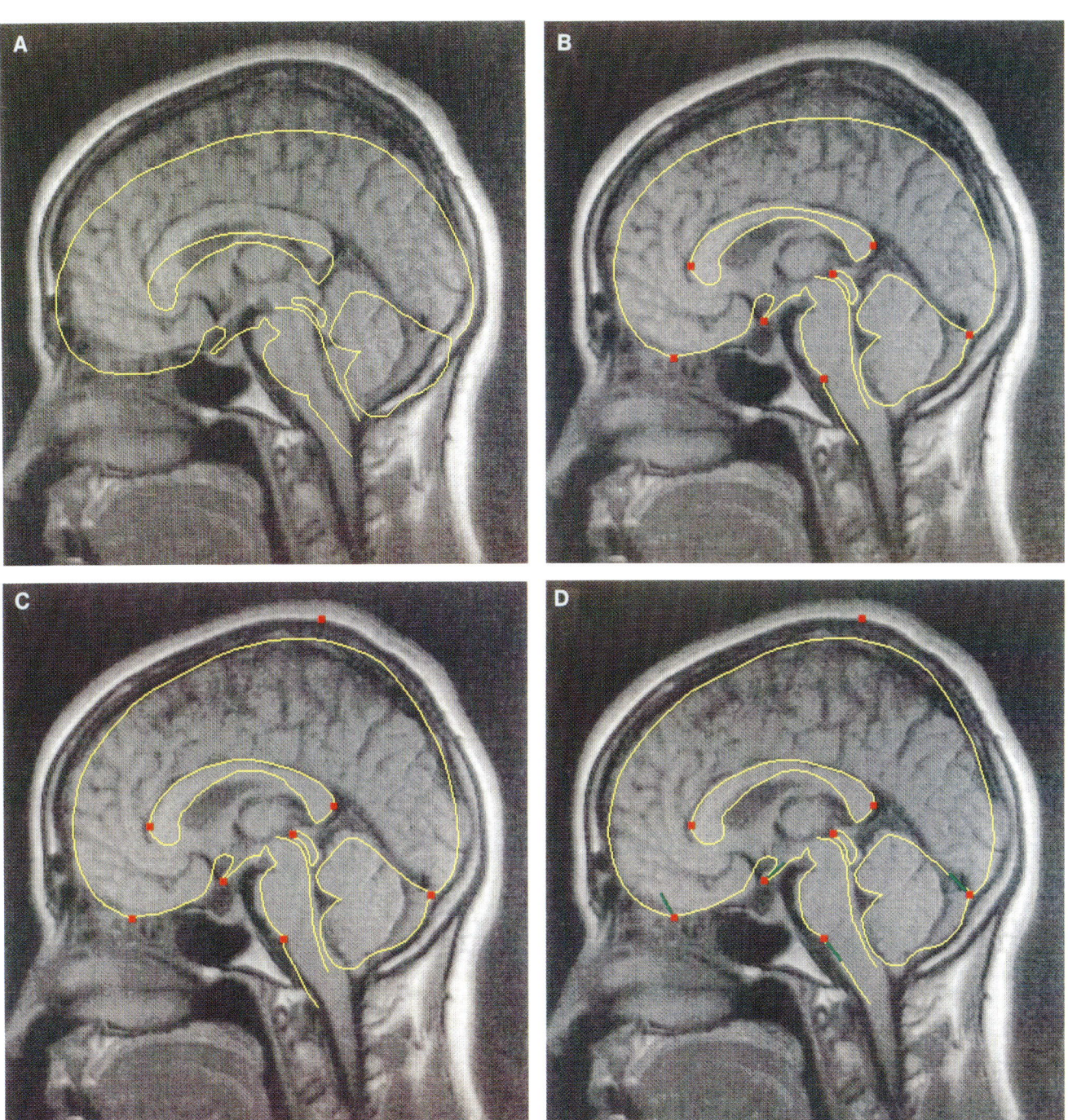

Plate 14 Digitizing images. (A) Start: arbitrary superposition of unwarped "average." (B) Eight-landmark fit, clearly missing the vault. (C) Better overlay using a new point at "vertex." (D) Improved fit, shearing the edgels indicated in Fig. 7D. (E) Equivalent deformation of Fig. 7D. (F) Another case, in which the splenium of the corpus callosum could not be located. (G) An average of 14 images unwarped in this wise is sharper than the images in Fig. 3 in the vicinity of the assigned edgels. Note that, even though the location of the vertex is mildly indeterminate, the average is sharp there. The frontal pole of the cortex apparently cannot be enregistered from these data.

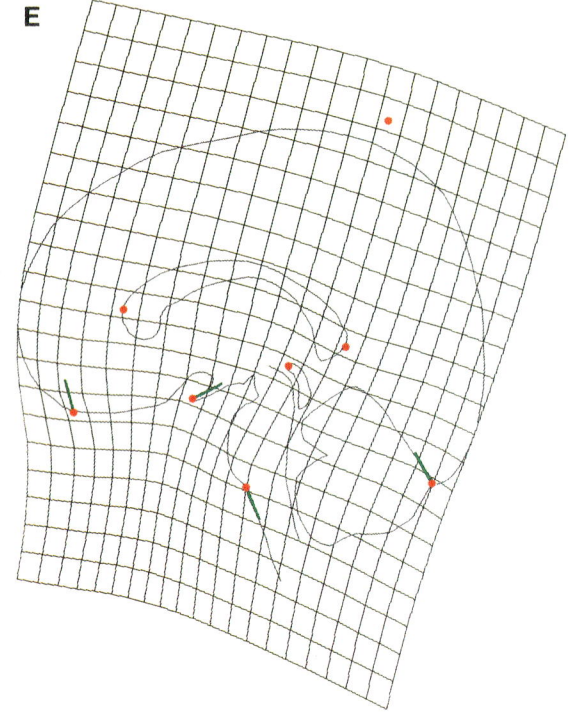

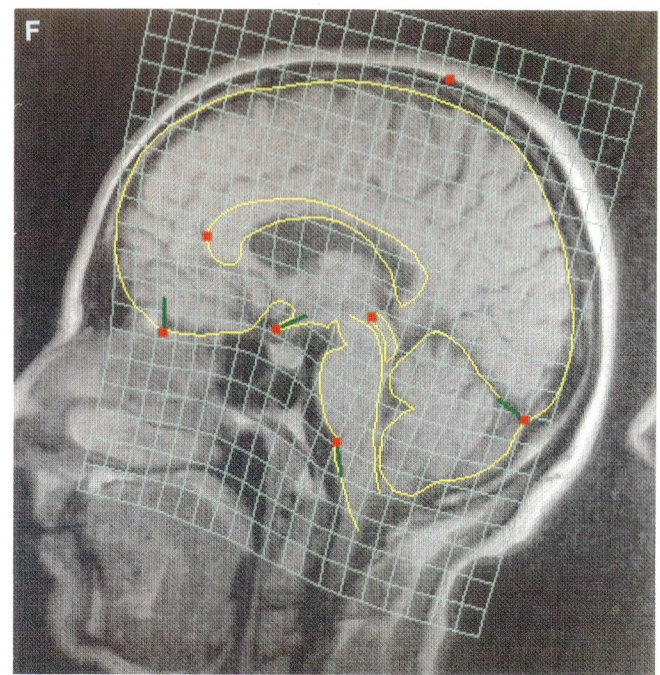

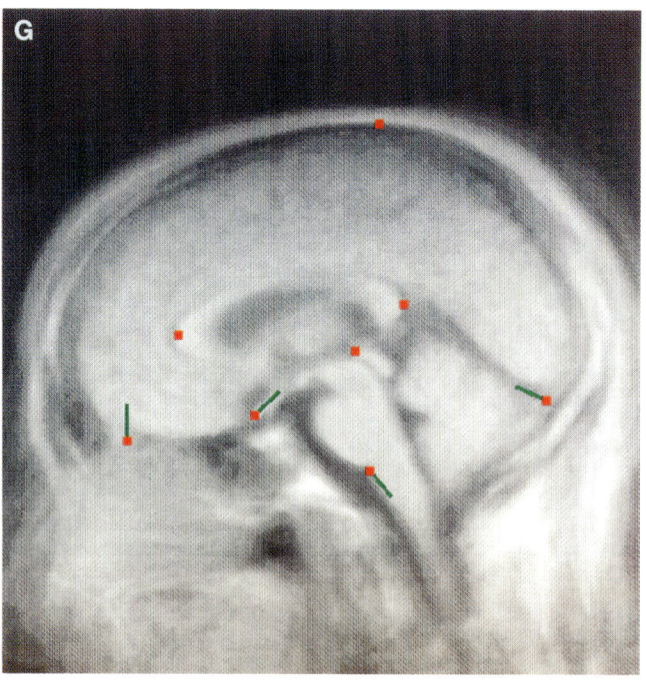

Plate 14 (*continued*)

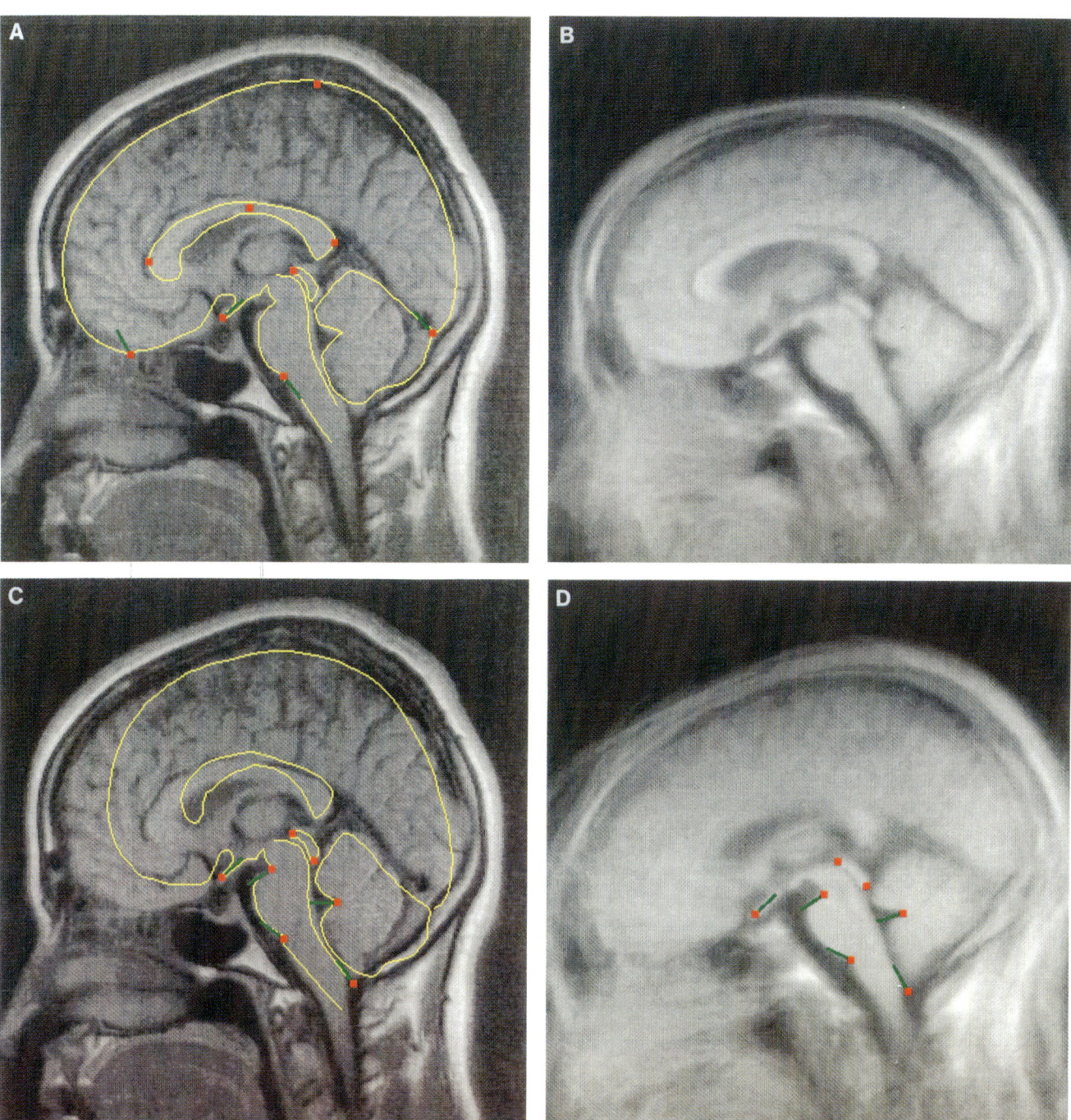

Plate 15 Extensions to improve the registration of specific organs. (A) Augmenting the scheme of Plate 14 by a point at the arch of corpus callosum. (B) Resulting average, sharper there than in Plate 14G. (C) Enriching the digitization of the pons and neighboring structures: additional edgels bisecting the angle of the fourth ventricle, aligning with the dorsocaudal margin of the brainstem, and tangent to the belly of the pons at its extrema. (D) The resulting averaged image, wildly out of alignment for distant cortical structures but much clearer for the pons per se. (E) A similar average ignoring the edgel information supplies less sharp contours. (F) Enriching the digitization of the cerebellum. An additional edgel is aligned with a striking sulcus. (G) Resulting averaged image. Dense local digitizing schemes like these may prove suitable for accumulating the archives of the neural circuitry database at the level of individual organs.

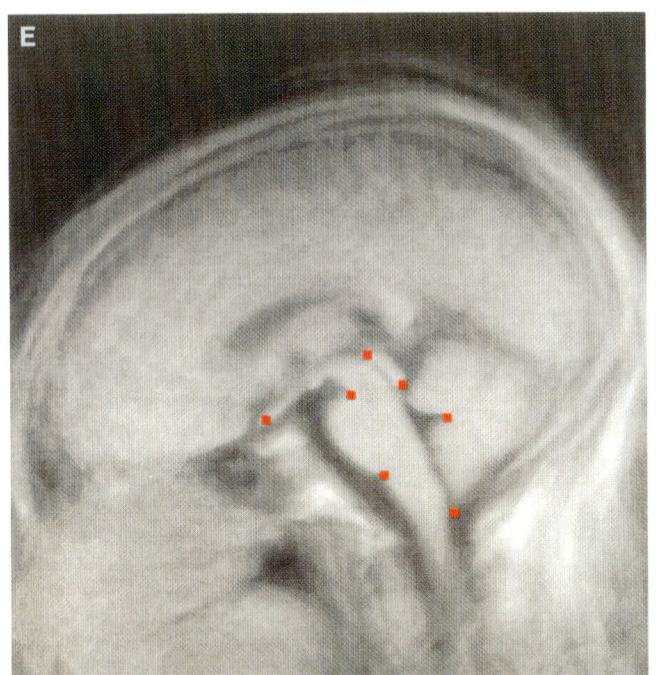

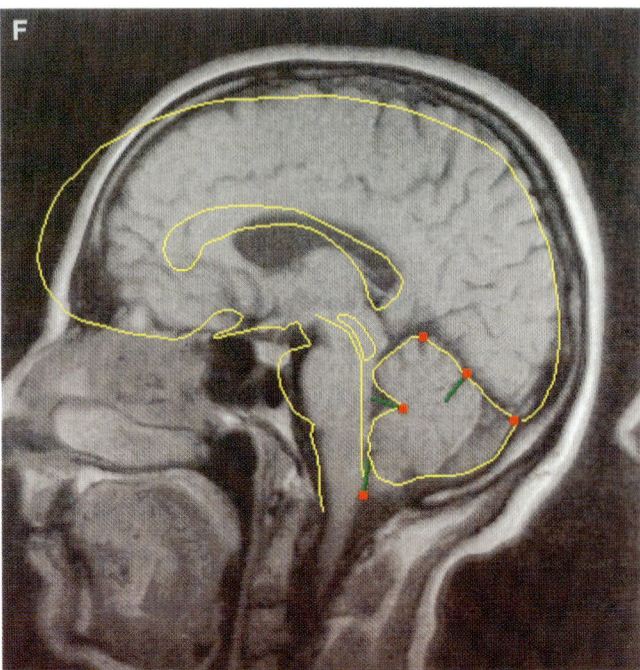

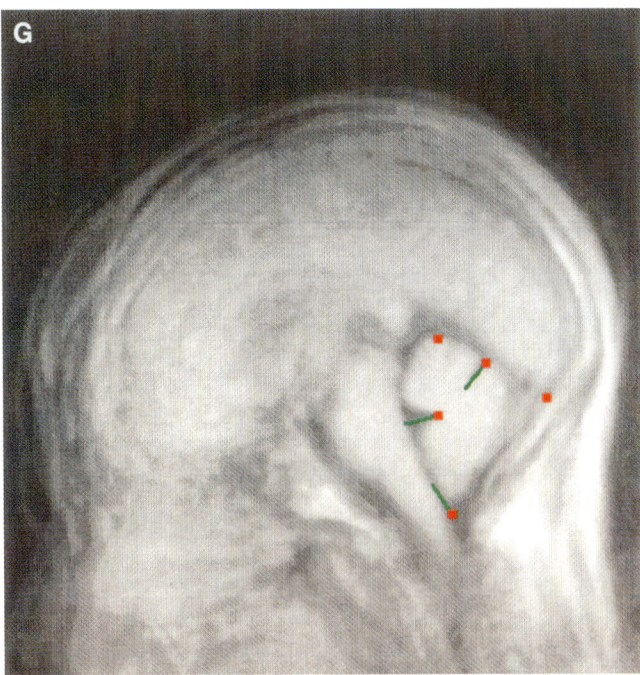

Plate 15 (*continued*)

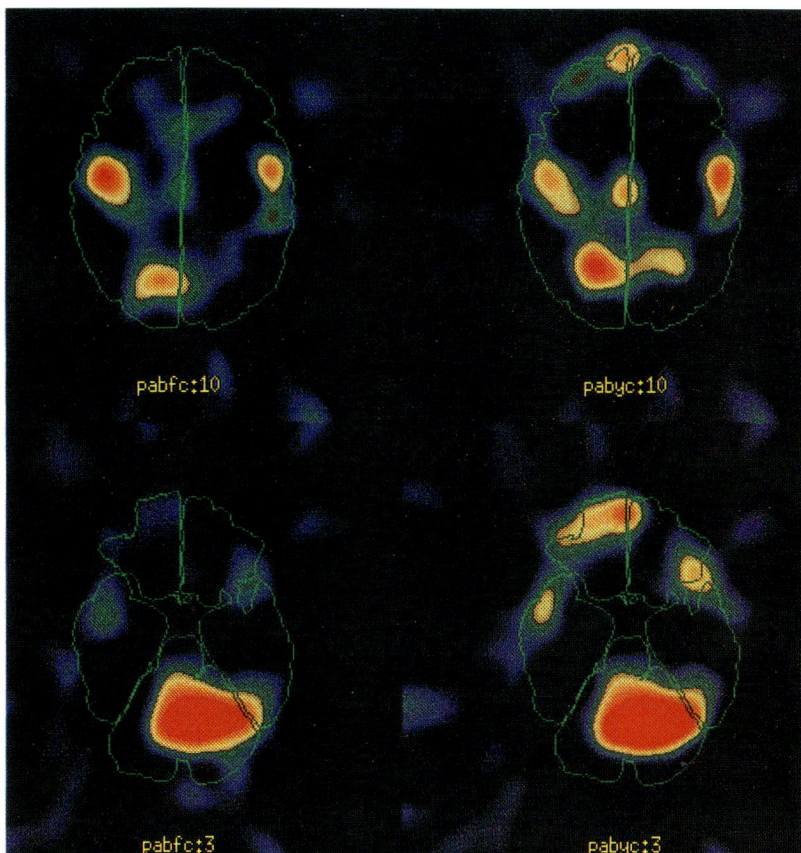

pabfc:10   pabyc:10

pabfc:3   pabyc:3

Plate 16 A demonstration of the importance of proper alignment of the images when performing comparisons with subtraction technique. The images represent an intraindividual subtraction between two images reading aloud and two reading silently and for which CBF has been measured with [^{15}O]butanol. A plane at the level of the cerebellum (lower row) and a plane at the level of the representation of the motor component of speech production (upper row) are shown. To the left, a proper alignment through the studies demonstrates areas of true activation, whereas in the right column one of the four images has been intentionally shifted by three pixels (7 mm). Prominent alias phenomena occur. A good fixation of the head during the study will secure a proper image alignment. From Ingvar *et al.* (1993).

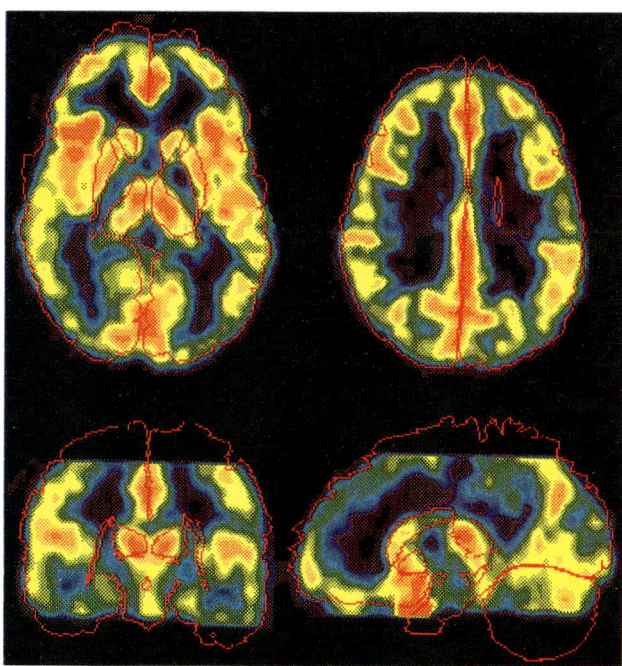

Plate 17 With good-quality functional images, it is possible to fit the CBA directly, especially when no gross structural disturbances are present. The CBA matching procedure can be performed by fitting the brain surface, ventricles, basal ganglia, and thalamus. This image represents an intraindividual summation image of seven measurements of cerebral blood flow.

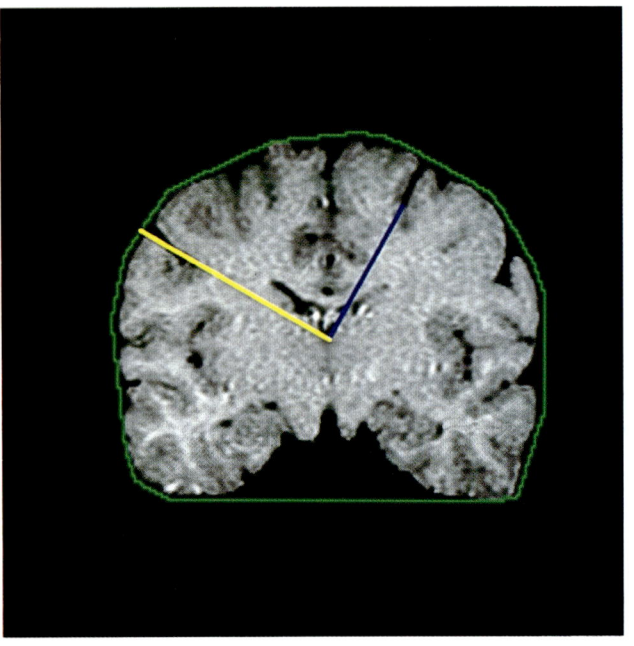

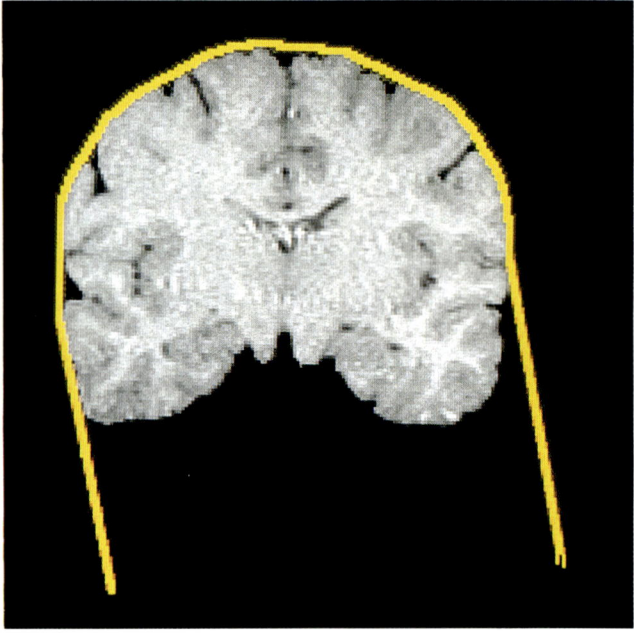

Plate 18 Basis for scaling. The blue line indicates the radial distance from the y axis to the valley of a sulcus. The yellow line represents the radial distance from the y axis to the convex hull, which avoids scaling to the underlying sulcus.

Plate 19 Convex hull generation in 2D. Illustration of a string wrapping the brain surface to create a convex hull.

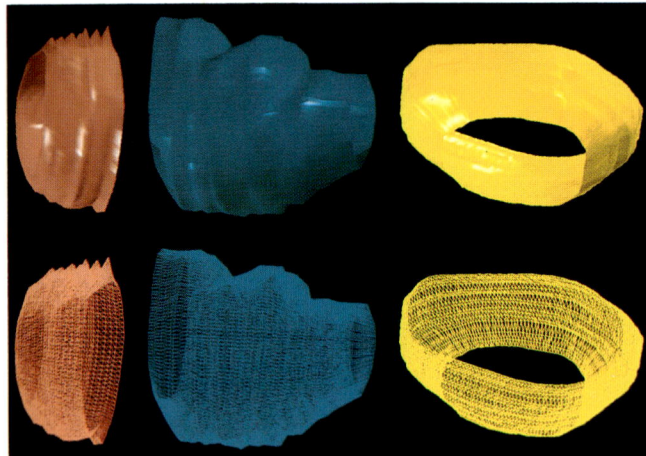

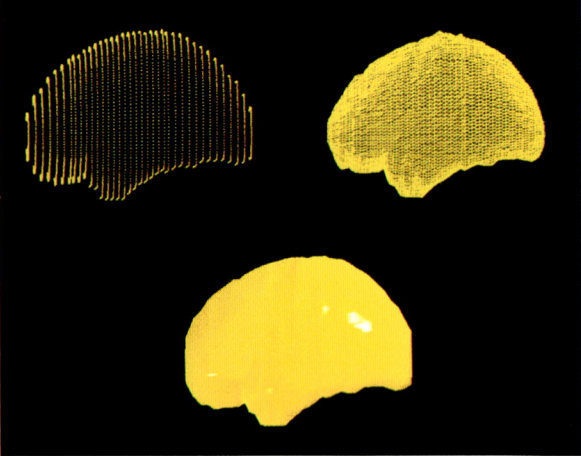

Plate 20 Convex hulls generated from the older Talairach atlas. Left, axial data; middle, coronal data; right, sagittal data. The upper row illustrates the wire frames of the convex hulls. The lower row illustrates the shaded surfaces of the convex hulls.

Plate 21 Convex hull generated from the newer Talairach atlas. Left upper, points used to generate the convex hull; right upper, wire frame of the convex hull; lower, shaded surface of the convex hull.

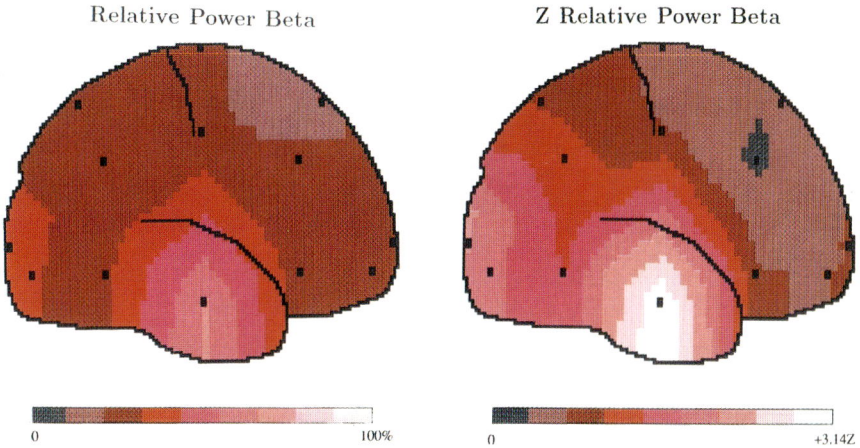

Relative Power Beta   Z Relative Power Beta

0   100%   0   +3.14Z

Plate 22 Right-hemisphere topographic QEEG maps obtained shortly after an infarct of the anterior temporal branch of the right anterior cerebral artery (Pt. No. 20006). Left, relative percentage power in the β frequency band; right, same data as above after Z transformation of relative β power.

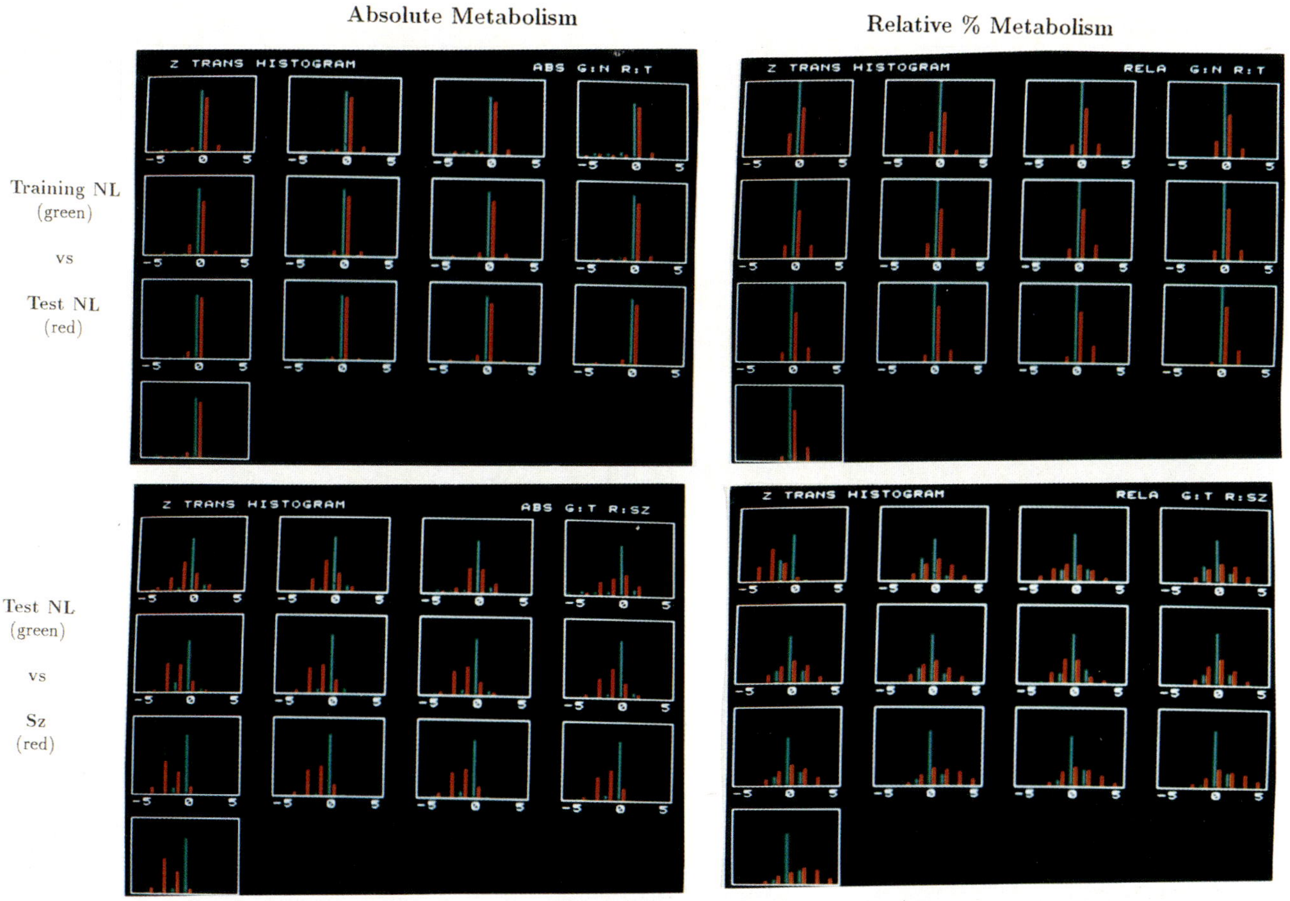

Absolute Metabolism   Relative % Metabolism

Training NL
(green)

vs

Test NL
(red)

Test NL
(green)

vs

Sz
(red)

Plate 23 Histograms of pixel Z scores for slice 2 (top row, left) through slice 14 (bottom row, left), showing the distribution of Z scores across a training group (N) of 25 normals used to establish normative pixel values, a test group (T) of 15 normals used to confirm the adequacy of the norms, and a group of 45 nonmedicated chronic schizophrenic patients (Sz). Top row, distribution of pixel Z scores for the training group (green) and test group (red), with absolute metabolism on the left and relative metabolism on the right; bottom row, distribution of pixel Z scores for the test group (green) and the schizophrenic patients (red), with absolute metabolism on the left and relative metabolism on the right.

Absolute Metabolism   Relative % Metabolism

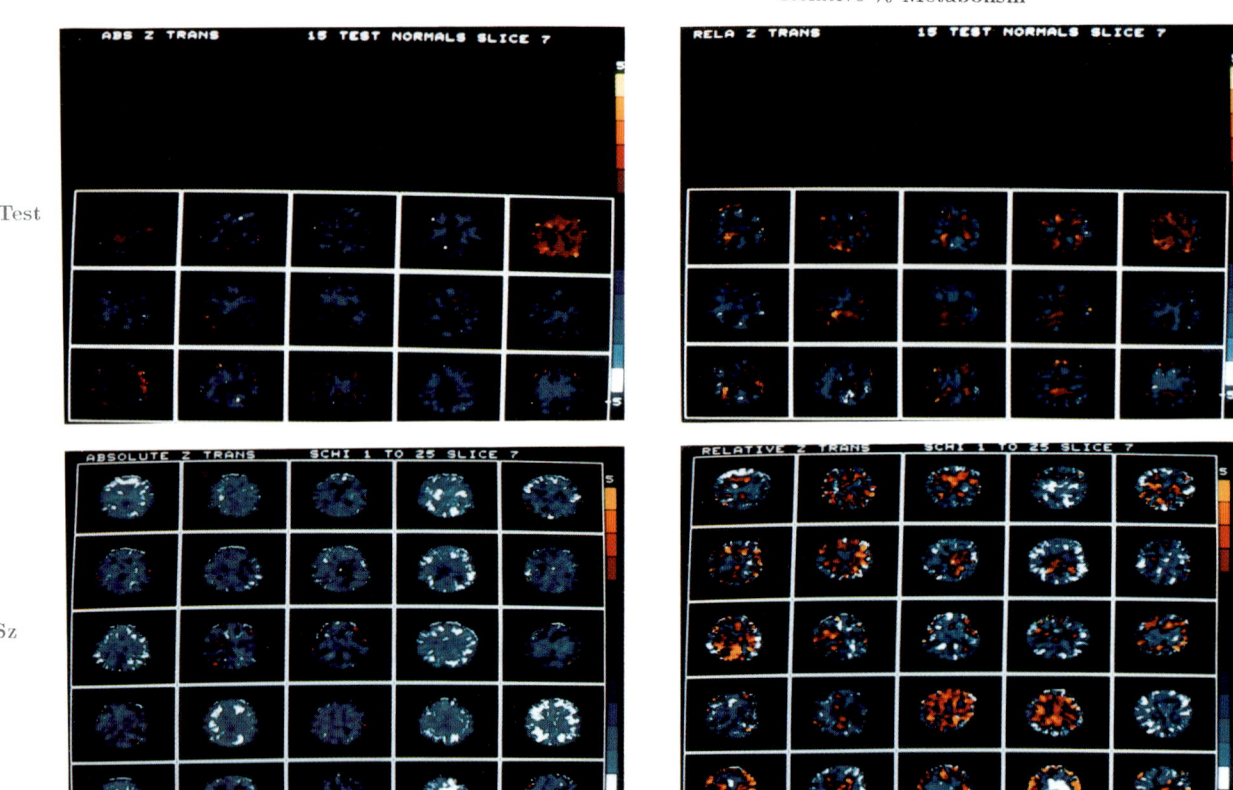

Plate 24 SPI of slice 7. Top row, SPI for 15 members of the test group of normals, with absolute metabolism on the left and relative metabolism on the right; bottom row, SPI for 25 of the group of 45 nonmedicated schizophrenics, with absolute metabolism on the left and relative metabolism on the right.

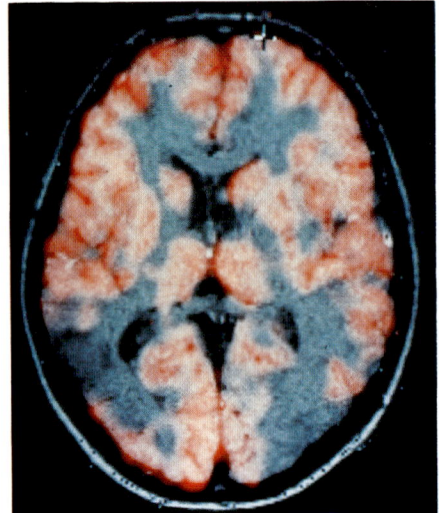

Plate 25 Merged MRI/PET (FDG) for bilateral occipital ischemia. The bilateral hypometabolism shown by PET is evident only on the MRI as a unilateral lesion. From Evans *et al.* (1992b).

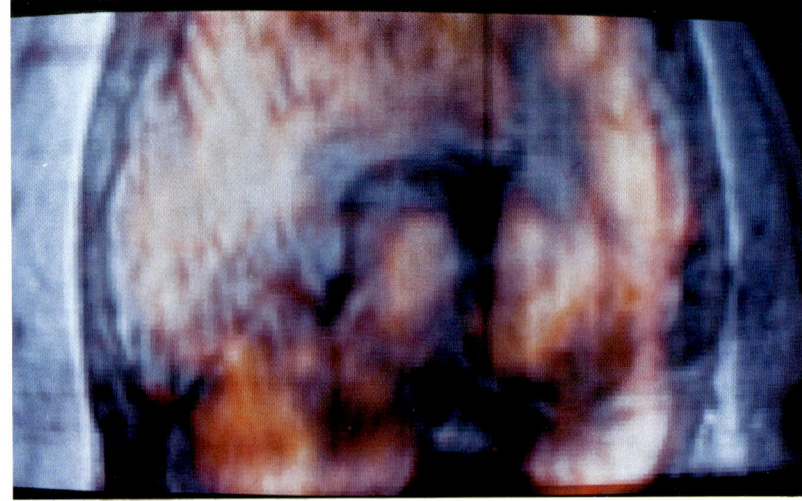

Plate 26 Merged MRI/PET dataset using 3D volume rendering for each dataset before opacity-weighted compositing. From Evans *et al.* (1991a). A 3D sector was first removed before rendering. The PET data show glucose metabolism from an FDG scan.

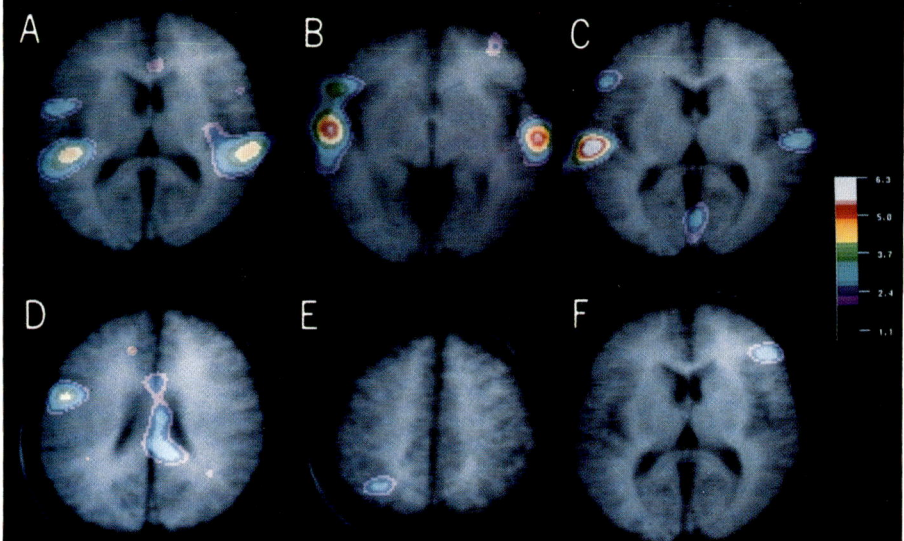

Plate 27 A series of merged MRI/PET datasets illustrating auditory processing, identified by local blood flow changes, in an average of 10 subjects. In B–E monosyllabic word pairs were presented to normal subjects. Images shown illustrate the response to bursts of noise frequency-matched to the word pairs (A); two cuts through the data obtained when the word pairs were presented (B and C); two cuts obtained when the subjects were asked to identify a change in final consonant (D and E); and one cut when they were asked to identify a change in pitch between the two words (F). Results show a lateralization of higher auditory processing. From Zatorre *et al.* (1992a).

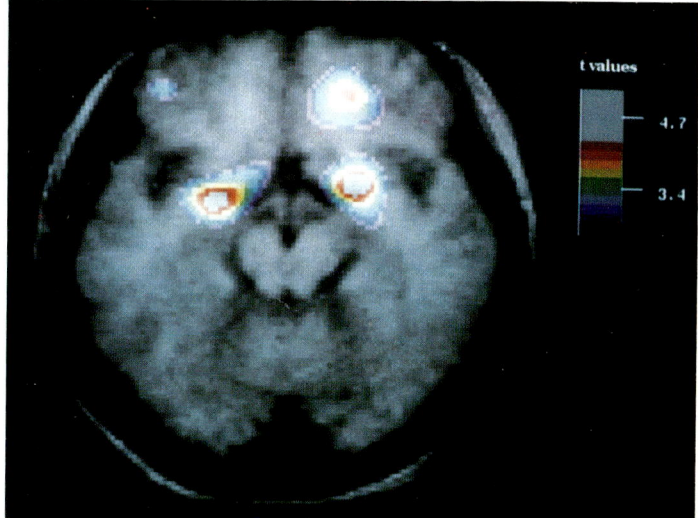

Plate 28 Olfactory processing shown in an average MRI/PET dataset obtained in 10 subjects. The images show the regions activated by strong olfactory stimulation. From Zatorre *et al.* (1992b).

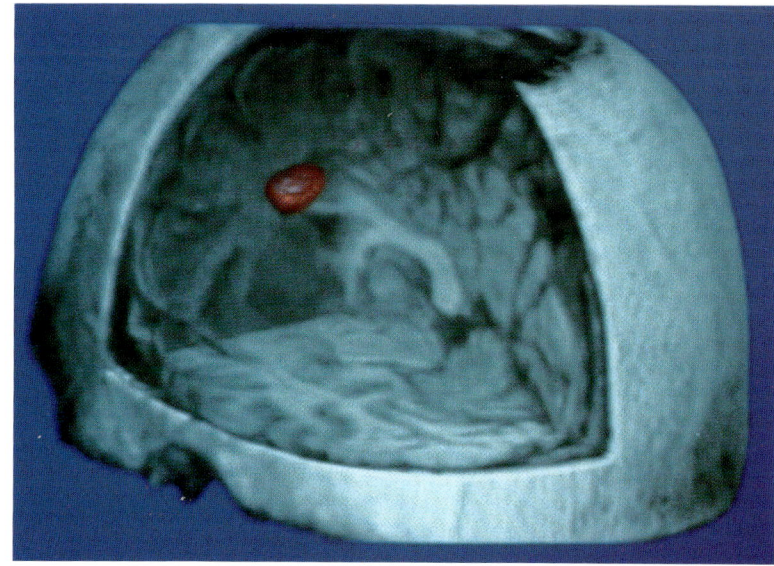

Plate 29 Gradient-enhanced volume rendering of MRI following removal of a 3D sector to expose a PET activation focus in the anterior cingulate gyrus. The focus was one of four identified in response to a painful stimulus. From Talbot *et al.* (1991).

Plate 30 Merged MRI and PET datasets showing extrastriate cortex activation during a visual stimulation task. The baseline condition, passively viewing a fixation cross on a monitor, and the activation condition, passively viewing complex line drawings of animals, both activated primary visual cortex. The changes observed bilaterally in associated visual cortex reflect processing of the complex line segments.

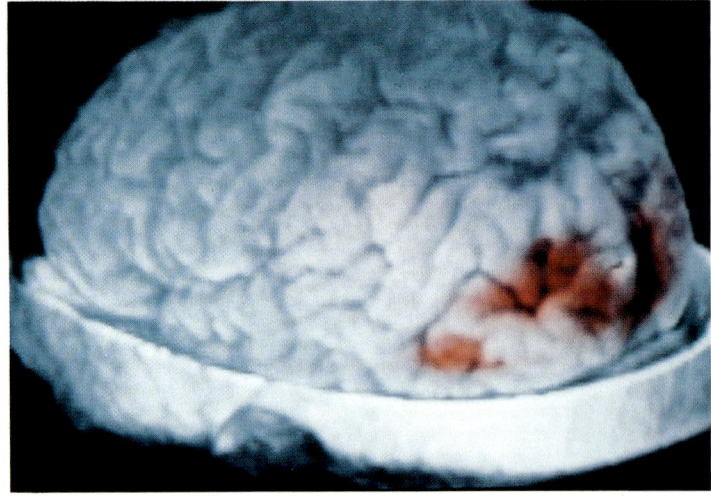

Plate 31 Interactive 3D interface for comparing activation data obtained from different experiments and stored as stereotactic coordinates. On the left, a 3D vector representation of the stereotactic VOI atlas can be manipulated in real time. Specific regional VOIs can be turned on and off at will. Focal activation coordinates are displayed as colored dots within the atlas. On the right, a triplane display shows orthogonal cuts through a raster image at any 3D point (shown as a cross) in stereotactic space. The image shown is the 305-brain composite, but any 3D image is allowed. The interface allows the user to jump to any focus in both vector and raster representations or to move a cursor around in real time. The three foci shown on the left are from the olfactory experiment illustrated in Plate 28. Two foci appear as red dots; the third appears as a white dot and is the currently active focus being plotted in the triplane display.

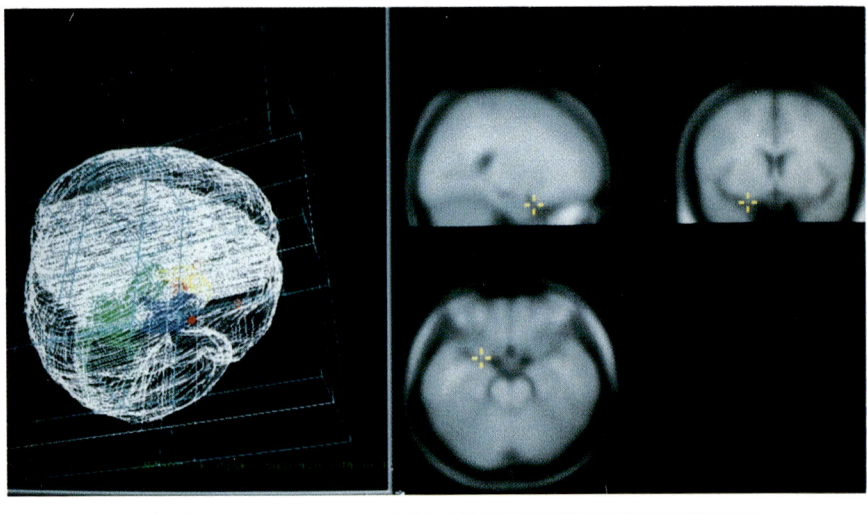

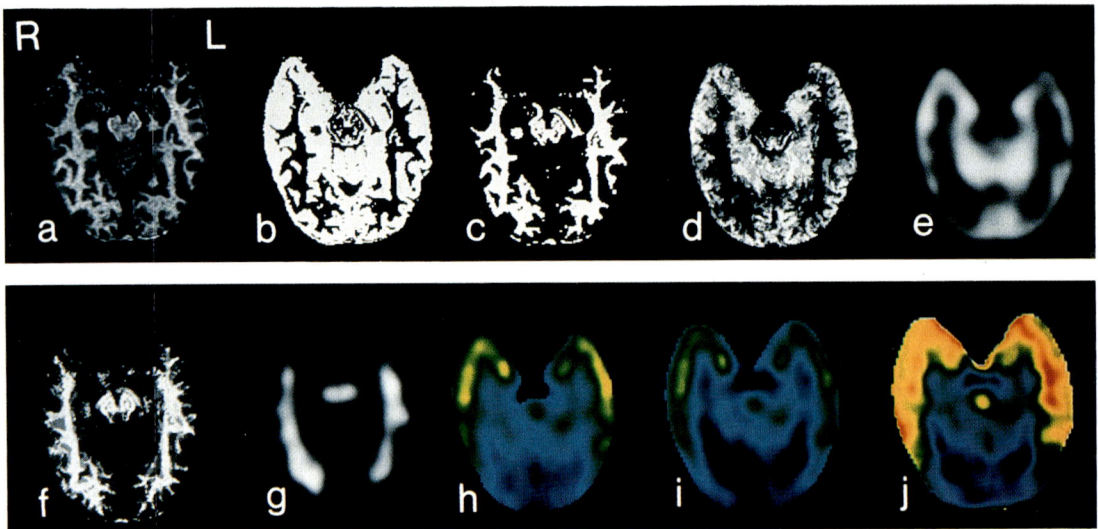

Plate 32 GM PET of μ opiate receptors in a patient with left-sided temporal lobe epilepsy using [^{11}C]carfentanil. Values in h–j are displayed to the same scale. (a) T_1-Weighted spoiled grass (SPGR) MRI image. (b) Segmented gray matter image. (c) Segmented white matter image. (d) Summed segmented gray matter images. (e) Convolved segmented gray matter images. Note that the density of gray matter tissue in the left anterior temporal lobe is lower compared with that in the right side. (f) Summed segmented white matter images. (g) Convolved segmented white matter images. (h) Observed PET image. Symmetric distribution of [^{11}C]carfentanil binding to μ opiate receptors in temporal lobe. (i) PET image of the gray matter, obtained by subtracting the convolved weighted summed white matter image g from the observed PET image. (j) GM PET image. Result of dividing image i by image e. The image shows a global increase in the apparent tracer concentration. More importantly, [^{11}C]carfentanil binding to the left anterior temporal lobe is now higher when compared with that to the right anterior temporal lobe. Reprinted with permission from Raven Press, New York.

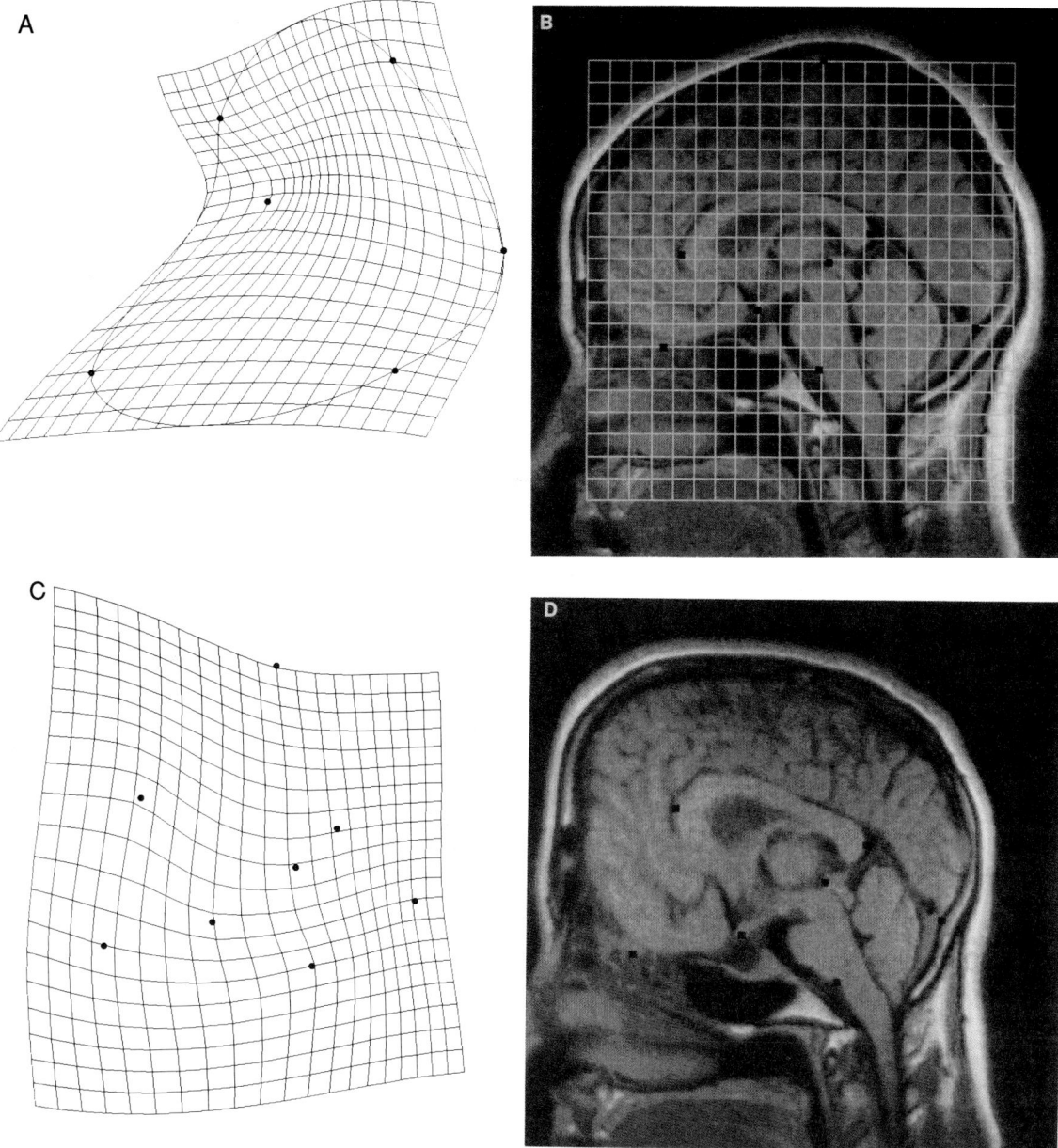

Figure 2 Warping other biological information along with landmarks. (A) Embedded information about outlines may be warped along with the landmarks. The landmarks need not be upon the outline. (Before deformation, this outline was a circle.) (B–D) Likewise, explicit pixel values may be carried along: (B) starting image with landmarks and grid; (C) grid transformation; (D) picture transformation (anatomically unrealistic, of course).

As plates, these maps have the *global minimum* of *bending energy*—summed squared second derivatives, integrated over all of R^2—of all surfaces of specified heights over specified locations of a base plane. As deformations, interpolating the homologous Cartesian coordinate in place of "height," they still minimize that integral, which is now interpreted as *information about localization of shape change* (variation of the affine derivative from point to point). In the vicinity of a mean form, bending energy is a quadratic form in the coordinates of the landmarks, supporting the extraction of energy-orthogonal modes of bending, the "principal warps," and likewise the "relative warps" orthogonal both in energy and in sample covariance.

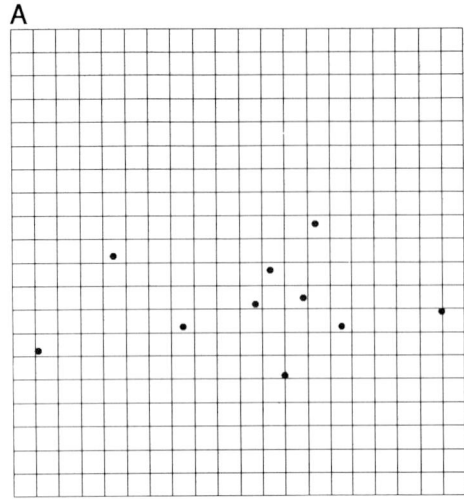

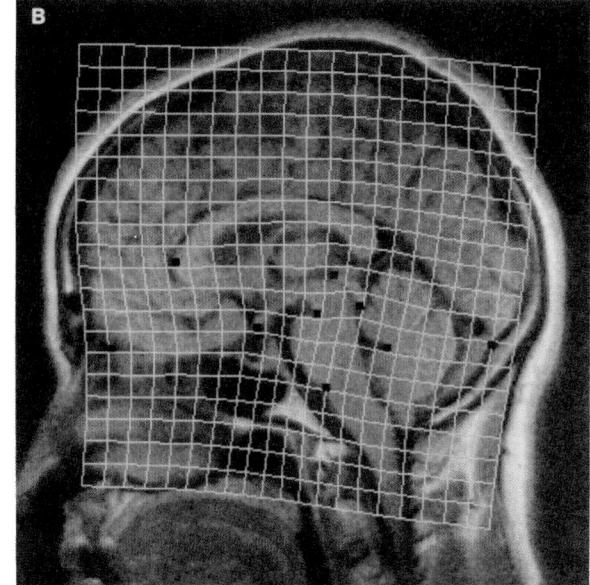

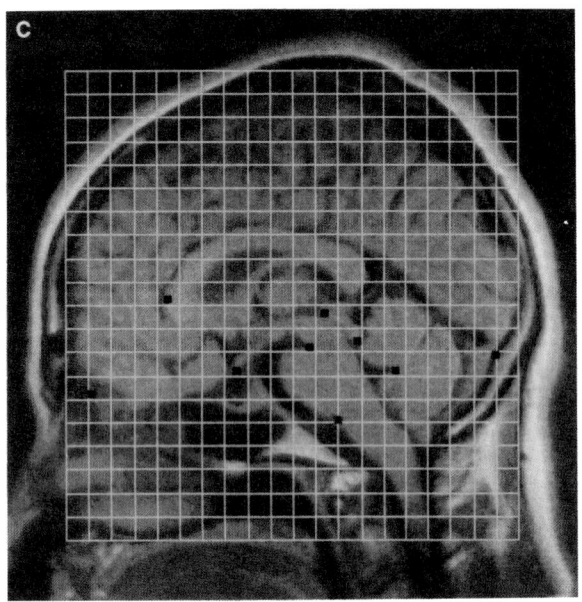

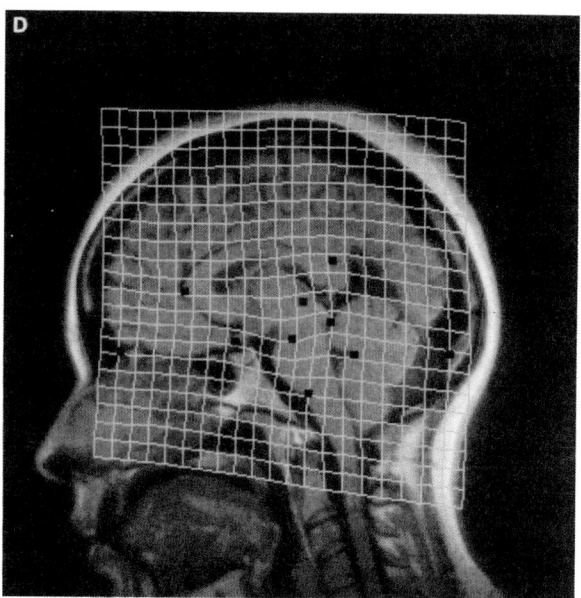

Figure 3 Construction of an averaged atlas by unwarping: ten landmarks. (A) Average of configurations of 10 landmarks over 14 normal midsagittal MRI scans (earlier computation), with a reference grid. Left to right, frontal pole of cortex, genu of corpus callosum, optic chiasm, top of pons, posterior commissure, bottom of pons, inferior colliculus, splenium of corpus callosum, tip of fourth ventricle, and posterior pole of cortex at tentorium. (B) Case DK1, with his landmarks and his deformation grid. (C) The corresponding unwarping. (D) Case ER3. (E) The corresponding unwarping. (F) Pixelwise average of all 14 unwarped images like C and E. (G) Whereas an average using only four landmarks preserves most of the large-scale information, our attention is inevitably drawn to the variability of edge sharpness even in the average using all 10.

cal structure of covariation and cross-prediction. Descriptions of image gradients, blobs, tracts, and the like are a combination of both languages, as the single image supplies information about both organ shape and organ location. The new morphometric methods make it possible to conceal all the details of this approach from the viewer of a visualization regardless of how much relevant spatial detail has been encoded.

The problem of image standardization itself is not new. The strategy of thin-plate splining that I shall review presently takes its place in a list of approaches that date from the Renaissance [see, for example, Dürer (1524)]. The most famous earlier declaration that biological shape ought to be measured as deformation is perhaps D'Arcy Thompson's "method of Cartesian transformations" (Thompson, 1917), but he

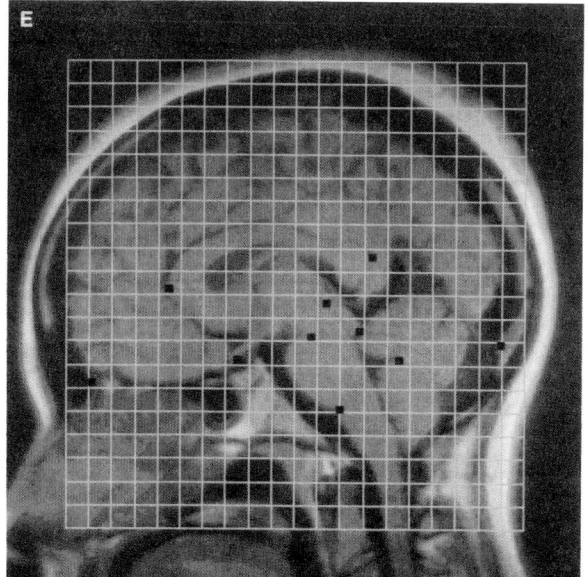

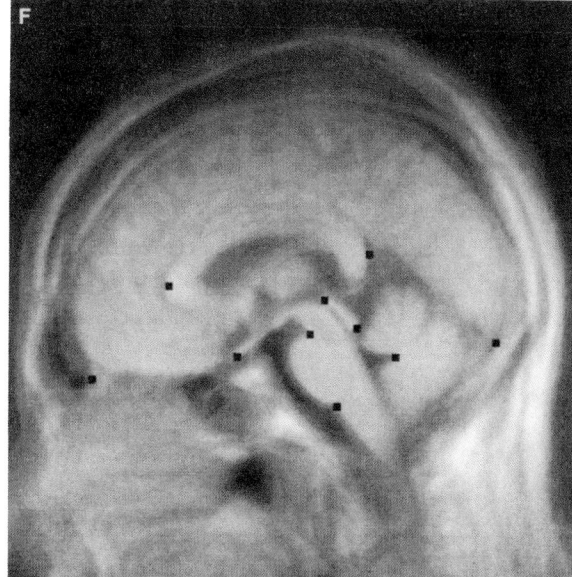

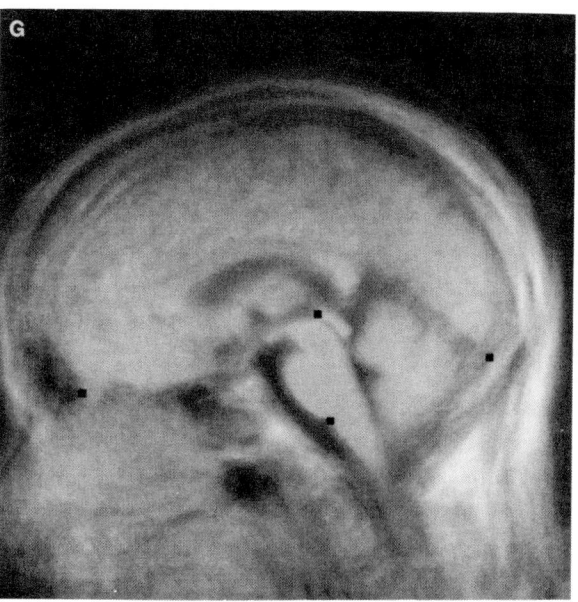

Figure 3   (*continued*)

had no particular insight into quantification. For a review of the vicissitudes of Thompson's insight in biomathematics, see Chapter 5 of Bookstein (1978). Analyses in Thompson's spirit have emphasized maps of arbitrary complexity (which accounts for the difficulty hitherto of actually reducing these sketches to quantity). Others have recommended simpler maps that, although algebraically tractable, are of limited flexibility: examples include Sneath (1967), Fox *et al.* (1985), and Greitz *et al.* (1991).

The fusion that I wish to review arose in the 1980s as a hybrid of two fields previously only distantly related. From image analysis, we have borrowed the idea of minimizing a generalized pictorial "energy" under constraints of fairly arbitrary form. Originally a surface interpolation technique (Duchon, 1975), the idea appears to have been discovered and generalized for image analysis by Terzopoulos (1983) and his students and colleagues. It has proven very fruitful for a great variety of applications, including several having nothing to do with our anatomical task at hand; some recent elaborations are assembled in Vemuri (1991). To these essentially graphical techniques for analyzing pictures two at a time, the morphometrician adds a concern with matters of variation, covariation, and averaging. Such techniques arise out of a quite different tradition, the main line of multivariate biometrical analysis running from Francis Galton (who discovered regression) through to the modern school of multivariate morphometrics. In this approach one could always describe the covariation of form with its causes and effects, but was often at a loss to say what those contrasts looked like: the biometrician, however efficient his approach to the finite-dimensional feature space of size and shape measurements, often lost sight of the form as a whole.

The two approaches—generalized "template matching" and generalized linear modeling of geometric features—were unified by the late 1980s in a surprisingly quick and peaceful methodological ad-

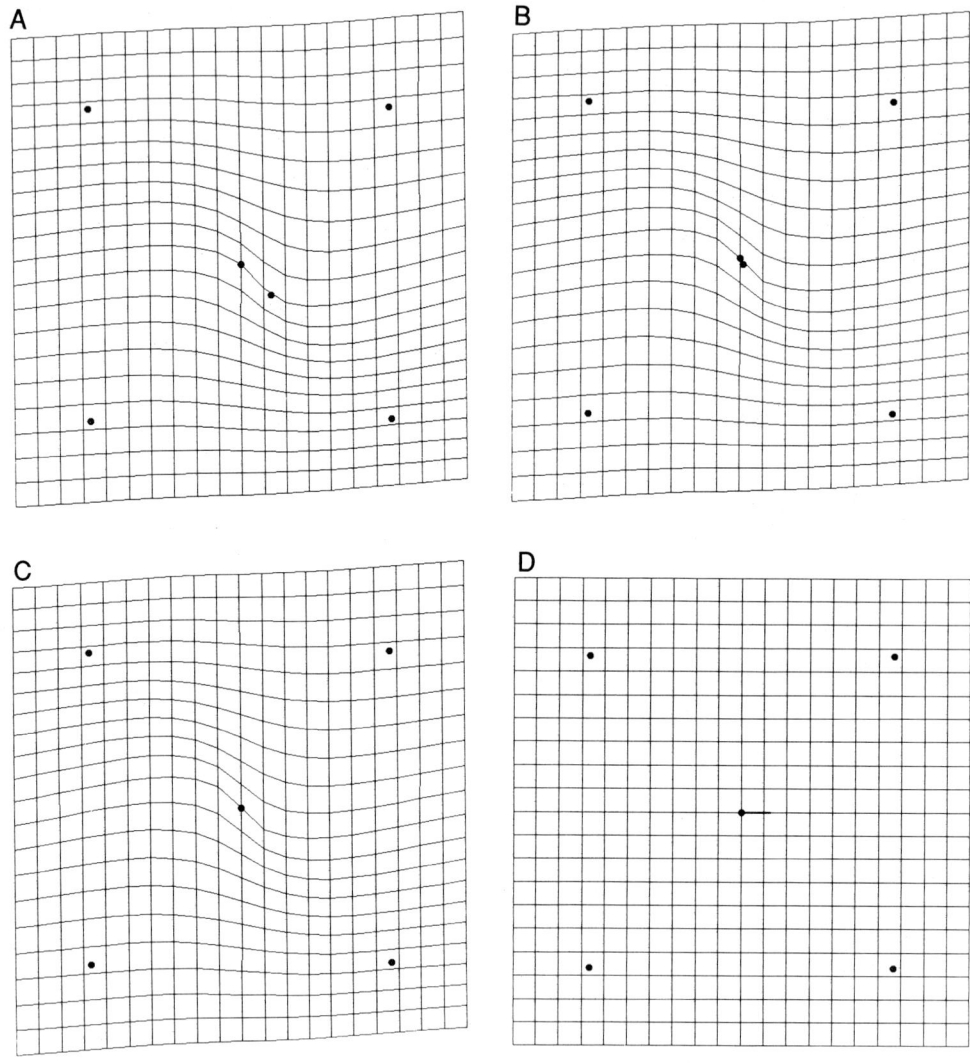

Figure 4 Shearing a single edgel. A quincunx of landmarks is fixed, and we vertically shear a sixth in the vicinity of the central one, using the ordinary spline machinery as in Figs. 1, 2, and 3. (A) Segment of length 10% of side of square, sheared downward by $45° = \tan^{-1} 1$. (B) Segment of length 1% of side of square, sheared downward by an angle $\tan^{-1} 2$. (C) Segment of length 0.01% of side of square (endpoints indistinguishable), sheared downward by an angle $\tan^{-4} 4$. Note that $4 = \log(0.0001)/\log(0.1)$. These are all nearly the same change: that is, the finite effect of changes in (infinitesimal) segment length is nearly proportional to the reciprocal of the logarithm of that segment length. (D–F) Limiting form of the map: (D) starting scene (five landmarks, one *edgel* of length unspecified); (E) deformation by a suitable multiple of the map underlying A, B, and C; and (F) equivalent physical thin metal plate (note intuition of "clamping" at center). (G) The positions of neighboring landmarks determine the "half-width" of the decay away from the edgel-shear in all directions. The "suitable multiple" (E) aligns the edgel graphic with shears of the underlying segment for all shears of moderate extent.

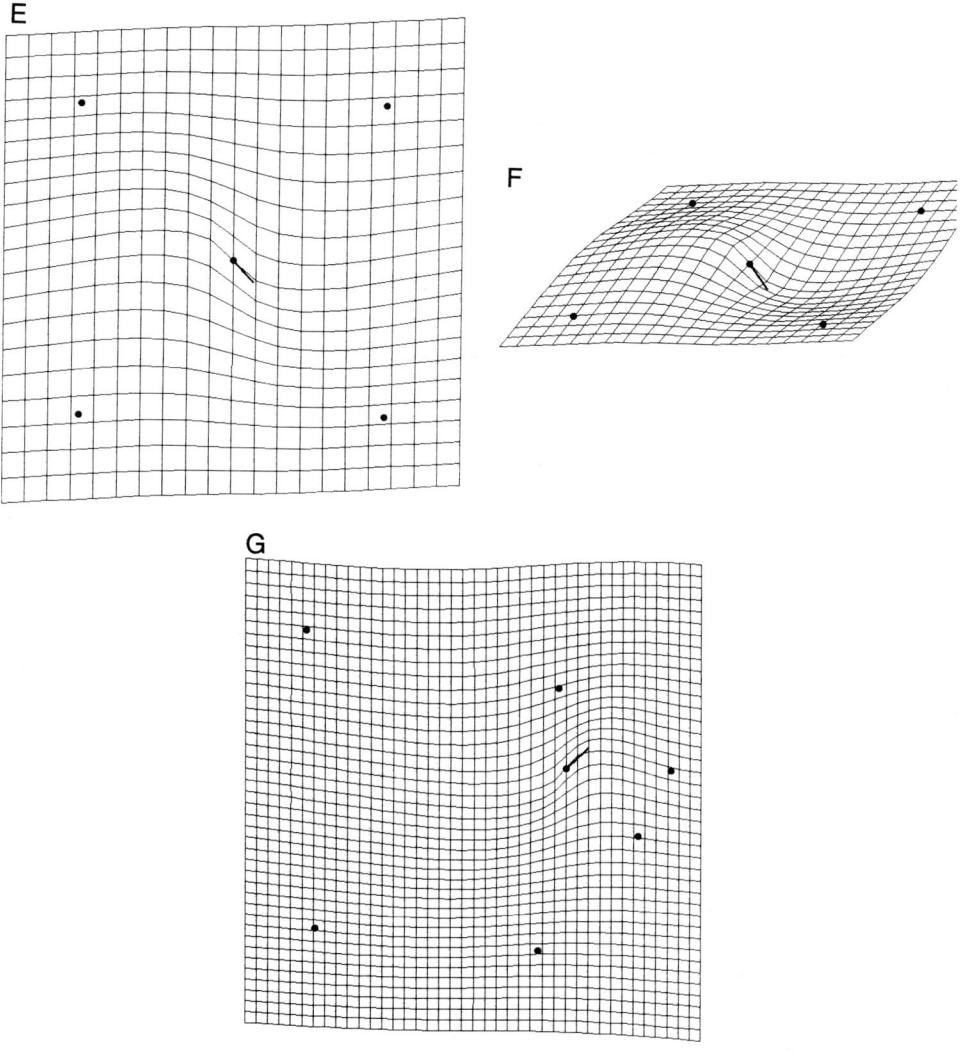

Figure 4 *(continued)*

vance. First, in independent developments by D. G. Kendall and myself, sets of landmark locations were turned into *statistical variables*—the sort of things that can be averaged and correlated—and then I found how well-suited thin-plate splines were for visualizing biometric features of those spaces. My monograph of 1991 is the first presentation of this new synthesis at adequate length.

But this essay is as different from a treatise as it can be: it transcribes an illustrated lecture reviewing all the main themes wholly in diagrams, without any equations. The argument will proceed in nine segments, each an extended figure caption to a series of many individual scenes. The extended figures, and their roles in the argument as a whole, are as follows.

Figure 1 introduces the formalism of thin-plate splines as either physical structures minimizing "bending energy" or interpolation functions for arbi-

trary lists of point correspondences. In the morphometric applications, points will always be landmarks, the correspondence of which from form to form is a matter of prior biological knowledge. Figure 2 shows how these transformations apply to biological images that include outline or gray-scale information, and Fig. 3 extends this in order to average 14 midsagittal MRI images after unwarping each according to a consistent set of anatomically reliable landmark points. But however redundant the information about global bending in point sets like these, still the information about local bending may be too scanty.

Figure 4, then, begins anew with the spline machinery, showing how an additional sort of spline basis element, the edgel, arises as a straightforward limit of point configurations. In the morphometric context, an edgel is a landmark with a biologically preassigned direction through it. Figure 5 shows how this ex-

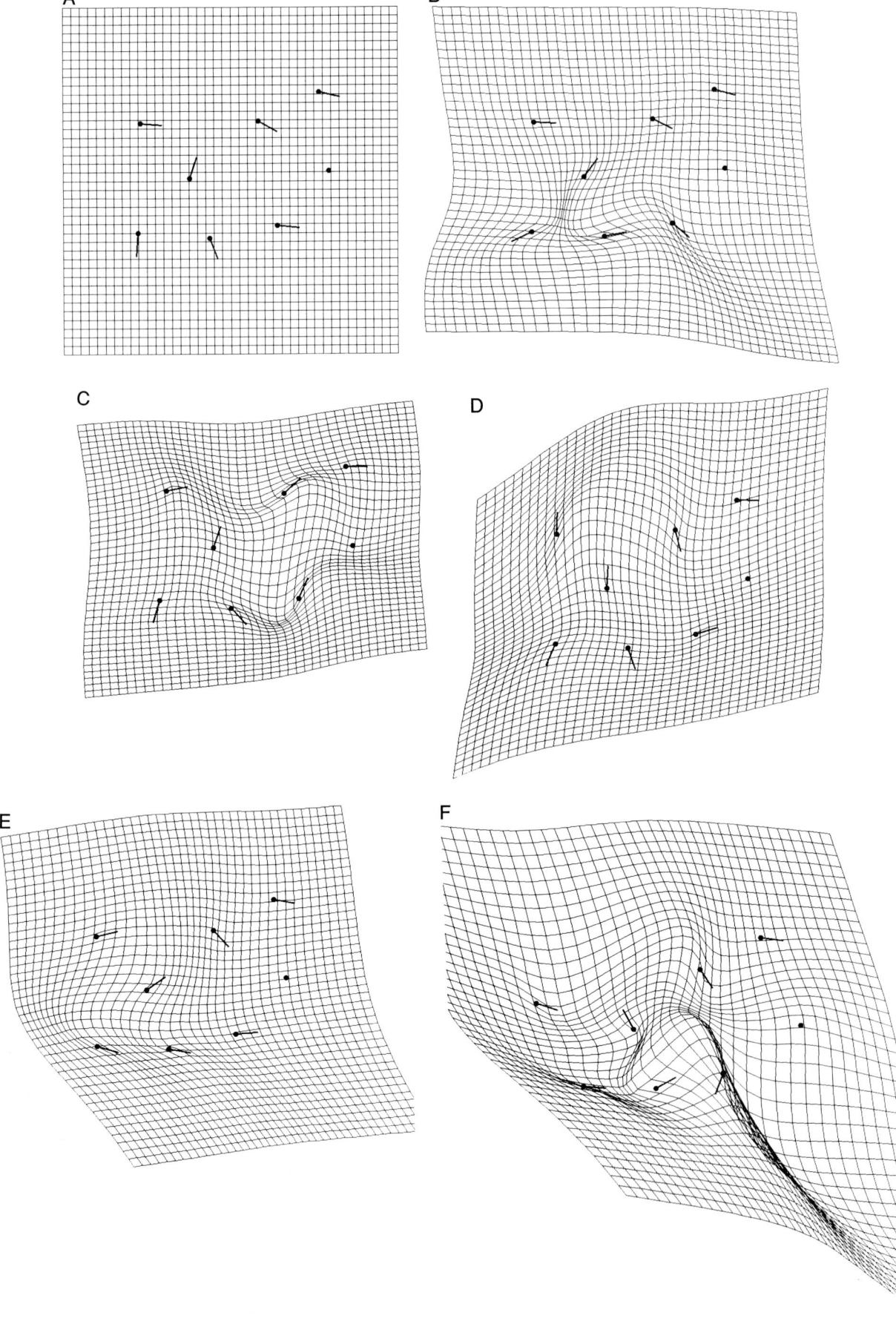

tended system of splining edgels along with points leads to a flexible family of image descriptors of arbitrary complexity. Returning to the context of medical images, Fig. 6 translates these features into a tentative language of outline shape changes and introduces some types of shape processes that may be reminiscent of familiar biological phenomena. Figure 7, using an outline schema from the averaged image in Fig. 3, shows how these edge features may be used to "digitize" (specify matching functions for) individual images more effectively than by points alone, and Plate 14 applies the extended technique to construct a more informative average image than that of Fig. 3 from the same 14 specimens. Plate 15 shows how to upgrade this technique "interactively" (digitize, average, redigitize, re-average, ...) so as to sharpen representation of specific organs—to calibrate both horizontal *and* vertical variations more effectively. In closing I shall comment on the import of these feature spaces, both horizontal and vertical, for medical image measurement in general and for the coherent archiving of neurological images in particular.

Except for the last three of these figures, all the material here has appeared somewhere earlier. My favorite reference for Fig.1, as for the technology of thin-plate splines in general, is Bookstein (1991), which represents the state of the art of landmark morphometrics up to, but not including, edgels. Sections 2.2 and 7.5 of that monograph include all the important equations. For an overview of the typical tactics of morphometrics as a statistical technique, see my chapters (Bookstein, 1990) in Toga's compendium. The averaged midsagittal MRI in Fig. 3 was previously published in Bookstein and Jaynes (1990) and in Appendix 1.3 of Bookstein (1991). Evans *et al.* (1991) have already published similar point-driven averaged unwarped images for three-dimensional data. The provenance of the quadrilateral of landmarks in the last panel of that figure—it is a multivariate statistical finding—is explained in Bookstein (1991a). The equations underlying the edgel splines and the grids of Figs. 4 and 5 are set out in Bookstein and Green (1992, 1992a), and the details of the extension to many edgels, in Bookstein and Green (1993), where these methods are further extended to incorporate more

general manipulations of the derivatives of maps at landmarks. These papers all describe the relation of the bending energy of edgels to that of landmarks in some detail. The particular single-edgel spline in Fig. 4 was prefigured in Timoshenko and Woinowsky-Krieger (1959). The analyses of Plates 14 and 15 are *not* meant to represent findings about neuroanatomy, but only to indicate the power of the splining technique for image standardization both horizontal and vertical.

II. Discussion: Visualization and Measurement

The problems we are pursuing originate in data that are already visualized. The source of information was a medical image, indicating a physical property (some sort of interaction with radiation) within each of a grid of little volumes inside a region of tissue. Our scientific concern is to investigate aspects of this sort of data many sets at a time. The visualization we seek is to concentrate certain features of particular interest out of the rather dilute, hard-to-compare information that is each original brain scan. To emphasize this task of concentration rather than the pursuit of arbitrary detail is to ask a question different from the question that the original visualization was designed to answer. The goal now is to retrieve not what is unique in each instance but what is common to all, what is most variable among them, what typically covaries with exogenous causes or effects, etc.

The data under discussion are, in general, vectors at each point of a domain organized on Euclidean principles—multispectral pixels or voxels: the vertical features to which I alluded in the Introduction. There is always additional information in the horizontal part of this imagined figure—the information about where the labeled locations and gradients of the ground plane actually lie with respect to the pixels and how their configurations covary with the height(s) of the surface(s) above them. The labels attach to the points and directions of the ground plane (or ground space, in the 3D applications), not the points of the imaginary data surfaces floating above them. These labels, which

---

Figure 5 Deformations using multiple edgels. (A) A scene of eight landmarks, seven with edgels. Edgels may be initialized at any orientation. (B–E) When the landmarks are fixed, as here, the bending energy of the equivalent (15-point) spline is nearly a quadratic form in the vector of shears of edgels away from their starting orientations, multiplied by an indeterminate (the reciprocal of the logarithm of the common segment "length"). The eigenvectors of this quadratic form specify coordinated shears of all the edgels at once that are most bent, least bent, or of stationary bending for fixed summed squared extent of shear. These are useful features for description of shape change in scenes with edgels. (B and C) Two highly bent principal edgel warps. (D and E) The two least bent principal edgel warps. (F) A fantasy on the same starting configuration of landmarks.

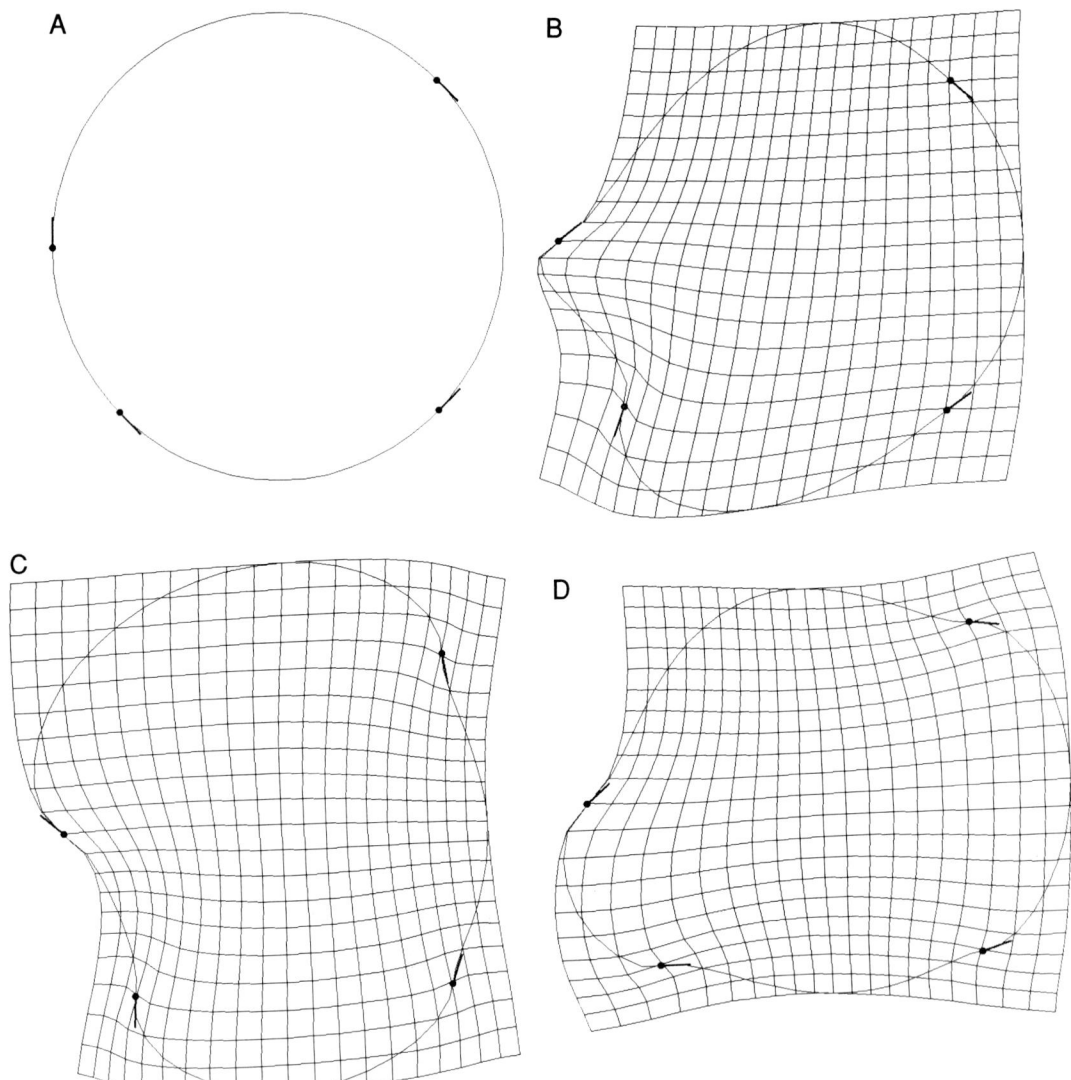

Figure 6 Principal edgel warps for outlines. In images with outlines, the principal edgel warps serve as an orthogonal basis for small rotations of the outline(s) around their sample mean orientations at the landmarks. We seem unfamiliar with these basis elements; for instance, we have difficulty naming them. (A) A circle with four unequally spaced edgels tangent to it. (B–G) Principal edgel warps 1 through 4 (most to least bent). Each of these may also be reversed in sign. (B) Sharpest warp, formation of a "nose." (C) Warp 2, left-to-right flattening. (D) Top-to-bottom flattening (opposite of C), with extrusions. (E) Warp 3, a droop to the lower right. (F) Warp 4, the gentlest of these warps, turning the circle into a version of Al Capp's infinitely gentle cartoon character, the Shmoo. (G) Opposite of the Shmoo warp, difficult to characterize: Taco Bell?

of course identify the landmarks and edgels of the earlier discussion, have their own metrics, including the versions of bending energy reviewed here, that complement the more usual metrics (perhaps manipulations of height, gradient steepness, curvature, or divergence) for the multivariate observations above them. Labeled points and directions move about in their Euclidean domain at the same time that images change above them, leading to decompositions of the variance "at" a point that are very interesting both scientifically and statistically.

For instance, a vertical analysis may be best if one wants to use the geometry of the labeled image rather as one uses a covariate in a classic experimental design. In this case, it is as if the shape of the configuration of labeled points—fluctuation in biological meaning of the basis for the vector space underlying the pixellated data—is to be treated as nuisance variation, control of which increases the precision with which other effects can be addressed. That is, one analyzes vertically—examining the gradients of the picture, for instance, or its correlations with physical or biological

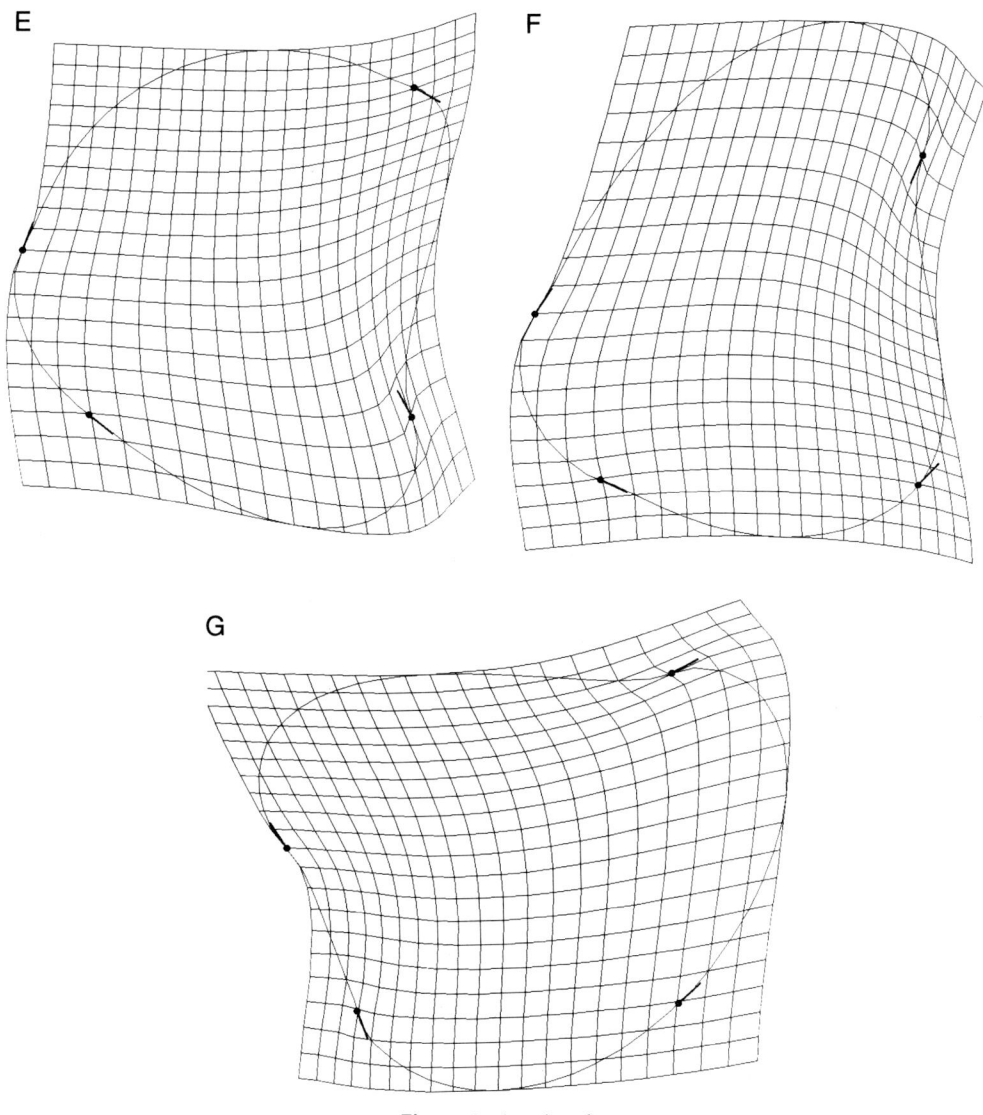

Figure 6 (*continued*)

processes—only after unwarping horizontally to a more focused feature space in which processes more nearly stay put to have their statistically standardized pictures taken. The experience of generations of anatomists shows how this maneuver improves the power of subsequent multivariate tactics, such as discrimination or analysis of covariance. When averaging pictures of brain activity over brains of different shape, for instance, the landmarks serve as guides to the correspondence of regions (the *Atlas*) prior to averaging. It is the atlas, not the squares of the grid of a PET reconstruction, that represents the true coordinate system for valid biometric analyses. In general, there is no way to simulate this procedure by vertical (pixelwise) operations that are even remotely linear.

This much is often conceded. Less often acknowledged is that in most applications this horizontal vari-

ation is not noise or nuisance but instead a signal in its own right. In the vicinity of their mean configuration, the labeled points and edgels induce a very powerful low-dimensional feature space. With the aid of a convenient basis for shape variation (recall Fig. 1 or Fig. 6), this information may be concentrated into linear features of its own. The variables of this block can be paired with less delicately crafted descriptors of the original vertical scalar or vector content for prediction of other images, such as later images of the same system, and for the joint evocation of shape and content as a bispectral signal in a detection or classification problem, such as locating tumors or quantifying their recession under treatment.

Visualization of vectors in this feature space of edge information at landmarks is at least as straightforward as visualization of changes in surfaces above the

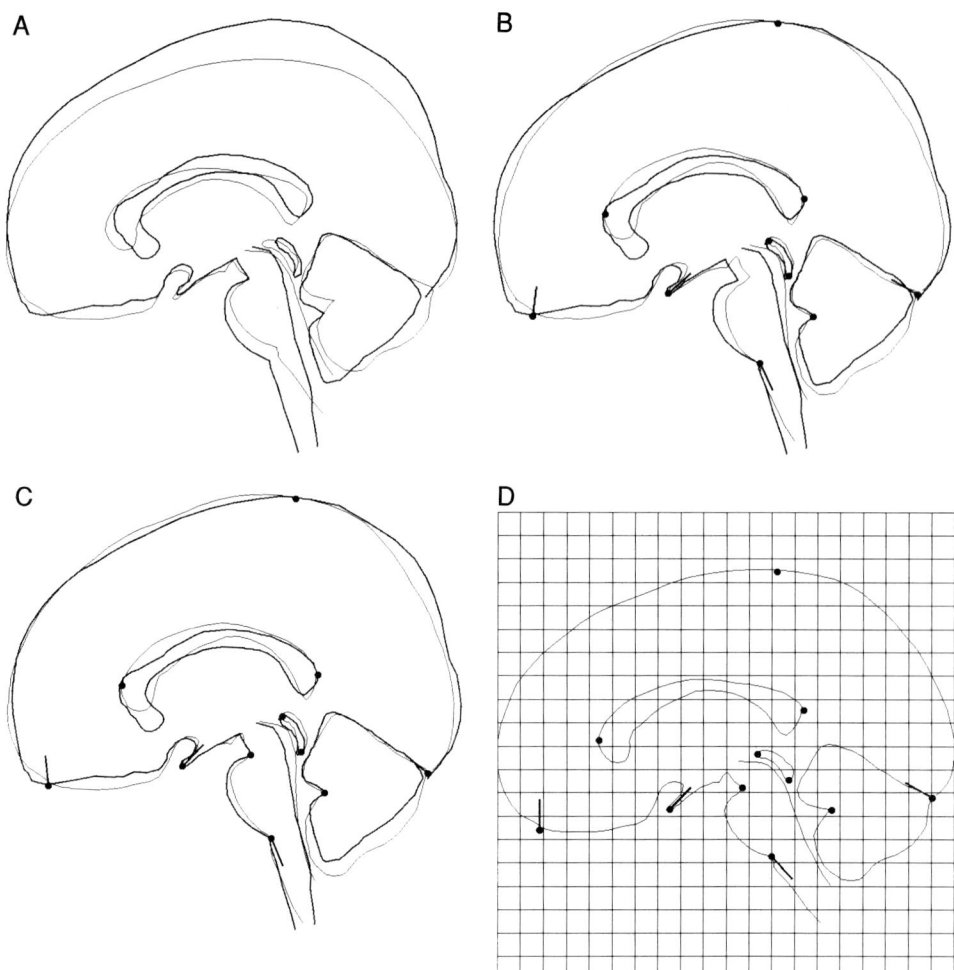

Figure 7 Digitizing outlines by edgel splines. (A) Some extended edges from the averaged image in Fig. 3F (light curves) and the homologous contours from one of the original 14 images (heavy curves). The upper margin of the cortical edge corresponds to the upper margin of white in Figs. 3F and 3G. (B) Overlay after warping the light curve in panel A to match 10 landmarks. (C) Better fit after adjusting four edgels (and one more landmark). (D) Schematic of eight of these features, with a reference grid, in the coordinate system of the averaged image (Fig. 3F). These will be used in Plate 14 for digitizing whole images. The vertex point will be adjusted upward to the bony calva to circumvent the variable obliteration of gray levels that owes to partial volume effects along the falx.

planes or volumes tagged by those points. The best diagrams are suggestive of the process explanations automatically familiar to any sentient organism that ever navigated a binocular landscape. We read these deformation grids as easily as we can read simulations of surfaces by gray-scale shading, the cues of barrels or pincushions, or any other pictorial metaphor of a spatial field. The combination of features of labeled point shape with features of the image at the average shape—the careful separation of vertical from horizontal variation in these mixed feature spaces, along with the careful, specialized visualization of the horizontal—is, in my view, the most powerful discipline available for scientifically effective analyses of biomet-

rical images. The averaging of biological images is made vastly more effective when the horizontal transformations are executed first in their own linearized domain. In practice, the two domains of linearization, and the resulting two complementary styles of visualization, are combined for composite analyses of changes over a deforming scene, as when a growing tumor changes texture while it deforms surrounding tissues. The same duality applies also in analysis of image variability, as of structure–function correlations, unrelated to physical dynamics. Whether the problem is dynamic or cross-sectional, the best visualizations of quantitative biometrics involve both horizontal and vertical operators.

The power for image analysis and scientific insight of the new methods that exploit labeled point and edgel data to enrich the conventional metaphor of measurement is thus immense, and mostly unexploited. Interactions of real nonlinear geometry with linear feature extraction are key to the solution of many presently intractable problems of pattern detection and display throughout functional neuroimaging and across the medical imaging sciences. The crux of this combination of vertical and horizontal descriptions is their careful separation to begin with: separation of change of image content from deformation of the index set of pixels or voxels. The separation proceeds best with the aid of a unique intermediate linearized structure, the nonstandard multivariate technology of shape space for labeled point and edge configurations. In its peculiar finite-dimensional elegance, this space affords two bases at once: one for linear features of the arbitrarily nonlinear transformations that we see in the real world and the other for the pictorial features of the normalized images that result from these very flexible models of deformation.

Acknowledgments

All the figures here were produced by the program "Edgewarp," designed and coded in C and XWindows by William D. K. Green, my collaborator in working out the limiting cases of the thin-plate spline and in all the other papers of this series. Our efforts were supported in part by USPHS Grants GM-37251 and NS-26529 to Fred L. Bookstein. The midsagittal brain images were supplied by John Mazziotta of UCLA, and their landmarks were originally digitized by Dan Valentino.

References

Bookstein, F. L. (1978). "The Measurement of Biological Shape and Shape Change," Lecture Notes in Biomathematics, vol. 24. Berlin: Springer-Verlag.

Bookstein, F. L. (1990). Morphometrics. Distortion correction. In "Three-Dimensional Neuroimaging" (A. W. Toga, Ed.), pp. 167–188 and 235–249. New York: Raven Press.

Bookstein, F. L. (1991). "Morphometric Tools for Landmark Data." New York: Cambridge University Press.

Bookstein, F. L. (1991a). Thin-plate splines and the atlas problem for biomedical images. In "Information Processing in Medical Imaging" (A. C. F. Colchester and D. Hawkes, Eds.). Lecture Notes in Computer Science, Vol. 511, pp. 326–342. Berlin: Springer-Verlag.

Bookstein, F. L., and Green, W. D. K. (1992). A feature space for edgels in images with landmarks. In "Proceedings of the Conference on Mathematical Methods of Medical Imaging," Vol. 1768, pp. 228–247. S.P.I.E., Bellingham, Washington.

Bookstein, F. L., and Green, W. D. K. (1992a). Edge information at landmarks in medical images. In "Visualization in Biomedical Computing 1992" (R. A. Robb, Ed.), Vol. 1808, pp. 242–258. S.P.I.E., Bellingham, Washington.

Bookstein, F. L., and Green, W. D. K. (1993). A feature space for edgels in images with landmarks. J. Math. Imaging Vis. **3:** 231–261.

Bookstein, F. L., and Jaynes, W. (1990). "Thin-Plate Splines and the Analysis of Biological Shape." Videotape.

Duchon, J. (1976). Interpolation des fonctions de deux variables suivant la principe de la flexion des plaques minces. RAIRO Analyse Numérique **10**, 5–12.

Dürer, A. (1524). "Vier Bücher von menschlicher Proportion."

Evans, A. C., Dai, W., Collins, L., Neelin, P., and Marrett, S. (1991). Warping of a computerized 3-D atlas to match brain image volumes for quantitative neuroanatomical and functional analysis. In "Proceedings of the Fifth Conference on Medical Imaging," Vol. 1445, pp. 236–246. S.P.I.E., Bellingham, Washington.

Fox, P. T., Perlmutter, J. S., and Raichle, M. E. (1985). A stereotactic method of anatomical localization for positron emission tomography. J. Comput. Assist. Tomogr. **9**, 141–153.

Greitz, T., Bohm, C., Holte, S., and Eriksson, L. (1991). A computerized brain atlas: Construction, anatomical content, and some applications. J. Comput. Assist. Tomogr. **15**, 26–38.

Sneath, P. H. A. (1967). Trend surface analysis of transformation grids. J. Zool. **151**, 65–122.

Terzopoulos, D. (1983). Multilevel computational processes for visual surface reconstruction. Comput. Vision, Graphics, Image Processing **24**, 52–96.

Thompson, D'A. W. (1917). "On Growth and Form." London: Macmillan.

Timoshenko, S. S., and Woinowsky-Krieger, S. (1959). "Theory of Plates and Shells," Second ed. New York: McGraw–Hill.

Vemuri, B. B. (Ed.) (1991). "Proceedings of the Conference on Geometric Methods in Computer Vision," Vol. 1570. S.P.I.E., Bellingham, Washington.

11

Accuracy and Precision in Image Standardization in Intra- and Intersubject Comparisons

Lennart Thurfjell,* Christian Bohm,† Torgny Greitz,‡ Lars Eriksson,‡,§ and Martin Ingvar§

*Centre for Image Analysis, Uppsala University, Uppsala, Sweden; †Department of Physics, University of Stockholm and Departments of ‡Neuroradiology and §Neurophysiology, Karolinska Institute/Hospital, Stockholm, Sweden

I. Introduction

The need for intra- and intersubject comparisons arises from a desire to extend the scope of examinations to multiple sets of neuroimaging data or to generalize individual results to groups of patients. These comparisons require, however, a preceding standardization to ensure image compatibility. The standardization process can in general be expressed as a transformation that brings the images into a form in which each pixel corresponds to the same anatomical entity. In the case of intrasubject comparisons, this can be accomplished by using a reproducible patient fixation system. Another way is by deriving appropriate rotations and translations from the image volumes themselves and then transforming the data into a standard orientation. In intersubject comparison, however, the process is more difficult because it requires removal of individual anatomy dependence from the data. This task can be accomplished by transforming the data into a standard anatomy.

II. Ideal Standardization Transformations

An ideal *intrasubject* standardization transformation should be able to transform images from different investigations of the same patient into a standard form. If the time interval between the different investi-gations is sufficiently small, temporal changes can be disregarded. If this is the case and the investigations are made with the same imaging equipment, such a transformation will at most be a general rigid transformation that can be expressed by a combination of a translation and a rotation. With different imaging equipments, the transformation must also include geometrical and intensity scalings.

The ideal *intersubject* standardization transformation is much more complex. This may also be the case for intrasubject standardization extending over long time periods. The corresponding transformations must therefore be able to handle quite general deformations with constraints introduced by the cranial bones, the falx, and the tentiorium, with different degrees of freedom in different parts of the brain. A unique mapping or transformation between the brains can be found when there is a unique correspondence between equivalent points in different brains, so that for each point in one brain a corresponding point can be found in the other. Furthermore, because all nearby points in the same or connected brain structures are mapped into nearby points, this transformation must at least be partly continuous. However, nearby points in unconnected brain structures, such as points on either side of a sulcus, need not be mapped into adjacent points. This means that all internal brain surfaces are potential discontinuity surfaces of the transformation. Moreover, it is clear that the relative size of adjacent structures may vary greatly. This implies that an

FUNCTIONAL NEUROIMAGING

otherwise smoothly changing deformation parameter may change character (implying a discontinuous derivative in the transformation) at structure boundaries, even if these are connected. This is especially true at the boundary of the ventricular system. Practical experiences show that the transformation required for standardization of the central brain structures is quite well behaved, whereas the corresponding transformation for the cortex exhibits frequent discontinuities. In limited areas the transformation may not even exist. These problems are, of course, more pronounced in pathological cases with expanding lesions.

III. Standardization Techniques

Numerous approaches for transforming individual data into an anatomy-independent coordinate space have been reported. All methods have the common characteristics that the standardization is achieved by matching the individual data with some sort of standard model. The transformations defined by this matching will then move the image elements from the dataset into new locations in an anatomy-independent standard space.

A. Characteristics

The process of image standardization can be divided into three steps: (1) defining common features in the image dataset and in the standard model, (2) finding the matching transformation and, (3) transforming the images to make the feature points coincide with the standard model. Matching features can, for example, be anatomical landmarks, external fiducial markers, corresponding contours of brain structures, or the complete brain surface. A suitable matching transformation can then be found, interactively or more or less automatically. The third step is normally accomplished by resampling the original data according to the defined matching transformation and is, apart from the interpolation technique used, essentially identical for all methods. Although the standardization principles are similar in different methods, there are a number of important features in the standardization process that can be used to characterize them. Some of these aspects will be described below.

1. Introducing Information from Other Modalities

The objective is usually the standardization of functional images. Many methods, however, have to rely on structural information that is not available in functional images. In such cases, an intermediate match-

ing is performed on a set of anatomy-rich images (e.g., MRI). The final matching is then obtained by determining the rigid transformation parameters (i.e., the intrasubject transformation) that bring the functional data volume into coincidence with the anatomy-rich dataset. This extra step is vital when high precision registration is desired.

2. Utilizing Fixation Systems

The need for intrasubject registration can be eliminated or at least reduced by using head fixation systems (Bergström *et al.*, 1981). Another method for intrasubject registration of PET and MRI data, which is less constraining for the patient, uses external fiducial markers attached to the patients head and visible in both types of images (Evans *et al.*, 1991). The matching of the data is then performed by bringing these points into coincidence by minimizing the mean-square distance between equivalent points. The advantage is obvious: the matching process is greatly simplified. The disadvantages include the extra effort required during patient setup and the inconvenience for the patient, which might influence the results from certain activation studies. However, this inconvenience is probably smaller than that caused by a fixation systems. With external fiducial markers, there is also a possibility of markers being altered between studies, thus introducing new errors. The fiducial head attachment can normally not be removed and reattached between scans and is thus not useful in cases in which repeated measurements on the same individual are performed.

A reproducible head fixation is usually preferred when repeated studies are performed in the same imaging device. This allows for direct comparison of all data in the study without a previous image registration, provided the fixation precision is sufficient. This is valuable because any image registration, even if it is perfect, will cause information loss through interpolation. But even if the precision of the fixation system is not sufficient, it will still limit the magnitude of the corrections and thus contribute to an improved result.

3. Including External Information

The inclusion of external information such as a well-designed set of standard templates or, even better, a standard atlas simplifies and stabilizes the fitting procedure. However, it presumes that the assumed external information is correct. Incorrect external information will spoil the result, sometimes quite drastically. This is, for example, the case when fiducial markers have been altered in between studies or when the standard model used is not appropriate for the data.

Most standardization methods depend on some kind of model. This standard model can be said to be internal when image properties inherent in the data are used in the matching process. This is, for example, the case when the standardization is achieved by a simple linear resizing. A more sophisticated approach using an internal model is the selection of one subject in a study as the standard. Data from other subjects are then transformed to match this standard. In this case, more complex transformations can be used. An external model, on the other hand, is used when external information is introduced. This is, for example, the case when the data are matched with an external standard such as a brain atlas or a standard template. When using an external model, the magnitude of differences between the images to be standardized and the anatomy standard will require different degrees of complexity in the transformations—complex differences in shape will require complex transformations in order to achieve an adequate standardization. A prerequisite is, of course, that large areas are not mapped into the same point. This may, for example, be the case if a monkey model is used to standardize human data. This categorization of models as either internal or external and how it can affect results under certain circumstances are further discussed in Section V.C.

4. Automatic versus Interactive Matching

Automatic procedures rely on the matching of characteristic features, fiducial points, that appear in the images to be processed. The first task in the matching process is to identify these features. The matching is then performed by minimizing the distances (or rather some function of distances) between the corresponding features in the respective images. Most methods assume rigid body motion and are thus applicable only for intrasubject standardization. In general, it can be stated that a fully automated method, when available, is always preferable because it is operator independent. However, implementing a fully automated procedure is not always possible and, when possible, is far from trivial. There are two major obstacles: (1) the definition of common features is difficult, especially when the images to be matched are of different types (e.g., MRI and PET), and (2) the problem of finding the best rather than just a good transformation (i.e., the global rather than a local minimum). Manual intervention is often required either during the operation itself or later to check the feasibility of the result. Further complications are added when dealing with functional images such as those obtained from PET because similar studies with different tracers can produce quite different images. The counting statistics

and also the stimulation used in the case of activation studies are other factors that can affect an automatic matching procedure. Some of these difficulties can be overcome by using different standards for different input data in order to simplify the definition of common features in the data to be matched. For example, PET images, obtained in a FDG study, can be standardized using a model consisting of an average image created from other PET images obtained using the same tracer. In the case of intrasubject registration involving PET, the matching process can be simplified by using data from transmission images (images reconstructed from transmission data used for attenuation correction in the reconstruction of emission images) if such images are available (Pelizzari et al., 1989). An automatic process will, in most cases, also require preprocessing of the data in order to get the data from the individual to conform with the standard model. This preprocessing often includes segmentation to isolate the brain and interpolations to get new voxel dimensions.

Interactive methods have several advantages. They are robust and can be applied to various types of input data, generally without any requirement for preprocessing. The main disadvantage is their inherent subjectivity and the risk for introducing systematic errors. However, the risk can be reduced by careful planning of the standardization procedure, for example, by setting up rules and by assuring that different actions in the matching process always are taken in the same order. There is also a possibility that these rules may serve as a starting point when constructing automatic systems based on expert system methodology.

5. Sensitivity to Anatomical Variations

Another important characteristic of a standardization method concerns its ability to compensate for pathological deformations. The simplest standardization approach is estimating the rotation and scaling to the correct size. A slightly better approach is to fix the orientation using landmarks such as the AC–PC line and to divide the data into different sections before resizing. These method can correct only for variations in size, although the latter approach has some ability to correct for global variations due to the partitioning of the data before resizing. Even better is to use more general transformations (e.g., a general second-degree polynomial in all three dimensions). Such methods can account for most types of normal variability such as a narrowing forehead, etc., but cannot compensate for local deformation due to pathology. The best alternative is then to use elastic matching based on the information from a large number of fix points or based on edge information. However, even this strategy is not always applicable (see Section II) and is, in any case, far from trivial to implement. But among the above-mentioned techniques, it is the one that best can account for pathological deformations.

B. Different Methods

In this section, some of the standardization methods reported in the literature will be described. The purpose is not to give a complete list of the existing methods, nor to categorize them according to the features described above, but to give an overview of different approaches. It is natural to group methods into those applicable only to intrasubject comparisons and into those also capable of intersubject standardization.

When registering data for intrasubject comparisons, a rigid transformation is assumed. It requires three translational and three rotational parameters to be determined. If the images are obtained using different modalities, a scaling parameter also has to be determined. The most common techniques are those that use landmarks or surfaces as matching features. Landmarks can be internal (Maguire *et al.*, 1991) or external (Evans *et al.*, 1991). A surface matching technique for registration of PET, CT, or MR images has been described by Pelizzari *et al.* (1989). A similar technique that uses a multiresolution approach (using images of different resolution) to speed up the matching process and multiple thresholds to minimize the influence of misplaced matching points (e.g., due to noise) has been described by Jiang *et al.* (1992). Principal axes (Faber and Stokely, 1988) can also be used as matching features. The principal axes depend only on the shape for binary objects. Two objects identical except for orientation and scale can be registered exactly using the principal axes method. However, in the registration of images from different modalities, difficulties in defining corresponding volumes will affect the precision.

Registration of data for intersubject comparisons is much more complex because it requires the transformation of individual data into an anatomy standard—a standard model. Many of the approaches for matching data from an individual with a standard model can be referred to as landmark-based methods, of which the most common is the Talairach proportional squaring model. In this method, a stereotactic origin is defined based on the identification of the AC–PC (anterior comissura–posterior comissura) line (Talairach and Tournoux, 1988). The AC–PC points normally cannot be directly identified in functional images. Fox *et al.* (1985) used an indirect method to

determine the AC–PC plane from a lateral skull X ray obtained at the time of the PET scans. Evans *et al.* (1992) point out the difficulties involved in the direct use of the AC and PC points and uses several other more easily located landmarks in correlated MRI data to estimate the AC–PC line. Friston *et al.* (1989) have described a method for estimating the AC–PC line directly from landmarks in 3D PET volumes. Most methods using AC–PC landmarks differ in the estimation of the AC–PC line but are otherwise essentially identical. An orthogonal coordinate frame based on the AC–PC line is established and the brain is divided into different 3D boxes. The standardization of the data is then achieved through linear resampling of the data in each box.

Bookstein (1991) has described a general landmark-driven method that also accounts for second-order variability. The technique uses a thin-plate spline function to warp one configuration of landmarks to another. This approach is general in the sense that data from a number of subjects in a study can be warped to match one selected individual, or the data can be warped to match an external standard.

A multiresolution algorithm for elastic matching of three-dimensional CT data with a voxel-based atlas has been described by Bajcsy and Kovacic (1989). The matching is performed in two steps. First, the input data and the atlas are globally aligned using translations, rotations, and linear scalings. After the global alignment, local elastic matching is performed using a coarse-to-fine strategy. Unlike the methods mentioned above, this method can be used in cases with pathological anatomies (producing reasonable large deformations). The algorithm uses local edge information in the matching process and will therefore be difficult to generalize to functional data. A further disadvantage is the requirement for sensitive preprocessing of the input data to conform with the atlas. Manual intervention is often needed. This preprocessing of the CT data includes resampling and interpolation to achieve cubic voxels of the same size as those of the atlas as well as removing the skull from the data in order to isolate the brain.

Friston *et al.* (1991) have developed a method in which a nonlinear resampling technique is used to match PET images to a standard template. The method was developed to be used in activation studies and is not applicable to studies in which differences between individuals due to anatomical or functional pathology are present. In such cases, the method would erroneously try to compensate for the structural differences in the data.

The CBA method described below (Section V) uses a contour-based approach for the individualization of the atlas brain. Stereotactic standardization is then achieved through a nonlinear resampling determined by the function adapting the atlas to the individual.

IV. Errors in the Standardization Process

Errors in the standardization process originate from different sources such as positioning errors, limited scanner resolution, instrument calibration, incorrect external information, normal variations in brain shape, and pathological deformations. These factors will introduce extra variations in the standardized images that ultimately will increase the errors in the localization of brain function. This is a very coarse classification of possible error sources and many of these sources of errors can be further subdivided. It has already been pointed out how incorrect external information can affect the results. This is further described in Section V.C. Some other errors will be illustrated with a few examples below. The influence of an error component is closely related to the resolution of the imaging method in question. Because errors often combine quadratically, smaller errors will not significantly affect the results.

A. Positioning Errors

There are many types of methodological errors that can be referred to as positioning errors. These include unaccounted fixation errors, misplacement of the reference plane in methods using the AC–PC line for reference, incorrect specification of landmarks in landmark-based methods, translation errors of the standard brain in the CBA method, bad registration of images from different modalities, and so on. Positioning errors will affect the standardization and will contribute to the blurring of average images. Larger positioning errors can cause ring artifacts in subtraction images. Small positioning errors, however, can enhance spurious areas in subtraction images that may then falsely be interpreted as, for example, metabolic differences in brain activation studies (Plate 16).

B. Errors due to CT and MR Calibration

It is sometimes profitable to include information obtained from other modalities. This may also lead to the introduction of new errors. The registration between the different datasets is an area with many potential problems. If a rigid match is used, errors in registration will belong to the class of positioning errors discussed above. Another, quite different source of error is in instrument calibration. The transfer of

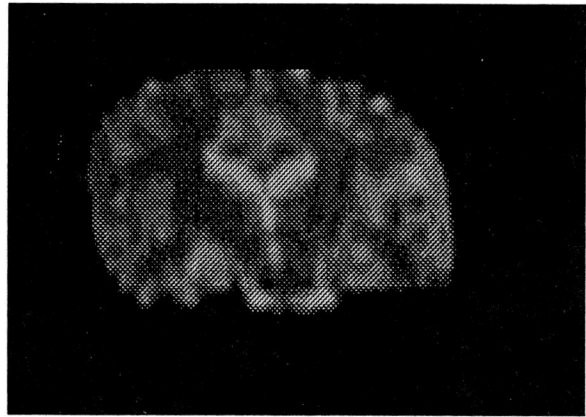

Figure 1 When transferring information between imaging modalities, it is important that a true representation of the Cartesian space is present. Often 3D information is based on a stack of 2D images. Here such a volume based on a set of transaxial MRI images is shown. In spite of perfect, in-plane reproduction, the stack of 2D images yielded an incremental shift in the coronal plane.

information between different methods is especially rewarding when used to correlate results obtained with an anatomy-rich method to images obtained with a method displaying less anatomic but more functional information. However, when transferring spatial information from images obtained with different techniques, it is important to check that the images are free from distortion. Special attention has to be paid to the artifactual deformities that may be produced by inhomogeneity of the magnetic field with MRI (Fig. 1). One way of avoiding this source of error is to check the field characteristics regularly, using a test phantom for calibration.

V. The Karolinska Computerized Brain Atlas (CBA)

The stereotactic standardization used in CBA is usually achieved by matching a transformed standard brain atlas to an anatomy-rich imaging modality such as CT or MRI. A nonlinear resampling determined by the inverse transformation will then adapt the individual to the atlas. There is no need for fiducial markers in the adaptation process, nor is any preprocessing of the data required. The transformations used account for differences in brain size as well as for second-order variability. If the atlas is first adapted to a set of CT or MRI images, the final matching to the functional data is done using the same curve-based approach to determine the rigid transformations bringing the two datasets into registration. The atlas is based on anatomical information derived from various sources in the literature. Structures were drawn on displayed digitized photos of one single cryosectioned brain fixated *in situ* soon after death. The anatomy database contains at present three-dimensional representations of the brain surface, the ventricular system, and the cortical gyri and sulci, as well as the Brodmann cytoarchitectonic areas. The major basal ganglia, including the thalamic nuclei, the brain stem nuclei, the lobuli of the vermis, and the cerebellar hermispheres, are also contained in the database (Bohm *et al.*, 1983, 1986; Greitz *et al.*, 1991).

A. Individualization of the Atlas

When using the CBA approach, the atlas is in a first step transformed to fit the patient under study. Two types of transformations are used: a patient-related *general* transformation, determined once for each patient, and an examination-*specific* transformation that compensates for the different positioning of the patient in the different examinations. The adaptation of the atlas is performed interactively by matching the selected atlas structures (normally the brain surface and the ventricular system) to the corresponding structures in a series of images of the patients brain. Subsequent adaptations to images from other examinations are then obtained by determining only the specific rigid (translations and rotations) parameters. The general adaptation can then be made to a set of high-resolution CT or MR images. The modified atlas is then transferred to the functional PET or SPECT images. However, with suitable tracers, the adaptation can be made directly to the functional images with acceptable precision (Plate 17). The transformation used in the adaptation of the atlas includes translations, rotations, and scaling factors in x, y, and z, as well as plastic deformations. The compound transformation is mathematically equivalent to a general second-degree polynomial in x, y, and z (Thurfjell *et al.*, 1993). In practice, the adaptation is performed in a series of successive adjustments of the transformation parameters: first the translation and rotation parameters are adjusted until the orientation is correct, and then the atlas is resized using the linear scalings. Finally, when the orientation and size of the atlas brain are correct, the second-order parameters are adjusted to account for normal variability in brain shape.

B. Accuracy and Precision in the CBA Method

The spatial accuracy and precision of the CBA standardization method has been investigated by measuring the spread of well-defined anatomical structures in reformatted MRI images of 26 healthy male volunteers

(Seitz *et al.*, 1990). All subjects were imaged by a Siemens Magnetom (0.5 T) MRI system using a fixation helmet (Bergström *et al.*, 1981). Sixteen transaxial images with a slice thickness of 10 mm and a separation of 6.75 mm were produced for each subject. The data were corrected for geometrical distortion using a correction function obtained from a phantom study and were stored as 256×256 images with 1.27 mm^2 pixels. The brain atlas was then adapted to fit each subject by interactive matching of the contours of the atlas structures with the corresponding contours as presented in a series of transaxial slices and in reconstructed coronal and sagittal planes. The selected atlas structures were the brain surface and the ventricular system. When a suitable fit was obtained, nonlinear resampling was used to transform the data into a standard space corresponding to the anatomy of the CBA database brain. This produced 14 transaxial slices with a separation of 6.75 mm.

All 26 spatially standardized images were then used to create an average MRI dataset (Fig. 2). The extent of blurring in this average image is a measure of the precision in the standardization process. The blurring is caused by both methodological errors and unaccounted morphological differences among the indi-

Table 1 Spread of Anatomical Structures in Individual Reformatted Magnetic Resonance Images of 26 Healthy Subjects

Anatomical landmarks	SD (mm) in reformatted image
Fornix at foramen	0.87 (x)
Monroi	2.04 (y)
Tip of fourth ventricle	1.12 (x)
	2.21 (y)
	2.57 (z)
Top of lateral ventricles	
Right	2.76 (z)
Left	2.78 (z)
Medial end of right central sulcus	2.83 (x)
	4.34 (y)
Medial end of left central sulcus	3.59 (x)
	4.49 (y)
Contour of hemispheres	
Right	
Frontal	1.59 (y)
Occipital	2.87 (y)
Lateral	1.85 (x)
Left	
Frontal	1.83 (y)
Occipital	3.23 (y)
Lateral	2.21 (x)

Source. From Seitz *et al.* (1990).

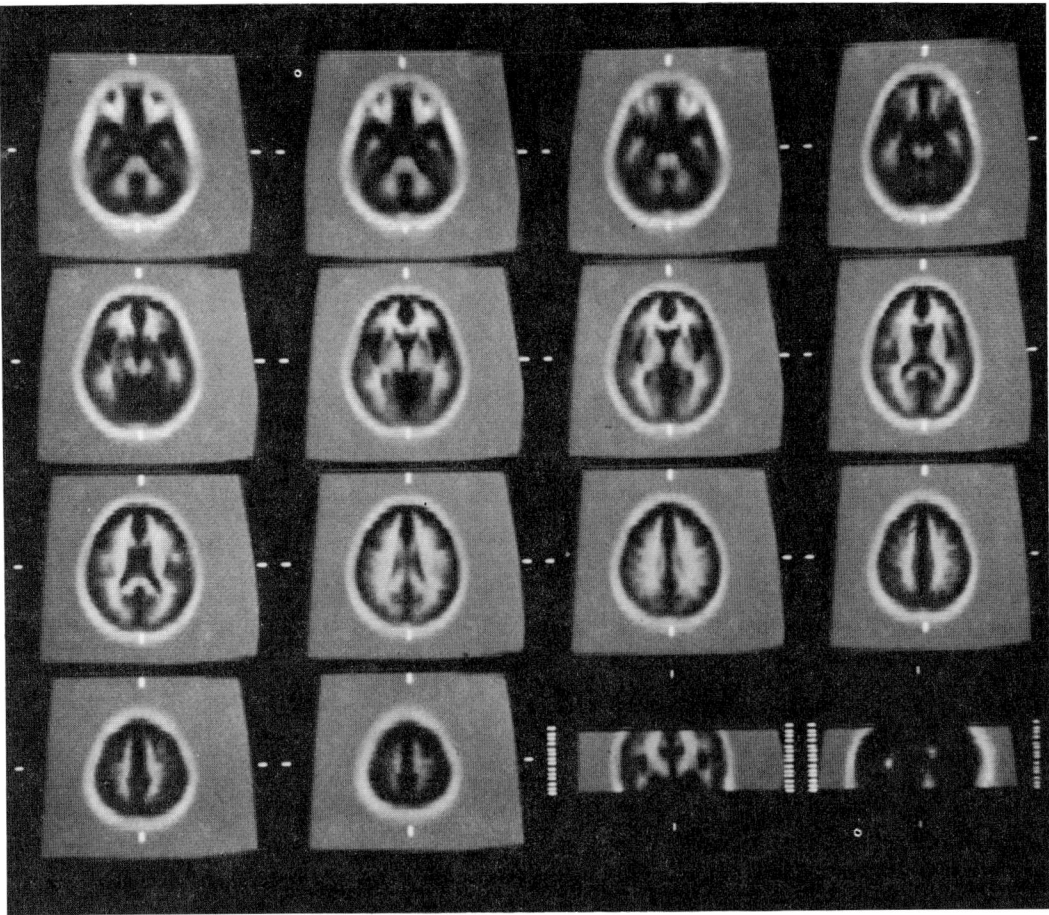

Figure 2 The mean MRI images from 26 spatially standardized MRI images of healthy volunteers. Details are visible, but some blurring occurs due to both methodological shortcomings and minor, local, anatomical differences that the CBA procedure does not account for. From Seitz *et al.* (1990).

viduals. The precision was further evaluated by measuring the spread of a number of well-defined anatomical landmarks. The location of these landmarks was also compared with the location of the same points provided by the CBA database. Measuring points were selected at the brain surface at maximum width, the maximum length of each hemisphere, the medial end of the central sulcus, the top of the lateral ventricles as presented in a coronal slice at the maximum width of the cerebral hemispheres, the fornix at the level of the foramen Monroi, and the rostral end of the fourth ventricle. The standard deviations (SD) of the landmarks in the reformatted MRI images are summarized in Table 1. These values gives a quantitative measure of the precision in the standardization process.

The reformation process of the CBA program seems to transform the anatomy of the individual brain into that of a standard brain with reasonable accuracy (Seitz *et al.*, 1990). The precision of the reformation

had an SD of about 1 mm for the dislocation of the midline structures and 2–3 mm for the dislocation of the outer and inner brain surfaces. The corresponding SD for most brain structures, including the cerebral sulci, were 1–4 mm in the x direction and 2–5 mm in the y direction. The spread of the peak rCBF values in a motor task experiment was 2–3 mm in the x direction and 5–6 mm in the y direction. That the spread of the activity maximum is greater than that of the corresponding anatomical structures (in this particular case, the central sulcus) is due mainly to the fact that the distribution of functional areas differs to a certain degree from that of the gross anatomical structures. The difference depends also on the more subjective way of selecting the functional maximum compared with an anatomical reference point. This discrepancy is likely to be present with any method of standardization.

If a certain anatomical structure is selected as a primary area of interest, a local adjustment of the atlas can be made to this structure (e.g., the thalamus), after a preceding global adaptation of the atlas. A local adaptation can also be performed on the neighboring structures, such as the central sulcus when the motor area is of interest or the lower, posterior surface of the frontal lobe when looking for an activation in the accumbens nucleus. In this way, a higher local precision around the area of interest can be achieved at the expense of a loss in precision in more remote areas.

C. Using Inaccurate External Information

It has been shown (Fujita *et al.*, 1993) that the CBA atlas can be adapted with greater precision to Swedish brains than to Japanese brains (cf. Seitz *et al.*, 1990). In fact, the original Friston method, employing a simple three-dimensional scaling technique (Friston *et al.*, 1989), gives—when applied to Japanese brains—a smaller standard deviation in the spread of the location and boundaries of anatomical structures than does the CBA method. The latter seems to allow for a more precise adaptation when applied to Swedish or European brains. The Friston method uses an internal model for defining a stereotactic origin and then resizing the data, whereas the CBA method uses an external model derived from a Swedish brain. In the CBA method, the Japanese brains must first be mapped so that their common anatomy is transformed to match the Swedish standard. Unfortunately, such transfor-

mations are difficult to implement and are not yet available in the CBA program. Therefore the result of a CBA transformation of Japanese brains will be slightly inferior to a simple linear scaling, i.e., the Friston method. The somewhat better results achieved with the Friston method were mostly obtained for structures located in, or very close to, the intercommissural plane, where the adaptation with the Friston method should be most accurate. The difference between the results achieved with the two methods is hardly noticeable and is sometimes reversed, especially for structures more remote from that plane, such as the central sulcus. The standard deviation for the x and y coordinates of the activated area in a motor task (Speech Kana-Rest) experiment using the CBA standardization was found to be 5–7 in the x direction and about 7.0 mm in the y direction (Fujita *et al.*, 1993). The point of maximum activity, subjectively determined, was selected. According to Seitz *et al.* (1990), the standard deviations of the spread of the peak rCBF values in a motor task experiment were 2–3 mm in the x direction and 5–6 mm in the y direction, i.e., considerably less, especially in the x direction. This again speaks for the difficulty in adapting the CBA atlas to Japanese brains. Two general observations have been made. One is that the occipital horns appear to be more greatly separated than those in the European brains. This fact has stressed the necessity of scaling x in the x direction, not from one side to the other, which is indeed possible, but from

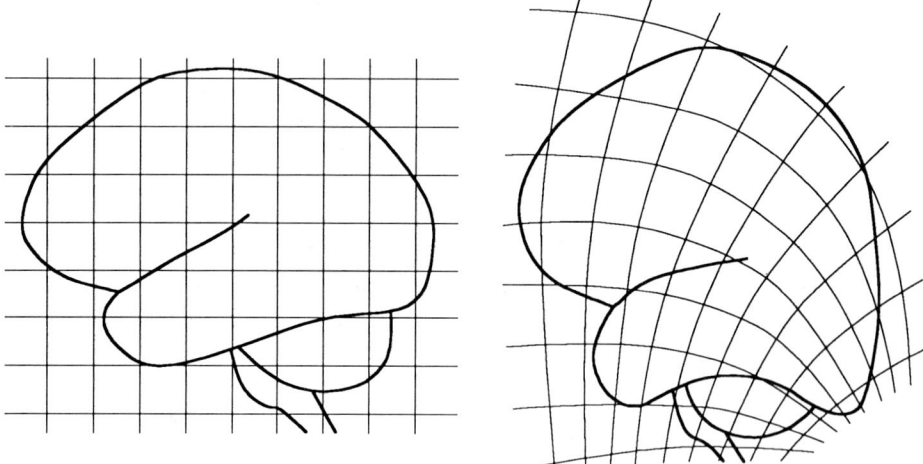

Figure 3 A freehand drawing of a suggested CBA routine to correct for some of the systematic anatomical differences between Swedish and Japanese brains. Such a routine would have to be supplemented with a procedure in which the occipital hornes can be shifted laterally in order to be a useful correction, allowing comparisons between datasets collected in the different countries. When performing standardization, it is, of course, better to have fewer differences between the anatomy standard and the brains that are going to be fitted.

the midline and toward both sides, increasing the more medial values and decreasing the more lateral ones. Also the propensity of the Japanese occipital lobes to hang down posterior to the cerebellum probably makes a special transformation necessary. From the work of d'Arcy Thompson, we have been inspired to suggest that such a transformation, in the sagittal plane, is something like that depicted in Fig. 3.

Our results raise the question of whether one should take the racial differences into consideration when using methods to "anatomize" functional images. It probably creates less problems when, for example, the East Asian institutions use their own standard brains. This means that different standard brains should be used in different parts of the world. However, when results from these different places are to be compared for scientific reasons, more sophisticated transformation methods might be applied on the mean images obtained, for example, when comparing Swedish and Japanese results.

VI. Discussion

Image standardization, making inter- and intrasubject comparisons possible, plays an increasingly important part in the quantification of neuroimaging data. We have discussed different characteristics of standardization methods and described some of the different approaches reported in the literature, each of which has its own merits in certain applications. None of these methods fulfill the criteria of the ideal standardization transformation described in Section II. However, by knowing the advantages and disadvantages of the method used and by carefully planning the study in advance, identifying the possible sources of error, and trying to minimize their influence, the standardization can still be performed, with introduced errors kept at a reasonable level.

In the future, image standardization techniques will certainly use much more complex transformations, enabling them to more closely approximate the ideal standardization. In the clinical situation, a database library of standardized images might become available. Such a library could contain mean images from a normal group as well as mean images of different pathological situations. The state of an individual could be compared with images in the database, for example, by subtracting the mean image from the normal group from the image of the patient, thus giving diagnostic aid to the radiologist (Greitz *et al.*, 1991). Whether this will be realized or not, it is clear that, when standardization methods become more

frequently used, there will be a strong demand for fully automated methods. An automatic matching procedure will, in this case, not be sufficient. Preprocessing of the data, such as image segmentation (e.g., isolation of the brain), must also be performed without requiring manual intervention.

References

Bajcsy, R., and Kovacic, S. (1989). Multiresolutional elastic matching. *Comput. Vision Graphics Image Process.* **46**, 1–21.

Bergström, M., Boethius, J., Eriksson, L., Greitz, T., Ribbe, T., and Widen, L. (1981). Head fixation system for reproducible position alignment in transmission CT and positron emission tomography. *J. Comput. Assist. Tomogr.* **5**, 136–141.

Bohm, C., Greitz, T., Kingsley, D., Berggren, B. M., and Olsson, L. (1983). Adjustable computerized stereotaxic brain atlas for transmission and emission tomography. *Am. J. Neuroradiol.* **4**, 731–733.

Bohm, C., Greitz, T., Blomqvist, G., Farde, L., Forsgren, P. O., Kingsley, D., Sjögren, I., Wiesel, F. A., and Wik, G. (1986). Applications of a computerized adjustable brain atlas in positron emission tomography. *Acta. Radiol.* **369**(Suppl.), 449–452.

Bookstein, F. L. (1991). Thin-plate splines and the atlas problem for biomedical images. In "Information Processing in Medical Imaging: Lecture Notes in Computer Science" (A. Colchester and D. Hawkes, Eds.), Vol. 511. Berlin: Springer-Verlag.

Evans, A. C., Marett, S., Torrescorzo, J., Ku, S., and Collins, L. (1991). MRI–PET correlation in three dimensions using a volume-of-interest (VOI) atlas. *J. Cereb. Blood Flow Metab.* **11**, A69–A78.

Evans, A. C., Marett, S., Neelin, P., Collins, K. W., Weiqian, D., Milot, S., Meyer, E., and Bub, D. (1992). Anatomical mapping of functional activation in stereotactic coordinate space. *Neuroimage* **1**, 43–53.

Faber, T., and Stokely, E. (1988). Orientation of 3-D structures in medical images. *IEEE Trans. Pattern Anal. Mach. Intell.* **10**(5), 626–633.

Fox, P. T., Perlmutter, J. S., and Raichle, M. E. (1985). A stereotactic method of anatomical localization for positron emission tomography. *J. Comput. Assist. Tomogr.* **9**(1), 141–153.

Friston, K. J., Passingham, R. E., Nutt, J. G., Heather, J. D., Sawle, G. V., and Frackowiak, R. S. J. (1989). Localisation in PET images: Direct fitting of the intercommissural (AC–PC) line. *J. Cereb. Blood Flow Metab.* **9**, 690–695.

Friston, K. J., Frith, C. D., Liddle, P. F., and Frackowiak, R. S. J. (1991). Plastic transformation of PET images. *J. Comput. Assist. Tomogr.* **15**(4), 634–639.

Fujita, H., Kanno, I., Greitz, T., and Eriksson, L. (1993). A comparison of two methods of standardizing 3D brain imaging data: The use of European standard brain on Japanese population. Manuscript in preparation.

Greitz, T., Bohm, C., Holte, S., and Eriksson, L. (1991). A computerized brain atlas: Construction, anatomical content and some applications. *J. Comput. Assist. Tomogr.* **15**(1), 26–38.

Greitz, T., Holte, S., Bohm, C., Eriksson, L., Seitz, R., Ericson, K., Nybäck, H., and Stone-Elander, S. (1991). A data base library as a diagnostic aid in neuroimaging. *Neuroradiology* **33**(Suppl.), 2–4.

Ingvar, M., Eriksson, L., Greitz, T., Stone-Elander, S., Dahlbom,

M., Rosenqvist, G., af Trampe, P., and von Euler, C. (1993). Methodological aspects of brain activation studies: Cerebral blood flow determined with [^{15}O]butanol and positron emission tomography. *J. Cereb. Blood Flow Metab.,* accepted for publication.

Jiang, H., Robb, R., and Holton, K. (1992). A new approach to 3-D registration of multimodality medical images by surface matching. *In* "Visualization in Biomedical Computing 1992," Vol. 1808, pp. 196–213. Chapel Hill: SPIE.

Maguire, G., Noz, M., Rusinek, H., Jaeger, J., Kramer, E., Sanger, J., and Smith, G. (1991). Graphics applied to medical image registration. *IEEE Comput. Graph. Appl.* **2**(2), 20–28.

Pelizzari, C., Chen, G., Spelbring, D., Weichselbaum, R., and Chen, C. T. (1989). Accurate three-dimensional registration of CT, PET, and/or MR images of the brain. *J. Comput. Assist. Tomogr.* **13**(1), 20–26.

Seitz, R. J., Bohm, C., Greitz, T., Roland, P. E., Eriksson, L., Blomqvist, G., Rosenkvist, G., and Nordell, B. (1990). Accuracy and precision of the computerized brain atlas program for localization and quantification in positron emission tomography. *J. Cereb. Blood Flow Metab.* **10**, 443–457.

Talairach, J., and Tournoux, P. (1988). "Co-Planar Stereotactic Atlas of the Human Brain: 3-Dimensional Proportional System—An approach to Cerebral Imaging." Stuttgart/New York: Thieme Verlag.

Thurfjell, L., Bohm, C., Greitz, T., and Eriksson, L. (1993). Transformations and algorithms in a computerized brain atlas. *IEEE Trans. Nucl Sci.* **40**(4), 1187–1191.

12

Three-Dimensional Surface-Based Spatial Normalization Using a Convex Hull

J. Hunter Downs III, Jack L. Lancaster, and Peter T. Fox

Biomedical Image Analysis Division, Research Imaging Center, University of Texas Health Science Center at San Antonio, San Antonio, Texas 78284

I. Introduction

Given its convoluted cortex, the brain presents investigators with a fundamental quandary of how to report locations of research findings. It is difficult to describe such locations relative to common and easily located structures, such as the central sulcus, for several reasons. Structures, visible in the images of one modality, may not be apparent in another modality. Additionally, because the shape and size of these structures are variable across subjects, measurements from one subject are inappropriate for another. However, the fundamental problem with using relative location descriptors is the lack of a standard frame of reference. To define a reference frame, the position and orientation of a brain within a coordinate system must be established. A localization technique based on a reference frame derived from an anatomically defined coordinate system resolves these problems. Size and shape of individual brains can then be adjusted to match a standard brain within the reference frame. This normalization process facilitates comparison of function localization across subjects and localizations, which are individually statistically insignificant, can be averaged together to provide a group statistic that is significant (Fox *et al.*, 1988).

II. Atlases

Talairach proposed a reference frame for neurosurgery as early as 1967 in his atlas based on the bicom-

missural (AC–PC) line. It was not used for image alignment, however, until Tokunaga and Takase (1977) proposed the use of the glabella–inion (GI) line as a baseline for tomographic scan orientation of CT studies and defined the relationship between the GI line and the AC–PC line. Using these relationships, Fox *et al.* (1985) established a method for transforming a set of PET brain slices into the Talairach coordinate system. About the same time, Vanier *et al.* (1985) established a technique for transforming CT brain slices into the Talairach coordinate system. Other techniques for transforming PET tomographic scan data into the Talairach coordinate system (Friston *et al.*, 1989, 1991; Minoshima *et al.*, 1992) have since been developed.

The original Talairach atlas is not without problems in defining a standard reference frame for the brain. For one, there is no standard brain; the atlas is actually an amalgamation of different brains. Second, there is no brain within the atlas adequately sampled in the slice direction. This is due, in part, to the fact that sampling was done with histologic sections, making it impossible to obtain slices through any one brain in transaxial, coronal, and sagittal orientations. This problem is less severe with the more recent atlas by Talairach (Talairach and Tournoux, 1988). In this later atlas, a single brain was accurately sectioned (sagittally) in both hemispheres and the sections photographed. From actual size prints of the photographs, the sagittal sections were outlined and then, using these outlines, outlines for the other two orientations, coronal and transaxial, were interpolated by point-

FUNCTIONAL NEUROIMAGING

to-point projection. One other significant difference between the earlier atlas and the more recent one is the definition of the origin of the coordinate system. In the earlier version, the origin was placed at the mid-point between the AC and PC. The newer version has the origin moved to the posterior margin of the AC (PMAC).

The Talairach atlases are not the only ones to which researchers have normalized their data. Other atlases tend to be designed as volume-of-interest (VOI) atlases. Bajcsy *et al.* (1983) created a computerized anatomy atlas using outlines digitized from a standard atlas. Bohm *et al.* (1983) and Greitz *et al.* (1991) created an atlas from photographed microtome sections and outlines of VOIs. Evans *et al.* (1988) designed a computerized VOI atlas in which 56 VOIs were defined in each hemisphere on a MRI scanned brain chosen as a standard. One interesting difference in the use of these atlases, compared with the use of the Talairach atlas, was the idea of transforming the atlas to fit the data rather than *vice versa,* as done with Talairach atlas applications. It should be noted, as Greitz *et al.* (1991) pointed out, that atlas-to-data and data-to-atlas transformations are merely inverses of each other and there is no reason why these transforms cannot be applied in either direction.

III. Spatial Alignment

Whatever the transformation direction, the first step in the transformation involves spatial alignment. As a matter of terminology, a distinction should be made between spatial registration and spatial alignment. Spatial registration is the process of orienting one dataset, which defines an object, to match the orientation of another dataset of the *same* object. In the field of brain imaging, this usually refers to a process whereby, to use the terminology of Bookstein (1989), landmarks or points with a biologically meaningful label are specified in each dataset and a transformation is designed that minimizes the positional difference between corresponding landmarks in the two datasets. Orienting a PET scan to match the orientation of an MR scan of the same patient (e.g., Pelizarri *et al.*, 1989) is an example of spatial registration. Spatial alignment, on the other hand, is the process of orienting a dataset along a set of axes defined by a *standard* object. In brain imaging, this usually implies orienting the image volume such that landmarks defining anatomically significant lines and planes are aligned with the three orthogonal axes (x, y, z,) in the transformed volume's digital matrix. An example of spatial alignment is using the anterior and posterior commissure

landmarks to define the bicommissural line that is then transformed, using some affine transformation, to align along the corresponding line within a standard atlas. When a 3D object's orientation relative to all three axes of the coordinate system has been defined, a reference frame has been established for that object.

The newer Talairach atlas reference frame is defined by using the interhemispheric sagittal plane, the location of the AC–PC line, and the posterior margin of the anterior commissure (PMAC). The interhemispheric sagittal plane is defined as the y–z plane in the Talairach coordinate system. The AC–PC line, which lies in the interhemispheric sagittal plane, is the y axis in the Talairach reference frame and, therefore, defines the orientation of the interhemispheric sagittal plane. The PMAC, located on the AC–PC line, is the origin of the Talairach reference frame. The z axis is then the line, in the interhemispheric sagittal plane, passing through the PMAC and orthogonal to the AC–PC line. Finally, the x axis is the line, passing through the PMAC, that is mutually orthogonal to the y and z axes (Fig. 1).

Using the Talairach reference frame, corresponding landmarks in the scan data are selected and an optimal transformation determined. To accomplish this, the scan data are transformed by rotation in a manner to accurately represent the interhemispheric sagittal plane as a single tomographic slice. This midsagittal slice is then used to determine the location of the AC–PC line. Methods for determining the location of the AC–PC line vary. Fox *et al.* (1985) estimated AC–PC line location based on a determined relationship between the line and the glabella–inion line, which was obtained from a lateral skull radiograph. In an effort to remove the necessity of the lateral skull radiograph required by this technique, Friston *et al.* (1989) applied a regression fit, using four points, the anterior and posterior commissures, the thalamic nuclei, and the occipital pole, to determine the AC–PC line location. Most recently, Minoshima *et al.* (1992) estimated the AC–PC line, from PET data, using four automatically detected landmarks: the frontal and occipital pole, the most ventral point of the anterior corpus callosum, and the subthalamic point. Determining the location of the PMAC is readily accomplished because this landmark is often defined in the AC–PC line fit. By recording the rotations required to orient the midsagittal, the orientation of the AC–PC line, and the location of the PMAC, a transformation that comprises three rotations and three translations is defined. Applying this transformation to the original scan data results in a new spatially aligned dataset in the Talairach reference frame.

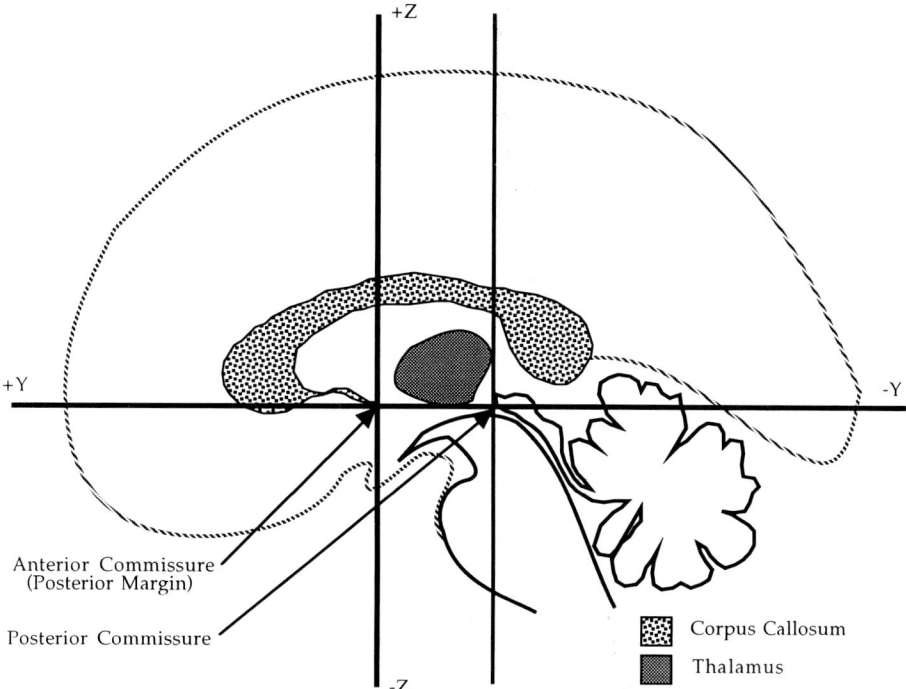

Figure 1   Reference frame of the Talairach atlas. This illustration is of the midsagittal plane. The y and z axes are illustrated. The positive x axis is oriented out of the page, arising from the intersection of the y and z axes.

It should be stressed that, whereas the majority of the spatial alignment methods have been directed toward PET spatial alignment, nothing constrains these methods to PET data only. Applications to other tomographic imaging modalities, such as MR and CT, are currently under investigation.

Software developed at the Research Imaging Center for spatial alignment provides a quick, standard method of image alignment. This software provides high-speed rendering of axial, coronal, and sagittal slice views that assist the user in manually aligning the midsagittal plane using rotation and translation tools provided for all views. Automated methods to perform this task are being researched and may use cross-correlation and Hough transform techniques (Brummer, 1991). Next, the software presents a sagittal view and asks the user to mark the points suggested by Friston *et al.* (1989) for fitting the AC–PC line. The line is then defined using a weighted least-squares fit of the marked points. Because alternative sets of points and weightings exist for AC–PC line definition, modification of the software is underway to provide a menu of the point sets to allow the user to mark the points with which they feel the line is most accurately delineated. Also, help screens with these points marked on images from various modalities are being implemented to assist the user in mark-

ing. Finally, the software will incorporate a method for automatically detecting the AC–PC line. After the AC–PC line has been identified, the program has all the parameters necessary for spatial alignment and can output the aligned dataset for use in image registration and fusion applications [Mazziotta's Merger 1 applications (Mazziotta *et al.*, 1991)] or the program can move onto spatial normalization tasks (Merger 2 applications).

IV. Spatial Normalization

Once aligned, a dataset can then be normalized. Normalization can be broken down into two distinct processes: a morphometrics task and a morphological transform or homology map (Bookstein, 1989). The morphometrics task is measuring and comparing the shapes of the dataset and the standard (Bookstein, 1990). The morphological transform alters the shape of the dataset to conform to that of the standard. In the neuroimaging field, normalization implies the transformation of a dataset of brain images such that chosen morphometric parameters match those of a standard such as an atlas.

The morphometrics task in neuroimaging is one of determining the parameters that define the shape and size of the brain and quantifying those parameters. The parameter set used for the data must have an equivalent set available for the atlas. Because morphometric parameters are usually readily available for an atlas, research has concentrated on which parameters best define the imaged brain. Research into which morphometric parameters should be used for brain shape description lead to a variety of parameter sets (Fox *et al.*, 1985; Vanier *et al.*, 1985; Friston *et al.*, 1989; Minoshima *et al.*, 1992). Minimally, it would seem that a parameter for measuring the size in the direction of each axis (x, y, z) would be necessary. Fox *et al.* (1985) used the length of the AC–PC line between the inner tables of the skull as a parameter for y-axis scaling, the perpendicular distance from the center of the AC–PC line to the inner table of the skull for z-axis scaling, and the width of each tomographic slice of a transmission scan template of the cranium for x-axis scaling. These morphometric parameters, in effect, encompass the maximum extent of the brain in each direction and form a slice-by-slice "bounding box" (Arvo and Kirk, 1989). The problem with the z-axis scaling in PET is that most scans do not encompass the entire head. Originally this was corrected with a lateral skull radiograph. It has since been proposed that dependencies on ancillary imaging techniques for the normalization of a scan be avoided (Mazziotta and Koslow, 1987, 1991). Recently, Minoshima *et al.* (1992) reported estimating the z-axis scaling for the Talairach atlas by matching the midsagittal contour with the atlas contour.

The morphological transformation between the dataset and the atlas has, in general, been handled by a linear transformation using scale factors determined from the ratio of the corresponding morphometric parameters. As a supplement to this standard linear transformation, Friston *et al.* (1991) used the cumulative distribution of counts for both the data and the atlas template image in a process known as histogram specification (Gonzales and Woods, 1992) to nonlinearly resample the data. As an alternative to this linear mapping, Bookstein (1987, 1989, 1990) investigated the use of the "thin-plate spline" mappings derived from landmark correspondences.

The fundamental problem with normalization methods to date is obtaining adequate morphometric parameters. The method of Fox *et al.* (1985) is adequate when transforming the data along the Talairach axes. However, there are potential misregistrations of data distant from the axes. Friston *et al.* (1991) point out that their plastic (nonlinear) transformation relies on the assumption that there not be significant regional differences between the data and the template.

In an effort to obtain better morphometric parame-

ters, research at the Research Imaging Center has focused on representations of the brain surface in 3D. In the process of collecting a large number of samples of the surface of the brain for use as morphometric parameters, one immediate obstacle must be overcome: the problem of local intersubject surface variability. Brain surface folding varies regionally between subjects, and finely sampling highly variable features of sulci while maintaining the primary shape attributable to gyri on the brain surface for scaling parameters can lead to dramatic anomalies in the normalization process (Plate 18). To avoid, quite literally, the pitfalls of finely sampling the brain's surface, methods that use the convex hull as a morphometric descriptor are under investigation at this institution.

The convex hull is the smallest convex set that contains a given dataset. A convex set is a set such that all points along a straight line connecting any two points within the set will be contained within the set (Farin, 1990). In an effort to visualize this in 2D, imagine tightly wrapping a string around the perimeter of an object, so that points touching the surface are connected by a straight line. The string connecting the points around the object guarantees that concave features will be avoided (Plate 19). In 3D, this can be visualized as wrapping a rubber sheet around the surface of the object in such a way that points in contact with the surface are connected with planes.

Preliminary research indicates that the brain has sufficient asymmetries in the sagittal and axial sections to make applying the convexity criterion in these directions potentially detrimental. For this reason, 2D convex hulls will be taken from slices cut along the brain's coronal axis. As a prerequisite step to the convex hull generation, the dataset must be spatially aligned with the Talairach atlas. After the dataset is aligned, a tool for effectively wrapping an object with a string is used to create a convex hull on each slice. Software to fully automate this task is under development. Each of the coronal slices in the series of 2D convex hulls—resulting from the wrapping—is radially sampled to determine the distance from the Talairach y axis to the edge of the hull. This set of distance measurements constitutes the morphometric descriptor for the dataset. To normalize the dataset to the scale of the Talairach atlas, ratios of the distances of corresponding morphometric sample points are computed. Each ratio is used to resample the pixels in the dataset along the ray corresponding to the ratio. This resampling, combined with interpolation, will effectively stretch (or shrink) the convex hull of the dataset to exactly match that of the Talairach atlas. An alternative for determining the morphometric descriptor set would be to make the sampling rays emanate from the Talairach origin rather than at specified increments along a specific Talairach axis; this will be the subject of a future investigation.

Initial research in the use of the convex hull as a morphometric descriptor concentrated on the appropriateness of the Talairach atlas for developing a standard convex hull. Both the old and the new atlases were evaluated. A 2D convex hull (convexity in the slice direction was ignored) of the older Talairach atlas was created for each of the three standard orientations. All three convex hulls have been judged to be inadequate, due to a lack of samples near the edges of the brain (Plate 20). However, the coronal based convex hull of the new atlas appears adequately sampled to be used as a morphometric descriptor (Plate 21).

Evaluation of the accuracy of normalizing brains scanned using MRI to the latest Talairach atlas serves as a starting point for testing of the convex hull normalization technique. Once the technique demonstrates an accceptable level of accuracy with MRI, PET images spatially aligned with the Talairach atlas and scaled to match a corresponding set of MR images from the same person, will be normalized using the convex hull of the MRI dataset. A longer-term goal is to make convex hulls, from spatially aligned PET, CT, and, potentially, SPECT images, with the intent of normalizing the images used to create them.

V. Future

The design of any technique used for normalization should consider the potential for evolution of the atlas reference frame. As atlas reference frames evolve into brain morphology models and begin to include such factors as age, sex, and race into the normalization process, two areas of concern must be addressed. The first deals with the issue of how to transform data normalized with older methods into newer brain morphology models. The second concern is the need for management of the model to include standardization, maintenance, and distribution. Although efforts are being made to address these concerns (e.g., Institute of Medicine Committee on a National Neural Circuitry Database, 1991), they remain as yet unresolved.

References

Arvo, J., and Kirk, D. (1989). A survey of ray tracing acceleration techniques. In "An Introduction to Ray Tracing" (A. S. Glassner, Ed.), pp. 201–262. San Diego: Academic Press.

Bajcsy, R., Lieberson, R., and Reivich, M. (1983). A computerized system for the elastic matching of deformed radiographic images to idealized atlas images. J. Comput. Assist. Tomogr. 7(4), 618–625.

Bohm, C., Greitz, T., Kingsley, D., Berggren, B. M., and Olsson, L. (1983). Adjustable computerized stereotaxic brain atlas for transmission and emission tomography. Am. J. Neuroradiol. 4, 731–733.

Bohm, C., Greitz, T., Seitz, R., and Eriksson, L. (1991). Specification and selection of regions of interset (ROIs) in a computerized brain atlas. J. Cereb. Blood Flow Metab. 11, A64–A68.

Bookstein, F. L. (1989). Principal warps: Thin-plate splines and the decomposition of deformations. IEEE Trans. Pattern Analy. Machine Intelligence 11(6), 567–585.

Bookstein, F. L. (1990). Distortion correction. In "Three-Dimensional Neuroimaging" (A. W. Toga, Ed.), pp. 235–249. New York: Raven Press.

Bookstein, F. L. (1990). Morphometrics. In "Three-Dimensional Neuroimaging" (A. W. Toga, Ed.), pp. 167–188. New York: Raven Press.

Brummer, M. E. (1991). Hough transform detection of the longitudinal fissure in tomographic head images. IEEE Trans. Med. Imaging 10(4), 74–81.

Evans, A. C., Beil, C., Marrett, S., Thompson, C. J., and Hakim, A. (1988). Anatomical–functional correlation using an adjustable MRI-based region of interest atlas with positron emission tomography. J. Cereb. Blood Flow Metab. 8, 513–530.

Evans, A. C., Marrett, S., Torrescorzo, J., Ku, S., and Collins, L. (1991). MRI–PET correlation in three dimensions using a volume-of-interest (VOI) atlas. J. Cereb. Blood Flow Metab. 11, A69–A78.

Farin, G. (1990). "Curves and Surfaces for Computer Aided Geometric Design." San Diego: Academic Press.

Fox, P. T. (1991). Physiological ROI definition by image subtraction. J. Cereb. Blood Flow Metab. 11, A79–A82.

Fox, P. T., Mintun, M. A., Reiman, E. M., and Raichle, M. E. (1988). Enhanced detection of focal brain responses using intersubject averaging and change-distribution analysis of subtracted PET images. J. Cereb. Blood Flow Metab. 8(5), 642–653.

Fox, P. T., Perlmutter, J. S., and Raichle, M. E. (1985). A stereotactic method of anatomical localization for positron emission tomography. J. Comput. Assist. Tomogr. 9(1), 141–153.

Friston, K. J., Passingham, R. E., Nutt, J. G., Heather, J. D., Sawle, G. V., and Frackowiak, R. S. J. (1989). Localisation of PET images: Direct fitting of the intercommissural (AC–PC) line. J. Cereb. Blood Flow Metab. 9, 690–695.

Friston, K. J., Frith, C. D., Liddle, P. F., and Frackowiak, R. S. J. (1991). Plastic transformation of PET images. J. Comput. Assist. Tomogr. 15(4), 634–639.

Gonzalez, R., and Woods, R. E. (1992). "Digital Image Processing." Reading: Addison–Wesley.

Greitz, T., Bohm, C., Holte, S., and Eriksson, L. (1991). A computerized brain atlas: Construction, anatomical content, and some applications. J. Comput. Assist. Tomogr. 15(1), 26–38.

Mazziotta, J. C., and Koslow, S. H. (1987). Assessment of goals and obstacles in data acquisition and analysis from emission tomography: Report of a series of international workshops. J. Cereb. Blood Flow Metab. 7, S1–S31.

Mazziotta, J. C., Pelizzari, C. C., Chen, G. T., Bookstein, F. L., and Valentino, D. (1991). Region of interest issues: The relationship between structure and function in the brain. J. Cereb. Blood Flow Metab. 11, A51–A56.

Mazziotta, J. C., Valentino, D., Grafton, S., Bookstein, F. L., Pelizzari, C., Chen, G., and Toga, A. W. (1991). Relating structure to function in vivo with tomographic imaging. In "Exploring

Brain Functional Anatomy with Positron Tomography'' (D. J. Chadwick and J. Whelan, Eds.), pp. 93–112.

Minoshima, S., Berger, K. L., Lee, K. S., and Mintun, M. A. (1992). An automated method for rotational correction and centering of three-dimensional functional brain images. *J. Nucl. Med.* **33,** 1579–1585.

Minoshima, S., Berger, K. L., Mintun, M. A., Taylor, S. F., and Koeppe, R. A. (1992). Automated stereotactic transformation of functional brain PET images. *J. Soc. Nucl. Med.* **33**(5), 1007. [Abstr.]

Pechura, C. M., and Martin, J. B. (Eds.) (1991). ''Mapping the Brain and Its Functions: Integrating Enabling Technologies into Neuroscience Research.'' Washington, D.C.: National Academy Press.

Pelizzari, C. A., Chen, G. T. Y., Spelbring, D. R., Weichselbaum, R. R., and Chen, C.-T. (1989). Accurate three-dimensional registration of CT, PET and/or MR images of the brain. *J. Comput. Assist. Tomogr.* **13**(1), 20–26.

Talairach, J., and Szikla, G. (1967). ''Atlas d'Anatomie Stereotaxique du Telencephale.'' Paris: Masson & Cie.

Talairach, J., and Tournoux, P. (1988). ''Co-Planar Stereotaxic Atlas of the Human Brain. New York: Thieme Medical.

Tokunaga, A., Takase, M., and Otani, K. (1977). The Gabella–Inion line as a baseline for CT scanning of the brain. *Neuroradiology* **14,** 67–71.

Vanier, M., Lecours, A. R., Ethier, R., Habib, M., Poncet, M., Milette, P. C., and Salamon, G. (1985). Proportional localization system for anatomical interpretation of cerebral computed tomograms. *J. Comput. Assist. Tomogr.* **9**(4), 715–724.

13

Statistical Probability Mapping of Brain Function and Structure

E. Roy John,*,† Jian-Zhou Zhang,*,† Jonathon D. Brodie,*
and Leslie S. Prichep*,†

*Department of Psychiatry, New York University Medical Center, New York, New York 10016;
and †Nathan S. Kline Research Institute, Orangeburg, New York 10962

I. Introduction

Quantitative analysis of brain *functions* as reflected in such electrophysiological measures as the electroencephalogram (EEG) and sensory evoked responses (ERPs) began more than 20 years ago. At first, replacing subjective inspection of massive amounts of raw electrophysiological waveshapes by objective numerical data seemed as though it must be advantageous. However, organizing the voluminous numerical output in such a way as to extract useful basic or clinical information posed its own difficulties. The initial attempts to overcome these difficulties, and to make more explicit the anatomical information potentially available from such data, used interpolation algorithms operating on quantitative values assigned to electrode positions on a spatial grid to construct topographic maps. These maps showed cranial distributions of momentary EEG voltages, integrated EEG power in some time interval, or, eventually, computed the power in spectral frequency bands using Fast Fourier Transform (FFT). Such topographic maps greatly enhanced the clinical utility of quantitative EEG (QEEG).

II. Topographic Mapping of Quantitative EEG (QEEG) Measures

A. Voltage and Power Maps

Focal abnormalities, such as the onset and growth of a voltage peak corresponding to an epileptic spike, could be localized by constructing voltage maps at successive time points. Focal slow wave excesses, corresponding to the effects of a space-occupying lesion, could sometimes be localized by mapping the power in a low-frequency range such as the delta band (1.5 to 3.5 Hz) integrated across some period of observation. Wide-band spectral analysis, using FFT, permitted maps to be made of the power in a given frequency band, integrated across some period of observation. Power maps offered clinical utility in the evaluation of cerebrovascular disease, dementia, and encephalopathies due to various diseases or agents.

B. Normative Databases

As clinicians tried to extend the utility of topographic mapping of brain electrical activity, they encountered more and more instances in which diagnostic conclusions were uncertain because of the absence of objective criteria defining when numerical observations, quantitative though they might be, were to be considered abnormal. This uncertainty placed grave limitations on the utility of QEEG for the detection of small brain tumors, the early confirmation of cerebrovascular incidents, or the assessment of closed head injuries. The method was used but rarely for the detection of early degenerative deterioration in elderly patients with organic brain syndrome and essentially not at all for developmental disorders such as attention-deficit hyperactivity disorder or for the evaluation of psychiatric patients. Gradually, widespread recognition emerged of the desirability of establishing normative databases. Parametric statistical methods permit-

FUNCTIONAL NEUROIMAGING

ted assessment of a set of electrophysiological measurements relative to such a reference database, yielding an objective definition of "abnormal" as "*statistically improbable in the healthy population*" (John *et al.*, 1977; Duffy *et al.*, 1981).

C. Statistical Probability Maps

The top of Plate 22 shows an interpolated head map of the relative (percentage) power in the beta EEG frequency band (12.5–25.0 Hz), from a patient with an infarct of an anterior temporal branch of the right anterior cerebral artery. The color scale is in microvolts squared. The bottom of Plate 22 shows a statistical probability, or "Z-score," map, which presents the same data after subtracting the normative amount of beta power expected in an average healthy person who is the same age as the patient from each point and dividing the difference by the standard deviation of the normative distribution. The color scale is in standard deviations from the normal mean value, where red hues are excesses and blue hues are deficits. Note that in the map shown at the bottom of Plate 22, only beta excesses appeared, so the color scale shown defines only the degree of excess.

Notice how dramatically the statistical probability map pinpoints the focal abnormality. At the short time after the cerebrovascular accident when these data were recorded, this patient was CT-scan negative. Functional abnormalities related to such brain injuries very often can be detected as much as 36 h before changes can be revealed by structural imaging methods. Statistical probability images further enhance sensitivity.

D. Advantages of Z-Transformation

The basic calculation rests upon computation of the Z score:

$$Z = \frac{(\text{observed value} - \text{predicted normative value})}{\text{standard deviation of normative distribution}}.$$

Utilization of the Z score can provide a method for enhancement of the signal-to-noise ratio of *clinically significant* information in a computer-generated image. Prior to use of the Z score, it is extremely important to examine the distribution of normative data and impose transformations to render the score Gaussian if it is not so initially (John *et al.*, 1988). In our experience, many distributions of biological numerical descriptors deviate appreciably from Gaussianity. Generalized methods for transforming such nonnormal distributions to Gaussianity have been published (Box and Cox, 1964). Once this has been achieved, Z scores can be legitimately computed

and powerful parametric multivariate statistical methods become valid to use.

The Z transformation affords numerous important advantages. *First,* expected values are essentially treated as background information and removed by subtraction, thereby highlighting deviations from the expected, which are potentially of clinical interest. *Second,* a normalized scale is thereby provided in which the dimensions and absolute values of measures are replaced by the common metric of *probability.* Composite features can be constructed such as the *Mahalanobis distances,* computed from covariance matrices across large sets of local features. Such composite measures not only serve to compress large datasets but also account for the expected intercorrelation between measures, thus providing a quantitative description of relationships among a set of anatomical loci. These descriptors of *brain organization* can be regarded as quantifying certain *global* aspects of brain images. *Third,* objective image analysis or *pattern recognition* can be implemented using spatial principal component analysis to construct image descriptors, multivariate discriminant functions to classify images, and uninstructed cluster analysis both to classify and to construct subtypes.

III. Statistical Classifiers Using QEEG

A. Diagnostic Discriminant Functions

These methods, applied to electrophysiological data, have extended the utility of QEEG from the domain of neurology to the domain of psychiatry. Statistical probability maps reveal that psychiatric patients are characterized by complex and anatomically extensive abnormalities that indicate severe disturbances of brain interrelationships, disruption of system organization rather than focal lesions (John *et al.,* 1988). The pattern of disturbed organization appears to be distinctive for different disorders. Salient features are shared by a high proportion of patients diagnosed with certain neurological disorders or illnesses in the major categories defined by DSM-IIIR (American Psychiatric Association, 1987). Thus, it has been possible to construct multivariate discriminant functions that can accurately classify patients as psychiatrically normal or abnormal, or suffering from learning disabilities, closed head injury without loss of consciousness, alcoholism, primary degenerative dementia or dementia of vascular origin, primary affective disorder, or schizophrenia (Prichep and John, 1992). Such classifiers rely heavily on Mahalanobis distances, which can be used to evaluate covariance matrices that characterize complex brain relationships.

The accuracy of many of these classifier functions is shown in Table 1 (Prichep and John, 1992).

B. Subtype Identification by Cluster Analysis

Further, within many of these diagnostic categories, cluster analysis identified subtypes with the same clinical symptoms but different evolutions of disease or response to treatment. Among the subtypes thus far identified have been learning disabled children who will and will not respond to methylphenidate (Prichep and John, 1990), unipolar versus bipolar depressed patients presenting in a state of depression (Prichep, 1987; Prichep et al., 1990a), depressed patients who will and will not respond to electroconvulsive shock (Roemer et al., 1991), obsessive compulsive disorder (OCD) patients who will and will not re-

spond to serotonin reuptake inhibitors (Prichep et al., 1993c), elderly patients who will and will not show progressive cognitive impairment over a 3- to 10-year period in the future (Prichep et al., 1993b), schizophrenic patients who will and will not respond favorably to haloperidol (Prichep et al., 1990b; Czobor and Volavka, 1991), and comatose head injured patients who will remain in a vegetative state or return to useful cognitive function (Thatcher et al., 1991).

Since the introduction of statistical probability mapping in electrophysiology, less than 15 years ago, QEEG has moved from being a research tool limited to a few university laboratories to becoming a technique with increasingly acknowledged clinical utility, utilized routinely in more than a thousand facilities in the United States and abroad. *The critical steps in this enhancement of the practical value of brain electrical activity*

Table 1   A. Neurometric QEEG Two Group Discriminants

Group			n		Mean discriminant accuracy (%) (initial discriminant/ independent replication)	
I	vs	II	I	II	I	II
N	vs	Dep	95	111	88/86	83/93
Uni	vs	Bip	65	32	84/87	88/94
N	vs	MHI	150	52	91/84	89/92
N	vs	Sz	149	57	96/99	90/82
Dep	vs	Sz	103	46	84/88	84/85[a]
N	vs	Alc	120	30	95/95	75/90[b]
Abn	vs	Alc	32–97	30	91/88	96/93[b]
N	vs	LD	158	175	89/79	72/71
Vas Dem	vs	Dem	93	13	94/82	92/85[b]
RitResp	vs	NonResp	16	12	81/81[b]	83/83[b]

B. Neurometric QEEG Multiple Group Discriminants

Group							n				Mean discriminant accuracy (%) (initial discriminant/ independent replication)			
I	vs	II	vs	III	vs	IV	I	II	III	IV	I	II	III	IV
N	vs	Dep	vs	Dem			85	87	125	—	84/85	84/80	84/71	—
N	vs	Dep	vs	Alc	vs	Dem	120	103	30	125	77/75	72/85	80/80	79/77

Note. Summary of discriminant results for two group (A) and multiple group (B) neurometric QEEG discriminant functions. The initial discriminant accuracy is indicated first (X), followed by the accuracy in the independent replication (Y), as X/Y. Group codes are as follows: N, normal; Dep, major affective disorder, depression; Uni, unipolar depression; Bip, bipolar depression; MHI, mild head injury; Sz, chronic schizophrenia; Abn, abnormal groups combined; Alc, alcoholic; LD, learning disabled; RitResp, responders to ritalin; NonResp, nonresponders to ritalin; Dem, dementia (SDAT); Vas Dem, dementia of vascular etiology. From Prichep et al. (1992).

[a] Medicated group used for replication.

[b] Jackknifed replication.

mapping were construction of normative databases, subtraction of predicted values from the images obtained from individual patients, and statistical evaluation of the resulting difference images.

IV. Statistical Probability Images (SPI) of PET Scans

A. Construction of a Normative Pixel Database

Potentially, images of regional glucose utilization or the regional density of receptor sites for specific neurotransmitters or pharmacological agents, visualized by appropriate radioisotopic labeling of key substances and positron emission tomography (PET), offers an incredibly powerful tool not only for basic clinical research but also for improving the routine management of the psychiatric patient in particular. Unfortunately, until the present this potential has not been translated to practical application. PET images, although computed from quantitative measurements, depend for their evaluation upon the subjective qualitative judgment of a skilled and experienced interpreter. No clinical utility for PET images that enables their use in selecting the treatment for individual patients has yet been developed. In order to reach this stage, if indeed PET (or its near neighbor SPECT) is ever to become a routine clinical adjunct, we consider statistical image analysis an indispensable next step. Accordingly, we undertook to develop a normative pixel database for regional cerebral glucose utilization, with normative data for every pixel in the PET image, and to develop methods for the generation of statistical probability images (SPI) of PET based upon pixel-by-pixel Z transformation.

In order to perform the proposed rescaling of pixel values required to construct SPI, the mean value and standard deviation of the distribution of glucose uptake must be established pixel by pixel from a normative set of reference PET images. Prior to extraction of these normative statistical parameters, it was necessary to develop a method for the *normalization of size and shape* of brain slices from PET scans of a large number of normal subjects and to put corresponding pixels in different images into spatial registration. Scans using ^{18}F-deoxyglucose (^{18}F-DG), obtained from a PET VI camera, were obtained from 40 normal subjects.[1]

---

[1] These data were obtained through research supported by NIS Grant No. N515638 and NINDS Grant No. MH42647 under the direction of J. D. Brodie, M.D., Ph.D.

B. Shape and Size Normalization— Pixel Z Scores

Our method for shape and size normalization and statistical pixel evaluation (John *et al.*, 1994c) is illustrated in Fig. 1. It consists of the following steps.

(0) *Edge detection*—along each line of data across the image of each slice, the variance of density is computed for a small sliding window of pixels. The *edge* is defined by a significant increase (decrease) in pixel density;

(1) Using the area defined as the loci inside the set of edges thus defined, the *centroid* is calculated. This area is then translated so the centroid is located at the origin of a set of standard reference axes and rotated so its midline coincides with the vertical axis;

(2) A *standard circle* of radius R, centered at the centroid, is then circumscribed around the slice;

(3) Along each of 720 radii, each successively rotated $0.5°$ from the vertical axis to an angle Θ_i, a line r_i is drawn to the edge of the slice. These lines are then linearly *stretched* by an amount R/r_i, thereby dilating each slice to the standard circle with radius R.

(4) Each pixel in the slice area can now be identified as the pixel at location r_{ij} (where r_{ij} indicates the jth interval along the radius r_i at angle Θ_i). Using the mean value of that pixel, $\bar{r}_{ij}$; and the standard deviation, σ_{ij}, of the corresponding distribution of pixel values in the normative database, we calculate the *pixel Z score*,

$$Z_{rij} = (r_{ij} - \bar{r}_{ij})/\sigma_{ij};$$

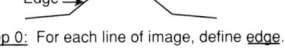

Edge → Step 0: For each line of image, define edge.

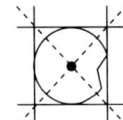

Step 1: Find center of edge-defined slices.

Step 2: Inscribe in standard circle.

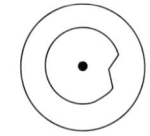

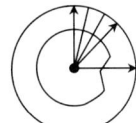

Step 3: For each of 720 intervals of $0.5°(\theta i)$, stretch $r(\theta i)$ to R, linearly expanding each interval by $R/r(\theta i)$.

Step 4: Divide each expanded radius $R(\theta i)$ into N intervals $\Delta rj(\theta i)$ and compute:

$$Z(\Delta rj, \theta i) = \frac{\Delta rj, \theta i - \overline{\Delta rj, \theta i}}{\sigma \Delta rj, \theta i}$$

Step 5: Construct probability image PET (SPI) using color heat scale which becomes more red to yellow for $Z > 0$ and more blue to white for $Z < 0$.

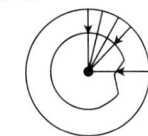

Step 6: Restore SPI image to original anatomical size shrinking at each of 720 $0.5°$ intervals by $r(\theta i) / R$.

Figure 1 Steps in shape normalization and pixel Z transformation of a PET image.

(5) The *SPI* is then constructed, color coding each pixel according to its Z score; and

(6) The slice can now be *shrunken* back to its original size and shape by linearly reversing the dilation, computing r_i/R. Alternatively, the standard circle representing all the slices from the whole brain can be stacked into a *standard cylinder*, from which sagittal or coronal slices can be computed.

V. Validation of Normalization Procedure

The precision of the resulting images depends upon the accuracy of pixel registration achieved by the size and shape normalization, and the adequacy of the normative distribution parameters. We tested this in three ways.

(1) The *total variance* was computed across the full set of about 45,000 pixels, representing 13 slices, for the sample of 40 normal subjects and for 45 chronic schizophrenics. For both sets of subjects, the intersubject variance across all subjects decreased about 8.5% after standard circle normalization, indicating that the individual scans were in better registration;

(2) An experienced PET interpreter marked a *reference point* (center of putamen) in each of a set of PET scans from 34 normals and 28 schizophrenic patients, from whom this point was reproducibly identified in two randomized visual identification sessions. The standard deviation of this reference point across the set of PET scans was 5.4 mm for the raw scans and 4.7 mm after standard circle normalization. This represents a 13% decrease in variance. The standard deviation of location is about one-half the solution of the PET VI.

The measurements were scaled with reference to a stereotaxic MRI atlas (Talairach and Tournoux, 1988). In order to identify specific anatomical regions of interest, we have modified this standard stereotaxic MRI atlas. We superimposed a grid on each coronal section, dividing the proportional scale into 10 horizontal intervals at each of 12 vertical levels. Each coronal slice was thus represented as 120 rectangles. Each rectangle is about 8×14 mm, or about $4\times$ of the standard deviation of localization in the standard circle. By slicing the Z-transformed PET images, stacked into the standard cylinder, into 16 coronal sections, about 16 slices $\times$ 10 horizontal intervals $\times$ 13 vertical levels = 2080 regions of interest can be defined. Each of these ROIs can be thought of as analogous to a volume element of a "Mercator" projection of the brain. If desirable, norms can be computed for each "voxel ROI" instead of for each pixel, as below.

(3) The mean and standard deviation were computed for every pixel in a "training" group of PET scans from 25 normal subjects. Using this pixel normative database, every pixel in each slice of the PET scans from a "test" group of 15 normal subjects was Z transformed. The *histogram of pixel Z scores*, representing 45,000 measures from each test subject, had fewer values significant at the $p < 0.01$ level than would be expected by chance. When the same test was performed using PET scans from 45 schizophrenic subjects, a high proportion of abnormal Z scores was obtained (see Plate 23).

VI. Absolute and Relative Metabolism

Z transformation in the test normal group and in the schizophrenic group were performed for two types of metabolic measures: *absolute metabolic rate* and *relative metabolic rate*, defined as the *percentage of total brain glucose* uptake represented by each pixel. Relative metabolic rate effects a normalization across brains, because total uptake is defined as 100%, independent of the absolute amount of glucose utilized. Absolute amounts can obviously vary from subject to subject due to factors quite extraneous to brain biochemical peculiarities. Such factors might include nonspecific influences like the level of arousal and attention, the time since the last ingestion of food and the overall level of blood glucose, and the permeability of the blood–brain barrier.

A. Pixel Z-Score Histograms of Normal and Schizophrenics

Plate 23 shows the histograms of the distribution of pixel Z scores for absolute metabolism in the left column and relative metabolism in the right column, for the training normal group (green) versus the test normal group (red) in the top row and the test normal group (green) versus the schizophrenic patients (red) in the bottom row. In each comparison, a separate histogram is shown for the pixel Z-score distribution of the relevant group of subjects, in all of the 13 slices from the top to the bottom of the PET scan (Zhang *et al.*, 1994).

B. Statistical Probability Images (SPI) of Normals and Schizophrenics

Plate 24 shows the Z-transformed SPI of PET slices from slice 7 in 15 normal members of the test group (upper arrays of slices) and in 25 chronic schizophrenics (lower arrays of slices), for absolute metabolic rate (left sets of arrays) and for relative metabolic rate (right sets of arrays). All SPI have been stretched to the standard circle, Z transformed, and color coded to reflect pixel deviations from mean normative values, and shrunk back to their original size and shape. Inspection of the SPI from the test normal group shows that most pixel values of these normal individuals were close to normative mean values, whereas those from the schizophrenic group show a high proportion of pixels whose metabolic rates were very deviant from the normal range.

C. Heterogeneity of Schizophrenic Population

Note the wide variety of different metabolic patterns in these patients. In general, the absolute value of glucose uptake is lower throughout the schizophrenic brain, as was evident from the distributions of pixel Z scores shown in Plate 23. Differences in the extent and anatomical distribution of this *hypo*metabolism can be seen from patient to patient. Note the different patterns of *relative metabolic* abnormality found in these patients. Compared to the *metabolic gradients* of the normal brain as defined by our training group and confirmed in our test group, the schizophrenic patients show brain regions in slice 7 that are significantly *hyper-* as well as *hypo*metabolic. In different subgroups of patients, different abnormal anatomical patterns appear. These schizophrenic patients display many different profiles of metabolic abnormality.

Using QEEG variables, we constructed a discriminant function that successfully separated normal from schizophrenic patients (Prichep *et al.*, 1993a). This discriminant relied heavily upon composite variables or Mahalanobis distances that quantified brain organization as reflected in covariance matrices of QEEG values. Schizophrenia is better reflected in measures of system organization rather than any measures of focal dysfunction. Cluster analysis of a group of 94 schizophrenics, using these discriminating QEEG variables, indicated the presence of five major clusters of patients in this population with different profiles of pathophysiology but similar clinical symptoms (John *et al.*, 1994a).

In each of these clusters, there were small numbers of patients for whom PET data, as well as QEEG and ERP data, were available. We are currently preparing an article that describes the QEEG, ERP, PET, and clinical features of members of each of these five schizophrenic subtypes (John *et al.*, 1994b).

The anatomically widespread patterns of PET and QEEG abnormalities in these patients, different in each subtype, suggest the need to develop complex descriptors of multimodal imaging data. Stratagems such as multimodal principal component analysis of composite electrophysiological–metabolic vectors, containing factor scores from spatial descriptors of both QEEG and PET abnormalities, should be explored. Extraction of factors with loadings on both pathophysiology and abnormal regional metabolism will not only elucidate relationships between functional correlates in the two modalities but also help to compress the mass of multimodal phenomenology to some salient aspects that can be more clearly comprehended. The richness of multimodal imaging will benefit us only if we develop multimodal as well as unimodal statistical descriptors.

References

American Psychiatric Association (1987). "DSM-IIIR: Diagnostic and Statistical Manual," Third ed., revised. Washington, D.C.: American Psychiatric Association.

Box, G., and Cox, D. (1964). An analysis of transformations. *J. R. Stat. Soc. Ser. B* **26**, 211–252.

Czobor, P., and Volavka, J. (1991). Pretreatment EEG predicts short-term response to haloperidol treatment. *Biol. Psychiat.* **30**, 927–942.

Duffy, F., Bartels, P., and Burchfield, J. (1981). Significance probability mapping. *Electroenceph. Clin. Neurophysiol.* **51**, 455–462.

John, E., Karmel, B., Corning, W., Easton, P., Brown, D., Ahn, H., John, M., Harmony, T., Prichep, L., Toro, A., Gerson, I., Bartlett, F., Thatcher, R., Kaye, H., Valdes, P., and Schwartz, E. (1977). Neurometrics: Numerical taxonomy identifies different profiles of brain functions within groups of behaviorally similar people. *Science* **196**, 1383–1410.

John, E., Prichep, L., and Alper, K. (1994a). Quantitative electrophysiological subtyping of schizophrenia. Submitted for publication.

John, E., Prichep, L., Brodie, J., and Zhang, Z. (1994b). Electrophysiological and metabolic characteristics of five subtypes of schizophrenic patients. Manuscript in preparation.

John, E. Prichep, L., Fridman, J., and Easton, P. (1988). Neurometrics: Computer assisted differential diagnosis of brain dysfunctions. *Science* **293**, 162–169.

John, E., Zhang, J., Brodie, J., and Bartlett, E. (1994c). Statistical evaluation of positron emission tomography: Image normalization, Z-transformation and MRI-identified 3D reconstruction. Submitted for publication.

Prichep, L. (1987). Neurometric quantitative EEG measures of depressive disorders. *In* (R. Takahashi, P. Flor-Henry, J. Gruzelier, and S. Niwa, Eds.), "Cerebral Dynamics, Laterality and Psychopathology" pp. 55–69. Amsterdam/New York/Oxford: Elsevier.

Prichep, L., and John, E. (1990). II. Neurometric studies of methylphenidate responders and non-responders. *In* "Perspectives on Dyslexia" (G. T. Pavlidis, Ed.), Vol. 1, Chap. 7, pp. 133–139. New York: Wiley.

Prichep, L., and John, E. (1992). QEEG profiles of psychiatric disorders. *Brain Topogr.* **4**(4), 249–257.

Prichep, L., John, E., Essig-Peppard, T., and Alper, K. (1990a). Neurometric subtyping of depressive disorders. *In* "Plasticity and Morphology of the Central Nervous System" (C. Cazzullo, G. Invernizzi, E. Sacchetti, and A. Vita, Eds.). London: M.T.P. Press.

Prichep, L., John, E., Mas, F., and Essig-Peppard, T. (1990b). Neurometric functional imaging. I. Subtyping of schizophrenia. *In* "Machinery of the Mind" (E. John, Ed.), pp. 460–470. Boston: Birkhauser.

Prichep, L., John, E., Alper, K., Rotrosen, R., and Mas, F. (1993a). Discriminating QEEG characteristics of chronic schizophrenic patients. Submitted for publication.

Prichep, L., John, E., Ferris, S., Reisberg, B., Alper, K., and Cancro, R. (1993b). Neurometric EEG correlates of cognitive deterioration in the elderly. *Neurobiol. Aging* **15**(1). In press.

Prichep, L., Mas, F., Hollander, E., Liebowitz, M., John, E., Almas, M., DeCaria, C., and Levine, R. (1993c). Quantitative electroencephalographic (QEEG) subtyping of obsessive compulsive disorder. *Psychiat. Res.* **50**, 25–32.

Roemer, R., Shagass, C., Dubin, W., Jaffe, R., and Katz, R. (1991). Relationship between pretreatment electroencephalographic coherence measures and subsequent response to electroconvulsive therapy. A preliminary study. *Neuropsychobiology* **24**, 121–124.

Talairach, J., and Tournoux, P. (1988). "Co-Planar Stereotaxic Atlas of the Human Brain." New York: Thieme Medical.

Thatcher, R., Cantor, D., McAlister, R., Geisler, F., and Krause, M. (1991). Comprehensive prediction of outcome in closed head injured patients. *Ann. N.Y. Acad. Sci.* **620**, 82–101.

Zhang, J., John, E., Brodie, J., Prichep, L., Rotrosen, J., Angrist, B., Wolkin, A., and Cancro, R. (1994). Statistical evaluation of positron emission tomography in schizophrenia: I. Absolute and relative metabolic z-score images. Manuscript in preparation.

14

Three-Dimensional Correlative Imaging: Applications in Human Brain Mapping

A. C. Evans,* D. L. Collins, P. Neelin, D. MacDonald, M. Kamber, and T. S. Marrett

McConnell Brain Imaging Center, Montreal Neurological Institute, Montreal, Quebec, Canada H3A 2B4

I. Introduction

A. Background

Numerous approaches to multimodality correlation have been reported. Despite numerous attempts to obtain matched image planes at acquisition time (e.g., Evans *et al.*, 1988; Meltzer *et al.*, 1990a), the majority of groups performing multimodality registration now favor a post hoc analysis, resampling one image volume to obtain a new set of image planes that are coincident with those of the other volume. The most popular approaches to date have employed surface matching (Pelizzari *et al.*, 1989; Levin *et al.*, 1989), homologous landmark matching (Evans *et al.*, 1989, 1991a; Hill *et al.*, 1991), or some form of solid modeling of the objects to be registered, using geometric properties of the derived object (e.g., principal axes) to define the required transformation (e.g., Alpert *et al.*, 1990). Recent developments (Collins *et al.*, 1992ab; Van den Elsen, 1992) suggest that a combination of all of these methods within a general feature-matching approach might be more robust against defects in the raw data resulting from incomplete object coverage, intensity distortion, geometric distortion, lack of contrast, and image noise. In the following sections, we describe

our point-matching registration and compare the results with surface-matching procedures.

1. Point Matching

Landmark-matching registration methods require the matching of a set of 3D points in one image with a homologous set in the other image. These points can be obtained from external fiducial markers attached to the head-holder or preferably to the head itself, or from internal anatomical landmarks.

External fiducials often consist of small capsules, visible in each modality, which are attached to the head but can also include more structured fiducial attachments, particularly for stereotactic surgery applications (Bergstrom *et al.*, 1981; Peters *et al.*, 1986, 1989; Kelly *et al.*, 1984; Kall *et al.*, 1987; Zhang *et al.*, 1990). Problems can arise with external fiducials in functional imaging, particularly in tracer uptake studies, because the fiducial signal must match that in each image to preserve dynamic range in the image data. Also, for correlative studies, the fiducials have stay in place during the setup procedure for both machines and, possibly, for some extended period between the functional and the anatomical scans.

The use of internal landmarks, identified by hand in each image, has the advantages that no special prescan procedures are required and that retrospective matching of data is possible. However, the applicability of the method rests on the ease with which

---

* To whom correspondence should be addressed.

image volumes can be searched to tag corresponding landmarks in each volume. Hence, its success is dependent upon the local implementation of the user interface as much as on fundamental considerations of algorithmic robustness, image contrast, and noise. The landmarks can also provide the raw data for image matching by nonlinear 3D warping of images from different subjects in studies of morphometric variability (Bookstein, 1991; Evans *et al.*, 1991b).

2. Surface Matching

A method that has gained acceptance recently in a number of centers is the "head and hat" approach for matching surfaces from the different modalities (Pelizzari *et al.*, 1989; Levin *et al.*, 1988, 1989; Neiw *et al.*, 1991). The surface of a 3D object that can be identified in both modalities, usually the brain surface, is extracted as a set of 2D contours by an automatic edge-finding operator applied to each slice. One set of contours, usually from the higher resolution data (MRI or CT), constitutes a rigid-body "head," whereas the other set is a rigid-body "hat." Fitting the hat on the head determines the best affine transformation between the two data sets. The algorithm achieves this by minimizing the volume between the two surfaces by an iterative nonlinear least-squares procedure, varying either six (three translation, three rotation) or nine (including anisotropic scaling) affine parameters.

B. MNI Implementation of Landmark-Matching Procedures

At the MNI, coregistration of MRI and PET is performed for every PET study. Between 1988 and 1993, over 500 such procedures were completed using the landmark-matching approach. PET data are acquired with a Scanditronix PC-2048B system with 15 slices and an intrinsic 3D resolution of $5 \times 5 \times 6$ mm (Evans *et al.*, 1991c). Phantom measurements indicated no significant geometric distortion over the imaging field of view. PET images are obtained using [^{18}F]fluorodeoxyglucose (FDG) for measurement of regional glucose metabolism (CMRGlc) (Phelps *et al.*, 1979), $H_2^{15}O$ for measurement of regional cerebral blood flow (CBF) (Herscovitch *et al.*, 1983), or [^{18}F]fluoroDOPA, a tracer for dopaminergic neurotransmission (Garnett *et al.*, 1983). Of the complement of PET/MRI corelated studies, approximately 400 have been studies of cerebral blood flow (CBF), predominantly in normal brain. For purposes of intersubject averaging in brain-mapping experiments (see Section II.A), in which anatomical variability prevents exact superposition of equivalent structures from different subjects, CBF images

have been reconstructed to a lower resolution, 18 mm, than that for single-subject analysis, for which the reconstructed resolution is typically 10 mm.

All MRI studies are performed on a Philips Gyroscan 1.5-T superconducting magnet system. Using 3D spin-echo acquisition, 64 nonoverlapped T_1-weighted ($T_R = 550$ ms, $T_E = 30$ ms) image planes are collected at 2-mm intervals over the whole brain. Measurements of the dimensions of an MRI calibration phantom indicate negligible geometric distortion through the central portion of the MRI imaging field (Peters *et al.*, 1988).

Correlative imaging takes place within the Neuro-Imaging Laboratory, a computational facility in close proximity to the MRI and PET scanning suites. Images are reconstructed on local VAX systems in each scanning suite and transferred via Ethernet to the Neuro-Imaging Laboratory. The 3D imaging systems used are a PIXAR-1, hosted by a SUN 3/180, or SGI 4D/35 and Indigo systems. To obtain registration of the MRI and PET image volumes, a 3D image processing package has been developed. This package allows the following.

- Arbitrary rotation, translation, and scaling of image volumes.
- Real-time triplane display through two volumes, independently controllable, and through the corresponding merged volume.
- Interactive identification of equivalent 3D points in two image volumes via cursor.
- Linear least-squares optimization to calculate the affine transformation, which minimizes the r.m.s. distance between two ensembles of paired points.
- Oblique sectioning through a volume using trilinear, quadratic, or cubic spline interpolation.
- Compositing of two image volumes by opacity weighting.

The registration procedure requires that two sets of equivalent points be defined, one in each volume, and is based on the *Procrustes* algorithm (Sibson, 1978; Golub and Van Loan, 1983), which finds the "best" solution in a least-squares sense by minimizing the r.m.s. distance among all paired points. During the procedure, any three cardinal planes can be selected through each of the MRI, PET and MRI/PET composite images and the nine resultant images, displayed simultaneously. Typically, 10–20 point pairs are tagged in 20–30 min, and the transformation that best matches the two-point ensembles is obtained by minimizing some distance norm, usually in a least-squares sense. The landmarks selected depend upon the tracer being used but generally include centers of obvious structures and features such as points of maximum curvature. For a typical CBF or CMRGlc study, in which tracer accumulates in gray matter, the landmarks selected include head of caudate, thalamus, frontal temporal and occipital poles, sylvian fissure, occipito–cerebellar junction, and the superior–lateral aspect of the parietal lobe. For tracers that provide less anatomical detail, such as fluoroDOPA, which accumulates significantly only in caudate and putamen, we combine points from the fluoroDOPA image and from the PET trasmission image. The transmission image, acquired immediately before the emission study, is in essence a CT scan of density but acquired with 511-keV gamma rays and a PET detector geometry. Although lacking the fine detail of true CT, such images identify petrous bones, sinus cavities, and skull landmarks that can be correlated with the MRI data. Validation studies below (see Section I.C) indicate that such procedures do not significantly degrade registration accuracy.

Plate 25 shows a single slice through a 3D example of matched MRI/FDG data, whereas Fig. 1 shows a composited fluoroDOPA + MRI image. Plate 26

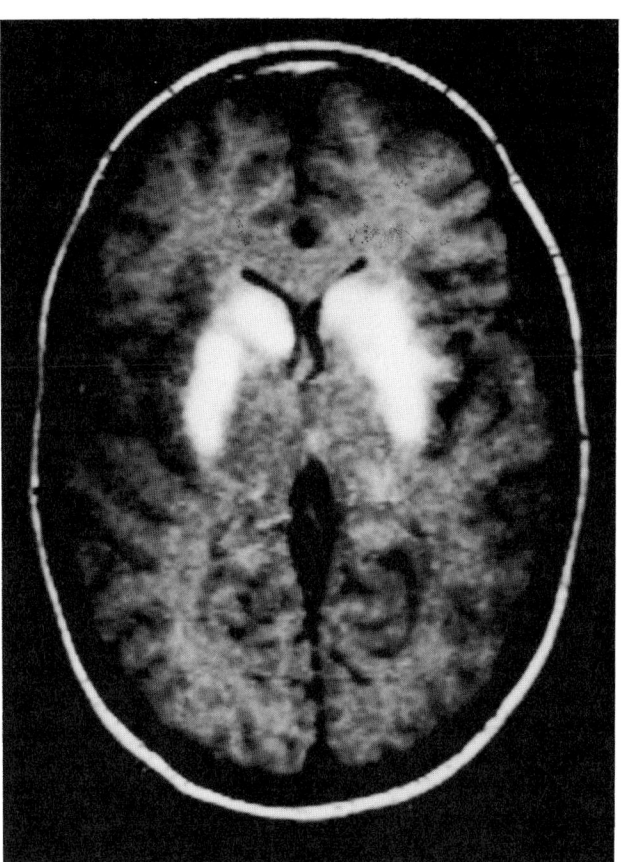

Figure 1 MRI/PET merged images showing ^{18}F-labeled fluoro-DOPA in normal brain (Evans *et al.*, 1992b).

shows a MRI/FDG composite after each image volume had been volume rendered (Drebin *et al.*, 1988) to enhance surfaces.

C. Validation of Point-Matching Registration Accuracy

In landmark-matching algorithms, the residual r.m.s. error between apparently homologous points is not a measure of registration accuracy because it also includes the error in identifying truly equivalent landmarks, referred to as the homology error. This error is often significantly larger than the true error in placing equivalent points in register. To measure the registration error alone, one may use attached fiducial markers but, because of looseness of the skin, it is difficult to fix the fiducial position between scans to the required tolerance of 1–2 mm. Hence, to determine the number of pairs the accuracy of point localization needed to obtain a given accuracy in registration, simulation studies were performed using random point ensembles. (Evans *et al.*, 1989, 1991a). Recently, we have extended these experiments using simulated 3D PET data and results from over 360 MRI/PET registrations performed in our laboratory to generate more realistic point ensembles and 3D transformations (Neelin *et al.*, 1993).

1. Simulated Images

Simulated PET images were generated as follows. Three-dimensional gradient-echo MRI data ($T_R = 75$ ms; $T_E = 14$ ms; flip angle, 60°; slice thickness, 3 mm) were collected over the whole brain. A model-based 3D tissue classification algorithm (Kamber *et al.*, 1992) was used to identify gray matter, white matter, CSF, and bone. Idealized PET images corresponding to blood flow or glucose metabolism were created by assigning gray : white : CSF voxel intensities a ratio of $4 : 1 : 0$. The volume was then sampled to generate planar projection PET data, taking ino account the 3D point spread function, sampling geometry, scatter, randoms, gamma-ray attenuation, and Poisson noise in the projections. (Ma *et al.*, 1993). Projection data were then reconstructed using filtered back-projection to generate a PET dataset registered by definition with the MRI. Applying a known realistic transformation to the MRI and performing the landmark identification procedure for registration yielded a direct measure of registration accuracy in the presence of realistic image contrast and noise characteristics. Table 1 shows the results obtained for 79 such simulated registrations, indicating an average registration error of 1.27 mm at the centroid and 2.83 mm at a distance of 75 mm from the centroid, (approximating the brain surface

Table 1 1D Errors in Registration of Simulated PET Images with MRI

	σ_x	σ_y	σ_z	Mean
Rotation error (°)	1.9	1.5	1.6	1.67 ± 0.08
Translation error (mm)	0.9	1.5	1.4	1.27 ± 0.06
Error at 75 mm (mm)	2.7	3.2	2.6	2.83 ± 0.13

Note. Standard deviations for 79 registrations.

distance). The corresponding r.m.s. error in identifying equivalent points averaged 4.9 mm in each dimension with no preferred direction.

2. Point Simulations

In a complementary study, a set of N points was taken to represent landmark positions identified in MRI. A random linear transformation was applied to generate corresponding PET landmarks and Gaussian noise, added to each coordinate to simulate homology errors (i.e., uncertainty in identifying these equivalent landmarks). The apparent inverse transformation was then determined and, after application of this transformation to the *noise-free* ensemble, the r.m.s. error in recovering the original landmark positions provided a measure or registration accuracy that could be assessed for different N and increasing levels of injected homology error. In contrast to earlier random point-ensemble simulations (Evans *et al.*, 1989, 1991), the landmarks and applied transformation were drawn from actual image registration procedures, either the 79 examples from section A or the 360 real MRI/PET registrations (mostly CBF studies; see Table 2). For each ensemble, a subset of N point pairs from 3 to a possible 16 was used for registration and the registration error measured on 4 of the omitted point pairs. For each N, 100 (for 8 FDG and 33 fluoroDOPA cases) or 20 (for 319 CBF cases) runs were performed at each noise level to generate stable estimates of registration error as a function of N. As shown in Fig. 2 for an

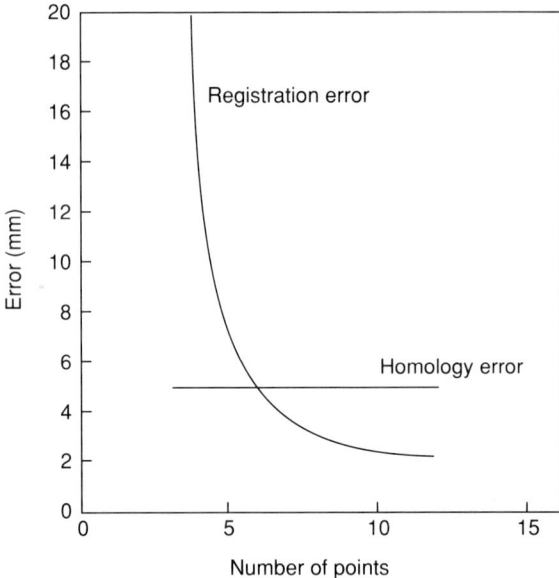

Figure 2 Registration error, σ_r, as a function of the number of landmark pairs, N, used in the *Procrustes* algorithm for a given uncertainty in identifying truly equivalent landmarks in each image volume, i.e., r.m.s. homology error = σ_h, set at σ_h = 5 mm. The registration error scales with input homology error, such that, for $N > 8$–10, σ_r is proportional to $\sigma_h/\sqrt{N}$.

injected homology error of 5 mm, registration errors falls rapidly with N at first and then adopts a $1/\sqrt{N}$ dependence after N of 8–10. Similar curve shapes were obtained for injected noise levels of 2.5, 5.0, 10, and 15 mm, the error scaling linearly with noise level.

These simulation results, for which both the registration error and the homology error are known, were then used to interpret the residuals obtained with real image data for which only the overall error is known, thereby extracting the registration error in real data. The ratio of overall error for real data to that of simulated data was constant with N for each class of image, confirming the adequacy of the simulation for predicting error propagation and allowing a direct estimate of typical homology and registration error in each case. Table 2 summarizes the results for our typical N of 16, indicating the registration error to be typically 1.1 mm at the centroid and typically 1.7 mm the brain surface (75 mm from the centroid). Interestingly, no strong dependence was observed on image type for registration error or for uncertainty in landmark identification, which was 4–4.5 mm (N.B. measurements are 1D; multiplying by $\sqrt{3}$ gives approximate 3D values).

Translational errors measured in Tables 1 and 2 are very similar, averaging 1.2–1.3 mm, but rotation errors are 40–50% bigger in Table 1 (typically 1.7°

Table 2 1D Error in Registration for Point Simulations

	Simulated PET	CBF	FDG	FDOPA
Simulations/point	7900	6380	800	3300
Homology error (mm)	4.66	4.14	3.92	4.51
Rotation error (°)	1.23	1.19	1.16	1.19
Centroid error (mm)	1.18	1.06	1.00	1.16
Error at 75 mm (mm)	1.81	1.66	1.61	1.73

Note. Values quoted are for 16 points. Distance measures are averages of each dimension.

versus 1.2°). This is partially due to a smaller N (mean of 14.4 versus 16) but also depends on the limited quality of the simulated images, for which imperfect tissue segmentation, particularly in cerebellum, degraded the resultant PET image. The use of an isotropic model for homology error may also be an oversimplification because in some cases (e.g., the frontal pole) the landmark is well defined in the radial direction but poorly defined in the tangenital direction. Such factors may adversely affect the rotational stability of the registration obtained from image-derived landmarks compared with point simulations. Nevertheless, the results overall indicate a typical 3D registration error of 2.5–3.5 mm, averaged over the whole brain when using 16 landmarks.

D. Comparison of Landmark Matching with Surface Matching

The landmark-matching method has the disadvantage of a manual step, needed to identify the landmarks. Landmark identification requires some anatomical training, although the problem rapidly becomes a pattern-recognition issue rather than a neuroanatomy issue. Anatomical definition from functional images is not straightforward, particularly when the tracer distribution is disrupted by pathology or when the tracer is confined to specific regions (e.g., with receptor/transmitter mapping of basal ganglia). As discussed above, it is possible to obtain additional anatomical information from the PET transmission scan acquired before (Evans *et al.*, 1991a) or simultaneously with (Ranger *et al.*, 1987; Thompson *et al.*, 1991) the emission study, to measure gamma-ray attenuation.

The strength of the surface matching is its potential for automatic operation or at least its operation by a trained technologist. Care must be taken to ensure that the extracted contours properly represent a continuous 3D surface and that the effects of variable image contrast (e.g., from "cold" lesions), noise, and reconstruction artifacts (e.g., intensity inhomogeneities, streaking) have been removed. This may require manual editing. Also, the method does not require a sophisticated user interface to extract the 2D contours and it can therefore be readily set up at remote sites. Problems can occur with missing data; for instance, the top of the head is missing in one set of contours. The iterative nature of the algorithm occasionally leads it to settle into a local minimum on the parameter surface that necessitates operator intervention to "nudge" the algorithm toward the global minimum. Pelizzari *et al.* (1989) quote registration accuracy for various permutations of two modalities (from MR, CT,

and PET) on the order of 0.7–2.5 mm in 2D images, dependent on the pixel size for the lower resolution dataset and the slice thickness. The 2D PET/MRI value of 2.5 mm is comparable to the 3D estimate obtained in our own simulation studies. Recently, Neiw *et al.* (1991) improved this method by automating the surface-detection operation, precomputing some of the geometric information relating surface points in each volume to the corresponding centroid, using a simulated-annealing algorithm for the parameter optimization that, although requiring much longer to converge, is less sensitive to problems related to local minima.

The head-and-hat algorithm minimizes the mean distance between hat points and the head surface. In MRI/PET correlation studies, the method yields residual r.m.s. distances between hat points and the heat surface on the order of 1–2 mm. The method differs from landmark-matching methods in that it minimizes a point-to-surface residual, whereas the *Procrustes* algorithm performs a point-to-point minimization. The methods therefore cannot be compared directly in terms of residual because, for example, a hat point may be moved parallel to the adjacent head surface without affecting its distance from that surface. The point-to-point mapping approach uses more specific constraints at the expense of requiring that equivalent points first be identified.

Pelizzari *et al.* (1991) recently compared a landmark-based method with this surface-matching procedure for PET/MRI correlation in three different types of PET image: (1) FDG CMRGlc reconstructed to 8-mm resolution, (2) H_2O CBF reconstructed to 20 mm, and (3) transmission reconstructed to 10 mm. They concluded that the methods produced very similar results in each case and that a 2-mm registration error represented a practical lower bound for both methods.

II. Intramodality Matching

It is often important to align datasets acquired at different times from a single subject to monitor and quantify disease progress (e.g., tumor growth and remission, proliferation of multiple sclerosis lesions, and surgical assessment from pre- and postoperative scans). Within the brain-mapping domain, it is essential to align the CBF images acquired from the same subject during different psychological states. Small misalignments will give rise to artifactual intensity features in the CBF difference images, which will confound the real stimulus-based changes being sought. Woods (1992) has recently employed a method that divides the two images voxel by voxel and iteratively adjusts three rotation and three translation parameters, one at a time, to minimizes the standard deviation of the voxel ratios. At the MNI, we have implemented a 3D multiscale cross-correlation approach to intrasubject alignment, which is discussed below (Section II.C).

It is also necessary to obtain optimal alignment of intramodal data but from different subjects so that, for instance, normal variability in anatomy or function can be measured. The definition of optimality will vary according to the application and implementation. It may involve the use of manually defined landmarks or automatic feature detection and may involve linear, piecewise-linear or full nonlinear deformation of the 3D images to achieve an optimal match, as discussed below. Of course, any transformation that is determined for one modality, such as MRI, can be applied in identical fashion to another modality, such as PET, if a previous cross-modality intersubject registration has been performed. We use this approach to map PET data into stereotaxic space via a correlated MRI dataset, which is transformed as discussed in the following section.

A. Stereotaxic Transformation

In this approach, 3D image data are linearly mapped into a standardized brain-based coordinate space such that all brains have the same extent in three orthogonal directions and each plane of the resliced volume can be directly compared with an anatomical atlas. The most commonly employed space is that developed by Talairach and colleagues (Talairach *et al.*, 1967; Talairach and Tournoux, 1988). Originally developed for use with pneumoencephalographic studies of brain stem and periventricular structures, this method has become central to brain-mapping studies for localization of activation foci (Fox *et al.*, 1985, 1988; Friston *et al.*, 1989, 1991). This stereotaxic transformation is based on the identification of the anterior–posterior commisural (AC–PC) line, extended to the cortical edge in the AP direction, and a set of perpendiculars to this line from the AC–PC points to the cortical edge. Strict application of the method (e.g., Lemoine *et al.*, 1991) requires the proportional scaling to be partitioned into three piecewise linear components in the AP direction (pre-AC, AC–PC, post-PC) and two in the CC direction (above/below AC–PC) and to be independent for each hemisphere. This is intended to overcome problems introduced by nonlinear morphometric variability among individuals. Most centers have either retained a single scale along each dimension or applied full nonlinear warping techniques to address the nonlinearity issue directly.

At the MNI, the Talairach space is used both for anatomical analysis with MRI data and for functional activation studies with PET, using a preregistered MRI image for defining the required transformation. Because the AC and PC points are close (approximately 25 mm apart) and difficult to identify reliably even on MRI, significant errors that are magnified at the cortex can be introduced. We therefore select a series of five well-separated midline landmarks that yield a least-squares fit approximation to the AC–PC line (Evans et al., 1992a). Validation studies in 37 young normal brains indicate an angular discrepancy of $-0.24° \pm 2.9°$ and a vertical translational error of 1.2 ± 1.0 mm.

Recently, we have implemented an automated method for mapping data into stereotaxic space, using general multiscale feature-matching techniques discussed in more detail below (Collins *et al.*, 1992ab). This strategy uses a 3D cross-correlation residual to match a single MRI volume to a 300-brain MRI composite already mapped to stereotaxic space (see below). When appropriate, the corresponding transformation is also applied to the previously registered PET.

B. Landmark-Driven Image Warping

A source of concern with intersubject comparison is the anatomical variability apparent in the transformed data after stereotaxic resampling with linear or piecewise linear algorithms. It is well known that the major sulci vary in position by 1–2 cm within a normal population (Talairach and Tournoux, 1988; Steinmetz and Seitz, 1991). Nonlinear 3D deformations offer the possibility of reducing this variability.

We have implemented a procedure for deforming 3D images under landmark-driven contraints, by application of the "thin-plate" spline procedure of Bookstein (1989). This method determines the continuous coordinate transformation that maps one set of 3D coordinates onto an equivalent set of homologous points. The procedure decomposes the overall deformation into a series of principal warps of decreasing geometric scale. In 2D, this is mathematically analogous to the bending energy required to deform a thin metal sheet so that a set of points on the sheet have a defined height above corresponding points on a flat surface. To assess the algorithm, we applied it to MRI from 16 young, normal subjects (Evans *et al.*, 1991b).

Using the landmark-tagging procedure, a set of anatomical features in each MRI study were matched to corresponding structures in a master MRI. Each point was also identified by its coordinates within the Talairach stereotaxic atlas for consistent reference among subjects, because a particular landmark could be identified in many ways (e.g., "center" of thalamus). A set of 26 points was identified in each MRI volume using the following rationale. Points at the extremities (frontal/occipital poles, brain vertex, pons/midbrain notch) were selected to constrain the overall size of the fitted atlas. Deep nuclei were identified by their approximate centroid as defined by the selected Talairach coordinates. These, combined with the anterior and posterior horns of the lateral ventricles, constrained the distortion of periventricular brain. Finally, a limited set of gyral/sulcal landmarks was selected to constrain the topology of the cortical mantle.

The landmark-driven 3D warping algorithm was then applied to each of the MRI volumes to bring it into registration with the master volume, using either the full nonlinear interpolation or the first three terms only, which define the affine component of the overall transformation. Figure 3 illustrates a single slice through the central region of the 16-brain average normalized intensity image using either linear or nonlinear transformation. The nonlinear transformation exhibits a sharper appearance and more detail than the linear version, reflecting the superiority of the nonlinear approach for bringing homologous structures in the neighborhood of individual landmarks into precise alignment.

C. Automatic Image Feature-Matching Strategy

A problem of some concern with interactive landmark-based approaches is the subjectivity of landmark choice (i.e., the dependence of the resultant deformation on the number and distribution of landmarks selected and the behavior of the algorithm in regions distant from any landmark). An alternative approach that avoids the need for potentially time-consuming landmark tagging but sacrifices explicitly defined point correspondence is that of feature matching (e.g., Bajcsy *et al.*, 1983, 1989). In this context, image features are local properties of the image intensity that can be extracted automatically by neighborhood operators (e.g., edges, zones of relatively homogeneous intensity, or particular shapes).

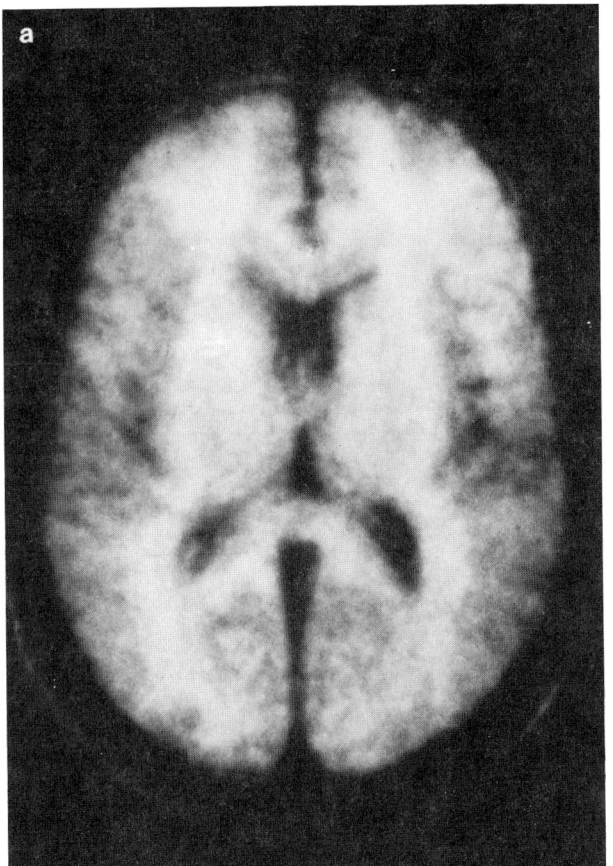 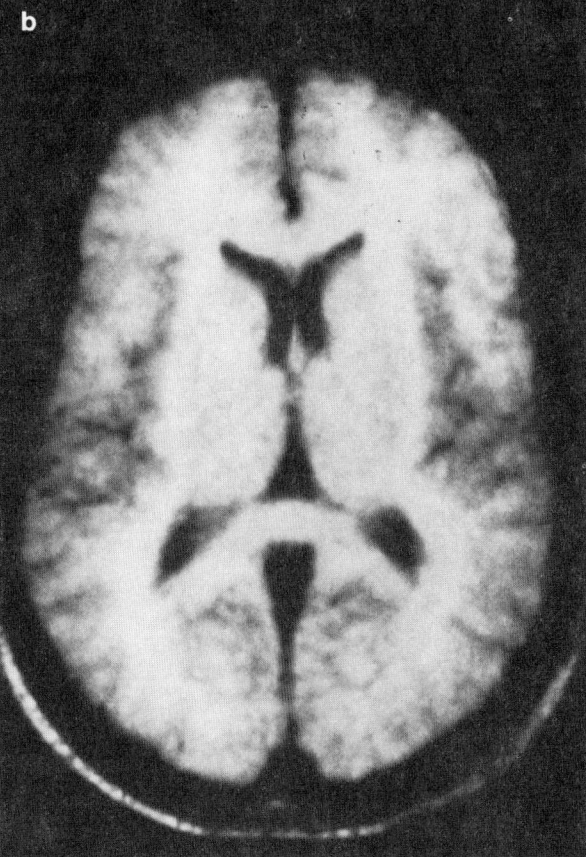

Figure 3 Comparison of the average MRI brain obtained from 16 subjects using linear (a) and nonlinear (b) models of anatomical variability.

Table 3 Simulation of Intra-subject Registration (20 Repeats, 17 Subjects)

	RMS error				Standard deviation		
	x axis	y axis	z axis	Average	x axis	y axis	z axis
Experiment 1							
Rotation (°)	0.0766	0.0958	0.0773	0.0832	0.0487	0.0612	0.0466
Translation (mm)	0.0959	0.1027	0.1081	0.1022	0.0576	0.0675	0.0639
Experiment 2							
Rotation (°)	0.0787	0.1010	0.0874	0.0890	0.0500	0.0640	0.0513
Translation (mm)	0.1055	0.1034	0.1218	0.1102	0.0628	0.0678	0.0760
Scale	0.0012	0.0011	0.0018	0.0014	0.0009	0.0007	0.0011

Note. Errors in affine parameters are for rotation and translation only (experiment 1) and with scaling (experiment 2).

We have implemented a 3D feature-matching procedure that employs repetitive evaluation of the feature cross-correlation function (FCCF) between two images (Collins *et al.*, 1992ab). The global maximum FCCF hypersurface, indicating the required transformation, is found by nonlinear optimization using the SIMPLEX algorthm. The algorithm operates in a multiscale loop, beginning with a heavily smoothed version of each image and successively sharpening the images at each iteration. The use of blurred images for obtaining approximate transformation parameters reduces the likelihood of encountering local minima during the search and is approximately four times faster than single-stage high-resolution optimization. At each stage, the original image is first convolved with a 3D Gaussian smoothing kernel before the best transformation is determined by maximizing the FCCF at scales (SD of Gaussian kernel) of 32, 16, 8, 4, and 2 mm. For affine transformation, the method uses only image intensity as a feature but for nonlinear image warping gradient vector fields are needed.

To measure intrasubject registration accuracy 20 random linear transformations (only translations and rotations) were applied to each of 17 MRI (T_1-weighted gradient echo sequence; 3 mm thick) volumes of the head from the normal volunteers (27 ± 3 years old) and the algorithm applied to recover the transformation. For each trial, two measures of registration error were calculated: the r.m.s. difference between input and recovered parameters and the r.m.s. registration error between 48 landmarks, manually identified in each volume. Over the 340 trials (see Table 3), the r.m.s. errors for rotation, translation, and landmark distance were less than or equal to 0.1°, 0.1 mm, and 0.2 mm, respectively. Adding anisotropic scaling to the simulations had a negligible impact on these values.

For intersubject registration, each dataset in turn was identified as the target, and the other 16 volumes were registered to it. Over the 272 trials, the linear transformation recovered by multiresolution registration yielded an r.m.s. landmark distance of 6.65 mm. Note that this measure is dominated by nonlinear anatomical variability and not by landmark homology error among MRI volumes . This value is in good agreement with the mean measure of anatomical variability of 6.52 mm in Table 4, determined with a different technique in different subjects (see Section III.B.1).

To compare this result to manual landmark registration, we submitted the 48 landmarks to the *Procrustes*

Table 4 r.m.s. Distance of the Regional 3D Center of Gravity from the Target Position Following Linear Warping of the VOI Atlas to Target Space, Indicating Residual Anatomical Variability not Handled by the Linear Model

Distance (R) (mm)	SD	Region
6.34	3.15	Superior frontal gyrus
7.69	2.27	Middle frontal gyrus
5.86	2.40	Inferior frontal gyrus
5.83	2.14	Precentral gyrus
5.05	2.35	Postcentral gyrus
4.50	1.91	Superior temporal gyrus
4.47	1.65	Middle temporal gyrus
5.19	2.07	Inferior temporal gyrus
5.38	2.19	Amygdala
5.22	2.26	Hippocampus
9.18	3.52	Head of caudate nucleus
7.14	2.99	Putamen
7.80	3.15	Globus pallidus
7.63	2.94	Thalamus
6.52	3.16	Total (N.B. 60 structures)

Note. A total of 60 regions (14 shown) and 16 subjects.

procedure (Section I.B). With an isotropic scale variable, the r.m.s. residual was 5.94 mm, whereas with anistropic scaling it was 5.79 mm. Although these values are smaller than the 6.65 mm obtained for the automatic approach, the comparison is biased because the points used to define the *Procrustes* transformation are the same as those used to measure the error. Nevertheless, the values indicate that the automatic feature-matching approach performs as requird.

III. Probabilistic MRI Atlas

The continued growth of quantitative functional neuroanatomy carried on within the standardized reference frame of Talairach has drawn attention to the inadequacies of the present methodologies. In particular, the current standard atlas of Talairach and Tournoux (1988) was derived from the postmortem sectioning of the brain of a single 60-year-old female. Slice separation is variable, typically 3 to 4 mm, and atlas data from orthogonal planes are inconsistent. Given (1) the known variability in human cortical anatomy, (2) the prevailing differences between local algorithmic variants of the stereotaxic transformation implemented at individual centers and the original piecewise–linear Talairach framework, and (3) that most brain-mapping studies are performed on young normal subjects, the precise anatomical localization for focal activation derived from PET using the Talairach atlas alone is problematic and can lead to overinterpretation of the results (Drevits *et al.*, 1992). These uncertainties and the availability at the MNI of a large database of MRI volumes obtained from young, normal subjects has lead to a program to construct a 3D probabilistic atlas of young, normal gross neuroanatomy, defined within stereotaxic space. Figure 4 shows a composite MRI dataset from 305 young normals (239 males; 66 females; age, 23.4 ± 4.1 years) after transformation of each MRI volume into Talair-

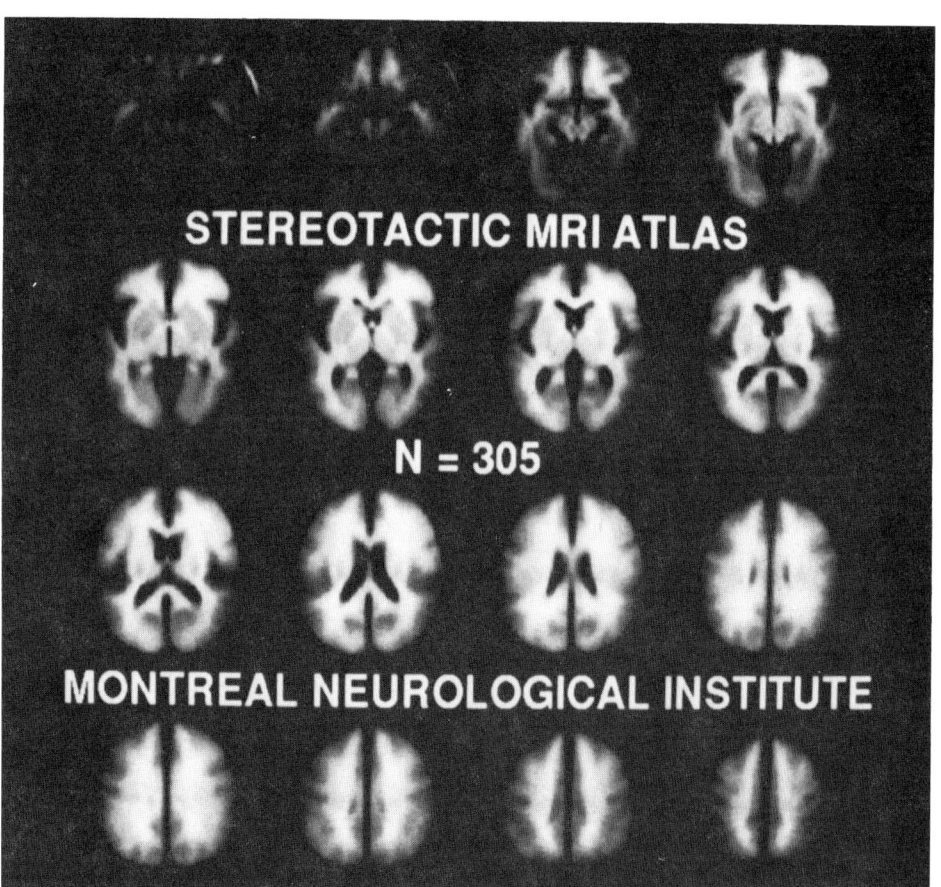

Figure 4 Mean MRI dataset drawn from 305 young normal volunteers. The dataset can be used as an anatomical atlas for locating functional activation data in Talairach space. It also provides a visual impression of local anatomical variability and an indication of how well a particular functional measurement can be localized.

ach space and intensity normalization. All subjects were right-handed and each MRI volume was acquired as 64 contiguous 2-mm-thick images (Evans *et al.*, 1992c). The transformed atlas is composed of 80 slices separated by 1.5 mm in Talairach coordinates. The average intensity MRI dataset obtained from the database illustrates the effect of anatomical variability in different brain areas and serves as a low-resolution, large sample atlas of gross neuroanatomy in Talairach space. The dataset has been distributed to over 30 centers for use alongside the Talairach atlas.

Although useful as a qualitative indicator of local anatomical variability, the composite MRI-intensity atlas is insufficient as a quantitative tool. For this purpose, the MRI intensity for each voxel in each MRI volume must be replaced by an anatomical label and a probability assigned for each voxel having a particular label. This requires a precise segmentation of each MRI volume into component structures, features, and tissue types. Manual labeling in addition to being prohibitively time consuming, would introduce intra- and interobserver variations in labeling strategy that would confound the overall goal. Completely automatic and accurate image segmentation at the regional level is as yet an unsolved problem. At the MNI, three overlapping projects are addressing the problem of anatomical variability, aiming to obtain the automatic labeling of 3D MRI datasets by tissue-type, by specific neuroanatomical volume, and by gyral/sulcal surface anatomy.

A. Tissue Classification

Preliminary tissue classification of double-echo MRI volumes into gray/white/CSF has yielded a 3D map of the likelihood of membership in a given tissue class. The classification algorithm employs the ID3 decision-tree classifier (Quinlan, 1986), operating on $3 \times 3 \times 3$ voxel neighborhoods and T_1-weighted and T_2-weighted intensity features for each voxel. This algorithm represents tissue classification rules in the form of a binary decision tree in which each tree node represents a test on a feature and each leaf represents a tissue class. A top-down divide-and-conquer strategy is used to grow the tree by recursively partitioning user-provided tissue training samples into progressively smaller subsets that eventually correspond to tissue classes (Kamber *et al.*, 1992). ID3 uses an entropy function that examines the feature values of each training sample to determine which continuous intensity feature best partitions the samples into two classes at every node until a minimum-entropy stopping criterion is reached. A error–cost complexity pruning algorithm (Breiman, 1984) is then applied to

reduce the total number of branches such that the cost of pruning, in terms of misclassified samples, is minimized. The pruned tree selected is the smallest tree with a misclassification rate within one standard error of the minimum.

The above segmentation procedure was applied to 12 3D spin-echo double-echo MRI datasets previously transformed into stereotactic space (Kamber *et al.*, 1992). The proportion of all datasets for which a voxel was assigned to a given tissue class represents a likelihood function for membership in that class when taken across the population. Figure 5 illustrates orthogonal planes through this stereotactic gray-matter probability mask. The data can be used, for example, as a constraint on subsequent classifications by rejecting a particular voxel classification that has a probability lower than some preset threshold (e.g., periorbital fat could not be classified as cerebral white matter). Alternatively statistical search strategies for identifying significant activation foci in a brain-mapping experiment can be confined to particular tissue classes (e.g., gray matter) by use of the appropriate probability mask.

B. Regional Segmentation

Tissue classification identifies only gross components of the brain and does not specifically label individual brain structures, such as caudate nucleus, automatically. For such segmentation, *a priori* information is needed to augment the intensity/gradient/texture features of the image, in the form of explicit geometric models or rules constraining the spatial relation of labeled structures. At the MNI, a 3D volume-of-interest (VOI) atlas has been constructed by the manual outlining of individual brain regions on 64 2-mm-thick adjacent MRI slices. Sixty structures in each hemisphere, including deep gray matter structures, major gyri, ventricles, and white matter zones, are identified. The data exist as a tesselated geometrical model that can be resliced along any 2D plane or warped in three-dimensions to fit an image volume. Usually the template is matched to MRI before being applied to a correlated PET image for functional measurement (Evans *et al.*, 1991a). We have employed this 3D model in two ways for regional segmentation of individual MRI datasets.

1. Landmark-Driven Matching of the VOI Atlas to Image

In this approach, the VOI atlas is deformed to match the individual image volume by manual identification of corresponding 3D landmarks in the VOI atlas and image, using the thin-plate spline algorithm

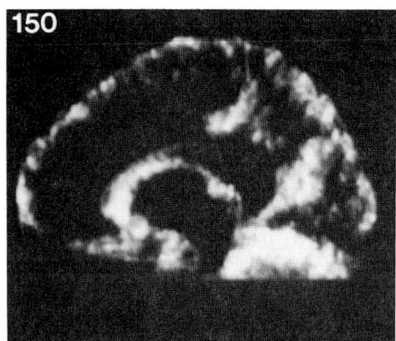
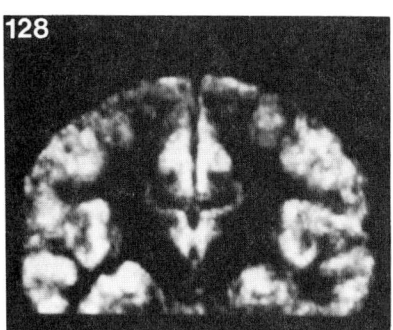
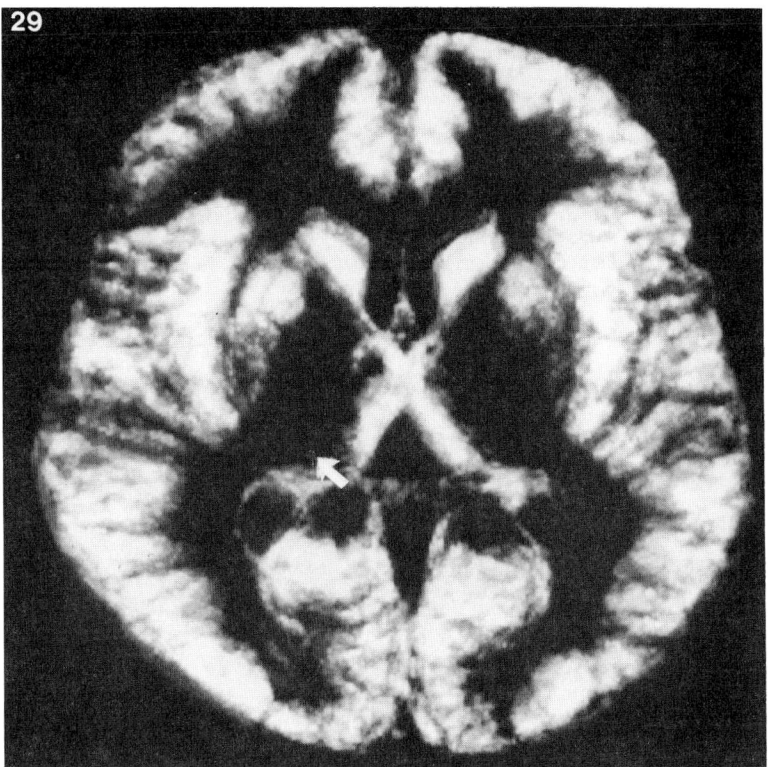

Figure 5   Gray matter probability map from 12 normal subjects. Three-dimensional tissue classification identified gray matter voxels in each subject. Transformation to a standardized coordinate space allowed a composite probability for each voxel. Similar maps have been derived for other tissue classes. From Kamber *et al.*, (1992).

(Bookstein, 1989). To investigate this procedure, the algorithm was applied in three dimensions to fit the VOI atlas to each of the 16 3D MRI datasets described in Section II.B (Evans *et al.*, 1991b). The same 26 landmarks used for warping individual MRI image volumes to fit a master MRI dataset were employed to wrap the VOI atlas, derived initially from that master MRI dataset, to fit each individual MRI volume. Figure 6 shows an illustrative slice through one of the matched VOI/MRI volumes at the level of the periventricular gray matter regions. As well as segmenting each MRI volume into labeled regions, the VOI atlas could be used to quantify nonlinearities in anatomical correspondence in the 16-brain dataset, as follows.

For each dataset, employing the 26 landmarks as before, the matched VOI atlas was inversely warped back to the master MRI space by the full nonlinear warp or by application of only the affine terms in the expansion. By restricting the number of terms in the warping algorithm to only affine transformations, including anisotropic scaling, the mapping operation was reduced to a linear model in which the solution was effectively a least-squares residual between master and target ensembles. Mapping the VOI atlas into

a single MRI volume by both linear and nonlinear solutions allowed a direct comparison of the two solutions for that volume. However, because each brain had different dimensions, the pooling of results across all subjects would not have been straightforward. Instead, by first fitting a volume with the nonlinear solution and then performing a numerical inverse solution but allowing only linear terms, all measurements were established in the master frame. This procedure was applied to the 16 datasets and the center of gravity for each of the structures in the VOI atlas used to assess the local inadequacy of the linear model.

In general, the warped atlas fit the central brain regions well owing to the number of landmarks identifiable in the periventricular regions (caudate, thalamus, anterior/posterior commissures, corpus callosum, lateral ventricles). In cortical regions the relative lack of identifiable landmarks limited the extent to which local cortical adjustments could be both initially specified and subsequently evaluated. The lack of specific cerebellar landmarks resulted in unsatisfactory fits of that region. Such problems must be dealt with by additional cerebellar constraints. The results in Ta-

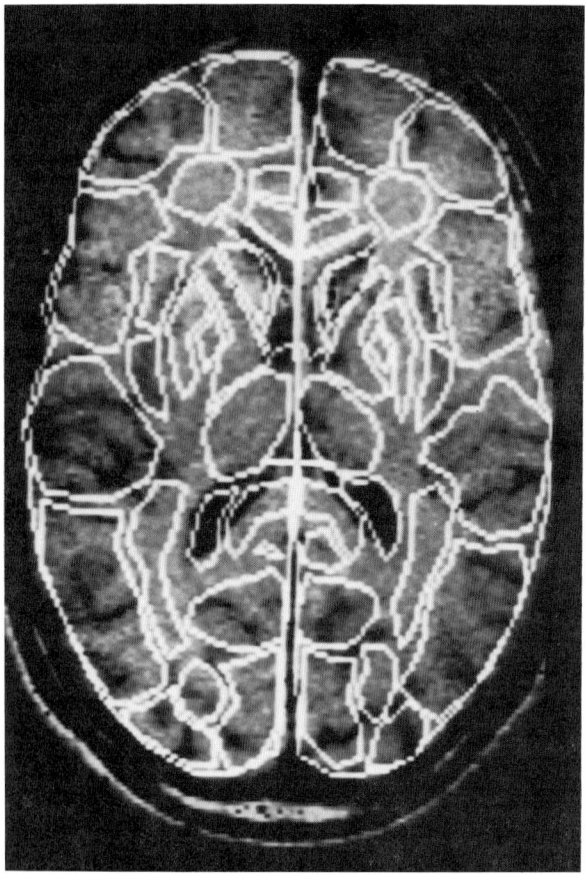

Figure 6 An example of the fit between a VOI atlas and a target MRI dataset in a plane passing through the basal ganglia.

ble 3 indicate a substantial component of normal anatomic variation cannot be accommodated within a linear model. The overall 3D center of gravity shift between linear and nonlinear models of 6–7 mm is considerable for applications that seek to localize specific structures with respect to other anatomical fiduciary markers based on principles of linear stereotaxy (e.g., biopsy or depth electrode placement).

2. Automatic Matching of Image to the VOI Atlas

We are presently developing a new procedure for automatic identification of individual brain regions (e.g., caudate, superior temporal gyrus) that combines multiscale image feature matching (Section II.C), the concept of stereotaxic space, and the VOI atlas. The VOI atlas and the MRI volume upon which the VOI atlas was originally defined are not resident in stereotactic space. Hence, mapping an individual MRI volume into this space by feature matching against the resident MRI also fits it to the VOI atlas. An inverse transformation fits the VOI atlas to the new MRI in its original space (Collins *et al.*, 1992ab). The multiscale nature of the feature-matching algo-

rithm facilitates the recursive application of the linear cross-correlation optimization to individual neighborhoods defined on a 3D grid with a dimension equal to the current scale. Hence, an overall nonlinear transformation is obtained by successive local linear transformations. Figure 7 shows application of the algorithm to recover the original shape of a 3D multiellipsoid brain phantom following application of a known deformation via a thin-plate spine 3D warp. Using a distance residual for 296 points distributed over all phantom surfaces as a measure of accuracy, the linear method yielded an r.m.s. registration error of 9.21 mm. The most recent version of the nonlinear algorithm reduced this value by 80%.

C. Cortical Surface Parameterization

The cortical surface is an area of particular interest in the brain mapping domain based on both its intrinsic neuroanatomical features and the relationship of functional neuroanatomy to the superficial gyral/sulcal patterns and to the underlying cytoarchitecture. The study of variability in cortical anatomy across the normal population merits special consideration, and new methods are being developed for this purpose. Many methods already exist for visualizing the cerebral cortex by extraction of isovalued surfaces, with

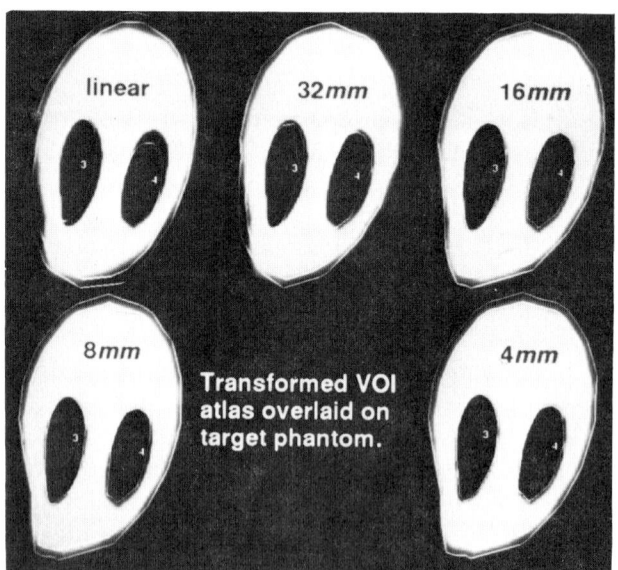

Figure 7 Results of the nonlinear registration/segmentation feature-matching algorithm using a simple multiellipsoid phantom. The original 3D phantom, composed of four separate ellipsoids, was first deformed to a pear shape using thin-plate spline warping based on manually defined landmarks. The automatic feature cross-correlation was then maximized at successively finer scales to register the original phantom with this new object. Using the object contours for clarity, a–e show the progress from a linear fit to a nonlinear fit at 32-mm, 16-, 8-, and 4-mm scales.

or without subsequent polygonalization. These techniques are susceptible to artifacts introduced by noise or signal inhomogeneities and do not enforce topological continuity (i.e., there can be holes in the surface). Moreover, the unstructured representation of the cortex as between 10^5 and 10^7 cuberilles or polygons is not best suited for point-to-point comparison of equivalent surfaces across a population. This goal has motivated attempts to use analytic representations to replace the isosurface. Such parametric representations are continuous, are relatively compact, and can often be expressed at different scales (i.e., resolutions) in a hierarchical fashion.

The problem of quantifying, as opposed to visualizing, the cortical surface an measuring its variability across subjects is difficult to express in mathematical terms because the boundaries of gyri and the extent of sulci are ill defined. Moreover, many secondary gyri have a highly variable manifestation or may be absent altogether. Even major sulci may have variable branching patterns. Van Essen and Maunsell (1980) advanced the notion of mapping the cortex, with examples in macaque and cat brains. Since then, various approaches have been made to apply such techniques with MRI data from the human brain. Gazzaniga *et al.* (1990) outline the cortex manually on successive cortical slices, whereas Carman *et al.* (1992) and Sereno and Dale (1992) have employed similar

surface tension models to define the cortical anatomy.

At the MNI, we have developed a procedure that combines the advantages of polygonal, parametric, and hierarchical representations with a fast converging elastic deformation model (MacDonald *et al.*, 1993). The vertices of a starting parametric surface, defined by a polygonal mesh, are moved toward a boundary surface, defined by a set of discrete boundary points, along a direction normal to the current parametric surface and for a distance controlled by a weighting factor for each boundary point. The weighting is linear such that zero weighting leaves the point unmoved and unit weighting moves directly to the boundary surface. The algorithm proceeds iteratively, adjusting all mesh points at each iteration, until equilibrium is obtained with all mesh edges of almost equal length. The simplicity of the model allows a simple control of the surface resolution, by subsampling of the boundary points, and hence the degree of sulcal detail apparent in the fitted surface. The boundary points are usually isosurface voxels obtained by intensity or gradient thresholding, but can also include additional manually defined boundary points reflecting specific surface targets with increased weighting. The mesh form of the parametric surface guarantees a continuous single surface topology and also allows a direct one-to-one mapping of the cortical surface to any simple parametric representation. Figure 8 illus-

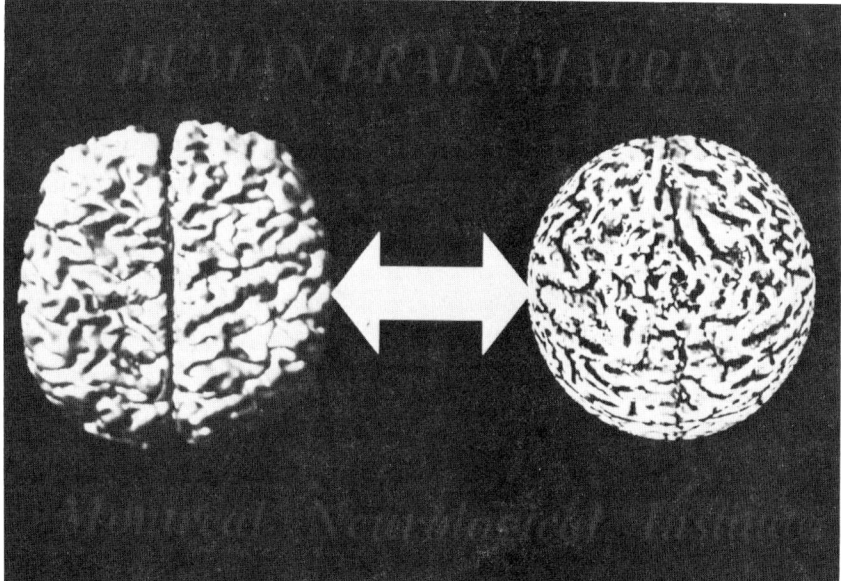

Figure 8 An example of cortical parameterization of "surface flattening." The surface is first extracted from 3D MRI data by intensity or gradient thresholding. The parameter surface, in this case a sphere, is expanded iteratively to overlay the extracted surface using a minimum distance criterion (see text). The one-to-one correspondence allows an inverse mapping of the cortex to the parameter surface. Dark areas on the parameter surface correspond to high negative curvature (sulcal floors), whereas light areas indicate high positive curvature (gyral ridges).

trates mapping from a 3D cortical manifold to a spherical projection, both viewed from above. Corresponding sulci and gyri are evident and can be identified by traditional cartographic lines of latitude and longitude. Application of this transformation to a large number of MRI datasets and morphometric analysis across a normal population require definition of specific orienting landmarks in native or parametric space. At present we use the existing Talairach transformation but this may be superceded by landmarks in the parametric space.

Similar procedures can be applied to each hemisphere separately to avoid the gross distortions involved in fitting the interhemispheric fissure. Since the deformation from the cortical surface to a simple parametric surface will also be severe in the vicinity of other major fissures, we are presently exploring the possibility of using the average cortical surface, drawn from a 305-brain MRI composite, as a starting surface instead of a sphere. The problem of surface modeling is then reduced to modeling local folding with respect to the average surface rather than to a simple object (i.e., a more realistic topology at the expense of a direct cartographic analogy).

IV. Applications and Summary

In this chapter, we have described various aspects of 3D correlative imaging in progress at the Montreal Neurological Institute, including both cross-modal and intra-modal registration with special reference to brain mapping applications.

The correlation of each subject's MRI and PET volumes provides a customized anatomical template for the functional image, which in brain-mapping studies, consists of a sparse map of CBF changes with no anatomical cues. Of course, the transformation of individual image volumes into stereotaxic space allows for their correlation with some form of knowledge base for anatomical interpretation. This may take the form of book containing an example or a schematic representation of a brain in stereotaxic space (Talairach *et al.*, 1967, 1988). In addition, a computerized atlas may be used to identify regions of this standardized brain space (e.g., Bohm *et al.*, 1991). Nevertheless, the differences between an idealized representation and the true underlying anatomy provided by MRI can sometimes be crucial to the interpretation of the data (Drevits *et al.*, 1992), especially in regions of high anatomical variability. The development of a true probabilistic atlas of gross neuroanatomy in young normals will complement the existing methods and

may provide a cautionary perspective on the interpretation of activation data.

The availability of correlated atlas or MRI data also offers the possibility of untangling the purely anatomical component from the variability in location of the response to a given stimulus observed among a population (Steinmetz and Seitz, 1991). The use of MRI is also vital in the interpretation of activation data obtained where there are likely to be morphological changes e.g., Alzheimer's disease, normal aging, space-occupying lesions. Plates 27–30 show examples of brain-mapping studies from our institution, illustrating the processing of auditory (Zatorre *et al.*, 1992a), olfactory (Zatorre *et al.*, 1992b), nociceptive i.e., pain (Talbot *et al.*, 1991) and visual (Evans *et al.*, 1992a) stimuli. The wealth of data accruing from brain-mapping experiments has resulted in a need for comparison of focal activations obtained with different experiments and different laboratories. In Chapter 9 of this volume, Fox *et al.* discuss the BrainMap database which allows for the literature searches of brain-mapping results. At the MNI a complementary approach uses many of the 3D imaging elements described here to allow interactive 3D display and analysis of the coordinates from many experiments. Plate 31 illustrates this interface.

The facility for assessing the functional status of a proposed operative site is likely to assume increasing importance as the technique become easier. In epilepsy surgery, it is often crucial to establish whether a seizure focus, often apparent in the functional image as a region of interictal hypometabolism, is in or near the motor strip. The use of correlated MRI data, in the form of a 3D surface rendering, usually can resolve this question prior to surgery. Conversely, in situations where the underlying anatomy is distorted from normal, the precise assessment of functional neuroanatomy is extremely difficult. Here, the use of functional brain-mapping techniques become important. For instance, the mapping of language or motor areas in the vicinity of vascular malformations or neoplastic lesions has already begun to figure in the surgeon's decision (Pardo *et al.*, 1986) and now combines MRI and PET in the process (Leblanc *et al.*, 1990, 1992). In the surgical setting, particularly where space-occupying lesions have distorted the normal anatomy, the addition of 3D vascular information from digital subtraction angiography can have a decisive effect on mapping of cortical responses (Peters *et al.*, 1986; Evans *et al.*, 1992b).

In this chapter it has been assumed for simplicity that CBF images are produced using PET techniques. Recent work in the functional MRI area, discussed in detail elsewhere in this book, have demonstrated focal vascular/perfusion changes in response to sensorimotor stimuli. The methods are based on magnetic susceptibility changes during stimulation, caused by (1) a focally increased blood volume as indicated by a paramagnetic vascular tracer (Belliveau *et al.*, 1991) or (2) noninvasively, by focal changes in the oxyhemoglobin:deoxyhemoglobin ratio (Kwong *et al.*, 1992). It has been suggested that intersubject averaging will not be necessary to obtain a significant signal from cognitive mapping paradigms using MRI since the experiment can be performed repeatedly within a single subject. The effects of task learning, habituation or attentional changes during extended scanning have yet to be studied rigorously. Even so, there remains a need to correlate intrasubject scans from different conditions where movements may have occurred and also a requirement to compare data from different subjects for common patterns of activation. In such cases, most of the discussion of linear or nonlinear intra-modal correlation presented in this chapter is applicable.

The intersubject comparison of 3D anatomical images is presently being used principally in studies of gross neuroanatomy and functional mapping of normal brain. However, as the field develops, it is likely to find increasing application in diagnostic settings. For instance, the use of normative data on the location of specific gyri and sulci, when expressed within a standardized brain space, may aid in the identification of cortical dysplasia as a basis for epileptogenesis, or for developmental problems in cognitive skills or language acquisition. The nonlinear mapping of presegmented brain models, in the form of raster volumes or 3D geometric atlases, onto individual datasets is an area of intense interest in many centers worldwide. The eventual goal in such cases is the automatic labeling of each structure within the brain according to some predefined anatomical heirarchy.

In conclusion, the study of human functional neuroanatomy with quantitative neuroimaging techniques and sophisticated computational analysis, brain mapping, has witnessed a remarkable growth in recent years. PET, MRI, and powerful 3D imaging techniques have revolutionized our ability to obtain quantitative anatomical and functional data from human brain studies and to synthesize these data into coherent models of large-scale neurocircuitry. While human neuroimaging has opened up exciting perspectives on the cognitive and sensorimotor processing, the limitations of spatial and temporal resolution are considerable. Combining PET and MRI studies with single cell recording, animal experiments, and

studies of impaired performance following focal lesions, these techniques provide a wealth of converging information on brain organization. Moreover, the temporal information about signal propagation during task performance provided by magneto- and electroencephalography (MEG and EEG) adds a crucial dimension to the interpretation of results. Increasingly, the integration of information from different neuroimaging modalities will become a routine, indeed mandatory, part of brain mapping.

Acknowledgments

The authors thank their colleagues, notably Drs. Terry Peters and Albert Gjedde and staff Weiqian Dai and Sylvain Milot, at the McConnell Brain Imaging Centre for many helpful comments and insights in the development of this work. We also thank Drs. John Crossman and David Hawkes from Guy's and Thomas' Hospitals, London, for their collaboration in the simulation studies.

References

Alpert, N. M., Bradshaw, J. F., Kennedy, D. N., and Correia, J. A. (1990). The principal axis transformation: A method for image registration. *J. Nucl. Med.* **31**(10), 1717–1722.

Belliveau, J. W., Kennedy, D. N., McKinstry, R. C., Buchbinder, B. R., Weisskopf, R. M., Cohen, M. S., Vevea, J. M., Brady, T. J., and Rosen, B. R. (1991). Functional mapping of the human visual cortex by magnetic resonance imaging. *Science* **254**, 716–719.

Bergstrom, M., Boethius, J., Eriksson, L., Greitz, T., Ribbe, T., and Widen, L. (1981). Head fixation for reproducible position alignment in transmillion CT and positron emisson tomography. *Comput. Assist. Tomogr.* **5**, 136–141.

Breiman, L., Freidman, J., Olshen, R., and Stone, C. (1984). "Classification and Regression Trees." Monterey, CA: Wadsworth.

Bajcsy, R., Lieberson, R., and Reivich, M. (1983). A computerized system for the elastic matching of deformed radiographic images to idealized atlas images. *J. Comput. Assst. Tomogr.* **7**(4), 618–625.

Bajcsy, R., and Kovacic, S. (1989). Multiresolution elastic matching. *Comput. Vision Graphics Image Process.* **46**, 1–21.

Bookstein, F. (1989). Principal warps: Thin-plate splines and the decomposition of deformations. *IEEE Trans. Pattern Anal. Machine Intelligence* **11**(6), 567–585.

Bookstein, F. (1991). Thin-plate splines and the atlas problem for biomedical images In "Lecture Notes on Computer Science 511: Information Processing in Medical Imaging" (A. C. F. Colchester and D. J. Hawkes, Eds.), pp. 326–342. Heidelberg: Springer-Verlag.

Carman, G. J. (1990). "Mapping of the Cerebral Cortex." Ph.D. thesis, Caltech.

Collins, D. L., Dai, W., Peters, T. M., and Evans, A. C. (1992a). Model-based segmentation of individual brain structures from MRI data In "Vis. Biomed. Comput. 1992, Proc. SPIE **1808**, 10–23.

Collins, D. L., Peters, T.M., and Evans, A. C. (1992b). Nonlinear multiscale image registration and segmentation of individual brain structure from MRI *Proc. IEEE Symp. Adv. Med. Image Process. Med.*, 105–110.

Drebin, R., Carpenter, L., and Hanrahan, P., (1988). Volume rendering. *ACM Comput. Graphics,* **22**(4), 65–74.

Drevits, W. C., Videen, T. O., MacLeod, A. K., Haller, J. W., and Raichle, M. E. (1988). PET images of blood flow changes during anxiety: Correction. *Science* **256**, 1696.

Evans, A. C., Beil, C., Marrett, S., Thompson, C. J., and Hakim, A. M. (1988). Anatomical–functional correlation using an adjustable MRI-based region-of-interest atlas with positron emission tomography. *J. Cereb. Blood Flow Metab.* **8**(4), 513–530.

Evans, A. C., Marrett, S., Collins, D. L., and Peters, T. M. (1989). Anatomical–functional correlative analysis of the human brain using three-dimensional imaging systems. *Proc. Int. Soc. Opt. Eng.* (*SPIE*): *Med. Imag. III,* 264–274.

Evans, A. C., Marrett, S., Torrescorzo, J., Ku, S., and Collins, L. (1991a). MRI–PET correlative analysis using a volume of interest (VOI) atlas. *J. Cereb. Blood Flow Metab.* **11**(2), A69–A78.

Evans, A. C., Dai, W., Collins, L., Neelin, P., and Marrett, S. (1991b). Warping of a computerized 3-D atlas to match brain image volumes for quantitative neuroanatomical and functional analysis. *Proc. Int. Soc. Opt. Eng.* (*SPIE*): *Med. Imag. V* **1445**, 236–247.

Evans, A. C., Thompson, C. J., Marrett, S., Meyer, E., and Mazza, M. (1991c). Performance characteristics of the PC-2048: A new 15-slice encoded-crystal PET scanner for neurological studies *IEEE Trans. Med. Imag.* **10**(1), 90–98.

Evans, A. C., Marrett, S., Neelin, P., Collins, L., Worsley, K., Dai, W., Milot, S., Meyer, E., and Bub, D. (1992a). Anatomical mapping of functional activation in stereotactic coordinate space. *NeuroImage* **1**(1), 43–63.

Evans, A. C., Peters, T. M., Collins, D. L., Henri, C. J., Marrett, T. S., Pike, G. B., and Dai, W. (1992b). 3-D Correlative imaging and segmentation of cerebral anatomy, function and vasculature. *Automedica* **14**(1), 65–80.

Evans, A. C., Collins, D. L., and Milner, B. (1992c). An MRI-based stereotactic brain atlas from 300 young normal subjects *In* "Proceedings of the 22nd Annual Symposium of the Society for Neuroscience, Anaheim," p. 408.

Fox, P. T., Perlmutter, J. S., and Raichle, M. E. (1985). A Stereotactic method of anatomical localization for positron emission tomography. *J. Comput Assist. Tomogr.* **9**(1), 141–153.

Friston, K. J., Passingham, R. E., Nutt, J. G., Heather, J. D., Sawle, G. V., and Frackowiak, R. S. J. (1989). Localization in PET images: Direct fitting of the intercommissural (AC–PC) line. *J. Cereb. Blood Flow Metab.* **9**, 690–695.

Friston, K. J., Frith, C. D., Liddle, P. F., and Frackowiak, R. S. J. (1991). Plastic transformation of PET images. *J. Comput. Assist. Tomogr.* **15**(1), 634–639.

Garnett, E. S., Firnau, G., and Nahmias, C. (1983). Dopamine visualized in the basal ganglia of living man. *Nature* **305**, 137–138.

Golub, G. H., and Van Loan, C. F. (1983). "Matrix Computations." Baltimore: Johns Hopkins University Press.

Herscovitch, P., Markham, J., and Raichle, M. E. (1983). Brain blood flow measured with intravenous H_2^{15} O. I. Theory and error analysis. *J. Nucl. Med.* **24**, 782–789.

Hill, D. L. G., Hawkes, D. J., Crossman, J. E., Gleeson, M. J., Cox, T. C. S., Bracey, E. E., Strong, A. J., and Graves, P. (1991). Registration of MR and CT images for skull base surgery using point-like anatomical features. *Br. J. Radiol.* **64**, 1030–1035.

Kamber, M., Collins, D. L., Francis, G. S., Shinghal, R., and Evans, A. C. (1992). Model-based 3D segmentation of multiple sclerosis lesions in MRI data. *Vis. Biomed. Comput. Proc. SPIE* **1808**, 590–600.

Kall, B., Kelly, P. J., and Goerss, S. (1987). Comprehensive computer-assisted data collection, treatment planning and interactive surgery. *Proc SPIE* **767**, 509–514.

Kelly, P. J., Kall, B., and Goerss, S. (1984). Functional stereotactic surgery utilizing CT data and computer generated stereotactic atlas. *Acta Neurochim.* **33**(suppl.), 577–583.

Kwong, K. K., Belliveau, J. W., Chesler, D. A., Goldberg, I. E., Weisskoff, R. M., Poncelet, B. P., Kennedy, D. N., Hoppel, B. E., Cohen, M. S., Turner, R., Cheng, H.-M., Brady, T. J., and Rosen, B. R. (1992). Dynamic magnetic resonance imaging of human brain activity during primary sensory stimulation. *Proc. Natl. Acad. Sci. USA* **89**, 5675–5679.

Leblanc, R., and Meyer, E. (1990). Functional PET scanning in the assessment of cerebral arteriovenous malformations. *J. Neurosurg* **73**, 615–619.

Leblanc, R., Meyer, E., Bub, D., Zatorre, R., and Evans, A. C. (1992). Language mapping with activation PET scanning *Neurosurgery,* **31**(2), 369–373.

Lemoine, D., Barillot, C., Gibaud, B., and Pasqualini, E. (1991). An anatomical-based 3D registration system of multimodality and atlas data in neurosurgery. *In* "Lecture Notes in Computer Science 511: Information Processing in Medical Imaging" (A. C. F. Colchester and D. J. Hawkes, Eds.), pp. 154–164. Heidelberg: Springer-Verlag.

Levin, D. N., Pelizzari, C. A., Chen, G. T. Y., Chen, C.-T., and Cooper. M.D., (1988). Retrospective geometric correlation of MR, CT and PET images. *Radiology* **169**, 817–823.

Levin, D. N., Hu, X., Tan, K. K., Galhotra, S., Pelizzari, C. A., Chen, G. T. Y., Beck, R. N., Chen, C.-T., Cooper, M.D., Mullan, J. F., Hekmatpanah, J., and Spire, J.-P. (1989). The brain: Integrated three-dimensional display of MR and PET images. *Radiology* **172**, 783–789.

Ma, Y., Rousset, O., and Evans, A. C. (1993). Three-dimensional MRI-based simulation of PET images. *Comput. Med. Imag. Graph* **17** (4/5), 365–371.

MacDonald, D., Avis, D., and Evans, A. C., (1993). Automatic parameterization of human cortical surfaces. *Annual Symp. Info. Proc. Med. Imag.* (*IPMI*).

Neelin, P., Crossman, J., Hawkes, D., Ma, Y., and Evans, A. C. (1992). Evaluation of MRI/PET registration using simulated PET brain images. *Comput. Med. Imag. Graph* **17**(4/5), 351–356.

Neiw, H. M., Chen, C.-T., Lin, W. C., and Pelizzari, C. A. (1991). Automated three-dimensional registration of medical images. *Proc. SPIE Med. Imag. III* **1445**, 259–264.

Pelizzari, C. A., Chen, G. T. Y., Spelbring, D. R., Weichselbaum, R. R., and Chen, C.-T. (1989). Accurate three-dimensional registration of CT, PET and/or MRI images of the brain. *J. Comput. Assist. Tomogr.* **13**, 20–26.

Pelizzari, C. A., Evans, A. C., Neelin, P., Chen, C.-T., and Marrett, S. (1991). Comparison of two methods for 3D registration of PET and MRI images. *Proc IEEE Eng. Med. Biol. Soc.* **13**(1), 227–228.

Peters, T. M., Clark, J. A., Olivier, A., Marchand, E. P., Mawko, G., Dieumegarde, M., Muresan, L. V., and Ethier, R. (1986). Integrated stereotaxic imaging with CT, MR imaging and digital subtraction angiography. *Radiology* **161**, 821–826.

Peters, T. M., Drangova, M., Clark, J. A., and Pike, G. B. (1988). Image distortion in MR imaging for stereotactic surgery. *In* "Proceedings of the SMRM Annual Meeting, San Francisco."

Peters, T. M., Clark, J. A., Pike, G. B., Henri, C., Collins, L., Leksell, D., and Jeppsson, O. (1989). Stereotactic neurosurgery planning on a personal-computer-based workstation. *J. Digit. Imag.* **2**(2), 75–81.

Quinlan, J. R. (1986). Induction of decision trees. *Machine Learning* **1**, 81–106.

Ranger, N. T., Thompson, C. J., and Evans, A. C. (1989). The application of a masked orbiting transmission source for attenuation correction in PET. *J. Nucl. Med.* **30**(6), 1056–1068.

Sereno, M. I., and Dale, A. M. (1992). A technique for reconstructing and flattening the cortical surface using MRI images. *Soc. Neurosci. Abstr.* **18**(1), 585.

Sibson, R. (1978). Studies in the robustness of multidimensional scaling: Procrustes statistics. *J. Stat. Soc. B* **40**, 234–238.

Steinmetz, H., and Seitz, R. J. (1991). Functional anatomy of language processing: Neuroimaging and the problem of individual variability. *Neuropsychologia* **29**(12), 1149–1161.

Talairach, J., Szikla, G., Tournoux, P., Prossalentis, A., Bordas-Ferrer, M., Covello, L., Jacob, M., Mempel, A., Buser, J., and Bancaud, J. (1967). Atlas d'Anatomie Stereotaxique du Telencephale.'' Paris: Masson.

Talairach, J., and Tournoux, P. (1988). Co-Planar Stereotactic Atlas of the Human Brain: 3-Dimensional Proportional System: An Approach to Cerebral Imaging. Stuttgart/New York: Thieme Verlag.

Talbot, J. D., Marrett, S., Evans, A. C., Meyer, E., Bushnell, M. C., and Duncan, G. H. (1991). Multiple representations of pain in human cerebral cortex. *Science* **251**, 1355–1358.

Thompson, C. J., Ranger, N., Evans, A. C., and Gjedde, A., (1991).

Validation of simultaneous PET emission and transmission scans. *J. Nucl. Med.* **32**, 154–160.

Van den Elsen, P., Maintz, J. B. A., and Viergever, M. A. (1992). Image fusion using geometric features. *Vis. Biomed. Comput. 1992, Proc. SPIE* **1808**, 172–186.

Van Essen, D. C., and Maunsell, J. H. R. (1980). Two-dimensional maps of the cerebral cortex. *J. Comparative Neurol.* **191**, 255–281.

Woods, R. P., Cherry, S. R., and Mazziotta, J. C. (1992). Rapid automated algorithm for aligning and reslicing PET images. *J. Comput. Assist. Tomogr.* **16**(4), 620–633.

Worsley, K. J., Evans, A. C., Marrett, S., and Neelin, P. (1992). Determining the number of statistically significant areas of activation in subtracted activation studies from PET. *J. Cereb. Blood Flow Metab.* **12**(6), 900–918.

Zatorre, R. J., Evans, A. C., Meyer, E., and Gjedde, A. (1992a). Lateralization of phonetic and pitch discrimination in processing of speech. *Science* **256**, 846–849.

Zatorre, R. J., Jones-Gotman, M., Evans, A. C., and Meyer, E. (1992b). Functional localization of human olfactory cortex with positron emission tomography. *Nature* **360**, 339–340.

Zhang, J., Levesque, M. F., Wilson, C. L., Harper, R. M., Engel, J., Lufkin, R., and Behnke, E. J. (1990). Multimodality imaging of brain structures for stereotactic surgery. *Radiology* **175**, 435–441.

15

Partial Volume Correction in Emission-Computed Tomography: Focus on Alzheimer Disease

Carolyn Cidis Meltzer* and J. James Frost†

*Department of Radiology, Divisions of *Neuroradiology and †Nuclear Medicine, The Johns Hopkins Medical Institutions, Baltimore, Maryland 21287*

I. Introduction

The utility of positron emission tomography (PET) and single photon emission computed tomography (SPECT) in the study of brain diseases lies in their ability to provide *in vivo* physiologic information on regional cerebral metabolism, blood flow, or neuroreceptor concentration. One limitation in the accuracy of quantitative measurements is that imposed by finite spatial resolution, which causes underestimation of the radioactivity concentration in small structures (Hoffman *et al.*, 1979; Kessler *et al.*, 1984), or when adjacent dilated cerebrospinal fluid (CSF) spaces produce significant partial volume effects (Mazziotta *et al.*, 1981). Diffuse or focal cerebral atrophy has been reported in normal aging (Coffey *et al.*, 1992; Tomlinson, 1992; Tanna *et al.*, 1991; DeCarli *et al.*, 1990; Jolles *et al.*, 1989; Shefer, 1972), as well as many neuropsychological disorders, such as Alzheimer disease (AD) (Tanna *et al.*, 1991; Wippold *et al.*, 1991; Kiddo *et al.*, 1989; Drayer, 1988; Coleman and Flood, 1987; Hubbard and Anderson, 1985; Brun and Englund, 1981; Terry *et al.*, 1981; Miller *et al.*, 1980; Wyper *et al.*, 1979; Shefer, 1972), epilepsy (Ashtari *et al.*, 1991; Hoedt-Rasmussen and Skinhoj, 1966), schizophrenia (Kelsoe *et al.*, 1988), Pick's disease (Tomlinson, 1992; LeMay, 1986), Creutzfeldt–Jakob (LeMay, 1986), alcohol dependence (Schroth *et al.*, 1988), traumatic brain injury (LeMay, 1986), Huntington's disease (LeMay, 1986), and AIDS (Gray *et al.*, 1991; Elovaara *et al.*, 1990).

Emission computed tomographic studies of these subject groups in comparison with normal controls may be confounded by increased partial volume averaging of widened sulci with expanded CSF spaces. In the absence of correction for greater partial volume effects, an underestimation of measured metabolic markers, receptor concentration, or blood flow measurements may artifactually accentuate group differences or suggest differences where none exist.

AD is a disorder for which study by PET and SPECT is profoundly affected by partial volume effects and, accordingly, will be the focus of this chapter. Furthermore, AD has been extensively studied with PET using [18F]fluorodeoxyglucose (FDG), with most groups reporting significant reductions in cerebral glucose metabolic rate (CMRGlc) in the temporal and parietal lobes (Nybäck *et al.*, 1991; Polinsky *et al.*, 1987; Jamieson *et al.*, 1987; Duara *et al.*, 1986; Chawluk *et al.*, 1985; Foster *et al.*, 1984; Friedland *et al.*, 1983). Frontal lobe hypometabolism (Duara *et al.*, 1986; Chawluk *et al.*, 1985) is variably found, particularly in severely affected patients (Cutler *et al.*, 1985; Chawluk *et al.*, 1985; Foster *et al.*, 1984). Widespread metabolic reductions are seen in later stages of AD (Cutler *et al.*, 1985), with relative sparing of the primary motor and sensory cortex (Nybäck *et al.*, 1991; Benson *et al.*, 1983). A similar distribution of metabolic abnormalities has been reported using SPECT (Jagust *et al.*, 1990; Jagust *et al.*, 1987). SPECT studies exhibiting a pattern of bilateral temporoparietal reduction in cerebral blood flow have demonstrated the greatest clinical diagnostic utility in differentiating AD from normal aging, multiinfarct dementia, and Pick's disease (Holman *et al.*, 1991; Battistin *et al.*, 1990; Bonte *et al.*, 1986, 1990; Frlich *et al.*, 1989; Jagust *et al.*, 1987), with a sensitivity of as much as 88% and a specificity of 87% reported (Holman *et al.*, 1991; Bonte *et al.*, 1990).

The pathological hallmarks of AD are neurofibrillary tangles and senile plaques. Many groups report a localization of these findings similar to regional PET abnormalities. Brun and Englund (1981) found a regional pattern of cortical degeneration in AD localized to the temporal lobe, with the exception of early mild cases. The occipital lobe showed little pathologic change until a very advanced stage of disease. Mountjoy *et al.* (1983) found a significant correlation between neuronal loss in temporal and frontal lobes and abundance of plaques and tangles. Furthermore, it has been recently suggested that neuronal loss may be a better marker of disease severity than plaques and tangles (Duyckaerts *et al.*, 1989). Although there is considerable variability in the degree of atrophy in individual patients (Miller *et al.*, 1980), overall cortical neuronal losses two- to threefold greater than those in normal aging have been reported (Shefer, 1972). The largest neuronal losses have been observed in the temporal, parietal, and frontal lobes, with relative sparing of the occipital lobe (Tomlinson, 1992; Coleman and Flood 1987, Mann *et al.*, 1985; Hubbard and Anderson, 1985; Mountjoy *et al.*, 1983; Terry *et al.*, 1981; Brun and Englund, 1981; Shefer, 1972). Terry *et al.* (1981) found large neurons reduced by 46% in the temporal lobes and 40% in the frontal lobes in AD patients over healthy controls. Whereas Tomlinson and Henderson (1976) failed to find a significant difference in neuronal counts between AD patients and aged controls, this study concentrated on areas thought to be relatively spared in AD, including pre- and postcentral gyri and the occipital lobe. Duyckaerts *et al.* (1985) suggested that a reduction in cortical length may be more important than loss of cortical thickness in the temporal lobes of AD patients.

Imaging parameters of atrophy have also been extensively investigated in AD. Increased computed tomographic (CT) measurements of ventricular volume (DeCarli *et al.*, 1990; Brinkman *et al.*, 1981; Wyper *et al.*, 1979) and sulcal enlargement, including focal temporal lobe atrophy (Kiddo *et al.*, 1989; George *et al.*, 1987), have been reported in AD brains. Considerable overlap exists between these measurements in individual AD patients and normal controls (Wippold *et al.*, 1991). Although volumetric rather than linear CT measurements provide better discrimination between AD and normals (Gado *et al.*, 1993), dementia severity

is not well correlated with CT volumetrics (Wippold *et al.*, 1991). Furthermore, an error of up to 16% for CT measurements of ventricular volume has been reported by Penn *et al.* (1978) based on phantom data, and Wyper *et al.* (1979) estimated a 20–30% error in ventricular volume measurements in patients using CT. Accurate sulcal measurements are even more difficult to obtain using CT because of beam-hardening artifacts (an important hindrance in imaging of the temporal lobe) and partial volume effects.

Magnetic resonance (MR) imaging has several advantages over CT in assessment of brain atrophy, including superior tissue contrast, lack of beam hardening, and multiplanar display capability. Accordingly, improved accuracy of MR over CT estimates of CSF space volumetrics has been demonstrated (Kohn *et al.*, 1991; Vannier *et al.*, 1991; Filipek *et al.*, 1989, 1987; Kelsoe *et al.*, 1988; Condon *et al.*, 1986a, 1986b). Filipek *et al.* (1989) calculated an error of 5.2% in volume measurements of a phantom studied with 3.1-mm contiguous high-contrast MR images. MR-based methods have found reduced regional brain volumes in AD patients compared with those in normals in the anterior temporal lobe and hippocampal formation, as well as increased ventricular and sulcal volumes (Jack *et al.*, 1992; Dahlbeck *et al.*, 1991; Seab *et al.*, 1988).

A regional correlation between focal hypometabolism and pathologic changes in AD has been observed (Fazekas *et al.*, 1989; Jamieson *et al.*, 1987; McGeer *et al.*, 1986). Fazekas *et al.* (1989) reported a similar regional pattern of hypometabolism and atrophy in 9 out of 28 AD patients studied with FDG–PET and CT. They concluded that focal atrophy was most likely to be associated with apparent local hypometabolism, but that regional hypometabolism did not predict the presence or absence of atrophy.

II. Partial Volume Correction

Recognition of a significant effect of cerebral atrophy on PET measurements, due to partial volume averaging of enlarged metabolically inactive CSF spaces, has been demonstrated in the past (Chawluk *et al.*, 1987). The recent literature has reflected attempts to evaluate and further to correct for this effect. Tissue atrophy may also affect PET measurements by altering attenuation properties of the organ imaged (Schlageter *et al.*, 1987). Because the attenuation effects of water (CSF) and brain tissue are very similar, this effect is likely negligible and may be disregarded.

Because emission computed tomography is more sensitive than MR or CT in the detection of AD, it is likely that the metabolic disturbance precedes structural atrophy (Fazekas et al., 1989; Wyper et al., 1979). This suggests that both neuronal dysfunction and tissue loss contribute to the finding of hypometabolism in AD relative to elderly normals with FDG–PET. Quantification of the effect of atrophy on PET measurements was assessed by Schlageter et al. (1987), who reported a significant negative correlation between global CMRGlc and CT measures of CSF volume. However, they concluded that partial volume effects due to atrophy accounted for no more than 13% of the variance in CMRGlc values.

Various approaches to the correction of PET studies for the effects of atrophy have been described. Both Herscovitch et al. (1986) and Chawluk et al. (1987) have used ventricular and sulcal volumes derived from CT to adjust whole-brain PET measurements of metabolism. The latter group reported a 16.9% increase in global CMRGlc in AD patients, compared with 9% in elderly controls. The correction of regional PET data for partial volume effects using quantitative CT density pixel values was demonstrated by Koeppe et al. (1989) in patients with olivopontocerebellar atrophy. In 1990, Chawluk et al. reported the elimination of a significant difference in glucose metabolism between AD patients and normals in the parietal lobe after application of regional CT-based partial volume correction. The error associated with CT morphometric measurements (Wyper et al., 1979; Penn et al., 1978) and lack of correction for axial resolution effects are limitations of these methods. Using MR-derived brain and CSF volumes, Tanna et al. (1991) reported higher values of 25.0 and 15.8% in whole-brain metabolic rates in AD patients and elderly normals, respectively. This study supported the greater sensitivity provided by MR over CT in separating AD from normals; however, it did not offer a means of quantifying the effect of such measurements on regional PET data.

In 1988, Videen et al. described a method for correcting regional PET data for effects of atrophy on a pixel-by-pixel basis using high-resolution CT or MR images. This was demonstrated in a two-dimensional brain phantom in which one hemisphere had simulated atrophy. Extension of this technique to the correction of PET data in three dimensions using MR was recently demonstrated in a phantom and in patient studies (Meltzer et al., 1990a). Meltzer et al. (1990a) used standard T_2-weighted MR images, which provide high contrast between brain tissue and CSF, to create binary images in which brain tissue pixels were assigned a value of 1 and CSF pixels a value of 0. A composite brain tissue image was obtained by summing a set of thin-section contiguous binary MR images, each weighted to the PET z-axis line-spread function. This

composite tissue image was then convolved to the in-plane resolution of the PET image. The original PET image was then divided by the convolved tissue image on a pixel-by-pixel basis, resulting in a corrected PET image in which count density represents activity per volume of brain tissue rather than spatial volume. Registration of the PET and composite binary MR image for the final division step was accomplished by subjective visual analysis of image overlay. A misregistration of one PET pixel (2.77 mm) was generally cleared recognized as such. (The effect of a one-pixel misregistration was calculated to average 7.8%.) The error introduced into correction data due to maximum missegmentation of brain and CSF was calculated at 3.6%.

A potential limitation of the binary correction method is that it does not take into consideration partial volume averaging between gray and white matter. Mazziotta et al. (1981) reported values of 1.41–1.81 for gray:white matter CMRGlc ratios at a full-width-at-half-maximum (FWHM) of 10–15 mm and estimated that this ratio would approach 3.5–4.0 with improved spatial resolution. There is equivocal pathological evidence of preferential gray matter losses in AD. Høedt-Rasmussen and Skinhøj (1966) reported decreased gray:white matter ratios in the presence of dementia. However, Miller et al. (1980) found no change in the proportions of gray and white matter in a postmortem study comparing brains from 12 elderly demented patients with those of age-matched normals. Prohovnik et al. (1989) demonstrated a diffuse reduction in gray matter relative weight in presenile but not senile-onset AD using ^{133}Xe inhalation method. This issue has also been addressed through imaging techniques. Using quantitative CT, Creasey et al. (1986) found that men with AD had significantly lower gray:white matter ratios than controls. The high-contrast resolution attainable with MR imaging makes it a potentially valuable tool for the in vivo determination of the relative proportion of gray and white matter in normals, as well as in aging and disease states (Lim et al., 1992; Chawluk et al., 1987). Rusinek et al. (1991), using inversion recovery MR image data, demonstrated a significant reduction in gray matter in the temporal, frontal, and occipital lobes in 14 AD patients when compared with 14 age-matched healthy controls, with no difference in white matter volume between the two groups.

A modification of the binary correction method to correct for potential differences in the gray/white matter proportions between groups has recently been described (Müller-Gärtner et al., 1992). This technique employs a spoiled grass (SPGR) MR pulse sequence to obtain high-contrast differences among gray matter, white matter, and CSF. Thus, pixels in the MR image are classified as one of three tissue components and proportionally weighted according to their relative contribution of each to the PET signal. Computer simulations indicated that cortical thinning of 3 mm without a change in actual tracer concentration would result in a 30% reduction in apparent tracer concentration in the PET image. The application of this trinary correction method to [^{11}C]carfentanil PET data was demonstrated in a 40-year-old male subject with left-sided temporal lobe seizures (Plate 32). Before correction, there is symmetric binding of [^{11}C]carfentanil to μ-opiate receptors in the right and left temporal lobes. After gray matter correction, there is relatively increased activity on the side of the seizure focus, as would be expected (Mayberg et al., 1988).

Both the binary and the trinary partial volume correction techniques make the assumption of zero activity from CSF in the PET image. If the actual amount of tracer in CSF spaces relative to brain tissue is indeed negligible is not known. Thus, the assumption of no significant signal contribution from CSF may be responsible for a small overcorrection of PET data. The ability to measure CSF tracer concentration in vivo is not possible in normal subjects due to the spatial resolution limitations of PET. However, in subjects with brain atrophy or hydrocephalus, activity in enlarged ventricles may be measurable with state-of-the-art PET scanners. Alternatively, CSF activity may be measured directly in animal studies.

III. Cerebral Metabolism in Alzheimer Disease

Initial implementation of the MR-based binary partial volume correction method on [^{11}C]carfentanil μ-opiate receptor PET studies of the temporal cortex in two AD patients and one young normal volunteer demonstrated average regional increases in count density of 11% in the normals and 39 and 48% in the patients (Meltzer et al., 1990a). Partial volume correction was thereafter performed on FDG–PET data of the temporal lobe in three AD and three elderly controls (Meltzer et al., 1990b). The average increase in temporal lobe activity after correction was shown to be 35% in the patients compared with 19% in the controls.

Recently, binary partial volume correction has been applied to FDG–PET data in 10 AD patients and 10 elderly controls. Two PET slices were analyzed, one selected for optimum sampling of the temporal and

occipital lobes, the other 32 mm superior for sampling of the frontal and parietal lobes. Increases in regional activity with partial volume correction in the AD patients compared with normals were 33 vs 25% temporal, 28 vs 27% frontal, 39 vs 32% parietal, and 23 vs 17% occipital. Before partial volume correction, the AD group exhibited significantly lower cortex-to-cerebellum ratios in the posterior temporal, parietal, and frontal lobes relative to the control group (Fig. 1). However, after correction there was no longer a significant difference between patients and controls in the posterior temporal region. This finding suggests that greater partial volume effects due to atrophy in the patients may substantially contribute to the apparent regional hypometabolism observed in uncorrected PET images.

IV. Future Directions

Partial volume correction in PET and SPECT, particularly in the study of aging and diseases of the elderly, is an important method and one for which recent progress has been made. Nonetheless, to fully validate and implement these methods for routine patient management and research applications, several components of the method will require further investigation.

First, more effort is needed in the optimization of MR image acquisition sequences to improve gray matter/white matter/CSF contrast. Because a major focus for application is in the elderly subject population, minimizing the acquisition time, and hence the potential for movement artifacts, is a critical constraint. Accordingly, a single acquisition protocol, such as the SPGR sequence, that permits subsequent segmentation of gray matter, white matter, and CSF is preferred over methods that require two or more acquisition sequences. If the MR tissue parameters differ significantly among normals and disease groups, the optimal acquisition protocol may need to be group specific. Furthermore, as partial volume correction is extended to peripheral structures such as the heart and non-CNS neoplasms, additional acquisition protocols will need to be developed.

Second, further development and validation of methods for gray matter/white matter/CSF segmentation is required. This is an active area of research and many proposed methods are already available, but their validation has not been accomplished. One can employ either realistic brain phantoms or direct in vivo/ex vivo imaging studies in experimental animals for validation; the latter methods, although the most

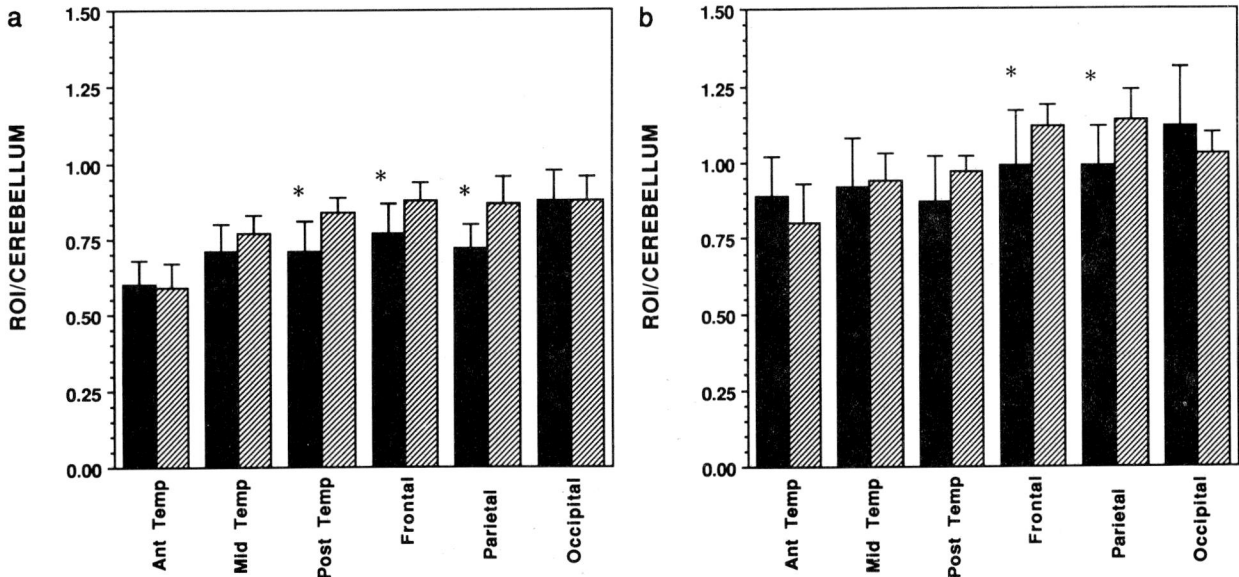

Figure 1 Comparison of regional (ROI/cerebellum) uncorrected (a) and corrected (b) PET data in AD (solid bar) patients and elderly (hatched bar) controls. *$p < 0.05$ (error bars indicate 1 s.d.)

rigorous, are the most technically demanding to execute. Human studies could conceivably be used for validation, but problems of registration and postmortem delay would be difficult to surmount. This is a complex problem whose solution for partial volume correction and volumetric analysis is likely to represent a compromise between precision and accuracy. A small but definable segmentation error, together with high precision, may be an acceptable compromise for the purpose of comparing data in normal subjects and various disease groups. A complicating factor may be found in diseases for which the MR imaging tissue parameters, and hence the gray matter/white matter/CSF contrast, are altered.

Third, more investigation and validation of methods to register PET, SPECT, and segmented MRI images are required, because the accuracy of the partial volume correction procedure is dependent on the accuracy of image registration (Phillips *et al.*, 1991; Meltzer *et al.*, 1990a). This is also an area of active investigation apart from partial volume correction, and several methods are available, including those which use MR- and PET-visible fiducials and those using various contour fitting algorithms. Independent validation of the registration algorithms will be required prior to the implementation of partial volume correction.

Fourth, further investigation of the effect of inhomogeneous distribution of tracer activity on the accuracy of the partial volume correction procedure is needed. As demonstrated previously (Müller-Gärtner *et al.*, 1992), the existing methods for partial volume correction are most accurate within a region of homogeneously distributed radiotracer, although the effect of inhomogeneity is not a major limitation. Further investigation of the effect of gray matter inhomogeneity can be accomplished through the use of physical and computerized brain phantoms. Furthermore, ancillary image processing methods, such as image filtering, can be developed and validated to further improve the partial volume correction in regions of focal inhomogeneity.

Fifth, additional studies are required to determine the correct values for white matter and CSF radioactivity concentration used in performing the partial volume correction. Previously it has been assumed that CSF has a negligible radiotracer concentration and that the concentration of white matter is homogeneous and can be obtained with high-resolution scanners by sampling the centrum semiovale. The CSF concentration could, in future studies, be determined in patients with CSF shunts by withdrawal and counting of CSF or in patients with enlarged ventricles using imaging alone. The constancy of radiotracer concentration within white matter seems reasonable, but can be validated for some receptor binding radiotracers by blocking the specific receptor binding in gray matter. In the case of the μ-opiate receptor, blockade of binding in normal volunteers results in a very homogeneous image, supporting the constancy of white matter nonspecific binding. Simulation studies using computerized brain phantoms generated from MR images may be subsequently used to determine the error propagation of inaccurate white matter or CSF concentration into the partial volume correction.

Finally, new algorithms and software programs will be needed to handle the large MR and PET or SPECT image datasets required for the partial volume correction and to rapidly perform the computations. State-of-the-art PET scanners acquire up to 47 slices, and for each slice one might use 5–10 MR images of 1-mm or smaller slice thickness to accurately sample the z-axis line spread function for each PET image. Kinetic acquisitions would further increase the size of the datasets. For the partial volume correction method to be accessible to large groups of investigators and clinicians, the time to complete all of the above steps must be kept to a minimum.

V. Summary

The capability of PET and SPECT to provide us with a greater understanding of neuropsychiatric disorders is hindered in cases of cerebral atrophy due to partial volume averaging of brain tissue with enlarged CSF spaces. In particular, this problem has confounded the interpretation of quantitative metabolic studies of AD, which compare patients with atrophy with normal controls. The importance of determining the degree to which differences in metabolic measures are due to increased partial volume effects rather than specific pathophysiologic effects of the disease is recognized. Various approaches to the quantitation and correction of this potential source of error have been presented. Results from an MR-based method for partial volume correction of regional PET data suggest that biochemical abnormalities as well as atrophic changes account for FDG hypometabolism in temporoparietal and frontal areas in AD. Although SPECT has been used primarily as a nonquantitative clinical tool in the study of AD, correction of SPECT image data for partial volume effects may improve the sensitivity and specificity for early disease detection.

Acknowledgments

This work was supported by U.S.P.H.S. Grants AGO88740, AG10624, and NS15080.

References

Ashtari, M., Barr, W. B., Schaul, N., and Bogerts, B. (1991). Three-dimensional fast low-angle shot imaging and computerized volume measurement of the hippocampus in patients with chronic epilepsy of the temporal lobe. *AJNR* **12**, 941–947.

Battistin, L., Pizzolato, G., Dam, M., Ponza, I., Borsato, N., Zanco, P. L., and Ferlin, G. (1990). Regional cerebral blood flow study with ⁹⁹ᵐTc-hexamethyl-propyleneamine oxime single photon emission computed tomography in Alzheimer and multi-infarct dementia. *Eur. Neurol.* **30**, 296–301.

Benson, D. F., Kuhl, D. E., Hawkins, R. A., Phelps, M. E., Cummings, J. L., and Tsai, S. Y. (1983). The fluorodeoxyglucose ¹⁸F scan in Alzheimer disease and multi-infarct dementia. *Arch. Neurol.* **40**, 711–714.

Bonte, F. J., Ross, E. D., Chehabi, H. H., and Devous, M. D. (1986). SPECT study of regional cerebral blood flow in Alzheimer disease. *J. Comput. Assist. Tomogr.* **10**, 579–583.

Bonte, F. J., Hom, J., Tintner, R., and Weiner, M. F. (1990). Single photon tomography in Alzheimer disease and the dementias. *Sem. Nucl. Med.* **20**, 342–352.

Brinkman, S. D., Sarwar, M., Levin, H. S., and Morris, H. H. (1981). Quantitative indexes of computed tomography in dementia and normal aging. *Radiology* **138**, 89–92.

Brun, A., and Englund, E. (1981). Regional pattern of degeneration in Alzheimer disease: Neuronal loss and histopathological grading. *Histopathology* **5**, 549–564.

Chawluk, J., Alavi, A., Hurtig, H., Dann, R., Rosen, M., Kushner, M. J., Silver, F. L., and Reivich, M. (1985). Altered patterns of regional cerebral glucose metabolism in aging and dementia. *J. Cereb. Blood Flow Metab.* **5**(Suppl. 1), S121–S122.

Chawluk, J. B., Alavi, A., Dann, R., Hurtig, H. I., Bais, S., Kushner, M. J., Zimmerman, R. A., and Reivich, M. (1987). Positron emission tomography in aging and dementia: Effect of cerebral atrophy. *J. Nucl. Med.* **28**, 431–437.

Chawluk, J. B., Dann, R., Alavi, A., Hurtig, H. I., Gur, R. E., Resnick, S., Zimmerman, R. A., and Reivich, M. (1990). The effect of focal cerebral atrophy in positron emission tomography studies of aging and dementia. *Nucl. Med. Biol.* **17**, 797–804.

Coffey, C. E., Wilkinson, W. E., Parashos, I. A., Soady, S. A. R., Sullivan, R. J., Patterson, L. J., Figiel, G. S., Webb, M. C., Spritzer, C. E., and Djang, W. T. (1992). Quantitative cerebral anatomy of the aging human brain: A cross-sectional study using magnetic resonance imaging. *Neurology* **42**, 527–536.

Coleman, P. D., and Flood, D. G. (1987). Neuron numbers and dendritic extent in normal aging and Alzheimer disease. *Neurobiol. Aging* **8**, 521–545.

Condon, B. R., Patterson, J., Wyper, D., Hadley, D. M., Teasdale, G., Grant, R., Jenkins, A., Macpherson, P., and Rowan, J. (1986a). A quantitative index of ventricular and extraventricular intracranial CSF volumes using MR imaging. *J. Comput. Assist. Tomogr.* **10**, 784–792.

Condon, B., Wyper, D., Grant, R., Patterson, J., Hadley, D., Teasdale, G., and Rowan, J. (1986b). Use of magnetic resonance imaging to measure intracranial cerebrospinal fluid volume. *Lancet* **1**(8494), 1355–1357.

Creasey, H., Schwartz, M., Frederickson, H., Haxby, J. V., and Rapoport, S. I. (1986). Quantitative computed tomography in dementia of the Alzheimer type. *Neurology* **36**, 1563–1568.

Cutler, N. R., Haxby, J. V., Duara, R., Grady, C. L., Kay, A. D., Kessler, R. M., Sundaram, M., and Rapoport, S. I. (1985). Clinical history, brain metabolism, and neuropsychological function in Alzheimer disease. *Ann. Neurol.* **18**, 298–309.

Dahlbeck, S. W., McCluney, K. W., Yeakley, J. W., Fenstermacher, M. J., Bonmati, C., Van Horn, G., and Aldag, J. (1991). The intertruncal distance: A new MR measurement for the hippocampal atrophy of Alzheimer disease. *AJNR* **12**, 931–932.

DeCarli, C., Kaye, J. A., Horwitz, B., and Rapoport, S. I. (1990). Critical analysis of the use of computer-assisted transverse axial tomography to study human brain in aging and dementia of the Alzheimer type. *Neurology* **40**, 872–883.

Drayer, B. P. (1988). Imaging of the aging brain. II. Pathologic conditions. *Radiology* **166**, 797–806.

Duara, R., Grady, C., Haxby, J., Sundaram, M., Cutler, N. R., Heston, L., Moore, A., Schlageter, N., Larson, S., and Rappaport, S. I. (1986). Positron emission tomography in Alzheimer disease. *Neurology* **36**, 879–887.

Duyckaerts, C., Hauw, J. J., Piette, F., Rainsard, C., Poulain, V., Berthaux, P., and Escourolle, R. (1985). Cortical atrophy in senile dementia of the Alzheimer type is mainly due to a decrease in cortical length. *Acta Neuropathol.* **66**, 72–74.

Duyckaerts, C., Llamas, E., Delaère, P., Miele, P., and Hauw, J.-J. (1989). Neuronal loss and neuronal atrophy: Computer simulation in connection with Alzheimer disease. *Brain Res.* **504**, 94–100.

Elovaara, I., Poutiainen, E., Raininko, R., Valanne, L., Virta, A., Valle, S-L., Lähdevirta, J., and Iivanainen, M. (1990). Mild brain atrophy in early HIV infection: The lack of association with cognitive deficits and HIV-specific intrathecal immune response. *J. Neurol. Sci.* **99**, 121–136.

Fazekas, F., Alavi, A., Chawluk, J. B., Zimmerman, R. A., Hackney, D., Bilaniuk, L., Rosen, M., Alves, W. M., Hurtig, H. I., Jamieson, D. G., Kushner, M. J., and Reivich, M. (1989). Comparison of CT, MR, and PET in Alzheimer dementia and normal aging. *J. Nucl. Med.* **30**, 1607–1615.

Filipek, P. A., Kennedy, D. N., Caviness, V. S., Klein, S., and Rapin, I. (1987). *In vivo* magnetic resonance imaging-based volumetric brain analysis in subjects with verbal auditory agnosia. *Ann. Neurol.* **22**, 410–411.

Filipek, P. A., Kennedy, D. N., Caviness, V. S., Rossnick, S. L., Spraggins, T. A., and Starewicz, P. M. (1989). Magnetic resonance imaging-based brain morphometry: Development and application to normal subjects. *Ann. Neurol.* **25**, 61–67.

Foster, N. L., Chase, T. N., Mansi, L., Brooks, R., Fedio, P., Patronas, N. J., and Di Chiro, G. (1984). Cortical abnormalities in Alzheimer disease. *Ann. Neurol.* **16**, 649–654.

Friedland, R. P., Budinger, T. F., Ganz, E., Yano, Y., Mathis, C. A., Koss, B., Ober, B. A., Huesman, R. H., and Derenzo, S. E. (1983). Regional cerebral metabolic alterations in dementia of the Alzheimer type: Positron emission tomography with 18F-fluorodeoxyglucose. *J. Comput. Assist. Tomogr.* **7**, 590–598.

Frlich, L., Eilles, C., Maurer, K., and Lanczik, M. (1989). Stage-dependent reductions of regional cerebral blood flow measured by HMPAO–SPECT in dementia of Alzheimer type. *Psychiat. Res.* **29**, 347–350.

Frost, J. J., Mayberg, H. S., Fisher, R. S., Douglass, K. H., Dannals, R. F., Links, J. M., Wilson, A. A., Ravert, H. T., Rosenbaum, A. E., Snyder, S. H., and Wagner, H. N. (1988). Mu-opiate receptors measured by positron emission tomography are increased in temporal lobe epilepsy. *Ann. Neurol.* **23**, 231–237.

Gado, M., Hughes, C. P., Danziger, W., and Chi, D. (1983). Aging, dementia, and brain atrophy: A longitudinal computed tomographic study. *AJNR* **4**, 699–702.

George, A. E., Stylopoulos, L. A., de Leon, M. J., Klinger, A., Kluger, A., and Miller, J. D. (1987). Temporal lobe CT diagnostic features of Alzheimer disease. *AJNR* **8**, 931.

Gray, E., Haug, H., Chimelli, L., Geny, C., Gaston, A., Scaravilli, F., and Budka, H. (1991). Prominent cortical atrophy with neuronal loss as correlate of human immunodeficiency virus encephalopathy. *Acta Neuropathol.* **82**, 229–233.

Herscovitch, P., Auchus, A. P., Gado, M., Chi, D., and Raichle, M. E. (1986). Correction of positron emission tomography data for cerebral atrophy. *J. Cereb. Blood Flow Metab.* **6**, 120–124.

Hoedt-Rasmussen, K., and Skinhoj, E. (1966). *In vivo* measurements of the relative weights of gray and white matter in the human brain. *Neurology* **16**, 515–521.

Hoffman, E. J., Huang, S. C., and Phelps, M. E. (1979). Quantitation in positron emission computed tomography. 1. Effect of object size. *J. Comput. Assist. Tomogr.* **3**, 299–308.

Holman, B. L., Nagel, J. S., Johnson, K. A., and Hill, T. C. (1991). Imaging dementia with SPECT. *Ann. N.Y. Acad. Sci.* **620**, 165–174.

Hubbard, B. M., and Anderson, J. M. (1985). Age-related variations in the neuron content of the cerebral cortex in senile dementia of the Alzheimer type. *Neuropathol. Appl. Neurobiol.* **11**, 369–382.

Jack, C. R., Petersen, R. C., O'Brien, P. C., and Tangalos, E. G. (1992). MR-based hippocampal volumetry in the diagnosis of Alzheimer disease. *Neurology* **42**, 183–188.

Jagust, W. J., Budinger, T. F. and Reed, B. R. (1987). The diagnosis of dementia with single photon emission computed tomography. *Arch. Neurol.* **44**, 258–262.

Jagust, W. J., Reed, B. R., Seab, P. J., and Budinger, T. F. (1990). Alzheimer disease: Age at onset and single-photon emission computed tomographic patterns of regional cerebral blood flow. *Arch. Neurol.* **47**, 628–633.

Jamieson, D. G., Chawluk, J. B., Alavi, A., Hurtig, H. I., Rosen, M., Bais, S., Dann, R., Kushner, M., and Reivich, M. (1987). The effect of disease severity on local cerebral glucose metabolism in Alzheimer disease. *J. Cereb. Blood Flow Metab.* **7**(Suppl. 1), S410.

Jolles, P. R., Chapman, P. R., and Alavi, A. (1989). PET, CT, and MRI in the evaluation of neuropsychiatric disorders: Current applications. *J. Nucl. Med.* **30**, 1589–1606.

Kelsoe, J. R., Cadet, J. L., Picar, D., and Weinberger, D. R. (1988). Quantitative neuroanatomy in schizophrenia. *Arch. Gen. Psychiat.* **45**, 533–541.

Kessler, R. M., Ellis, J. R., Eden, M. (1984). Analysis of emission tomographic scan data: Limitations imposed by resolution and background. *J. Comput. Assist. Tomogr.* **8**, 514–522.

Kiddo, D. K., Caine, E. D., LeMay, M., Ekholm, S., Booth, H., and Panzer, R. (1989). Temporal lobe atrophy in patients with Alzheimer disease: A CT study. *AJNR* **10**, 551–555.

Koeppe, R. A., Rosenthal, G., Gilman, S., Lopez, R., Junck, L., and Gebarski, S. S. (1989). Correction for effects of tissue atrophy in PET studies using quantitative anatomic imaging. *J. Cereb. Blood Flow Metab.* **9**, S197.

Kohn, M. I., Tanna, N. K., Herman, G. T., Resnick, S. M., Mozley, P. D., Gur, R. E., Alavi, A., Zimmerman, R. A., and Gur, R. C. (1991). Analysis of brain and cerebrospinal fluid volumes with MR imaging. I. Methods, reliability, and validation. *Radiology* **178**, 115–122.

LeMay, M. (1986). CT changes in dementing diseases: A review. *AJNR* **7**, 841–853.

Lim, K. O., Zipursky, R. B., Watts, M. C., and Pfefferbaum, A. (1992). Decreased gray matter in normal aging: An *in vivo* magnetic resonance study. *J. Gerontol.* **47**, B26–B30.

Mann, D. M. A., Yates, P. O., and Marcyniuk, B. (1985). Some morphometric observations on the cerebral cortex and hippocampus in presenile Alzheimer disease, senile dementia of Alzheimer type and Down's syndrome in middle age. *J. Neurol. Sci.* **69**, 139–159.

Mayberg, H. S., Sadzot, B., Meltzer, C. C., Fisher, R. S., Lesser, R. P., Dannals, R. F., Lever, J. R., Wilson, A. A., Ravert, H. T., Wagner, H. N., Bryan, R. N., Cromwell, C. C., and Frost, J. J. (1991). Quantification of mu and non-mu opiate receptors in temporal lobe epilepsy using positron emission tomography. *Ann. Neurol.* **30**, 3–11.

Mazziotta, J. C., Phelps, M. E., Plummer, D., and Kuhl, D. E. (1981). Quantitation in positron emission tomography. 5. Physical–anatomical effects. *J. Comput. Assist. Tomogr.* **5**, 734–743.

McGeer, P. L., Kamo, H., Harrop, R., McGeer, E. G., Martin, W. R. W., Pate, B. D., and Li, D. K. B. (1986). Comparison of

PET, MRI, and CT with pathology in a proven case of Alzheimer disease. *Neurology* **36**, 1569–1574.

Meltzer, C. C., Leal, J. P., Mayberg, H. S., Wagner, H. N., and Frost, J. J. (1990a). Correction of PET data for partial volume effects in human cerebral cortex by MR imaging. *J. Comput. Assist. Tomogr.* **14**, 561–570.

Meltzer, C. C., Leal, J. P., Cromwell, C. C., Müller-Gaertner, H., Mayberg, H. S., Wagner, H. N., and Frost, J. J. (1990b). Partial volume correction of regional cerebral glucose metabolism in Alzheimer's disease. *Radiology* **177**(P), 217.

Miller, A. K. H., Alston, R. L., and Corsellis, J. A. N. (1980). Variation with age in the volumes of grey and white matter in the cerebral hemispheres of man: Measurements with an image analyser. *Neuropathol. Appl. Neurobiol.* **6**, 119–132.

Mountjoy, C. Q., Roth, M., Evans, N. J. R., and Evans, H. M. (1983). Cortical neuronal counts in normal elderly controls and demented patients. *Neurobiol. Aging* **4**, 1–11.

Müller-Gärtner, H. W., Links, J. M., Prince, J. L., Bryan, R. N., McVeigh, E., Leal, J. P., Davatzikos, C., and Frost, J. J. (1992). Measurement of radiotracer concentration in brain gray matter using positron emission tomography: MRI-based correction for partial volume effects. *J. Cereb. Blood Flow Metab.* **12**, 571–583.

Nybäck, H., Nyman, H., Blomqvist, G., Sjögren, I., and Stone-Elander, S. (1991). Brain metabolism in Alzheimer dementia: Studies of ^{11}C-deoxyglucose accumulation, CSF monoamine metabolites and neuropsychological test performance in patients and healthy subjects. *J. Neurol. Neurosurg. Psychiat.* **54**, 672–678.

Penn, R. D., Belanger, M. G., and Yasnoff, M. D. (1978). Ventricular volume in man computed from CAT scans. *Ann. Neurol.* **3**, 216–223.

Phillips, R. L., London, E. D., Links, J. M., and Cascella, N. G. (1990). Program for PET image alignment: Effects on calculated differences in cerebral metabolic rates for glucose. *J. Nucl. Med.* **31**, 2052–2057.

Polinsky, R. J., Noble, J., Di Chiro, G., Nee, L. E., Feldman, R. G., and Brown, R. T. (1987). Dominantly inherited Alzheimer disease: Cerebral glucose metabolism. *J. Neurol. Neurosurg. Psychiat.* **50**, 752–757.

Prohovnik, I., Smith, G., Sackeim, H. A., Mayeux, R., and Stern, Y. (1989). Gray-matter degeneration in presenile Alzheimer disease. *Ann. Neurol.* **25**, 117–124.

Rusinek, H., de Leon, M. J., George, A. E., Stylopoulos, L. A., Chandera, R., Smith, G., Rand, T., Mourino, M., and Kowalski, H. (1991). Alzheimer disease: Measuring loss of cerebral gray matter with MR imaging. *Radiology* **178**, 109–114.

Schlageter, N. L., Horowitz, B., Creasey, H., Carson, R., Duara, R., Berg, G. W., and Rapoport, S. I. (1987). Relation of measured brain glucose utilization and cerebral atrophy in man. *J. Neurol. Neurosurg. Psychiat.* **50**, 779–785.

Schroth, G., Naegele, T., Klose, U., Mann, K., and Petersen, D. (1988). Reversible brain shrinkage in abstinent alcoholics, measured by MRI. *Neuroradiology* **30**, 385–389.

Seab, J. P., Jagust, W. J., Wong, S. T. S., Roos, M. S., Reed, B. R., and Budinger, T. F. (1988). Quantitative NMR measurements of hippocampal atrophy in Alzheimer disease. *Magn. Reson. Med.* **8**, 200–208.

Shefer, V. F. (1972). Absolute numbers of neurons and thickness of the cerebral cortex during aging, senile and vascular dementia, and Pick's and Alzheimer diseases. *Neurosci. Behav. Physiol.* **6**, 319–324.

Tanna, N. K., Kohn, M. I., Horwich, D. N., Jolles, P. R., Zimmerman, R. A., Alves, W. M., and Alavi, A. (1991). Analysis of brain and cerebrospinal fluid volumes with MR imaging: Impact on PET data correction for atrophy, part II. aging and Alzheimer dementia. *Radiology* **178**, 123–130.

Terry, R. D., Peck, A., DeTeresa, R., Schechter, R., and Horoupian, D. S. (1981). Some morphometric aspects of the brain in senile dementia of the Alzheimer type. *Ann. Neurol.* **10**, 184–192.

Tomlinson, B. E. (1992). Ageing and the dementias. *In* "Greenfield's Neuropathology" (J. H. Adams and L. W. Duchen, Eds.), Fifth ed., pp. 1284–1410. New York: Oxford University Press.

Tomlinson, B. E., and Henderson, G. (1976). Some quantitative cerebral findings in normal and demented old people. *In* "Neurobiology of Aging" (R. D. Terry and S. Gershon, Eds.), Vol. 3, pp. 183–204. New York: Raven Press.

Vannier, M. W., Brunsden, B. S., Hildebolt, C. F., Falk, D., Cheverud, J. M., Figiel, G. S., Perman, W. H., Kohn, L. A., Robb, R. A., Yoffie, R. L., and Bresina, S. J. (1991). Brain surface cortical sulcal lengths: Quantification with three-dimensional MR imaging. *Radiology* **180**, 479–484.

Videen, T. O., Perlmutter, J. S., Mintun, M. A., and Raichle, M. E. (1988). Regional correction of positron emission tomography data for the effects of cerebral atrophy. *J. Cereb. Blood Flow Metab.* **8**, 662–670.

Wippold, F. J., Gado, M. H., Morris, J. C., Duchek, J. M., and Grant, E. A. (1991). Senile dementia and healthy aging: A longitudinal CT study. *Radiology* **179**, 215–219.

Wyper, D. J., Pickard, J. D., and Matheson, M. (1979). Accuracy of ventricular volume estimation. *J. Neurol. Neurosurg. Psychiat.* **42**, 345–350.

16

Visualization and Warping of Multimodality Brain Imagery

Arthur W. Toga

Laboratory of Neuro Imaging, Department of Neurology, University of California, Los Angeles,
School of Medicine, Los Angeles, California 90024

I. Introduction

Visualizing biomedical data is often a prerequisite to its understanding; *to see it is to know it*. Visualization enables us to extract meaningful information from complex datasets. Although the brain is the most complex of organs, its multidimensional composition lends itself to a variety of computerized visualization techniques concerned with representation, manipulation, and display. If we can visualize a structure, we can identify it. By employing the techniques of image processing, image synthesis, and computer graphics, we combine the utility of image and number, enabling us to statistically measure the visual representation. Further, such statistical analyses can be extended to compare and correlate a given view of brain with data from other modalities and other subjects.

Comparing images across modalities and subjects requires positional and shape transformations to make them occupy the same coordinate space. For example, accurate interpretation of PET or other views of functional anatomy can be improved by correlations with standardized templates. MRI can be used to identify the anatomy on an individual basis, and stereotactic atlases can be used as a common reference coordinate system. In addition, the atlas templates can aid in the segmentation of anatomic structures. The development of more generalized representations requires the ability to compare brains from different subjects and depends on the goodness of fit between datasets.

However, no single representation, whether it be an average or an atlas, can prove accurate even within a homogeneous population of subjects. Thus it is necessary to warp one brain to conform to another and to quantitate the degree of deformation necessary to make them coincident.

This chapter discusses the use of visualization techniques combined with geometric transformation methods to elucidate the relationship between modalities and between subjects.

II. Visualization

Visualization of neurobiological data enables us to create high-quality images from combined datasets to gain insight into the structure and function of brain. These combined datasets can be serial sections depicting anatomy or physiology, two or more modalities from the same subject, or ultimately data from multiple modalities from multiple subjects. The techniques used to process this information into comprehensible displays also must provide access to the quantitative nature of the data. Morphometry and densitometry are necessary elements of useful visualization schemes. Because our ultimate objective requires the warping of brain datasets, we will incorporate those aspects of visualization that help synthesize new information from multiple sources as well as present it quantitatively.

FUNCTIONAL NEUROIMAGING

Regardless of its source, organizing data into volumes can make visualization easier. A complete collection of brain slices can be reconstructed into a volume, whether it comes from tomographically or physically sectioned methods. Volume visualization has received considerable interest in recent years, resulting in several publications entirely devoted to it. The interested reader should consult Friedhoff and Benzon (1989); Kaufman (1991); Robb (1985); Toga (1990); and Udupa and Herman (1991). Advanced topics in medical volume visualization can be found in Hohne *et al.* (1990) and Levoy *et al.* (1990).

A. Surfaces and Volumes

To visualize a volume dataset, two approaches can be used. The first, termed volume rendering (Drebin *et al.*, 1988), projects volume primitives directly for shading and viewing. The second method computes explicit geometric primitives (Herman and Liu, 1979; Toga *et al.*, 1989) such as polygon meshes prior to the viewing and shading stages. It is termed surface rendering.

Representing the surface as explicit geometry is efficient when it is used with the conventional computer graphics approaches for shading and viewing. Further, it greatly reduces the necessary data storage and provides a data structure that can be measured. However, it requires the calculation of an intermediate surface representation. Volume rendering, on the other hand, does not compute an intermediate surface representation, instead it utilizes classification schemes to segment the data into components for inclusion (or exclusion) in a given view. Whereas surface rendering assumes that the data consists of surfaces that can be extracted and visualized, volume rendering does not assume any existing structure. Surface-rendered models (by themselves) do not retain any information deep to the surface, whereas volume representations maintain the entire dataset, allowing any part of the data to be viewed. Maintenance of the entire dataset also enables densitometric measurements. The utility of each approach is primarily dependent upon the type of data and the intent of the visualization. Numerous algorithms have been developed to take advantage of the relative strength and weaknesses of each (Elvins, 1992).

Both approaches are designed to communicate information about the datasets. Combining some of the characteristics of each can provide comprehensive and understandable displays that contain information suitable for morphometric and densitometric measurement. Warping multiple modalities and multiple

subject datasets will require such a combined approach.

B. Manipulation

Manipulating the location, orientation, and display primitives of a dataset is used to enhance our understanding of it as well as make it comparable to other datasets. Moving the position of the datasets within a coordinate system is called geometric transformation and can be accomplished using matrix algebra (Foley *et al.*, 1990; Newman and Sproull, 1979; Pavlidis, 1982). These movements include, but are not limited to, translation, rotation, scaling, and perspective. Ignoring the issues of stereotaxy, multiple modality, and multiple subject comparisons, certain locations and orientations are more illustrative than others. Similarly the display primitives and attributes of the display such as points, contours, wireframe mesh, solid modeling, Phong or Gouraud shading, opacity, and color can greatly influence the viewers comprehension of the material (Toga, 1990). Experimentation on the use of geometric transformations and variations of display primitives is often necessary to obtain the most satisfactory results.

Interactive manipulation of data is extremely useful in targeting specific loci or comparing the similarity (or disparity) between two (or more) datasets. Computational speed and storage size limitations will dictate the degree of interaction and type of data that can be manipulated in this way. But the usefulness of this approach in clinical settings is obvious.

C. Display

Visualizing measured quantities within a meaningful spatial framework is the intent of digital image display. Choosing the most appropriate method of presentation requires a diverse skill set that includes artistic, psychophysical, and statistical considerations. Because the goal of display is to describe, summarize, and in some instances interact with the data, great care is necessary in its design. An excellent treatise on this and related subjects was written by Tufte (1983, 1990). For our purposes we must use an image composition that conveys several important characteristics about the datasets simultaneously. These include spatial, densitometric, correlative, and sometimes temporal information. Assuming 3D, the location and orientation of the reconstructed data, as well as the shape, size, and relationship between substructures within the model, describe the spatial features of the dataset (Plate 33). The intensity or magni-

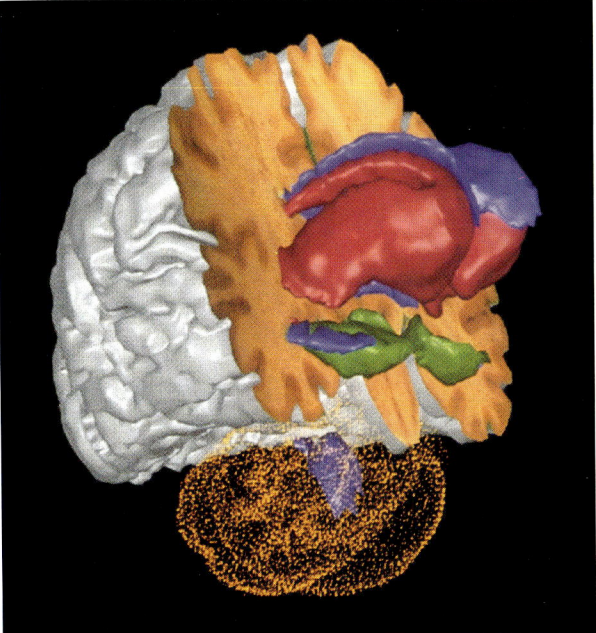

Plate 33 Combined surface and volume rendering of reconstructed human brain. This figure illustrates the use of perspective and specific orientations to enhance the viewer's appreciation of the depth and relative size of substructures. Different display primitives, including color and opacity help distinguish among anatomic regions. The anatomic regions were segmented using contours and surface rendered. A cut plane was introduced to display densitometric information (see text on texture mapping) contained in the original histological dataset. Thus this figure utilizes aspects of both approaches to volume visualization. A rostral–lateral view of the brain in which the cortex is surface rendered and Phong shaded, the ventricles are displayed as solid blue structures, the cerebellum is shown in yellow points, and the basal ganglia rendered solid red is used. A cut plane utilized an arbitrary color scale mapping of the original histological imagery. The data come from a single modality and a single specimen.

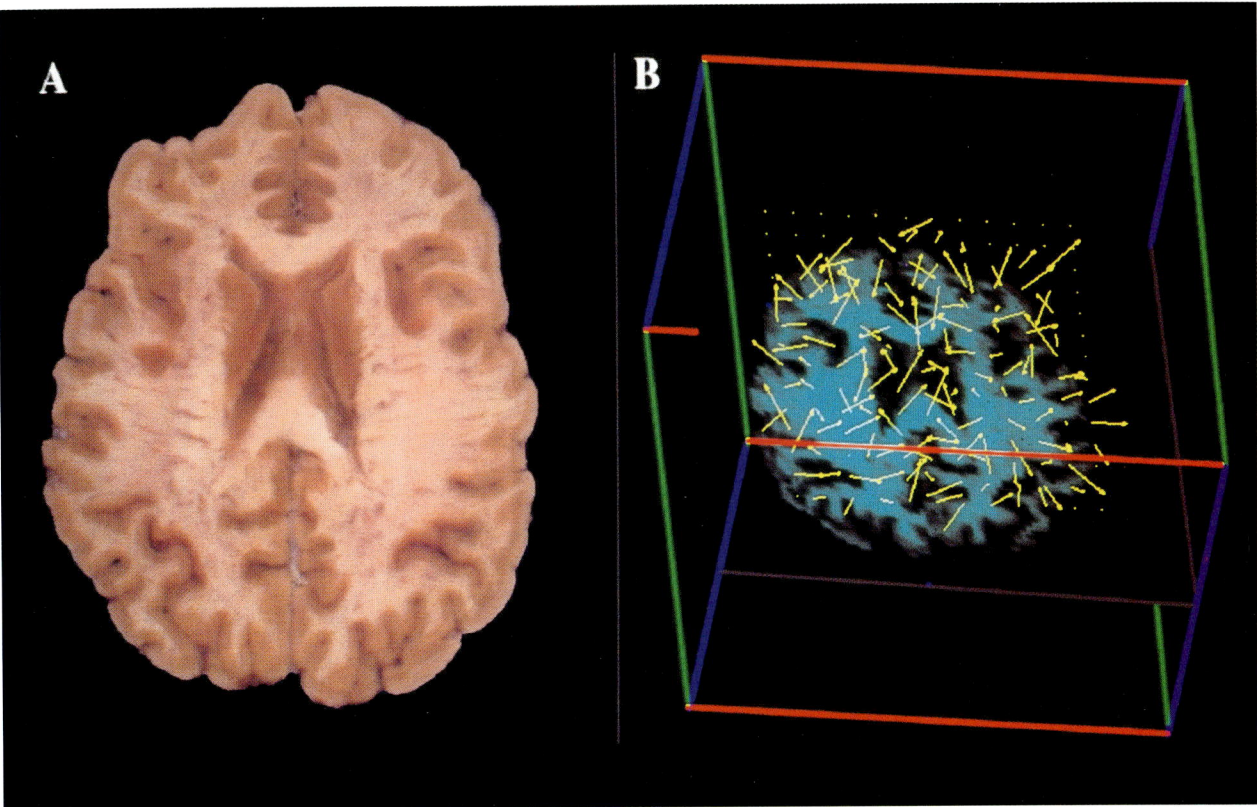

Plate 34 Surface model and vector displacement image of warped human brain. Human brains were reconstructed from serial sections of histological material collected with a cryomacrome at $1024^2 \times 24$ bits by 500 sections. The datasets were downsampled by reducing the resolution to 512. A 256×256×128 grid was placed on the volume, and the warping algorithm was executed as described in the text. (A) A resampled horizontal section through the original volume. (B) Cut plane through the warped volume. The displacement of grid points is illustrated with vectors, which describe the direction and magnitude of the displacement. The magnitude of each grid point displacement is illustrated as five times the actual magnitude. Data between grid points were interpolated. Note the fact that, although there are some trends in the warping, there is also considerable variation in the displacements.

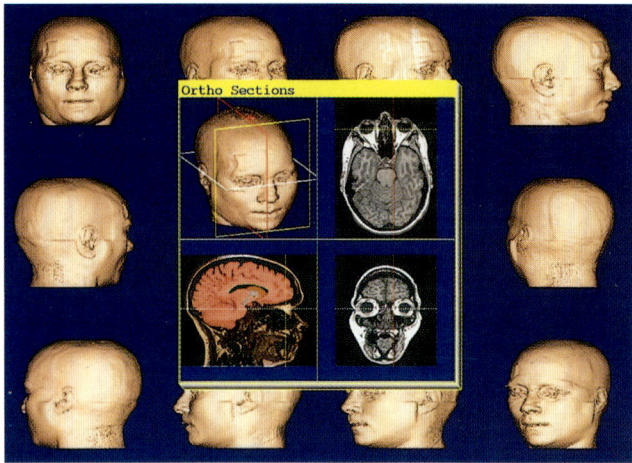

Plate 35 Intersecting orthogonal sections through points selected interactively on the rendered surface.

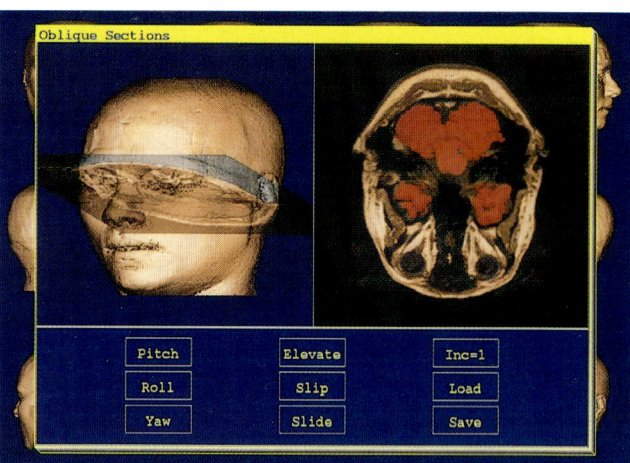

Plate 36 Oblique plane selected and shown transparently through the rendered surface.

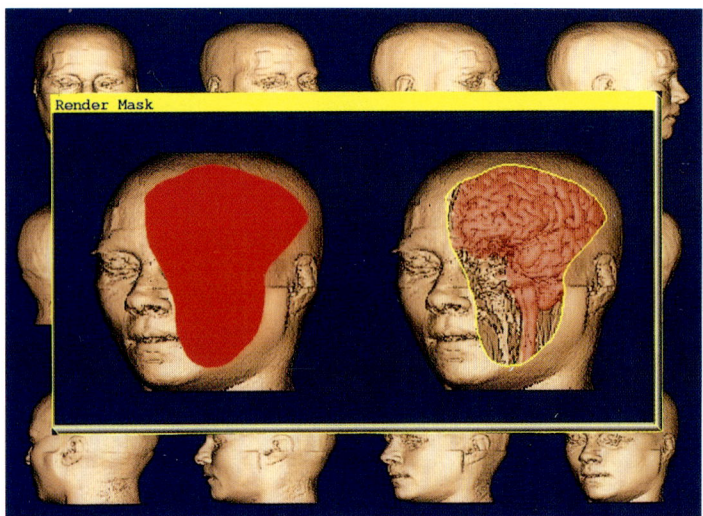

Plate 37 Interactively traced region to visualize underlying internal structures.

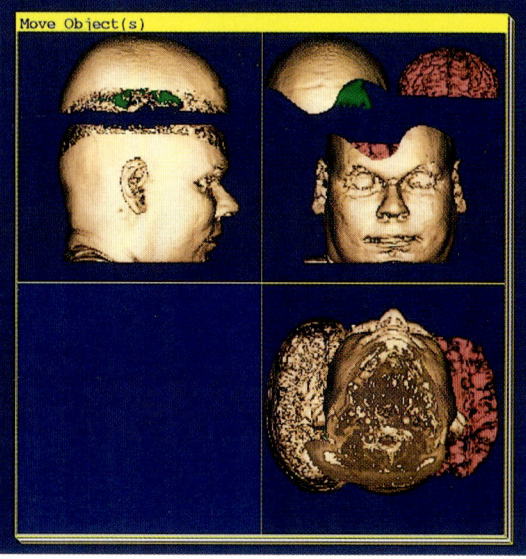

Plate 38 Interactive multiple object manipulation in volume rendering.

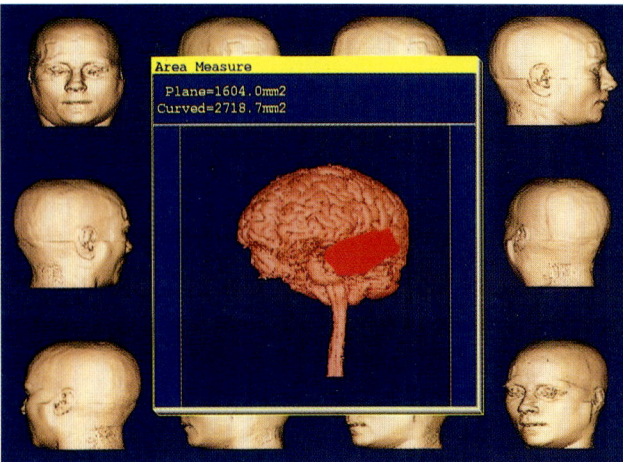

Plate 39 Interactive definition and measurement of surface area on rendered volume.

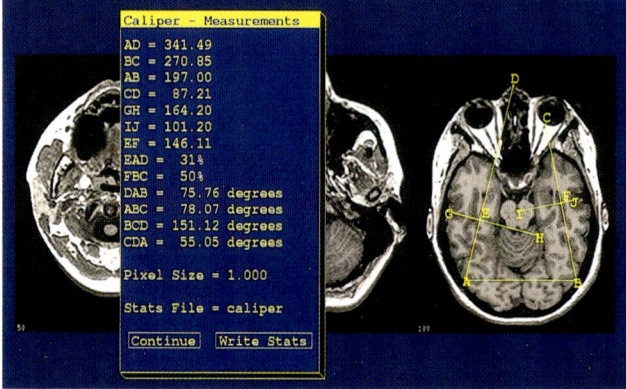

Plate 40 Caliper tool for measuring geometric information in anatomic images (distances, angles, etc.).

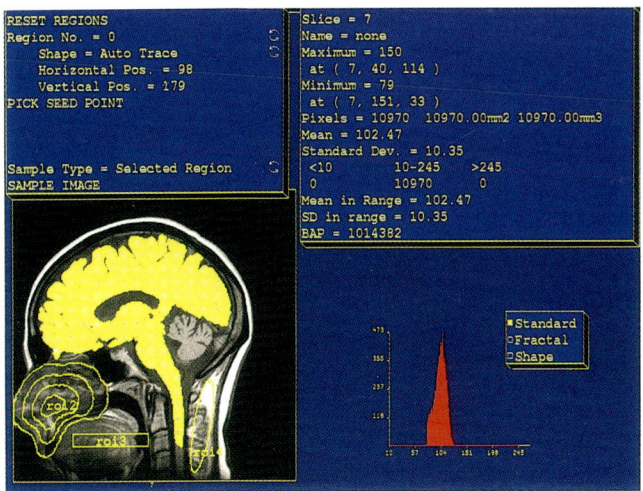

Plate 41   Region-of-interest definition and measurement.

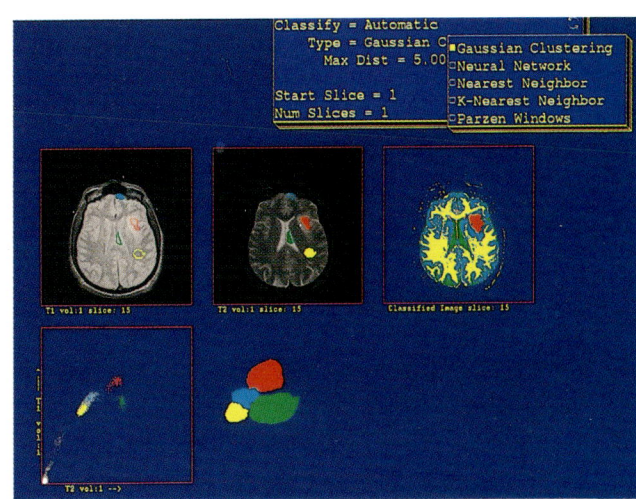

Plate 42   Tissue classification by multispectral analysis of T_1-weighted and T_2-weighted MR images.

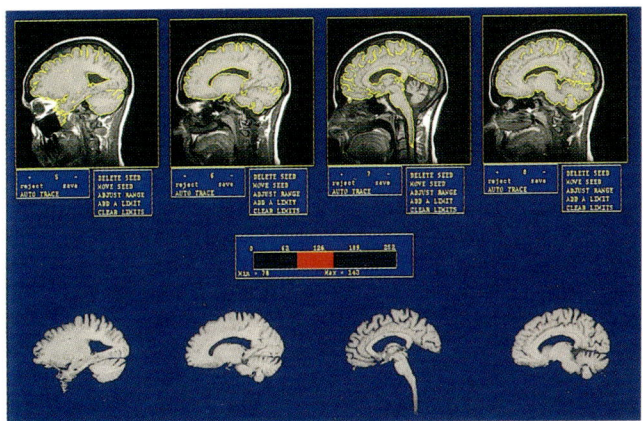

Plate 43   Semiautomated 3D segmentation by region growing.

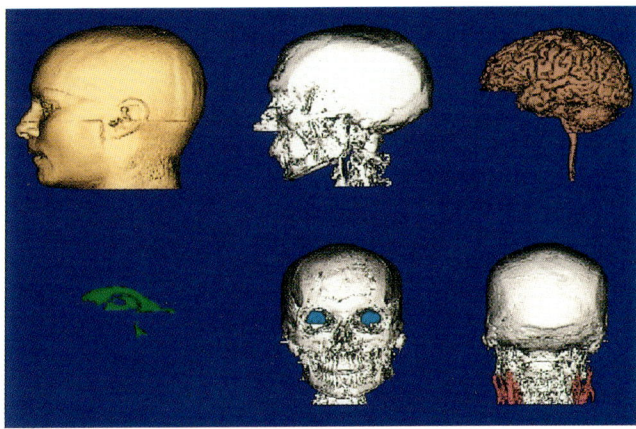

Plate 44   Automated 3D segmentation of multiple structures by math morphology.

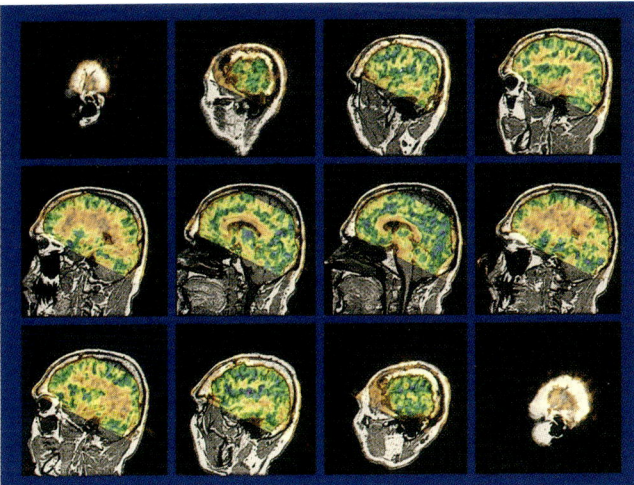

Plate 45   A 3D registered PET dataset transformed to match a 3D MR dataset using color diffusion ("colorwash").

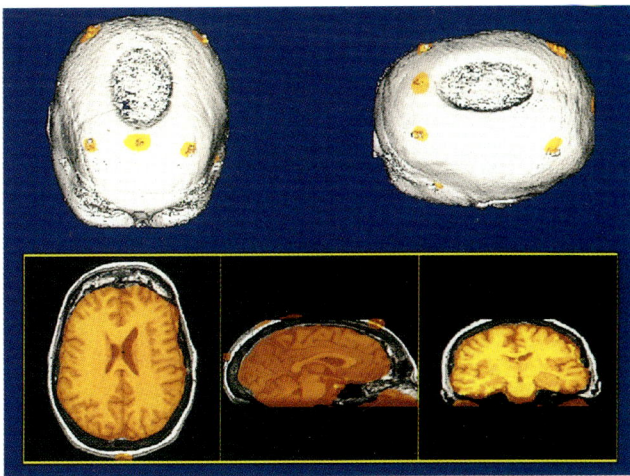

Plate 46   Two 3D surface views and three orthogonal section views of registered MRI and SPECT images with markers. Markers are in good registration in all three orthogonal planes.

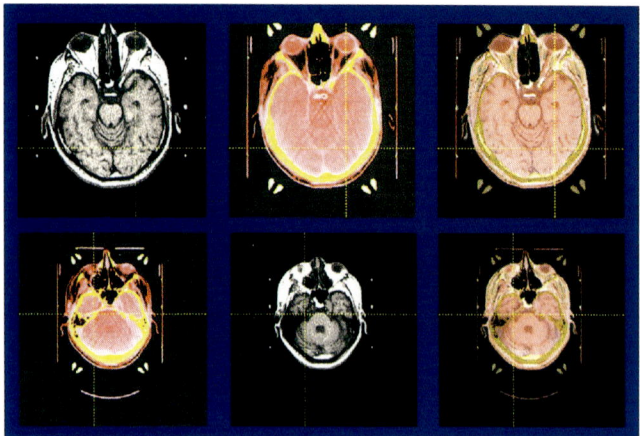

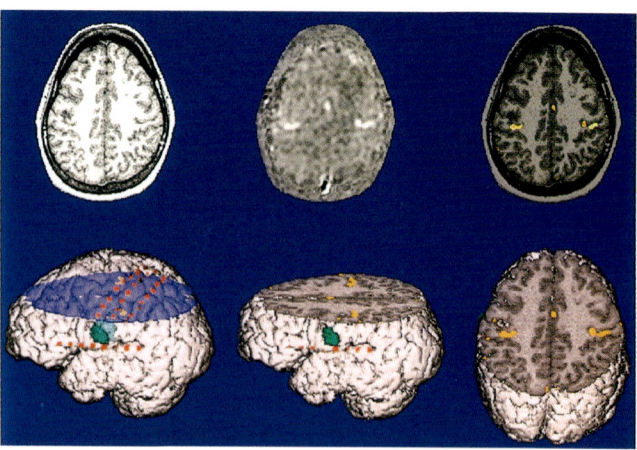

Plate 47 A 3D registration of MR and CT head images. (a) MR image, (b) corresponding registered CT image, and (c) fused image of MR and CT using the color diffusion technique. Both bone from CT and brain from MR are visible in fused image.

Plate 48 A 3D registration of T_1 and T_2 MR head images. Different sections through brain are shown with comparison of fused sections before and after registration.

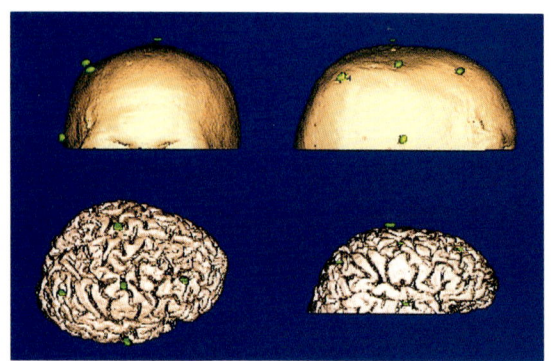

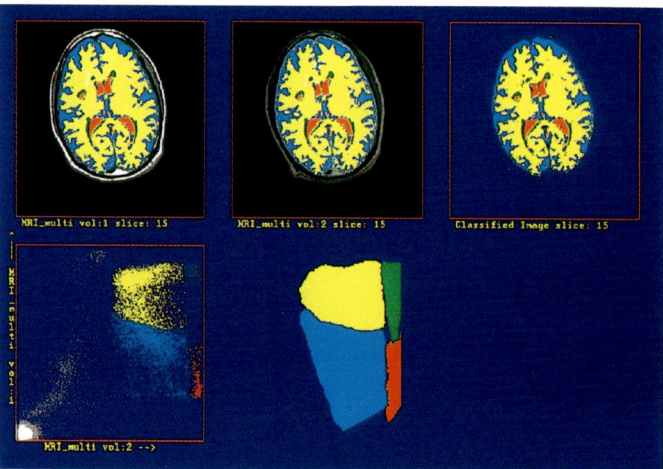

Plate 49 Volume renderings of 3D acquired MRI data of an epilepsy patient used for neurosurgical planning, showing computation and display of position of EEG electrodes on scalp and brain surfaces.

Plate 50 Lesion detection in multiple sclerosis (MS) using multispectral classification techniques.

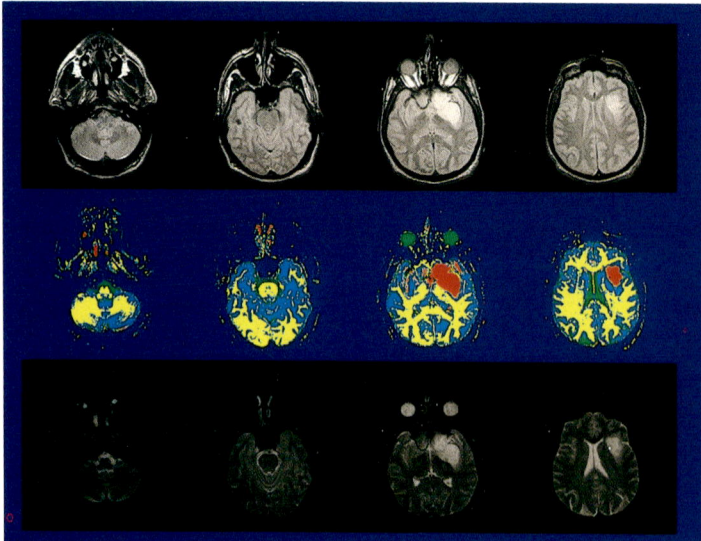

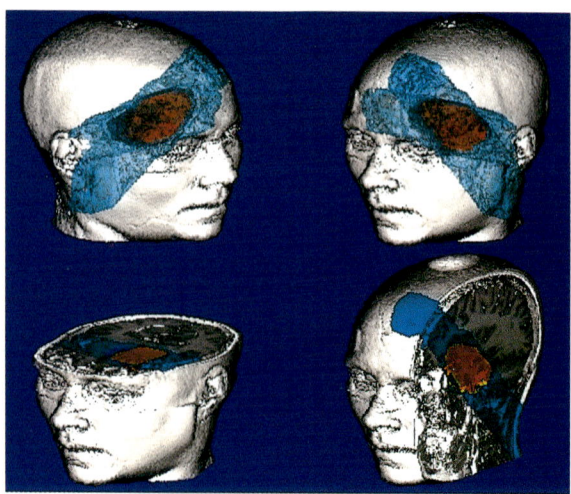

Plate 51 Multispectral classification of various brain structures, including a brain tumor.

Plate 52 Volume rendering for visualization of dose distribution in relation to anatomy in radiation treatment planning.

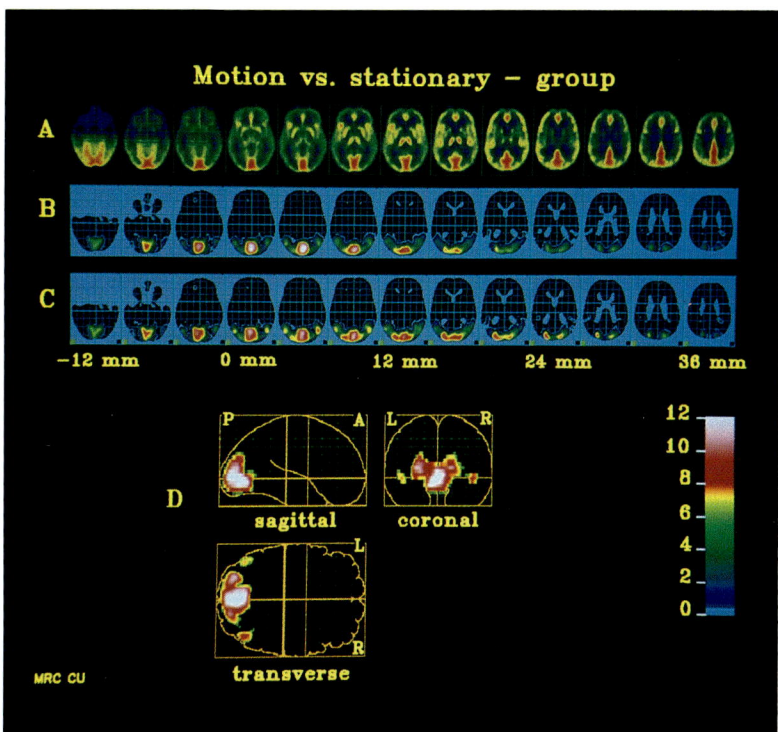

Plate 53 Data averaged from a group of 12 subjects. Above are transverse images of the brain after stereotaxic normalization, with the distances in millimeters from the intercommissural (AC–PC) plane as indicated. (A) Anatomical features obtained by averaging all blood flow scans from all subjects. (B) The arithmetical difference between adjusted mean blood flows for moving and those for stationary stimuli. (C) The SPM[t]s derived from the formal pixel-by-pixel comparison of the adjusted mean blood flows and variances for each of the two conditions. The color scale on the right applies to row C and reflects the Z score of each pixel in the SPM[t] images. (D) The orthogonal projections of the statistical comparison at the threshold of $p < 0.000001$, corrected for multiple comparisons (a mean Z value of 6.1). The areas showing significant increases in blood flow are on the lateral occipital surfaces at the junction of areas 19 and 37 of Brodmann (V5), the V1/V2 complex, and an area arising in the cuneus on each side and extending superiorly. From Watson *et al.* (1993).

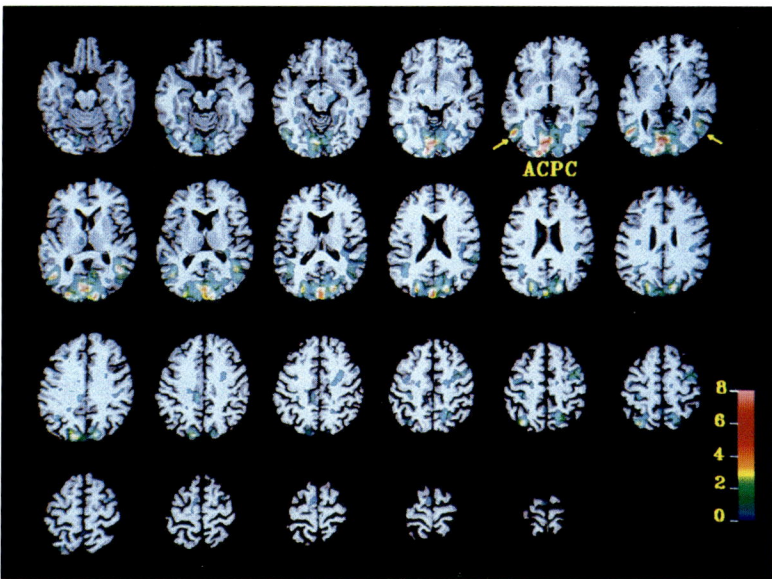

Plate 54 Data from a single subject in which the MR images and SPM[t] images have been coregistered and superimposed. Axial slices at 4-mm intervals are depicted, parallel with the AC–PC plane, indicated by the letters ACPC. The SPM[t] images have a set color scale for their pixels' Z values, indicated on the right of the figure. V5 is present on each side, and its relationship with an underlying sulcus may be seen. At the AC–PC level, there is activation along the calcarine sulcus, reflecting activity in the V1/V2 complex. On both sides there is also significant activation inferiorly in the lingual gyri and superiorly, arising from the cuneus and continuing upward. From Watson *et al.* (1993).

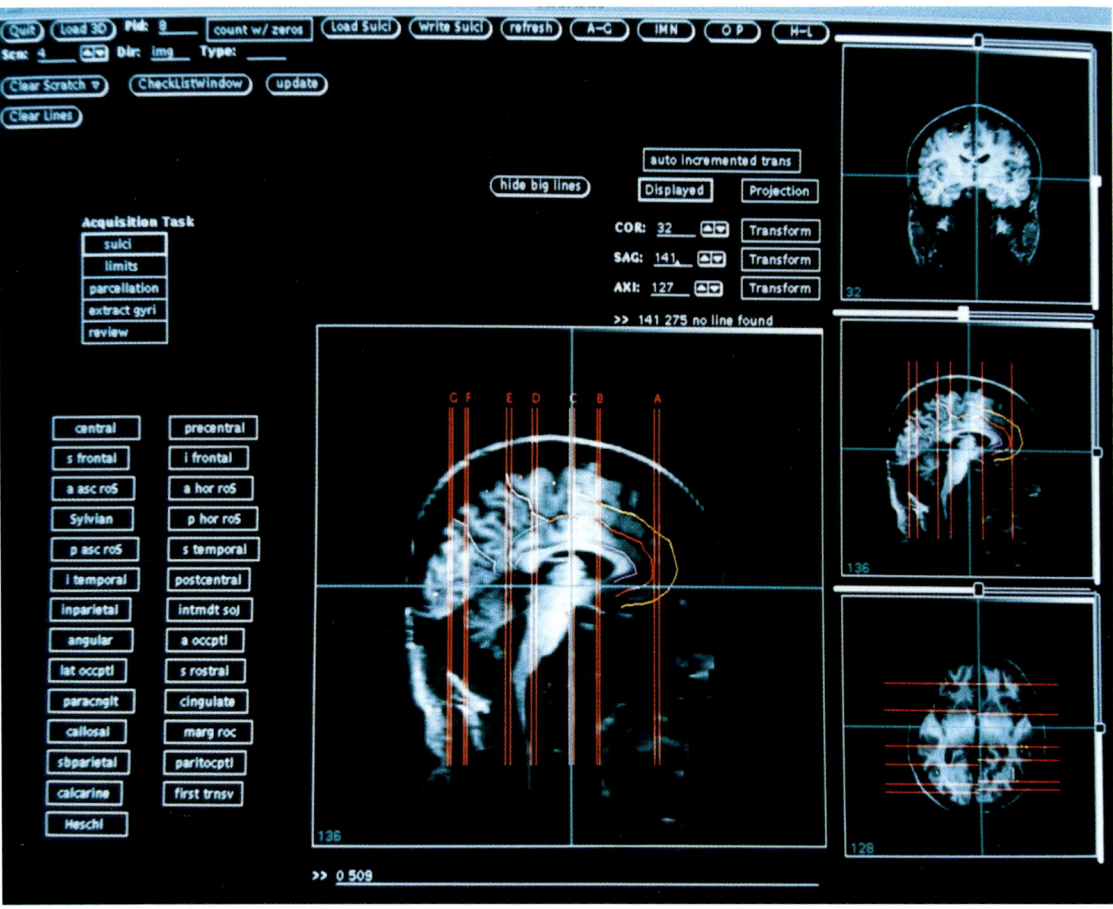

Plate 55 Overview of cortical parcellation software. The interface includes coronal, sagittal, and axial views of the volumetric image data, as well as interactive capabilities for the demarcation of the limiting planes, sulcal trajectories, and extraction of parcellation units.

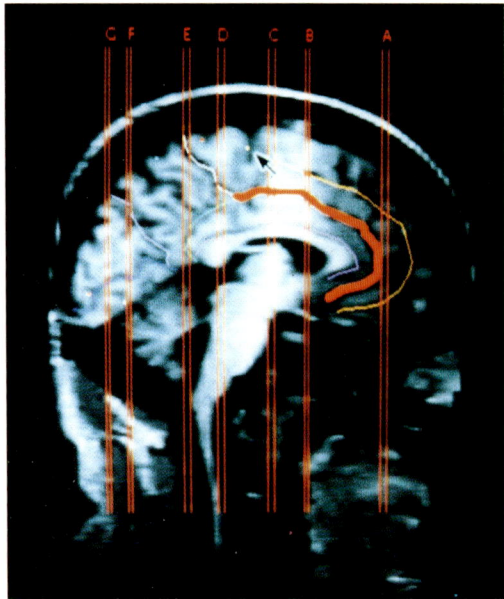

Plate 56 Enhanced sagittal view using the parcellation software. Sulcal trajectories, which are identified directly on this sagittal view, are shown as colored lines. The cingulate sulcus is highlighted by a bold red line. Cross-reference marks for sulci identified in other views are shown as colored dots (see arrow for precentral sulcus). The limiting planes are shown as vertical line pairs labeled A–G (the spacing of the line pairs indicates the original coronal slice thickness).

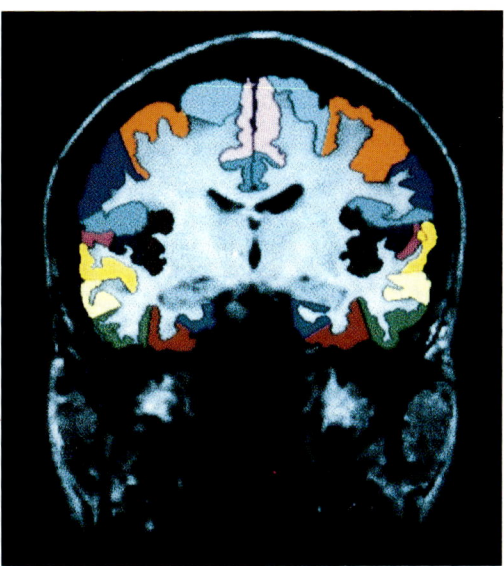

Plate 57 Coronal view during the review process in which each extracted cortical area is given a unique color code. The following anatomic regions are displayed in this figure (starting medially at the superior margin of the corpus callosum and working superiorly and around): anterior cingulate gyrus, *CGa*, turquoise; supplementary motor cortex, *SMC*, violet; inferior frontal gyrus/pars triangularis, *F3t*, aquamarine; precentral gyrus, *PRG*, coral; postcentral gyrus, *POG*, medium blue; central operculum, *CO*, sky blue; insula, *INS*, sienna; planum temporale (on left only), *PT*, sea green; Heschl's gyrus, *H1*, navy; planum polare, *PP*, violet red; anterior superior temporal gyrus, *T1a*, gold; anterior middle temporal gyrus, *T2a*, khaki; anterior inferior temporal gyrus, *T3a*, lime green; anterior temporal fusiform gyrus, *TFa*, indian brown; and anterior parahippocampal gyrus, *PHa*, blue.

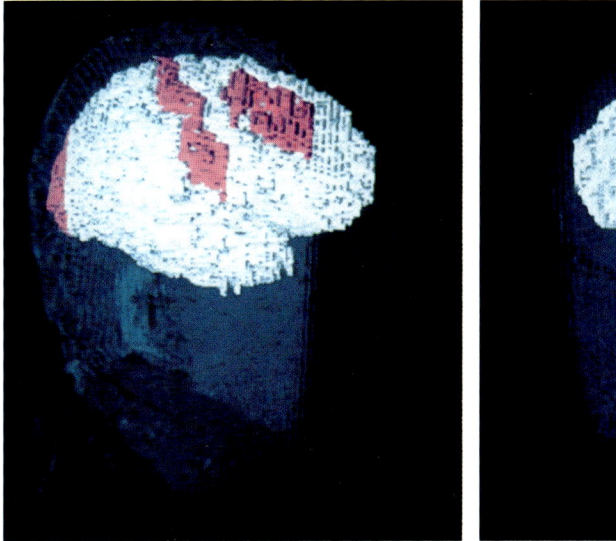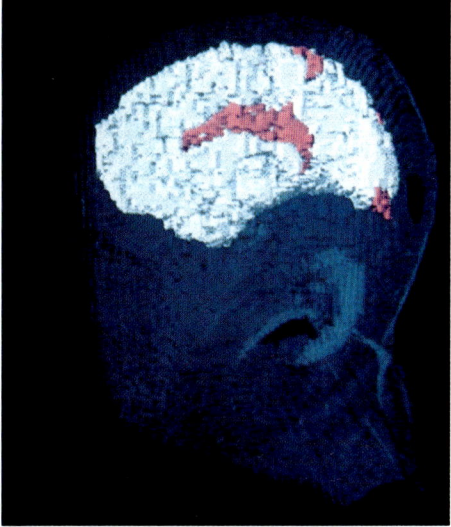

Plate 58 Three-dimensional surface-rendered views of selected cortical parcellation units. This example includes visualization of occipital pole, *OP*; anterior and posterior cingulate gyrus, *CGa, CGp*; postcentral gyrus, *POG*; and middle frontal gyrus, *F2*. The head surface has been rendered in a translucent fashion to yield orientation information, yet not obscure the cortical anatomy. Only the right cerebral hemisphere is included, so that the medial view demonstrates the medial surface of the brain.

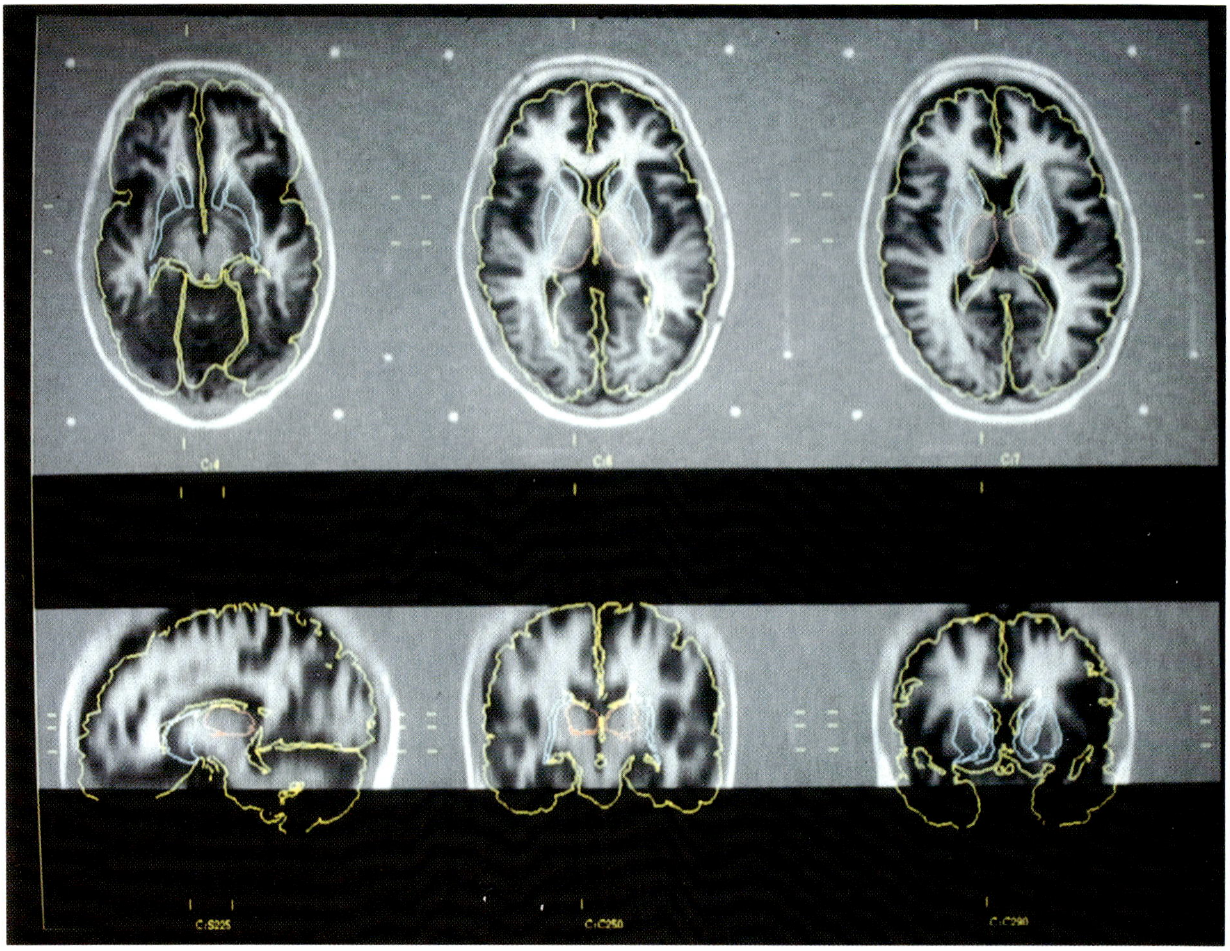

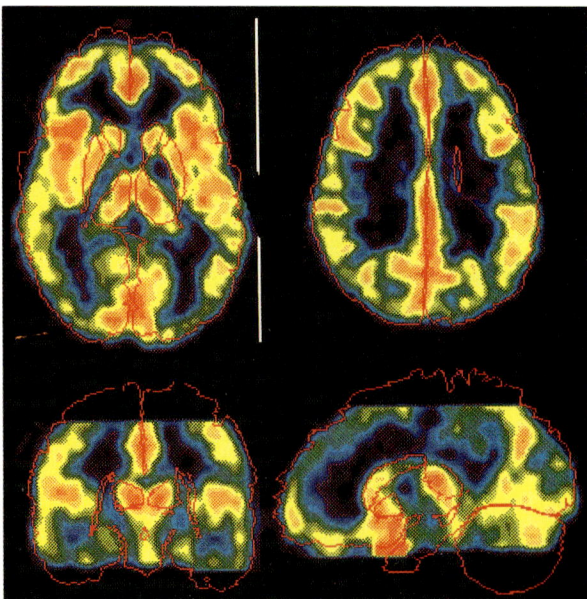

Plate 59 The CBA has been adapted here to a set of MRI images using the brain surface and the ventricular system as reference structures. The basal ganglia have been outlined after the adaptation.

Plate 60 In PET and other types of functional imaging, the anatomical information is combined with functional data. The CBA tool helps in identifying the functional information obtained from different structures. The figure shows an example of a direct adaptation of the atlas to a PET flow study with [^{15}O]butanol.

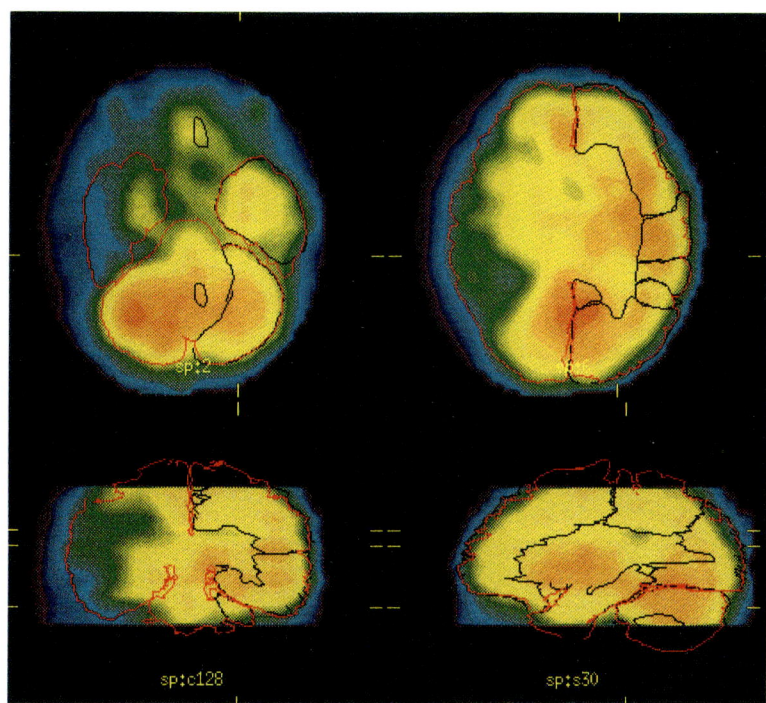

Plate 61 The CBA adapted to a SPECT image set from a case with cerebrovascular disorder of the left hemisphere. The anatomical delimitations as given by the CBA for the right frontal, temporal, parietal, and occipital lobes, as well as the right cerebellar hemisphere, are depicted in the image. The resulting crossed cerebellar diaschisis is visible in the top left image. The figure illustrates clearly that the lower the resolution, the greater the necessity for a proper anatomical guidance. The dataset for this figure was generously provided by Dr. Erik Ryding, Department of Clinical Neurophysiology, University Hospital, Lund, Sweden.

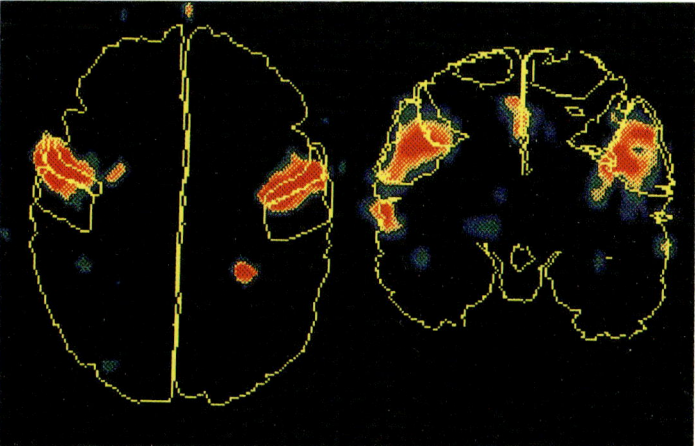

Plate 62 The resulting CBA images from the exploratory statistical procedure when subtracting reading aloud from reading silently. A horizontal and a coronal image of the activation of Brodman area 4 in the cerebral cortex. Data from Ingvar *et al.* (1993).

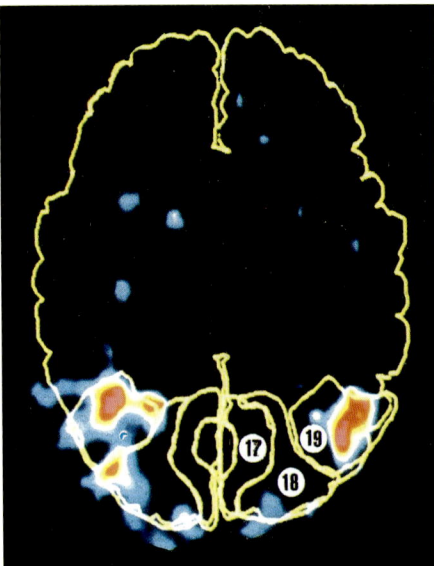

Plate 63 Exploratory *t* map displaying the cerebral activation encountered in patients with snake phobia. The secondary visual areas in area 19 displayed the most prominent activation. Data provided courtesy of Drs. Fredriksson and Wiik, the Department of Psychiatry, Karolinska Hospital, Stockholm.

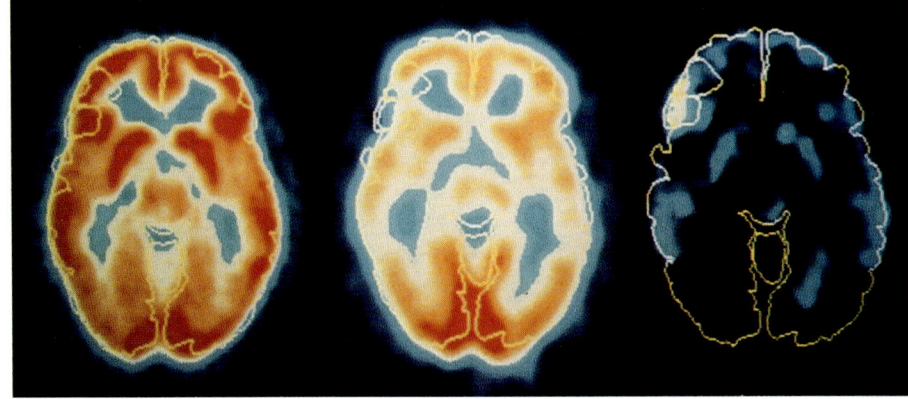

Plate 64 An epileptic focus is demonstrated by subtracting the image of the patient displaying a glucose metabolic rate as measured with FDG from the mean image of a group of normal individuals.

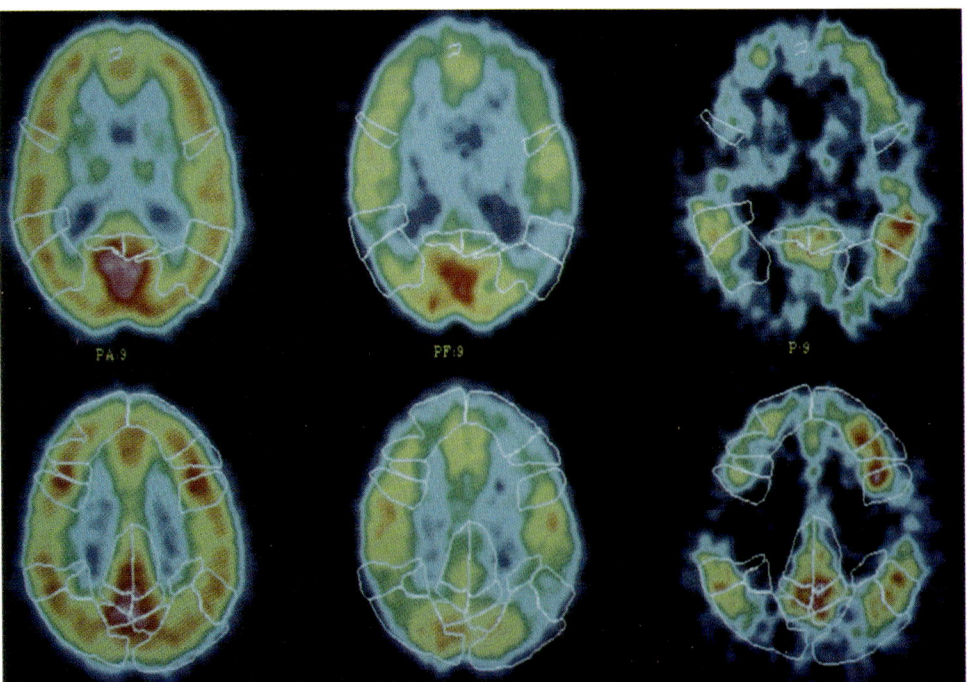

Plate 65 In this plate, the cerebral metabolism rate for glucose in a group of individuals (left column) has been compared with a similar dataset from a group of patients with Alzheimer's disease (middle column). The low metabolic rate in the parietal cortex in the Alzheimer group is clearly shown when a subtraction procedure is performed (right column).

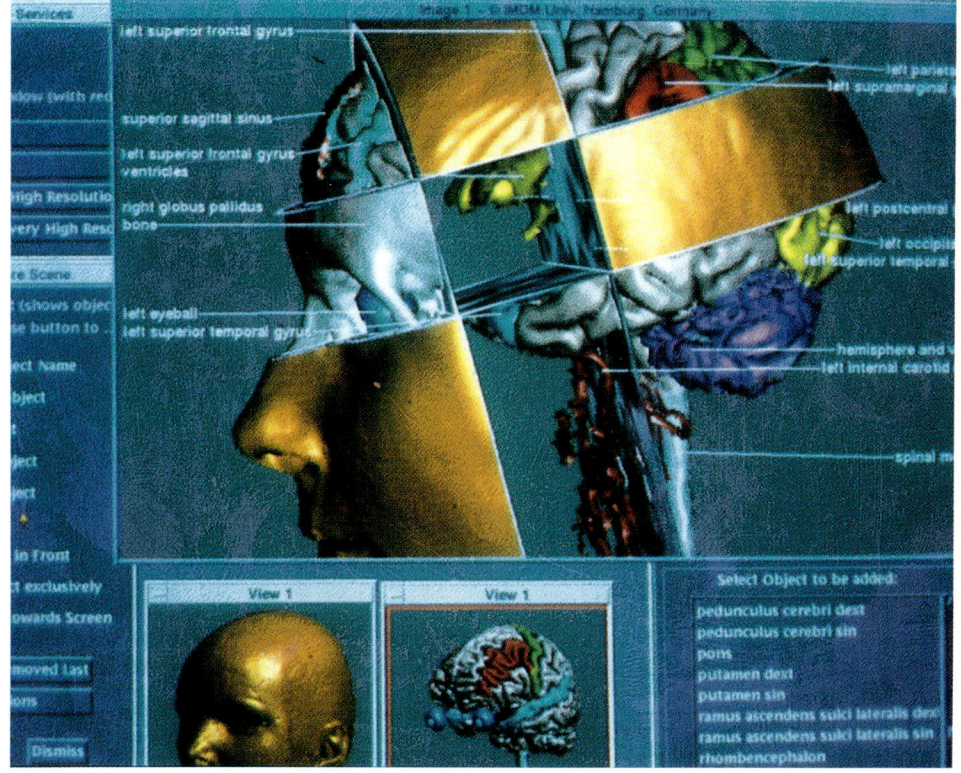

Plate 66 Three-dimensional digital anatomic atlas of the head from the Institute of Mathematics and Computer Science in Medicine (IMDM) at the University of Hamburg, Germany. This illustration demonstrates the user interface for the atlas, through which the viewer can access exploration tools via a mouse and generated annotated views with orientation, size, and resolution according to specific needs. The object description in the knowledge base can be used interactively to select specific objects in the scene. Reproduced with permission.

Plate 67 The application of a deformable electronic anatomic atlas of the brain in two dimensions is demonstrated. (A) Single slice from an MR study of the brain in a normal individual with spin density, T_1-weighted, and T_2-weighted images. This represents the MR brain atlas. (B) The template is matched to a patient study by first global and then local deformations. The top row of images shows the original template (atlas slice), the result of globally deforming the slice to match a patient MR scan and then locally deforming the slice to minimize the local differences. The bottom row shows difference images between the deformed atlas image and the study being matched. At first, the differences are major. After global deformation, the differences are small but are still noticeable at the boundaries of the brain. In the final image, the local differences vanish. (C) As a consequence of the atlas matching procedure based on deformable templates, an automatic segmentation of the brain slice is available. This is shown on the right with the corresponding manual segmentation of the same slice on the left. Near perfect segmentation was obtained automatically through atlas matching by deformable templates.

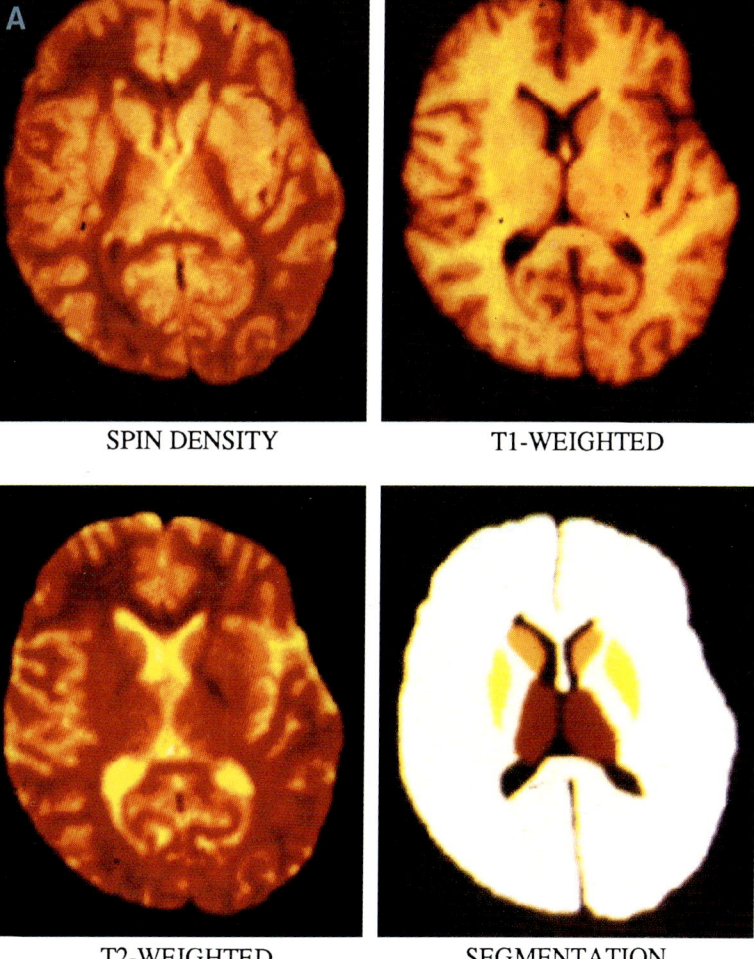

SPIN DENSITY   T1-WEIGHTED

T2-WEIGHTED   SEGMENTATION

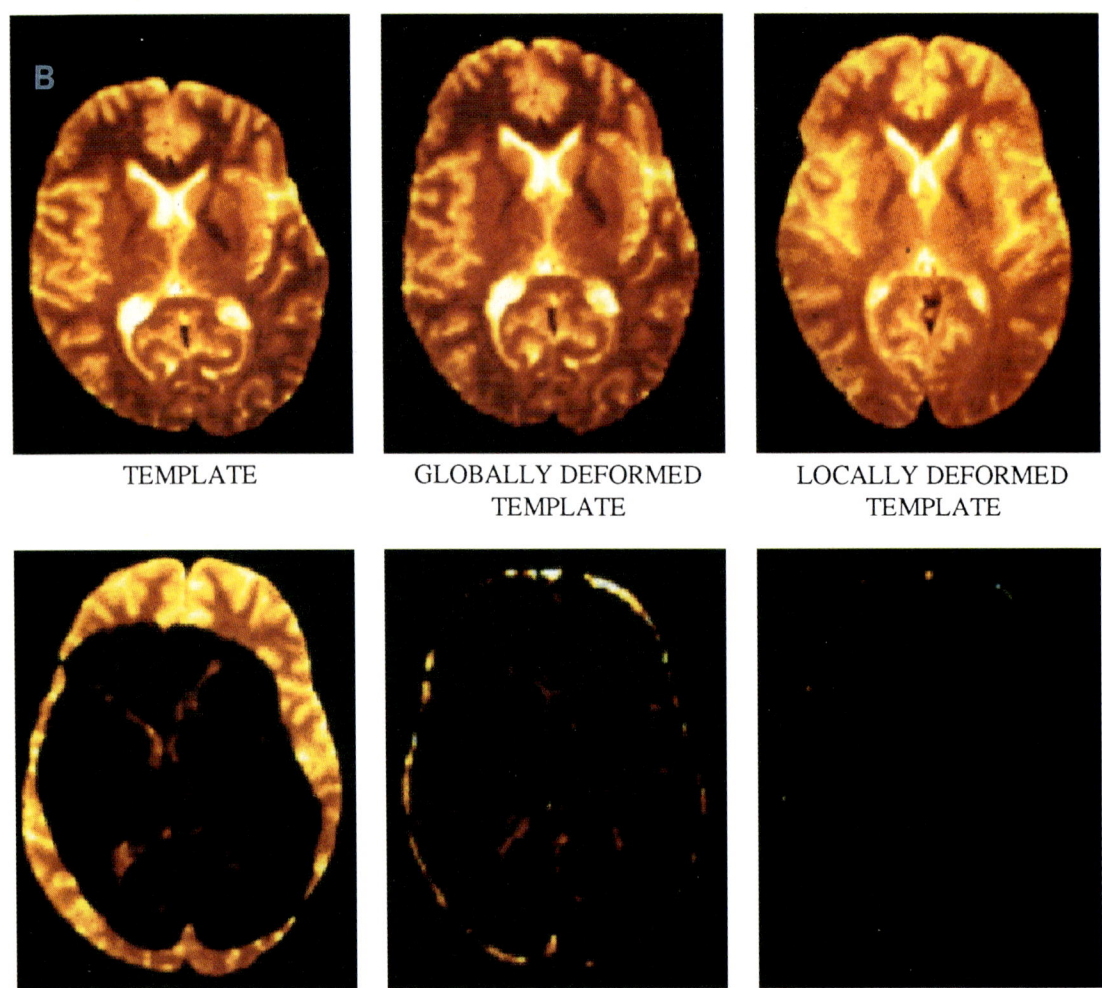

TEMPLATE GLOBALLY DEFORMED
TEMPLATE LOCALLY DEFORMED
TEMPLATE

DIFFERENCE IMAGES BETWEEN THE ABOVE IMAGES AND
THE STUDY BEING MATCHED

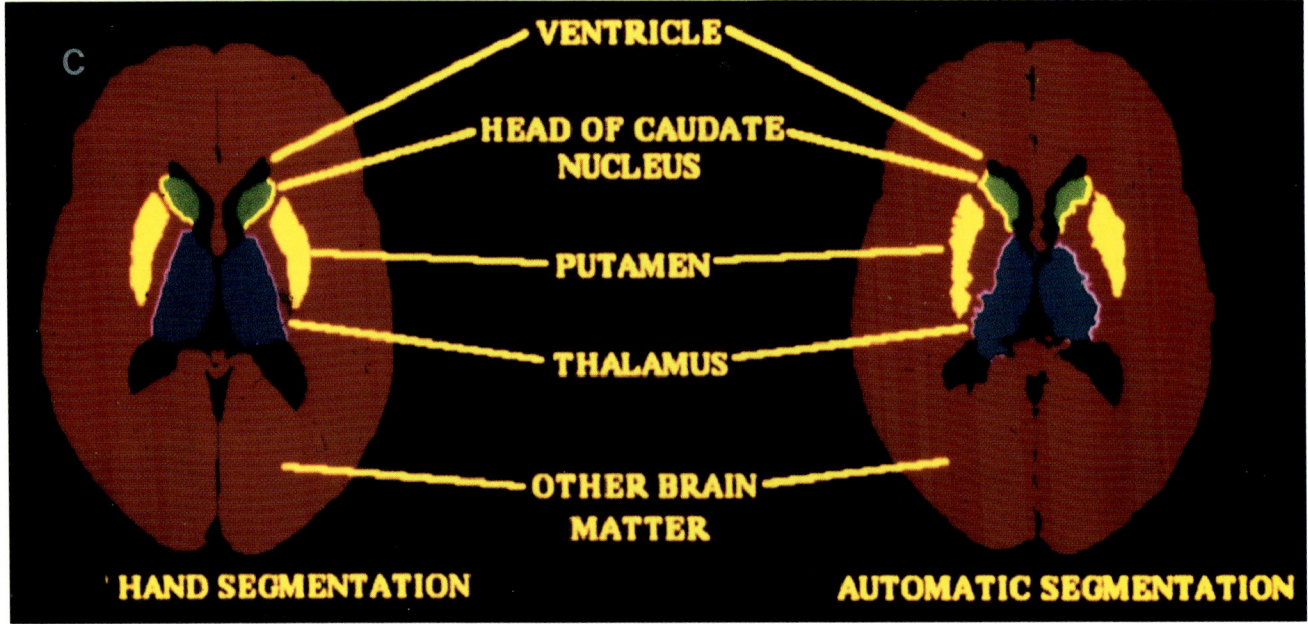

Plate 67 (*continued*)

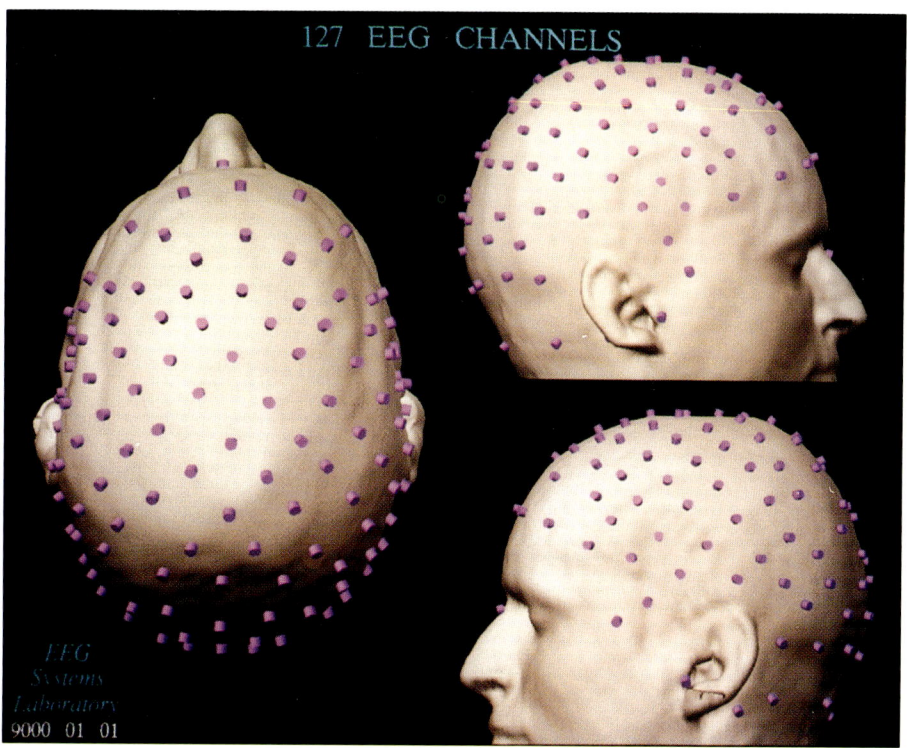

Plate 68 EEG–MRI registration. Graphic display of EEG–MRI alignment obtained from processing of 76 horizontal MRI slices. Three views of the same subject's head are shown.

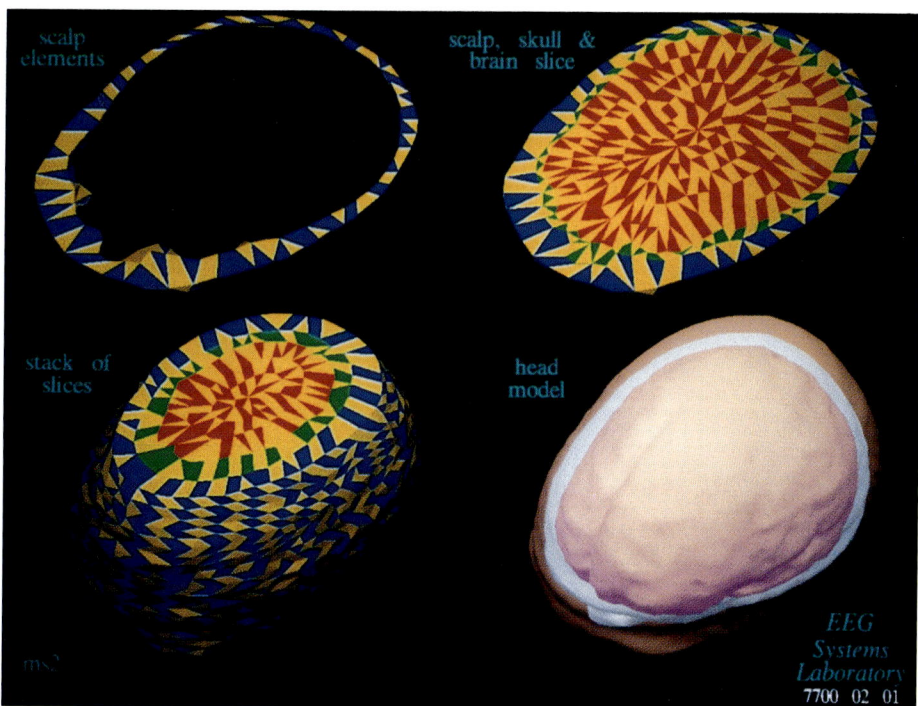

Plate 69 Construction of finite element head model. Finite elements corresponding to scalp, skull, and brain tissues are shown in blue, green, and red, respectively (with alternating elements shown in yellow). The upper left shows a single ring of scalp. At the upper right skull and brain, elements have been added within one slice bounded by two consecutive horizontal MR images. The lower left shows all slices except the topmost horizontal slice. At the lower right, the constructed scalp, skull, and brain surfaces are rendered transparent.

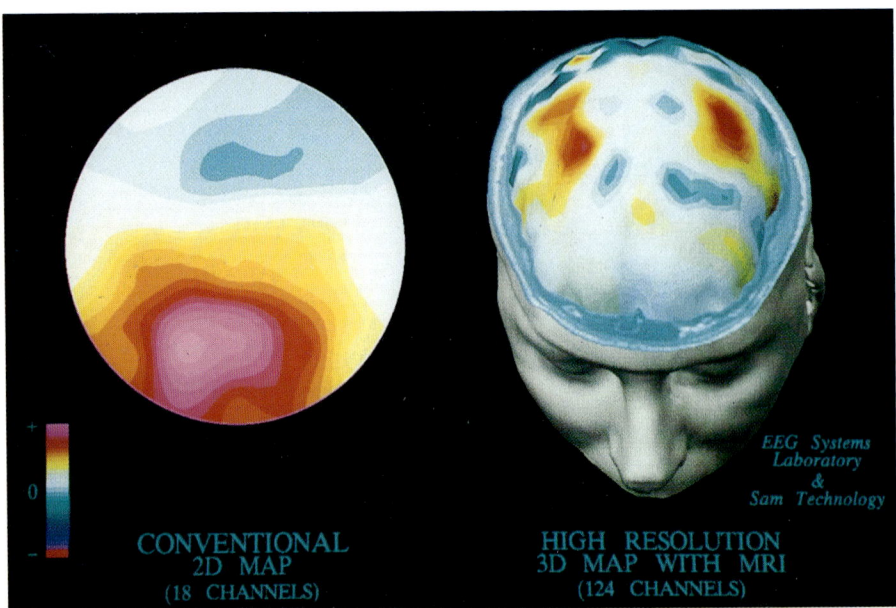

Plate 70 High-resolution somatosensory EPs. A high-resolution, 122-channel topographic map of the steady-state evoked potentials elicited by repetitive electrical stimulation of the left-hand middle finger and right-hand index finger (right) contains more useful localizing information than a more conventional topographic map of the same data sampled at 18 standard electrode locations from the 10-20 system (left). In the high resolution map, it is clear that the left and right somatosensory cerebral cortices, corresponding to the right and left hands, respectively, have been activated.

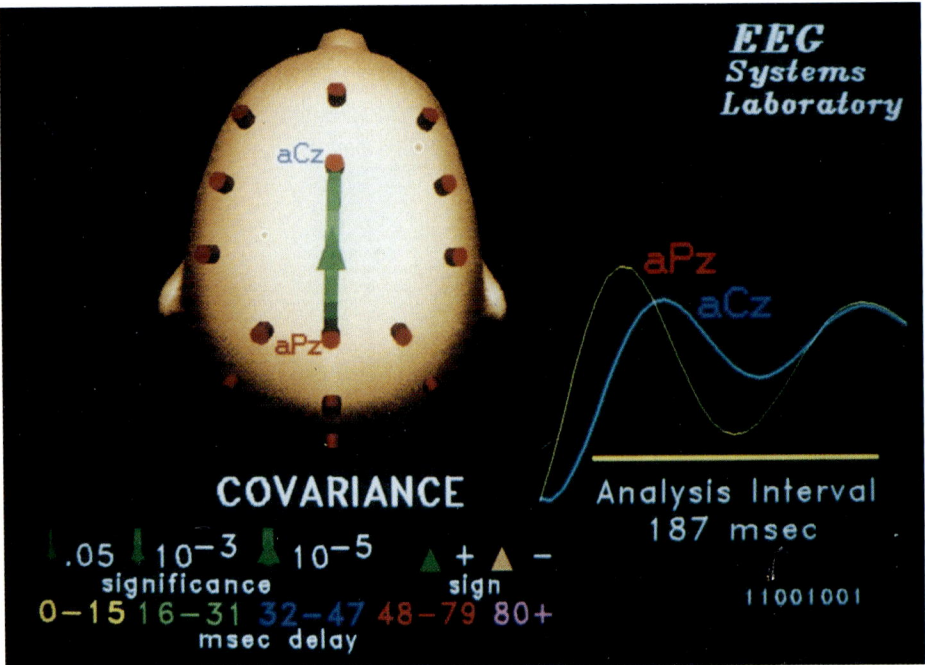

Plate 71 Illustration of the evoked potential covariance (EPC) method of characterizing activity in distributed neuronal networks. The (EPC) line on the top view of a model head (left) is computed from the evoked potential segments recorded from scalp positions aPz and aCz (right). The evoked potentials were spatially sharpened with a Laplacian derivation and then filtered to extract activity in a 4-to 7-Hz band; the EPC analysis interval was 187 ms wide. The width of an EPC line indicates the significance of the covariance between the two EP segments, with the scale appearing above the word "significance." The color of the arrow indicates the sign of the covariance (same color as line, positive; skin color, negative). The arrow points from the leading to the lagging electrode, unless there is no delay, in which case a bar is shown. The EPC between aPz and aCz is significant at $p < 10^{-5}$. The aPz waveform leads the aCz waveform by about 16–31 ms (green line), and the covariance is positive (green arrow). From Gevins *et al.* (1989a).

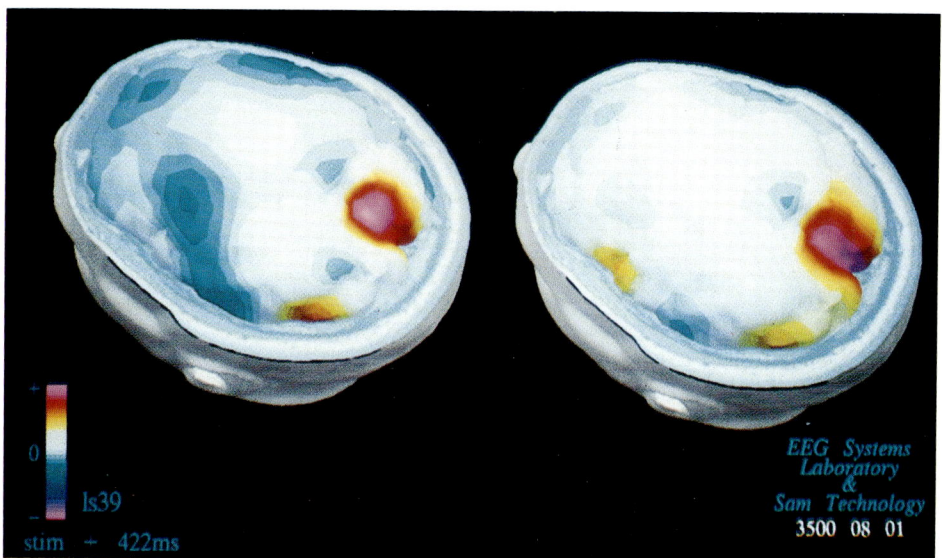

Plate 72 High-resolution evoked potentials (EPs) of linguistic encoding. Deblurred potentials from one subject corresponding to an EP peak 422 ms after the first visual stimulus (encoding) in tasks that required either a semantic (left) or a grammatic (right) judgment in response to the second stimulus (processing). In the semantic condition, the subject had to decide if the encoding and processing stimuli were antonyms; in the grammatic condition the subject had to decide if the encoding stimulus (a pronoun) and the processing stimulus (a verb) formed a grammatically correct sentence. Because the first stimulus was an open class (content) word in the semantic condition and a closed class (function) word in the grammatic condition, these deblurred EPs may reflect neural activity involved in the encoding of open and closed class words. The distinguishing feature is the higher voltage over a circumscribed area of left prefrontal cortex, in the region of Broca's area, in the grammatic condition. This effect was also evident in the averaged data of the nine subjects in the experiment.

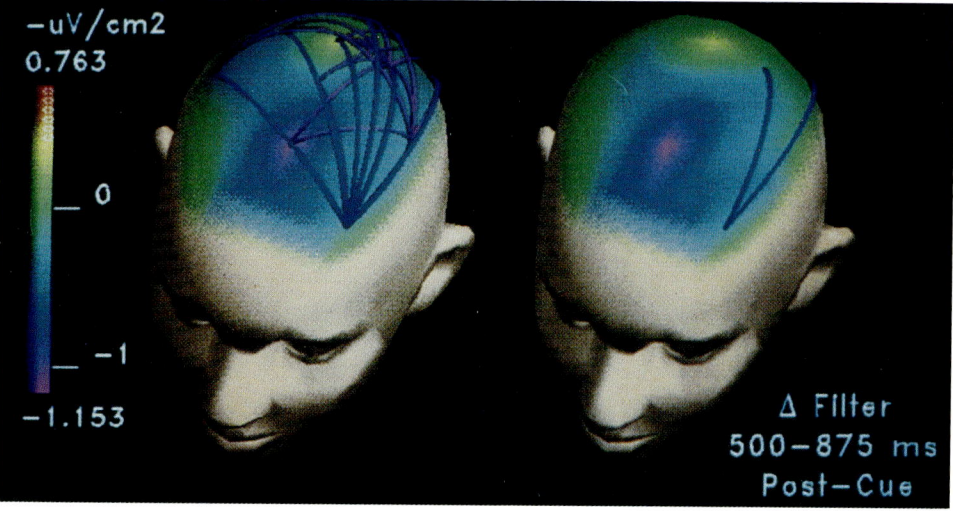

Plate 73 Preparatory evoked potential covariance patterns preceding accurate and inaccurate responses. EPCs involving left frontal, midline precentral, and left central, and parietal electrode sites are prominent in patterns preceding accurate performance (left). The number and magnitude of EPCs are smaller preceding inaccurate responses (right).

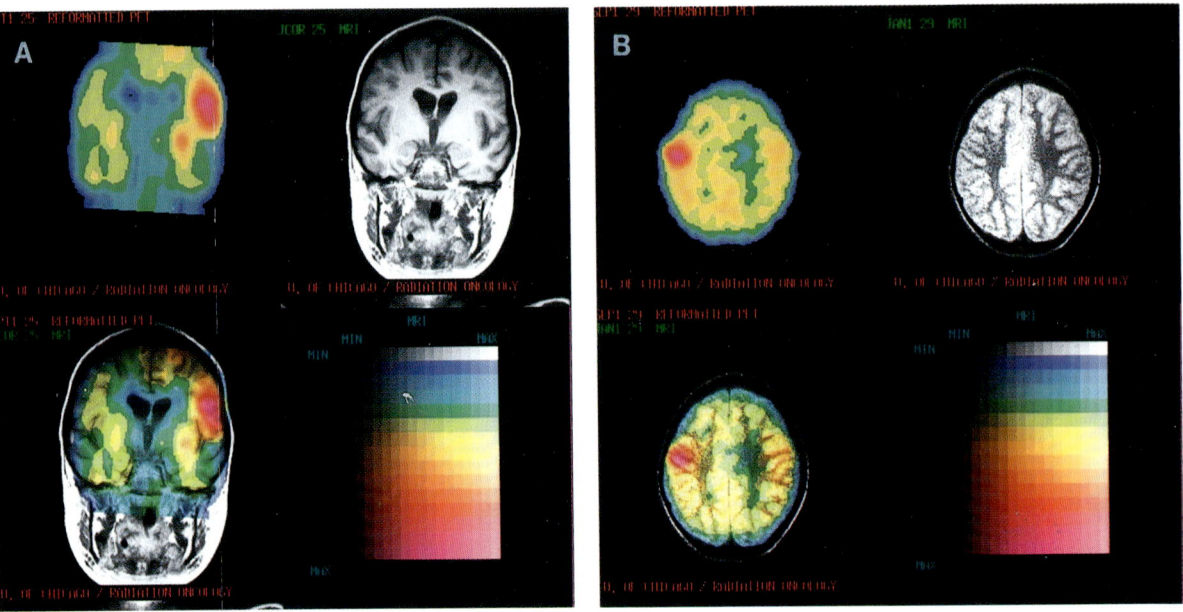

Plate 74 Registered PET data along the plane of an MRI slice for the same patient as that in Fig. 4. (a) Coronal MRI plane; (b) axial MRI plane.

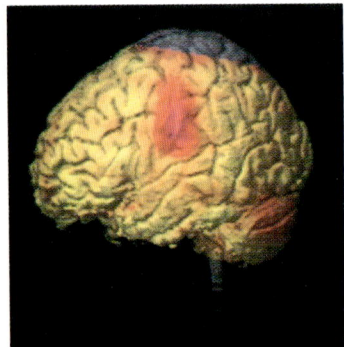

Plate 75 A 3D MRI/PET brain model showing a hypermetabolic focus (red) along the motor and sensory cortex.

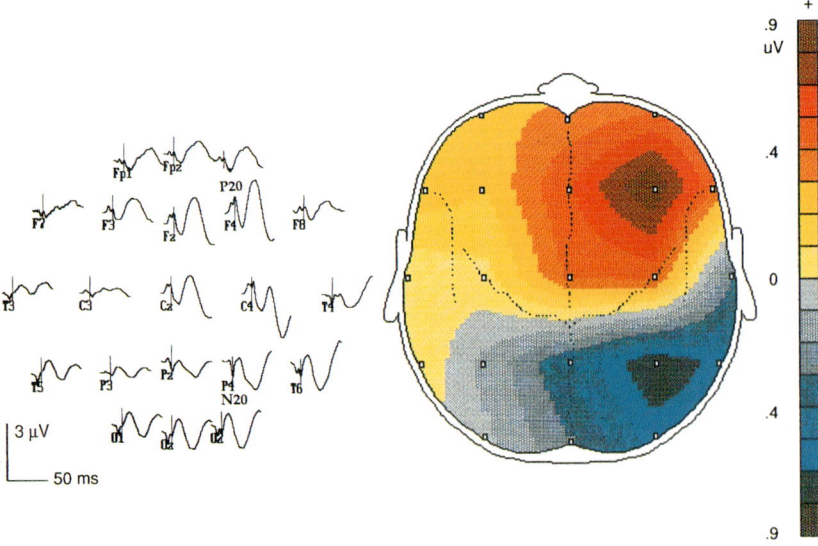

Plate 76 The average waveforms from the 10-20 electrode system in response to left median nerve stimulation at the wrist. The initial scalp response (N20) is a negative peak at the contralateral parietal scalp and a positive peak at the contralateral frontal scalp (left). The scalp distribution at that instant of time (right) is consistent with a horizontally oriented dipole located near the central sulcus.

tude of a response is conveyed by the value of the pixel or voxel. These values can be transformed to represent a physiological measurement or pseudocolored to enhance their differences. Correlating multiple modalities assumes the datasets are in register following the necessary geometric transformations. Display of the correlations can be in the form of superpositioning multiple datasets, each with different color assignments (Mazziotta *et al.*, 1991), texture mapping (see below) one modality upon another (Payne and Toga, 1990), or a statistical representation of the relationship between datasets (Toga *et al.*, 1986). Changes over time are best displayed as animations (Toga *et al.*, 1991) but also can be visualized as a static image of rate of change.

III. Warping

Warping is a subspecialty of image processing that deals with geometric transformation techniques (Wolberg, 1992). These transformations redefine the spatial relationship between points in an image(s). The degree of such transformations can be from simple repositionings to severe deformations (Fig. 1). For the purposes of multimodality and multisubject brain comparisons, warping is defined as those geometric transformations that alter the shape and does not include simple repositionings. The degree of warping is determined by the data source(s) and the application. Similarly, the implementation (density based or spatially based) of the warping is dependent on the type of data and its resolution. For example,

if anatomic or extrinsic landmarks are easily obtained, spatially based algorithms may be employed. These require the identification of several points in each dataset. The location and number of points are crucial to the goodness of fit. In other cases, density-based warping algorithms can maximize the cross-correlation coefficients between datasets without the identification of landmarks. The remainder of this section will describe several algorithms for spatially and densitometrically based warping.

A. Spatially Based Warping

Point- and contour-based algorithms are dependent upon explicitly defined geometry and sometimes manually identified locations. These approaches can be used across modalities for which no assumption about similar density patterns can be made. However, coincident landmarks must be identifiable.

1. Points

In point-based warping, a set of landmark points is specified and the image is warped by carrying out vector displacements of these landmarks. These displacement vectors in a 2D or 3D image are either explicitly specified or computed by identifying the landmarks on the test image with another corresponding set of landmark points from a reference image. Voxels (3D) other than the landmarks are obtained by interpolation. Often it is important to maintain the surface smoothness in the test image while warping; in this case, the deformation is computed through a homology map (Bookstein *et al.*, 1985). This maps the

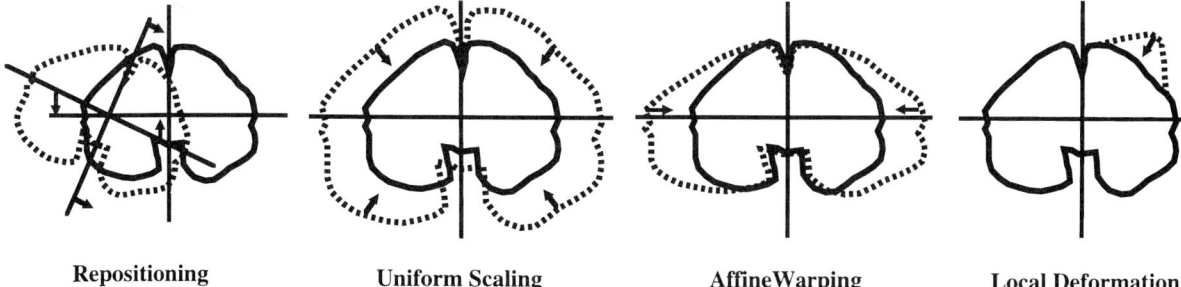

Repositioning   **Uniform Scaling**   **AffineWarping**   **Local Deformation**

Figure 1 Continuum of geometric transformations. For illustrative purposes this figure is shown in two dimensions, although the same approach can be applied in 3D. Repositioning datasets can be performed using the principle axes and center of mass. The least intrusive transformation concerns translation of one image into register with another. Rotational corrections may add interpolative error, in part, due to the discreteness of digital datasets. Noninteger uniform scalings can add interpolative error also. Transformations along axes can be applied linearly (affine) or nonlinearly (not shown). Local deformations are performed on a point-by-point or imposed grid system (see text). As the transformations become more complex, they may improve the goodness of fit. However, warping one dataset to map to another is an approximation at best, because interpolative error and other compromises are always necessary. Algorithms designed to perform these functions can be spatially based or density based. They can be applied to within or between modalities and subjects.

landmarks and smooth curves of one form to those of another. Another approach would be to obtain the desired image warp by a polynomial of a predetermined order and degree through a least-squares minimization technique. If the set of landmarks in the test image are represented as $\{L_i : 0 \leq i \leq n\}$, those in the reference image are represented as $\{L_i^* : 0 \leq i \leq n\}$, and if the coordinates (x, y, z) in the original image are mapped to the point (x^*, y^*, z^*) in the warped image through the polynomials P, Q, and R such that

$$x^* = P(x, y, z); \quad y^* = Q(x, y, z); \quad z^* = R(x, y, z), \quad (1)$$

then the coefficients of P, Q, and R are obtained by minimizing the Euclidean norm $\| (L_{ix}^*, L_{iy}^*, L_{iz}^*)$, $[P(L_i), Q(L_i), R(L_i)] \|$, where $\| \vec{a}, \vec{b} \| = \{(a_x - b_x)^2 + (a_y - b_y)^2 + (a_z - b_z)^2\}$. Olivio et al. (1991) have used this technique to achieve image distortion correction in 2D by using two second-degree polynomials of the form

$$
\begin{aligned}
P(x, y) &= p_0 + p_1 x + p_2 y + p_3 x^2 + p_4 xy + p_5 y^2 \\
Q(x, y) &= q_0 + q_1 x + q_2 y + q_3 x^2 + q_4 xy + q_5 y^2.
\end{aligned} \quad (2)
$$

Kenny et al. (1990) have used a similar method for registration of lung images. They manually located the corresponding pairs of landmarks (or control points) in the test and reference images and then applied a nonlinear polynomial mapping to warp the test image. If the number of landmark pairs is the same as the number of unknown coefficients, then an exact system of equations is obtained with a unique solution, but the solutions are sensitive to the accuracy in the choice of the landmark pairs resulting in instability. Kenny et al. (1990) suggested locating more landmark pairs than necessary to get an exact system in order to achieve an overdetermined system that could be solved by computing the pseudoinverse of the coefficient matrix.

2. Contours

In this method an image is warped so that its boundary matches another without reference to densitometric information. This method has been used for atlas template matching with experimental data (Toga, 1991). One approach is to treat the 2D image as an elastic sheet and warp it by the application of elastic forces along the image plane at a selected set of points in the image. The elastic forces can be derived automatically from elastic potential energy stored in the image when deformed to match the contour. The expression for elastic strain energy derived by Terzopoulos et al. (1987) could be used to compute this

potential energy, and subsequently the elastic force can be derived as the gradient of this potential. If $\vec{r}$ denotes the coordinates of the points of a space curve Ω, and $s(\vec{r})$, $\kappa(\vec{r})$, and $\tau(\vec{r})$ denote the length, curvature, and torsion, respectively, of the curve Ω, then the strain energy $E(\vec{r})$ is given by

$$E(\vec{r}) = \int \{\alpha(s - s^0) + \beta(\kappa - \kappa^0) + \gamma(\tau - \tau^0)\} d(\vec{r}), \quad (3)$$

where α, β, and γ are constants determining the amount of resistance to stretching, bending, and twisting, respectively (Terzopoulos et al., 1987).

3. Morphing and Minimum Distance Fields

Morphing refers to the process of changing the shape and form of one object to take on the characteristics of another. This approach utilizes the surface model and hence is spatially based also.

Surfaces may come from interactive techniques, such as outlining (Leventhal and Ware, 1972), or automatic ones like isosurface creation (Lorensen and Cline, 1987). But manipulating surfaces using either direct or implicit methods presents a number of problems. To address these problems, we have developed an approach that uses *distance fields*—the scalar fields derived from the synthesized triangle-based surface models from either anatomic or physiologic datasets (Payne and Toga, 1992). To apply these implicit surface methods to a given surface model, it must first be represented by scalar fields. The distance field represents the distance from a surface as a signed magnitude.

Surface models' distance fields have been used to remove surfaces (Payne and Toga, 1990) and interpolate between the upper and the lower boundaries of a structure (Toga et al., 1989). The distance fields also can be applied to averaging and interpolation of two or more surface models. This function is especially useful in studies in which the topology of markers across laminae needs to be assessed. By interpolating at successive intervals, an animation of a continuously deforming surface can be visualized. Other applications include smoothing and filtering (i.e., a low-pass Gaussian) a model that may contain high-frequency noise or artifacts, computing a model that is a fixed distance larger or smaller than the source, and blending several substructures into a single joined structure.

4. Flattening

Altering the geometry of the cortex can improve the analysis of both morphometric and densitometric features. One approach to this is to flatten convoluted or complex surfaces without introducing additional error. However, artifacts can be introduced when spherical (and close to spherical) structures are mapped onto planar surfaces. This is often referred to as the mapmaker's problem (Schwartz and Merker, 1986), which involves planar representation of curved surfaces. But these methods have traditionally been restricted to relatively smooth convex curved surfaces such as the surface of the earth. They cannot be applied to the task of cortical flattening because of the complex and locally nonconvex nature of the cortical surface. However, with algorithm modifications, the same underlying principle can be used for the complex polyhedral surface that is the cortex. The planar representation of an arbitrary shaped polyhedral surface can be obtained by finding piecewise continuous maps that would match, with minimum possible deviation, the minimum distance between any two points computed along the surfaces. Schwartz $et\ al.$ (1988) have used the cost function

$$L = \frac{1}{c} \sum_{i<j}^{i=N} \frac{(d_{ij} - \tilde{d}_{ij})^2}{\tilde{d}_{ij}}, \quad (4)$$

where

$$c = \sum_{i<j}^{i=N} \tilde{d}_{ij} \quad (5)$$

and d_{ij} and $\tilde{d}_{ij}$ are the distances between the ith and jth point along the original curved surface and along the planar representation, respectively. The fundamental step in this algorithm is to compute minimum distances between the nodes of the discretized approximation of the curved surface computed along the surface. Sharir and Schorr (1986) published an algorithm for computing the shortest paths along convex polyhedral spaces. Mitchell $et\ al.$ (1987) describes an algorithm for computing the shortest path between two points on arbitrary polyhedral surfaces. Wolfson and Schwartz (1989) have implemented an algorithm that is computationally more expensive (exponential time), but it is simpler in its implementation. However, it can take considerable time if the distances are computed over the whole surface. In addition, the authors only consider patches of about 10 nodes at a time. Although this performs well for visual cortex because their integral mean curvature is not very large, it has yet to be tested on larger cortical areas. The algorithm developed by Mitchell $et\ al.$ (1987) incorporates more nodes for computing the distance matrix and hence may be more accurate in its planar representation.

B. Density-Based Warping

Density-based algorithms do not explicitly define any geometry and make the assumption that density patterns among the datasets are similar. Density-based warping can be applied to both 2D and 3D images. Density-based elastic warping is preceded by principal axis alignment followed by a global affine transformation (see Fig. 1). The principal axis alignment brings the two volumes in rough spatial register, and the global affine matching achieves finer rotational, translational, and anisotropic scaling corrections. Readers unfamiliar with these alignment and matching strategies should consult Hibbard and Hawkins (1988).

Elastic deformations allow different parts of the volume to go through different amounts of stretching, contraction, etc., in order to match volumes densitometrically. This process is iterative and is terminated when the displacements fall below a predefined threshold (Bajcsy $et\ al.$, 1983; Bajcsy and Kovacic, 1989). A 3D grid is placed on the test image and a normalized image cross-correlation similarity function is computed for each grid point over spherical domains in the two images (Toga $et\ al.$, 1990, 1991). This similarity function is treated as the elastic potential, the gradient of which gives the elastic force vector to be applied at each grid point. A system of partial differential equations corresponding to elastic equilibrium are then solved to find the elastic displacements of the grid points, resulting in the elastic warp of the image.

Let D_{ijk} be the spherical domain in the reference image centered around the coordinates of the grid point g_{ijk} in the test image, and let there be N voxels $\{v_i : 1 \le i \le N\}$ in this spherical domain. Let c_i be the normalized cross-correlation between the projections for the point g_{ijk} in the test volume and those for the voxel v_i in the reference image. This discrete set of correlation values, c_i is then approximated by a quadratic function of the form

$$C_{\text{approx}}(x, y, z) = a_0 + a_x x + a_y y + a_z z + a_{xx} x^2 \\ + a_{yy} y^2 + a_{zz} z^2 + a_{xy} xy + a_{yz} yz + a_{zx} zx \quad (6)$$

in the least-squares sense over the domain D_{ijk}; i.e., the coefficients $a_0, a_x, a_y, a_z, a_{xx}, a_{yy}, a_{zz}, a_{xy}, a_{yz}$, and a_{zx} are obtained by minimizing

$$\sum_{l=1}^{N} [c_l - c_{\text{approx}}(x_1, y_1, z_1)]^2, \quad (7)$$

where (x_l, y_l, z_l) is the coordinate of the lth voxel in the domain D_{ijk}. The elastic force vector $\vec{F}_{ijk}$ for this grid point, g_{ijk}, is then found as the negative gradient of this approximation, $c_{\text{approx}}(x, y, z)$, computed at

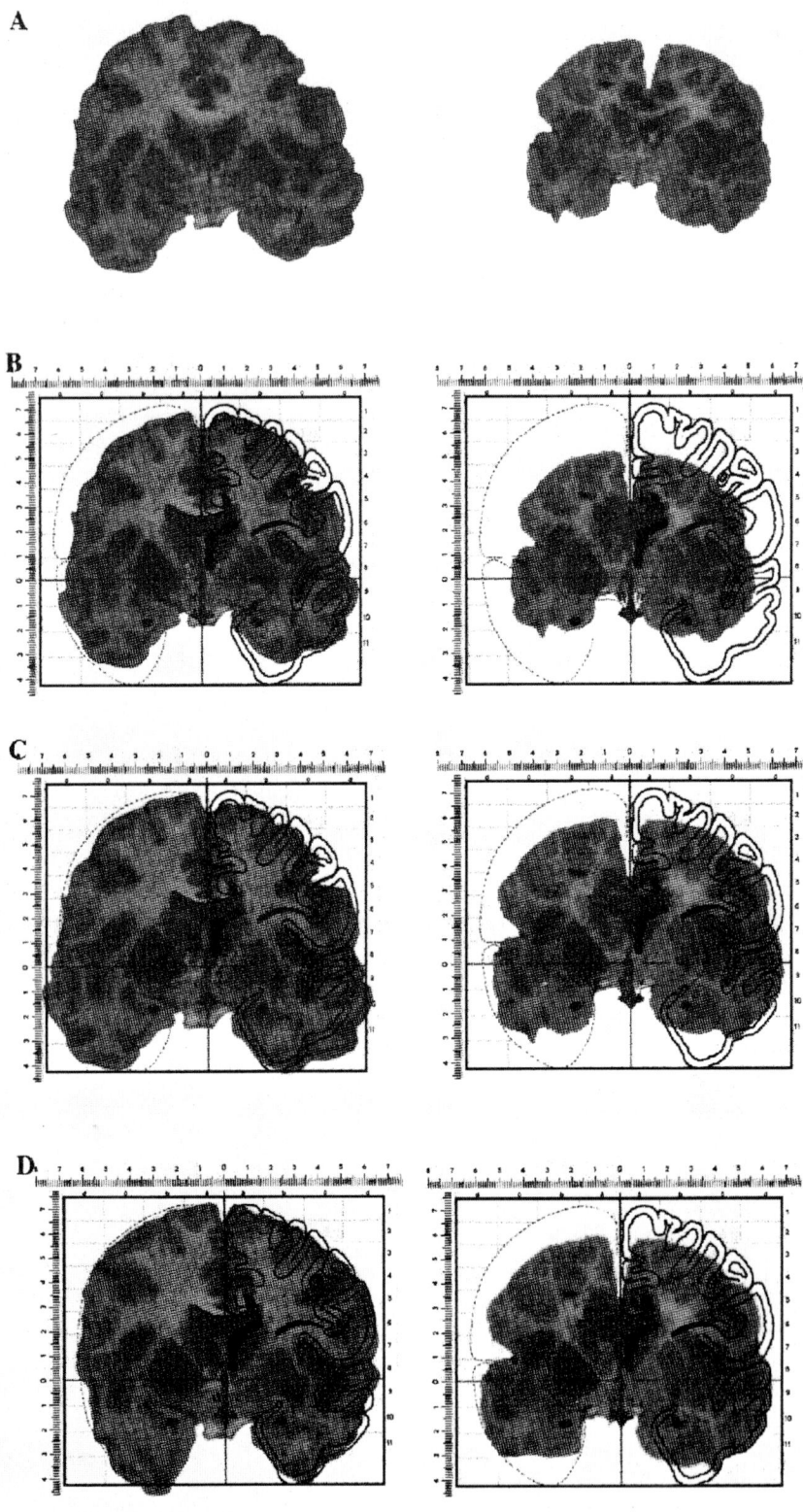

Figure 2 Human brain warped to Talairach-like atlas. The left column shows an adult human brain with varying degrees of warping to map to the corresponding plate, similar to that found in the Talairach atlas. The right column shows the brain from a neonatal subject. These specimens were taken postmortem and acquired using a cryomacrotome technique to produce extremely high-resolution (<500 μm) serial sections through the entire neuroaxis. The dataset was reconstructed to a 3D volume, resampled, positioned,

the grid point. Once these forces are computed for each of the grids, the displacement $\vec{u} = (u_x, u_y, u_z)$ of a grid point under a force, $\vec{F} = (F_x, F_y, F_z)$, is found by solving a set of partial differential equations representing elastic equilibrium (Bajcsy and Kovacic, 1989; Broit, 1981).

IV. Applications

Having surveyed several different approaches to visualization and warping, some examples and applications will be described. Warping a brain to an atlas, warping one modality to another, and warping multiple brains each have different objectives and different requirements of the visualization and warping algorithms.

A. Brain to Atlas

We use neuroanatomic labels to communicate; digital atlases use coordinate space to quantitate. Equating the relationship between neuroanatomic labels and a Cartesian (or polar) coordinate system is one of the by-products of warping to a digital atlas. In addition, segmentation of neuroanatomic structures within 3D datasets using anatomic templates such as the Talairach and Tournoux (1988) stereotactic atlas of the human brain helps make functional measurements between subjects comparable. Fitting anatomic templates to data will greatly increase the number of structures that can be defined. It also provides a common reference system (Bajcsy et al., 1983; Bohm et al., 1991; Wilson and Mountz, 1989) for multisubject comparison and ultimately the development of a database of normative data (Evans et al., 1991). Clinical usefulness has been tested also. Clark et al. (1991) presented initial, encouraging results for a statistical model that assessed the probability that an individual PET was normal or similar to those of patients with Huntington's disease.

Warping a brain to an atlas can be accomplished by sequentially mapping 2D sections through the dataset to an atlas template, assuming the sections are oriented identically. Alternatively, the reconstructed 3D volume can be positioned, warped, and resampled to correspond with the atlas templates (Toga, et al., 1994). Typically the spatial resolution of the atlas is significantly less than that of the experimental dataset, so the loss of accuracy due to resampling is not problematic. The warping can be performed to any degree as described in Fig. 1 and can be either spatially (Toga et al., 1989) or density based (Bajcsy et al., 1983). What must be considered, however, is the suitability of the atlas for the dataset under study. Normal morphometric variability can be obscured by overzealous warpings to effect a better fit. Figure 2 illustrates the use of different degrees of warping of an adult and a neonatal brain to map to the Talairach atlas.

B. Brain to Brain

To facilitate the statistical comparison of two brain datasets of the same modality, it is useful to either place them in the same coordinate space as defined with an atlas or warp one so that it maps to the other while maintaining a measure of deformation necessary to achieve coincidence. The development of an average or otherwise representative model may require that individual contributors be warped relative to one another. As discussed in earlier sections of this chapter, there are several approaches to the solution of these problems. To illustrate their implementation, density-based local deformations were imposed on a 3D volume dataset of high-resolution histology. This dataset was chosen so that noise introduced by the algorithm would be obvious because of the quality of original data.

First, the datasets are histogram equalized and filtered to eliminate any high-frequency or artifactual contamination of the warpings. Then the volume to be warped is subjected to principle axes and center of mass repositionings. Overall scaling and affine transformations may be applied next. A 3D grid of 256^3 points is placed on the volume, and the elastic forces are computed at each point. Forces are derived using the cross-correlation function between the two volume datasets. As described above mathematically,

---

and warped. Planes of the section were resampled to correspond to the atlas templates and superpositioned. (A) Resampled and segmented coronal sections taken from adult (left) and neonatal (right) brain datasets. Image segmentation of brain was performed manually. (B) Superpositioning of atlas template after the section was translated and rotated to the correct position. (C) Affine warpings, using landmarks, were applied to each section to improve the goodness of fit. (D) Local deformations were applied to each section. Note the degree of fit improves as the amount of warp increases. Note also that the mapping of the neonate is poorer than that of the adult due to the extreme difference in anatomical configuration. The extent of imposed deformation was limited.

the image similarity function is computed as a least-squares polynomial approximation of the image correlation in the spherical region around the grid point. The elastic force is computed as the negative gradient of this similarity function. The process continues iteratively until the maximum node displacement falls below a predetermined stop point, in this case 0.5 pixels. The results of this procedure are shown in Plate 34. The lack of resolution compared to original datasets (see Fig. 2a) is due to the use of widely spaced grid points. The execution time of the algorithm is about 2.5 h per iteration at a grid resolution of 16 pixels on a dataset iwth 256^3-pixel resolution. The program was run on an IBM RS6000 with 32 MB of memory.

C. Modality to Modality

The most common application of modality to modality warpings is between MRI and PET. The objective is to enable quantitative assessment of structure–function relationships (Andreasen *et al.*, 1992). In order to provide better anatomic localization, several methods for incorporating MRI data with PET images have been developed. Surface fitting techniques match the inner table of the skull form MRI data with the inner table surface observed in PET scans (Pelizzari *et al.*, 1989). Evans *et al.* (1991) employed multiple landmarks, and transformations including translation, rotations, and scaling were used to minimize the root-mean-square among corresponding points. Fox *et al.* (1985) utilized a stereotactic method to equate data from MRI and PET (and CT). The geometric transformations described in this approach included translation, rotation, and proportional corrections. Measurements and corrections were referenced to stereotactic atlases.

The mapping of one modality to another, once both have been warped to coincidence, can be accomplished in a variety of ways. Surface-based methods include direct mapping of function using false coloring without shading (Kehtarnavaz *et al.*, 1984). This type of visualization is difficult to appreciate. Flattening surfaces (Schwartz *et al.*, 1988) (see above) can aid in the visualization of multimodality maps. Employing color space (hue, saturation, and value) in specific ways permits the mapping of function upon structure while preserving shading cues (Heffernan and Robb, 1984). Texture mapping function on anatomically defined polygonal surfaces can utilize shading and color to indicate depth and magnitude (Payne and Toga, 1990). Plate 33 shows an example of texture mapping a cut-plane surface within a surface-rendered 3D model. This approach can utilize data from any number of modalities. Mazziotta *et al.* (1991) and Evans *et*

al. (1992) visualize multiple modalities by assigning function to a color scale and structure to a gray scale in a voxel-rendered model.

V. Conclusions

Visualizing reconstructed data, warping one dataset to another, and multimodality mappings all have the ability to accentuate or hide the variability that is included within the datasets. Possible sources of variability include error introduced during acquisition, sampling, segmentation, or measurement; normal individual differences; and pathological deviations. The degree to which visualization and warping alters the dataset is affected by the sources of variability, the assumptions of the algorithms, and the product of their execution (Fig. 3).

As described in this chapter, visualizing and warping datasets can alter their positional, structural (scaling, affine, and local), and functional (densitometric) descriptions. These procedures reduce the impact of

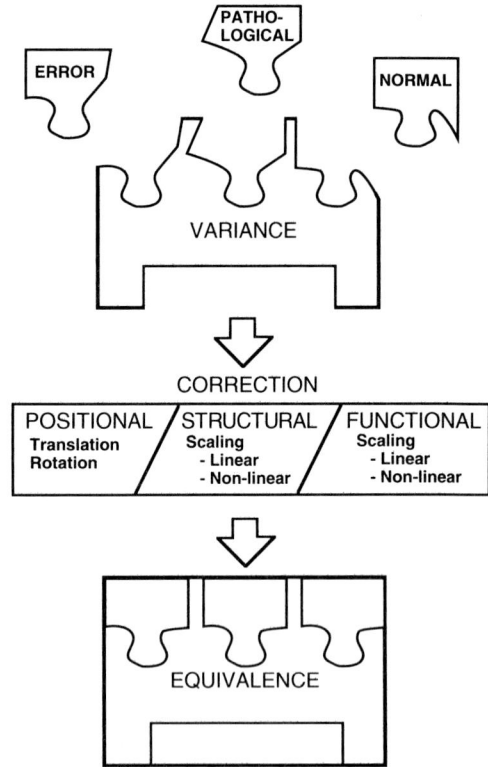

Figure 3 Sources of variance. Datasets all vary to one degree or another prior to the effects of warping and visualization algorithms. The power of warping and visualization can remove variance regardless of its source. These effects can be imposed on structural or functional datasets. Classification of the variance source as well as measurement of its magnitude should be a component of the data analysis and manipulation.

variability and assess its degree. Although this variability may cause problems for the definition of representative models, descriptions of morphometric variability, or descriptions of homogenous subpopulations, it is crucial that the source of this variability be considered when selecting the degree of warping and the type of visualization.

Acknowledgments

I am indebted to the staff of the Laboratory of Neuro Imaging, without whom this work would not have been possible. Specifically, I want to thank Karen Ambach for her help in all things, Pranab Banerjee for his mathematical and programming expertise, Andrew Lee for his graphical patience, and Brad Payne for his visualization proficiency. This work was supported, in part, by the National Science Foundation (DIR No. 89-08174) and the National Institutes of Health (R01-RR05956).

References

Andreasen, N. C., Cohen, G., Harris, G., Cizadlo, T., Parkkinen, J., Rezai, K., and Swayze, V. W. (1992). Image processing for the study of brain structure and function: Problems and programs. *J. Neuropsych.* **4**, 125–133.

Bajcsy, R., and Kovacic, S. (1989). Multiresolution elastic matching. *Comput. Vision Graphics Image Process.* **46**, 1–21.

Bajcsy, R., Lieberson, R., and Reivich, M. (1983). A computerized system for the elastic matching of deformed radiographic images to idealized atlas images. *J. Comput. Assist. Tomogr.* **7**(4), 618–625.

Bohm, C., Greitz, T., Seitz, R., and Eriksson, L. (1991). Specification and selection of regions of interest (ROIs) in a computerized brain atlas. *J. Cereb. Blood Flow Metab.* **11**, A64–A68.

Broit, C. (1981). "Optimal Registration of Deformed Images." Ph.D. dissertation. Philadelphia: University of Pennsylvania.

Bookstein, F. L., Chernoff, B., Elder, R. L., Humphries, J. M., Jr., Smith, G. R., and Strauss, R. E. (1985). "Morphometrics in Evolutionary Biology." The Academy of Natural Sciences Of Philadelphia.

Clark, C. M., Ammann, C., Martin, W. R., Ty, P., and Hayden, M. R. (1991). The FDG/PET methodology for early detection of disease onset: A statistical model. *J. Cereb. Blood Flow Metab.* **11**(2), A96–A102.

Dann, R., Hofordm, J., Kovacic, S., Reivich, M., and Bajcsy, R. (1989). Evaluation of elastic matching system for anatomic (CT, MR) and functional (PET) cerebral images. *J. Comput. Assist. Tomogr.* **13**(4), 603–611.

Drebin, R., Carpenter, L., and Hanrahan, P. (1988). Volume rendering. *Comput. Graph.* **22**(4), 65–74.

Elvins, T. T. (1992). A survey of algorithms for volume visualization. *Comput. Graph.* **26**(3), 194–201.

Evans, A. C., Beil, C., Marrett, S., Thompson, C. J., and Hakim, A. (1988). Anatomical–functional correlation using an adjustable MRI based region of interest atlas with positron emission tomography. *J. Cereb. Blood Flow Metab.* **8**, 513–530.

Evans, A., Marret, S., Torrescorzo, J., Ku, S., and Collins, L. (1991). MRI–PET correlation in 3 dimensions using a volume of interest (VOI) atlas. *J. Cereb. Blood Flow Metab.* **11**, 169–178.

Evans, A. C., Marrett, S., Neelin, P., Collins, L., Worsley, K., Dai, W., Milot, S., Meyer, E., and Bub, D. (1992). Anatomical mapping of functional activation in stereotactic coordinate space. *NeuroImage* **1**(1), 43–54.

Foley, J. D., van Dam, A., Feiner, S. K., and Hughes, J. F. (Eds.) (1990). "Computer Graphics Principles and Practice." Reading, MA: Addison–Wesley.

Fox, P. T., Perlmutter, J. S., and Raichle, M. E. (1985). A stereotactic method of anatomical localization for positron emission tomography. *J. Comput. Assist. Tomogr.* **9**, 513–530.

Friedhoff, M., and Benzon, W. (1989). "Visualization." New York: Harry N. Abrams.

Friston, K. J., Frith, C. D., Liddle, P. F., and Frackowiak, R. S. J. (1991). Plastic transformation of PET images. *J. Comput. Assist. Tomogr.* **15**(4), 634–639.

Heffernan, P. B., and Robb, R. A. (1984). A new procedure for combined display of 3-D cardiac anatomic surfaces and regional functions. *Proc. IEEE Comput. Cardiol.*, 111–114.

Herman, G. T., and Kiu, H. K. (1979). Three dimensional display of human organs from computed tomograms. *Comput. Graph. Image Process.* **9**(1), 1–21.

Hibbard, L., and Hawkins, R. (1988). Objective image alignment for three-dimensional reconstruction of digital autoradiograms. *J. Neurosci. Methods.* **26**, 55–74.

Hohne, K. H., Fuchs, H., and Pizer, S. M. (Eds) (1990). "3D imaging in Medicine, Algorithms, Systems, Applications." Berlin: Springer-Verlag.

Kaufman, A. (Ed.) (1991). "Volume Visualization." Los Alamitos, CA: IEEE Computer Society Press.

Kehtarnavaz, N., Philippe, E. A., and DeFigueirado, R. J. P. (1984). A novel surface reconstruction and display method for cardiac PET imaging. *IEEE Trans. Med. Imag.* **3**(3), 108–115.

Kenny, P. A., Dowsett, D. J., Vernon, D., and Ennis, J. T. (1990). A technique for digital image registration used prior to subtraction of lung images in nuclear medicine. *Phys. Med. Biol.* **35**(5), 679–685.

Levinthal, C., and Ware, R. (1972). Three-dimensional reconstruction from serial sections. *Nature* **236**(5344), 207–210.

Levoy, M., Fuchs, H., Pizer, S. M., Rosenman, J., Chaney, E. L., Sherouse, G. W., Interrante, V., and Kiel, J. (1990). Volume rendering in radiation treatment planning. In "Proceedings of the First Conference on Visualization in Biomedical Computing."

Lorensen, W., and Cline, H. (1987). Marching cubes: A high resolution 3D surface reconstruction algorithm. *Comput. Graph.* **21**, 163–169.

Mazziotta, J. C., Valentino, D., Grafton, S., Bookstein, F., Pelizzari, C., Chen, G., and Toga, A. W. (1991). Relating structure to function *in vivo* with tomographic imaging. In "Exploring Brain Functional Anatomy with Positron Tomography." Chichester: Wiley.

Newman, W. M., and Sproull, R. F. (1979). "Principles of Interactive Computer Graphics." New York: McGraw–Hill.

Mitchell, J. S. B., Mount, D. M., and Papadimitriou, C. H. (1987). The discrete geodesic problem. *SIAM J. Comput.* **16**(4), 647–668.

Olivio, J. C., Kahn, E., Halpern, S., and Fragu, P. (1991). Image registration and distortion correction in ion microscopy. *J. Microscop.* **164**, 263–272.

Pavlidis, T. (1982). "Algorithms for Graphics and Image Processing." Maryland: Computer Science Press.

Payne, B. A., and Toga, A. W. (1990). Surface mapping brain function on 3D models. *Comput. Graph. Appl.* **10**(5), 33–41.

Payne, B. A., and Toga, A. W. (1992). Distance field manipulation of surface models. *Comput. Graph Appl.* **12**(1), 65–71.

Pelizzari, C. A., Chen, G. T. Y., Spelbring, D. R., Weichselbaum, R. R., and Chen, C. T. (1989). Accurate three-dimensional registration of CT, PET and/or MR images of the brain. *J. Comput. Assist. Tomogr.* **13,** 20–26.

Robb, R. A., (Ed.) (1985). "Three-Dimensional Biomedical Imaging." Boca Raton, FL: CRC Press.

Sharir, M., and Schorr, A. (1986). On shortest paths in polyhedral spaces. *SIAM J. Comput.* **15**(1), 193—215.

Schwartz, E. L., and Merker, B. (1986). Computer-aided neuroanatomy: Differential geometry of cortical surfaces and an optimal flattening algorithm. *IEEE Comput. Graph. Appl.* (March), 36–44.

Schwartz, E. L., Merker, B., Wolfson, E., and Schaw, A. (1988). Applications of computer graphics and image processing to 2D and 3D modeling of the functional architecture of visual cortex. *Comput. Graph. Appl.* **8,** 13–23.

Talairach, J., and Tournoux, P. (1988). "Co-Planar Stereotaxic Atlas of the Human Brain." Stuttgart: Thieme.

Terzopolous, D., Platt, J., Barr, A., and Fleischer, K. (1987). Elastically deformable models. "Comput. Graph." **21,** 205–214.

Toga, A. W., Santori, M. S., and Samaie, M. (1986). Regional distribution of flunitrazepam binding constants: Visualizing Kd and Bmax by digital image analysis. *J. Neurosci.* **6**(9), 2747–2756.

Toga, A. W. (1990). "Three-Dimensional Neuroimaging." New York: Raven Press.

Toga, A. W. (1991). A digital three-dimensional atlas of structure/function relationships. *J. Chem. Neuroanat.* **4**(5), 313–318.

Toga, A. W., Samaie, M., and Payne, B. A. (1989). Digital rat brain: A computerized atlas. *Br. Res. Bull.* **22,** 323–333.

Toga, A. W., and Payne, B. A. (1991). Animating the 3D structure and function of the brain. *Comput. Med. Imag. Graphics* **15**(5), 285–291.

Toga, A. W., Absher, J. R., Banerjee, P. K., and Santori, E. M. (1994). Neuroanatomic variability of rat brains. Submitted for publication.

Toga, A. W., Banerjee, P., and Payne, B. A. (1991). Brain warping and averaging. *J. Cereb. Blood Flow Metab.* **11,** S560.

Toga, A. W., Banerjee, P. K., and Santori, E. M. (1990). Warping 3D models for interbrain comparisons. *Neurosci. Abstr.* **16,** 247.

Tufte, E. R. (1983). "The Visual Display of Quantitative Information." Cheshire, CT: Graphics Press.

Tufte, E. R. (1990). "Envisioning Information." Cheshire, CT: Graphics Press.

Udupa, J. K., and Herman, G. T. (Eds.) (1991). "3D Imaging in Medicine." Boca Raton, FL: CRC Press.

Wilson, M. W., and Mountz, J. M. (1989). A reference system for neuroanatomic localization on functional reconstructed cerebral images. *J. Comput. Assist. Tomogr.* **13**(1), 174–178.

Wolberg, G. (1990). "Digital Image Warping." Los Alamitos, CA: IEEE Computer Society Press.

Wolfson, E., and Schwartz, E. (1989). Computing minimal distances on polyhedral surfaces. *IEEE Trans. Pattern Anal. Machine Intelligence* **11**(9), 1001–1004.

17

Visualization Methods for Analysis of Multimodality Images

Richard A. Robb

Biomedical Imaging Resource, Mayo Foundation, Rochester, Minnesota 55905

I. Introduction

Much of what we know about brain function and brain disease has been derived from images—images produced by various instruments, which extend the range of human investigation into realms beyond that which is naturally accessible. The traditional disciplines of biological and medical science are significantly grounded in the observation of living structures and in the measurement of various properties of these structures (e.g., their functions). Images are a direct measurement of structure and often of function. Ever since the discovery of X rays, physicians, surgeons, and life scientists have been using images to diagnose and treat disease and to better understand basic physiological function. The imaging modalities used in modern medicine are based on a variety of energy sources, including light, electrons, lasers, X rays, radionuclides, ultrasound, and nuclear magnetic resonance. These various modalities provide largely complementary information. However, the full scientific and medical value of these images, although profoundly significant, remains largely unexploited. This is due primarily to the lack of objective, quantitative methods to fully visualize and synthesize the intrinsic information contained in the multimodality images. The need for resolution of this problem has become increasingly important and pressing as advances in imaging and computer technology have enabled more complex objects and processes to be imaged and simulated.

The process of forming an image involves the mapping of an object, some property of an object, or both into or onto what is called image space. This space is used to visualize the object and its properties and may be used to quantitatively characterize its structure, its function, or both. Imaging science may be defined as the study of these mappings and the development of ways to better understand them, to improve them, and to productively use them. The challenge of imaging science is to provide advanced capabilities for acquisition, processing, synthesis, visualization, and quantitative analysis of biomedical images in order to significantly increase the faithful extraction of the useful information that they contain and to render them useful clinically. The ANALYZE software system has been developed to effectively meet this need.

II. Background

The Biomedical Imaging Resource at the Mayo Clinic has been involved since the early 1970s in the design and implementation of computer-based techniques for the display and analysis of multidimensional biomedical images (Robb, 1988). The Resource constitutes a unique and technologically advanced facility for support of multimodality, multidimensional biomedical imaging investigations. It is associated with a comprehensive array of biomedical laboratories and patient clinical facilities within the Mayo Clinic and maintains a variety of extramural research collaborations nationally and internationally. The Resource has a multidisciplinary professional and skilled technical staff who have an established record in pioneering imaging research and who are committed to development, evaluation, and dissemination of new and improved technology, techniques, and systems for scientific visualization and multidimensional biomedical image display and analysis.

The algorithms and programs developed through this program have been integrated into a comprehensive software system called ANALYZE (Robb, 1990; Robb and Hanson, 1990), useful in a variety of multimodality, multidimensional biomedical imaging and scientific visualization applications. The ANALYZE system features integrated, complementary tools for fully interactive display, manipulation, and measurement of multidimensional image data. It has been applied to data from many different imaging modalities, including CT, MRI, PET, and SPECT. The software runs efficiently on standard UNIX workstations without the need for special-purpose hardware. The ANALYZE software system is written entirely in the C programming language and utilizes several features of the UNIX operating system to facilitate its modular architecture. The system comprises over 60 individual programs, each representing a particular imaging function or related set of functions, all of which are built from a base of 12 libraries. In total, the ANALYZE program contains over 500,000 lines of source code for all programs and libraries.

III. Selected Features of the ANALYZE Software System

Only a few of the ANALYZE modules will be described and illustrated, particularly those that pertain to functional neuroimaging. These will emphasize display, measurement, segmentation, registration, and fusion capabilities. More complete details on the ANALYZE system can be found in the References.

A. Two-Dimensional Displays

Images from an image database can be displayed directly from the acquired image information, or new images can be generated from this image information using both two-dimensional and three-dimensional functions. Several tools for interactive 2D image display are available in the ANALYZE system. These

include interactive display of multiple images with variable size control; interactive intensity windowing; rapid generation of orthogonal images from image volumes (i.e., multiplanar reformatting); display as a cube with control of size, intensity range, angle of view, and interactive dissections along orthogonal planes; generation and display of arbitrary oblique planar images through volume images with interactive control of the orientation of the plane using standard flying commands (e.g., pitch, roll, and yaw); generation of parallel oblique images for image volume reformatting along an arbitrary axis; interactive generation of "curved" images, radial image sections, or both through regions traced on orthogonal images; and rapid display of images in cine movie loops using multiple simultaneous panels with interactive control of speed and stop/start points.

Examples of two of these many capabilities for 2D display are shown in Figs. 1 and 2. Figure 1 shows multiplanar orthogonally reformatted images, including transverse, coronal, and sagittal images. The multiplanar images can be processed before display using intensity windowing, thresholding, smoothing, inverting, contouring, and rotating. Figure 2 illustrates computation and display of oblique planes that are interactively generated by "flying" through the volume image, that is, moving the oblique plane relative to its current position with well-defined flying maneuvers, such as pitch, roll, yaw, elevate, slip, and slide. Sequences of oblique images can be written to a new image file to obliquely reformat an entire image volume prior to subsequent analysis.

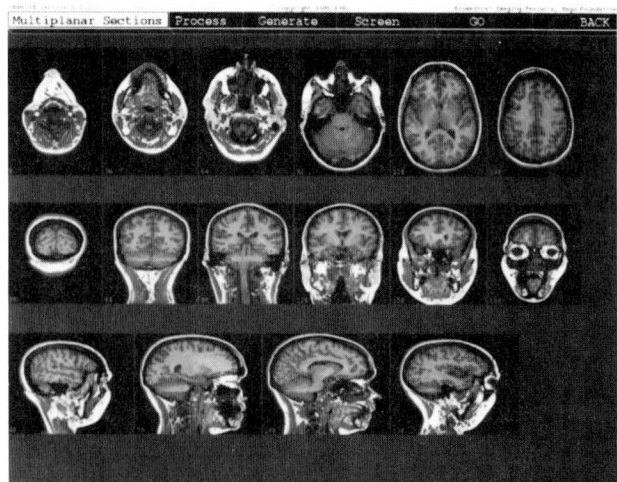

Figure 1 Multiplanar reformatting of a 3D MRI volume image of the head into transaxial (top row), coronal (middle row), and sagittal (bottom row) sections.

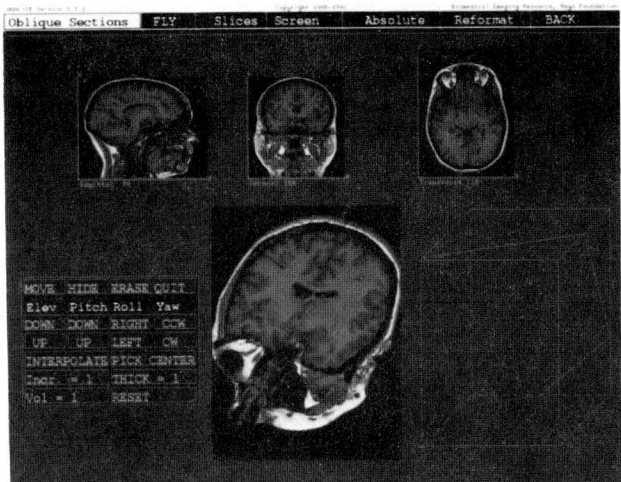

Figure 2 Oblique section computed and displayed through a 3D MRI of the head.

B. Three-Dimensional Displays (Volume Rendering)

One of the most powerful and versatile modules within the ANALYZE system for fully 3D display is volume rendering (Drebin *et al.*, 1988; Höhne and Bernstein, 1986; Levoy, 1988; Robb and Barillot, 1989). This program contains several algorithms that are based on ray casting. To render an image, the output pixel values are assigned appropriate intensities based on the algorithm and visualization parameters used to cast rays through the voxels in the volume image. There are two classes of rendering algorithms used: reflection (surface) algorithms and transmission (projection) algorithms. Examples of a few of these algorithms are shown in Fig. 3.

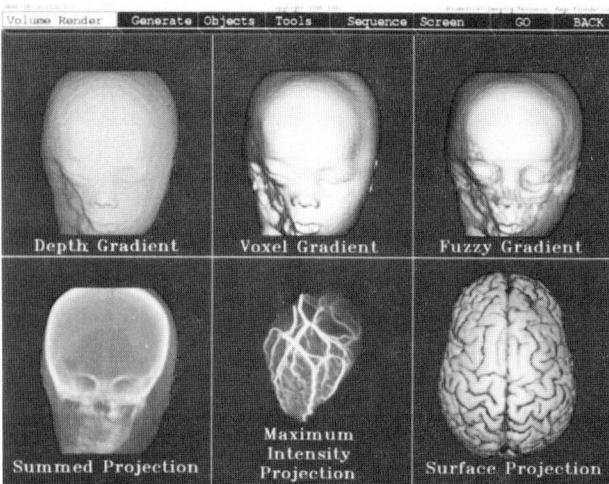

Figure 3 Display from different volume rendering algorithms.

In many visualization applications, it is often desirable to view and manipulate individual structures within the volume image (Robb and Hanson, 1990). A unique and powerful method has been developed in ANALYZE to allow interactive specification of individual structures for display and manipulation within the rendered volume image. This method classifies sets of voxels in the original volume image into user-defined objects, assigning variable names and attributes to each of the objects. This capability is realized using an auxillary data structure called an *object map*.

This construct forms a one-to-one mapping between the voxels in the original volume image and objects defined by segmentation. Sets of common values in the object map define complete "objects" without requiring spatial connectivity; that is, object maps can define multiple disjoint structures composing a single object, or objects can simply be a set of spatially unrelated voxels. This latter notion is important to functional imaging, as it permits visualization of "functional objects" (e.g., blood flow, electrophysiology, and temperature). The object map therefore provides direct classification of the voxels in the volume image into distinct representations of structures, functions, or both. Multiple object maps can be created for a single volume image.

The construction of an object map involves either prerendering segmentation of structures from the volume image or the interactive editing and specification of structures directly on the rendered image. Prerendering segmentation of structures can be accomplished by several ANALYZE programs, including manual and semiautomated image editing, 2D and 3D math morphology, and multispectral feature space classification. Structures in the object map can also be defined directly from rendered images in the volume rendering program using both manual and semiautomated (e.g., supervised region growing) methods applied in full 3D.

Once structures have been defined in an object map, attributes can be assigned to each individual structure, including visibility, color, spatial position, and orientation. These attributes can be effectively used to simultaneously display fused multimodality images. Visibility controls the inclusion or exclusion of the object voxels in the ray casting process. The color attribute assigns a specific color to the object and the number of color shades used to represent the surface of the object, with the number of shades available for all objects equitably divided across all objects to produce the most effective rendered display. An opacity attribute can be assigned to each object to produce multicolored transparent displays of the multiple objects.

Spatial position attributes can be assigned to each independent object, allowing for independent spatial manipulation of individual structures in the volume image. Translation and rotation provide for the positioning of an object at any specific 3D location within the volume rendering space. Individual objects can be mirrored across any of the orthogonal volume image axes. Increments can be established for each of the translation and rotation values used in conjunction with sequence generation to produce rendered sequences of spatial manipulations.

Volume rendering in ANALYZE provides a powerful 3D visual metaphor for analysis of multidimensional, multimodality images, and structure–function relationships. In particular, the ANALYZE volume rendering program provides tools that directly interact with the rendered image in three categories: display tools, manipulation tools, and measurement tools. The display tools use the 3D rendered image as a reference for resectioning the original volume image. Orthogonal sections in the transverse, coronal, and sagittal planes can be interactively computed and displayed using a cursor to indicate the point of intersection for the orthogonal planes on the rendered surface, as depicted in Plate 35. The rendered image can further be used as the visualization reference for the orientation of an arbitrarily oriented oblique plane passing through the volume image. Interactive maneuvers for plane orientation can be selected as the display of the plane updates its intersection with the rendered image. The rendered surface and the image on the oblique plane can be made transparent, so as to visualize the internal structures sectioned with the oblique plane as intersecting with the surface, shown in Plate 36. The display of the rendered surface can be used to define subregions to be selectively rendered with different parameters. After definition of a traced region on the surface, rendering parameters can be altered to render only the portion of the volume image inside of the trace as in Plate 37. Combined renderings of multiple objects using different algorithms can be accomplished with this feature (e.g., a transmission rendering of an object inside of a surface rendering of another object).

The manipulation tools apply transformations to the structures in the rendered image. Region growing can be invoked by selecting a seed point on a structure in the rendered image, with the voxels subsequently deleted from the volume image or saved to an object map. Structures can be manually traced, and all voxels found in the traced region throughout the 3D volume image can be found and deleted from the original volume image. Contours can be extracted from the currently rendered surface and stored in a contour

file for further analysis, bridging the gap between the volumetric description of the structure and a geometric description. All spatial manipulations and attribute control of objects can be done interactively using the workstation's mouse and a multipanel, multiviewpoint display of the rendered structures, as shown in Plate 38. Interactive manipulations are important to various imaging applications, including neurosurgical simulation and planning.

C. Measurement

Several tools are available in ANALYZE for direct measurement on the rendered image (Robb and Hanson, 1990). Points can be selected from the rendered surface, with the 3D coordinates and voxel value stored to a file. Distances can be measured between any two points selected on the rendered surface, including both the linear distance between the points and the curvilinear distance along the surface between the two points as projected from the current source position. The surface area anywhere on the rendered image can be measured by drawing a trace directly on the rendered image, depicted in Plate 39. Volume of any rendered object can be measured simply by selecting a point on a particular structure in the rendered image. The program counts the connected voxels to the seed point using a 3D region growing method.

The ANALYZE system contains several other tools for mensuration and quantitative analysis of image features. A magnifying glass can be used for magnification of any square region of the screen, as shown in Fig. 4. The size of the area being magnified, the magnification factor, histograms, and numeric pixel

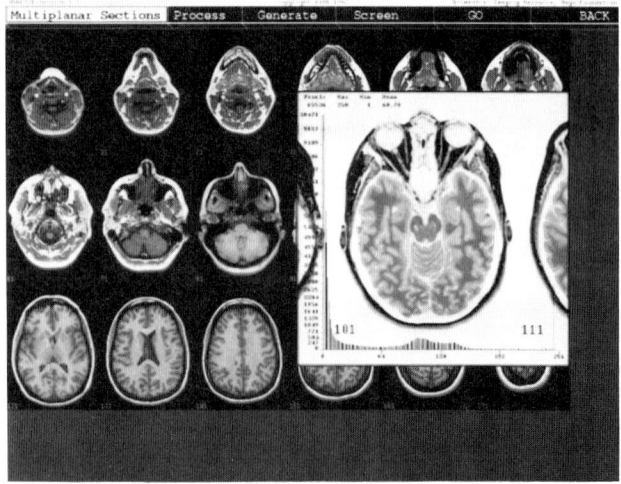

Figure 4 Magnifying glass for viewing and displaying regional detail, including inverse gray scale, histograms, and actual numeric values.

values can be computed and displayed for the region selected. A caliper tool, shown in Plate 40, can be used to measure linear segment distances and angles between specified lines. The shape and lengths of the line segments can be interactively manipulated by selecting the points along the lines to provide geometric measurement of anatomic structures within the image.

The Region of Interest (ROI) program can be used to interactively define and sample selected regions. Multiple regions can be defined using analytic shapes (e.g., rectangles and ellipses), by tracing a free-form area on the image or by using semiautomated boundary definition. Image information within these regions can be interactively sampled by user selection or can be sampled automatically by region name. Information provided by the area sampling includes the maximum and minimum values, mean and standard deviation of the values, the calibrated area within the region, the integrated brightness–area product, and a plot of the histogram of the sampled data, depicted in Plate 41. Measurements on these regions can be performed and then saved for further analysis. Other measurements provided by the ROI program are fractal signatures and shape measures for selected regions. These measures provide complementary information about tissue composition and morphology. Additionally, measurement of the volumes of arbitrary three-dimensional structures can be obtained using several techniques, including a fast probabilistic model.

D. Segmentation and Classification

The "calculus of imaging science" involves segmentation (differentiation) and fusion (integration) of images. ANALYZE has powerful tools for solving this calculus. Segmentation of features from multimodality images may be accomplished using several kinds of approaches (Collins *et al.*, 1992; Griffin *et al.*, 1992; Kamber *et al.*, 1992; Kübler and Gerig, 1990; Pizer *et al.*, 1990; Schiemann *et al.*, 1992; Vincken *et al.*, 1992), including both anatomical and functional segmentation. Three of the more powerful methods in ANALYZE, which operate in both 2D and full 3D, are multispectral analysis, region growing, and math morphology.

Multispectral analysis provides capabilities for segmentation of structure, function, or both. The multispectral classification program in ANALYZE provides both a set of manual tools for exploring and classifying two-spectrum images and a set of automated feature space classification algorithms that operate on images of any number of spectra. Multispectral images consist

of voxels that are actually vectors of values, usually reflecting measurements of different physical attributes of the same object obtained from multiple imaging modalities, such as correlated MRI/CT or CT/PET/MRI. Multispectral images may also represent derived measures from a single original volume image, such as gradients or texture features for each voxel. Just as scalar images may be segmented by defining extents of the gray scale used to represent different tissue types or organs, multispectral images can be segmented by defining different regions of the feature space associated with different tissue types. The promise of multispectral analysis is that the dimensionally expanded feature space will allow differentiations to be made that are impossible in any of the component images alone.

The manual tools in the multispectral program include display of the single-channel component images, along with a vector histogram of the two-channel image, a linked cursor that shows the same location in both channel images, the ability to sample the channel images and observe the location of the sampled pixels in the measurement plane, and the ability to define regions of the measurement plane and observe the regions of the channel images that meet that measurement criterion, as depicted in Plate 42. The automated algorithms include five common classification techniques, including Gaussian clustering, neural network, nearest neighbor, *k*-nearest neighbor, and Parzen windows, which differ in complexity and basic approach. These algorithms offer a variety of trade-offs in accuracy, computation time, and suitability to particular situations. All the automated algorithms assume that certain voxels have been defined by the user as belonging to certain classes, and these voxels are used as samples of these classes. Unassigned voxels are then classified (or left unclassified) based on the estimated likelihood of their belonging to each of the defined classes. Both the manual and automated modes allow classification of the entire multispectral volume image, storing results as either a "classification image" or an object map.

ANALYZE also features a robust 3D region growing program for spatial (anatomic) segmentation of volume images. In this method, the user selects a seed point and then interactively manipulates the threshold range about the selected seed pixel. As the region growing takes place, pixels that fall outside of the threshold range (above and below) are selected for boundary pixels, with a neighbor-connectivity constraint imposed to insure a continuous boundary, as demonstrated in Plate 43.

The 3D Morphology program applies 1D, 2D, or 3D mathematical morphological transformations

(Haralick *et al.*, 1987) and object topology operations. Transformations are chained together for application to any given volume image and can be saved for application to other volume images. The transformations available include Threshold, Erode, Dilate, Max, Min, Open, and Close. The 3D structuring elements available are Rectilinear, 6-Connected, 18-Connected, and 4-Connected. A variety of chained transformations provide automated, multistep processing. One of these powerful processes, called "successive inclusion," was used to automatically segment the several 3D structures shown in Plate 44 from the same MRI volume image of the head. Other mathematical and modeling approaches (Bookstein and Green, 1992; Brechbühler *et al.*, 1992; Waters, 1992) supplement the segmentation process by providing useful analytical and/or physical representations of object surfaces.

E. Registration and Fusion

Multimodality images obtained from medical imaging systems such as CT, MR imaging, PET, and SPECT generally provide complementary characteristic and diagnostic information. Synthesis of these image data sets into a single composite image containing these complementary attributes in accurate registration and congruence would provide truly synergistic information about the object(s) under examination. There have been several approaches developed to address this problem (Boesel and Bresler, 1992; Chen and Pelizzari, 1989; Henri *et al.*, 1992; Hill *et al.*, 1992; Höhne *et al.*, 1992; Levin *et al.*, 1989; van den Elsen *et al.*, 1992). We have developed a new method (Jiang and Robb, 1992) that produces effective correlation using parametric Chamfer matching. The method is fast, accurate, and reproducible. Surfaces are initially extracted from two different images to be matched using semiautomatic segmentation techniques. These surfaces are represented as contours with common features to be matched. A distance transformation is performed for one surface image, and a cost function for translation, rotation, and scaling to accommodate images of different position, orientation, and size. The matching process involves searching this multiparameter space to find the best fit to minimize the cost function. The local minima problem is addressed by using a large number of starting points. A pyramid multiresolution approach is employed to speed up both the distance transformation and the multiparameter minimization processes. Robustness in noise handling is accomplished using multiple thresholds embedded in the multiresolution search. The algorithm can register both partially overlapped and fragmented surfaces. Manual intervention is generally not

necessary. Preliminary results suggest registration accuracy on the order of the voxel size used in the registration process. Computational time scales with the number of matching elements used, with about 5 min typical for 256^3 images using a modern desktop workstation.

The fusion program in ANALYZE has been applied to several sets of simulated data to test robustness of the registration algorithm (Jiang *et al.*, 1992), but it has also been used with multimodality volume image data obtained from clinical patient studies. Using appropriate color-wash superposition displays and interactive linked cursors, pixel-to-pixel correspondence can be evaluated.

An MR head image of dimensions $256 \times 256 \times 123$ with voxel size $0.98 \times 0.98 \times 1.50$ mm^3 and a PET brain image from the same patient, dimensions $128 \times 128 \times 15$ and voxel size $2.0 \times 2.0 \times 6.5$ mm^3, were selected for registration, as shown in Fig. 5. Note the orthogonal differences in orientation (sagittal for the MR, transverse for the PET) between the two datasets. This represents no difficulty for the registration process, as long as appropriate corresponding surfaces can be obtained. The brain was segmented from both images and used as the common object for registration. The MRI brain is used for the base surface and the PET brain is used for the match surface. The threshold is set to 2.0% of the match surface dimension for the highest level of resolution. In this case, the PET brain surface is completely contained within the MR brain surface. The registration result is displayed in Plate 45. General orientation and specific internal anatomic landmarks are in good registration (within one pixel).

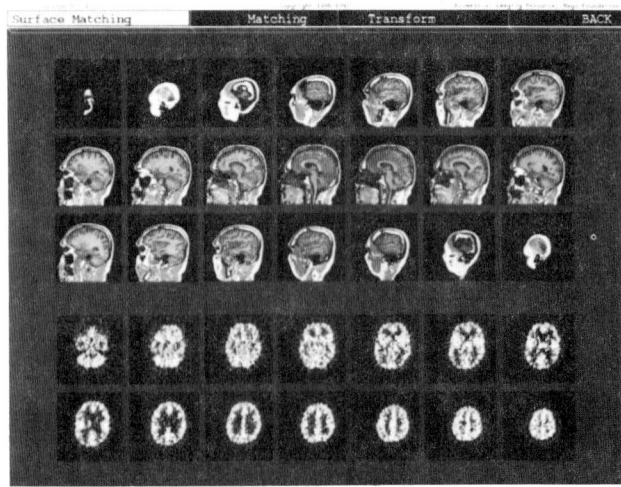

Figure 5 Original MR (top) and PET (bottom) head images used for registration.

An MR head image of dimensions $256 \times 256 \times 124$ with voxel size $0.781 \times 0.781 \times 1.2$ mm^3 and a SPECT brain image from the same patient, dimensions $64 \times 64 \times 48$ and voxel size $3.56 \times 3.56 \times 3.56$ mm^3, were selected for registration. The brain was segmented from both images and used as the common object for registration. The patient was scanned with special markers attached to the skin surface that can be seen in both MR and SPECT images, so that the registration accuracy can be evaluated to some degree by observing how accurately the markers overlap. The registration results are displayed in Plate 46. All the external markers and internal anatomic landmarks are in good registration.

An MR head image of dimensions $256 \times 256 \times 26$ with voxel size $0.938 \times 0.938 \times 3.0$ mm^3 and a CT head image from the same patient, dimensions $512 \times 512 \times 10$ and voxel size $0.674 \times 0.674 \times 3.0$ mm^3, were selected for registration. The patient was scanned in a stereotaxic head frame with markers visible in both MR and CT images. Registration accuracy can be evaluated visually by observing the alignment of the markers, using a linked cursor, as shown in Plate 47. These and prominent anatomic landmarks are in good registration.

Another important example of the use of image volume registration is in cerebral function mapping using evoked response experiments. Plate 48 depicts matching of T_1-weighted and SPGR Flash MR images of a patient suffering from tumor-related seizures. The images were obtained during controlled fist and jaw clenching, distinct symptoms of the patient's seizures. As shown in the top row of Plate 48, the enhanced region of cerebral activity captured in the functional image can be directly mapped onto the anatomically-detailed image using the chamfer surface matching algorithm. The functional regions (evoked response) can be accurately imbedded in the 3D acquired volume of the entire brain, and color-coded for display in selected anatomical planes intersecting the functional regions, as shown in the bottom row of Plate 48. The 3D volume images also indicate the positions of the tumor and subdural electrodes (matched to the MR images from CT scans) placed to identify the location of the motor strip.

These registration results for patient data look very promising. Examination by qualified experts (radiologists) suggests that all obvious landmarks are in good registration with visually confirmable accuracy. Determining a statistically significant value for the registration accuracy in such studies is nearly impossible, however, without extensive applications to a large number of datasets. The registration accuracy depends on statistical characteristics, such as spatial sampling, noise level and type, percentage of surface overlap, and complexity of surface features. Ongoing validation of the algorithm will take these factors into consideration.

IV. Some Applications

Several of the methods and tools available in ANALYZE are useful in functional neuroimaging applications. They include neurosurgery planning (Ehricke *et al.*, 1992; Hill *et al.*, 1992; Jack *et al.*, 1989; Kikinis *et al.*, 1992; Mohan *et al.*, 1988), lesion detection and analysis in multiple sclerosis (Kamber *et al.*, 1992; Kermode *et al.*, 1990), and tissue classification, measurement, and treatment (Bourland, 1990; Bourland *et al.*, 1992; Kikinis *et al.*, 1992; Mohan *et al.*, 1988; Sherouse *et al.*, 1990). MRI has proven useful for detailed visualization of soft tissue structures often unrevealed by other imaging modalities. For instance, MRI can be used to image the white vs gray matter in the brain, the cerebral spinal fluid, plaques, and tumors.

New scanning modes in MRI are beginning to provide isotropic 3D image datasets at high spatial resolution. Figure 6 shows volume rendered images from a 3D acquired MRI scan of a head for visualization of brain structure. The editing tools in ANALYZE have been used to segment the brain from other tissues, which is then rendered to visualize its position relative to other head structures. Such faithful detail in reconstruction of the brain surface has provided impetus for use of volume rendering in the planning of neurosurgery.

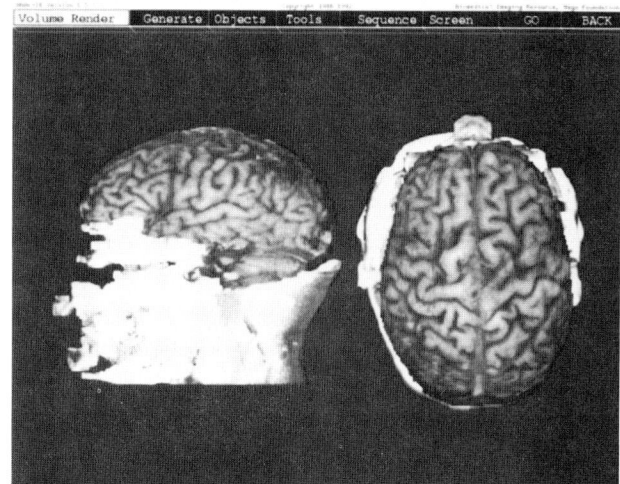

Figure 6 Automated segmentation and realistic rendering of the brain required for effective neurosurgical planning applications.

Plate 49 depicts a clinical neurosurgery application for volume rendering of 3D acquired MRI image volumes. In selected epilepsy patients, an EEG is performed to map the electrical activity of the brain to identify the portion of the brain generating the seizure focus activity. Once the electrodes at the seizure foci have been determined, markers (fat beads) are placed in the position of these electrodes, and the patient is scanned using the 3D MRI procedure. Using volume rendering, the markers can be shown on the skin surface (top images) and projected onto the surface of the brain (bottom images) for visualization of the precise region of the brain producing the seizure activity. The neurosurgeon can use these renderings to plan a surgical approach to the treatment of the disease, including minimizing brain tissue resection and its associated effects.

Plate 50 illustrates the application of multispectral classification to analysis of lesions in a patient with multiple sclerosis (MS). T_1-weighted and T_2-weighted MRI volume images of the head (upper left and middle) are used to generate a 2D feature space (lower left) from which several structures can be identified and automatically segmented, including gray matter (blue), white matter (yellow), CFS (red/green), and a single MS lesion (red/green spot at left center).

Plate 51 shows application of successive 3D image processing steps to isolate and measure a central nervous system tumor. The T_1-weighted (top row) and T_2-weighted (bottom row) MRI images were first spatially registered using surface matching and then used to form a feature space in which multispectral analysis was used to isolate the cluster corresponding to tumor tissue. The voxels corresponding to this cluster (red) were then automatically segmented from other structures in the brain, permitting the volume of the tumor to be accurately measured.

Plate 52 depicts an application in 3D radiation treatment planning. Using 3D MRI head scans and computed 3D distributions of dose simulated from multiple port X-ray beams, accurate treatment plans can be designed, viewed, and modified. Transparency images from multiple angles of view (upper row) and cut-away images from different orientations (lower row) can be rendered to visualize the paths of multiple beams used in conformal radiation treatment. The opacity of low dose objects has been set low, with the opacity of the high dose areas set high, allowing the red high dose surface to be visualized through the enveloping layers of low dose. These applications and others will be enhanced by the development of new and continuing improvement of current methods for

effective and efficient visualization and analysis of multimodality images.

V. Summary

Major segments of the biological sciences and the practice of medicine are based on the study and knowledge of the relationships of anatomic structure to biological function. Traditionally, this knowledge has been gained either indirectly or by inference and, in the final analysis, by direct surgical vivisection or postmortem examinations. Direct visualization and study of anatomic structure and function of internal organ systems in humans have, up to the present, been the preserve of the surgeon and pathologist. The revolutionary capabilities provided by multiple new 3D imaging modalities for obtaining similar information noninvasively, nondestructively, and painlessly can now provide this data to the internist, surgeon, and researcher for direct reproducible examinations of individual patients or experimental subjects without disturbing the physiology of the organ system under study or altering its normal integration into the physiology of the body as a whole.

The variety of disease processes and abnormalities affecting all regions of the human body are so numerous and different that each imaging modality possesses attributes that make it uniquely helpful in providing the desired understanding and discrimination of the disease or abnormality, and therefore no single method has prevailed to the complete exclusion of others. This is particularly true in neuroimaging, in which the imaging methodologies are largely complementary. The effective synthesis of these multimodal images would provide a powerful new armamentarium of clinical diagnostic and biomedical research capabilities that could significantly advance the practice of medicine and the frontiers of biological understanding.

However, the ability to visualize, synthesize, extract, and measure information in 3D biomedical images has not been fully developed. This is somewhat of a paradox, because on the one hand the new 3D imaging capabilities promise significant potential for providing greater specificity and sensitivity (i.e., precise objective discrimination and accurate quantitative measurement of body tissue characteristics and functions) in clinical diagnostic and basic investigative imaging procedures than ever possible before, but, on the other hand, the momentous advances in computer and associated electronic imaging technology that have made these 3D imaging capabilities possible have not been concomitantly developed for full exploitation of these capabilities. The ANALYZE software system was developed to fulfill this need.

ANALYZE continues to be refined and extended to facilitate comprehensive, detailed quantitative investigations and evaluation of 3D biomedical images. Under development are customized applications for simulation and planning of surgical procedures employed in many aspects of neurosurgery and for interactive design and manipulation of 3D treatment plans in radiation therapy. New user interfaces with comprehensive database management capabilities are being developed. Arguably the two most important problems inhibiting major progress in biomedical imaging are automated segmentation of features of interest and accurate fusion of information from multiple modality images. New algorithms for this imaging "calculus" are being developed, implemented, and evaluated in ANALYZE. All of these capabilities will combine, in an evolutionary way, to provide increased sensitivity and specificity in quantitative analyses of tissues, organs, and complete biological systems from multimodality images, leading to more effective diagnosis and treatment of disease.

Acknowledgments

The author is grateful to his colleagues in the Mayo Biomedical Imaging Resource, without whom this work would not be possible. The author would also like to acknowledge the important contributions of many imaging collaborators at the Mayo Foundation and at other national and international medical institutions. Special thanks to Gina Croatt for her assistance in the preparation of this manuscript.

References

Boesel, R. W., and Bresler, Y. (1992). A new paradigm for optimal multi-parameter image visualization. *In* "Proceedings of the Second Conference on Visualization in Biomedical Computing, Chapel Hill, NC," pp. 347–361.

Bookstein, F. L., and Green, W. D. (1992). Edge information at landmarks in medical images. *In* "Proceedings of the Second Conference on Visualization in Biomedical Computing, Chapel Hill, NC," pp. 242–258.

Bourland, J. D. (1990). "A Finite-Size Pencil Beam Model for Three-Dimensional Photon Dose Calculations." Doctoral dissertation. Chapel Hill, NC: University of North Carolina at Chapel Hill.

Bourland, J. D., Camp, J. J., and Robb, R. A. (1992). Volume rendering: Application in static field conformal radiosurgery. *In* "Proceedings of the Second Conference on Visualization in Biomedical Computing, Chapel Hill, NC," pp. 584–587.

Brechbühler, C., Gerig, G., and Kübler, O. (1992). Surface parameterization and shape description. *In* "Proceedings of the Second Conference on Visualization in Biomedical Computing, Chapel Hill, NC," pp. 80–89.

Chen, G. T. Y., and Pelizzari, C. A. (1989). Image correlation techniques in radiation therapy treatment planning. *Comput. Med. Imag. Graphics* **12**, 235–240.

Collins, D. L., Peters, T. M., Dai, W., and Evans, A. C. (1992). Model based segmentation of individual brain structures from MRI data. *In* "Proceedings of the Second Conference on Visualization in Biomedical Computing, Chapel Hill, NC," pp. 10–23.

Drebin, R., Carpenter, L., and Harrahan, P. (1988). "Volume Rendering: SIGGRAPH '88," pp. 65–74.

Ehricke, H.-H., Daiber, G., Sonntag, R., Strasser, W., Lochner, M., Schad, L. R., and Lorenz, W. J. (1992). Interactive 3D graphics workstations in stereotaxy: Clinical requirements, algorithms and solutions. *In* "Proceedings of the Second Conference on Visualization in Biomedical Computing, Chapel Hill, NC," pp. 548–558.

Griffin, L. D., Colchester, A. C., Robinson, G. P., and Hawkes, D. J. (1992). Structure-sensitive scale and hierarchical segmentation of grey-level images. *In* "Proceedings of the Second Conference on Visualization in Biomedical Computing, Chapel Hill, NC," pp. 24–32.

Haralick, R. M., Sternberg, S. R., and Zhuang, X. (1987). Image analysis using mathematical morphology. *IEEE Trans. Pattern Anal. Machine Intelligence* **9**, 532–550.

Henri, C. J., Cukiert, A., Collins, D. L., Olivier, A., and Peters, T. M. (1992). Towards frameless stereotaxy: Anatomical–vascular correlation and registration. *In* "Proceedings of the Second Conference on Visualization in Biomedical Computing, Chapel Hill, NC," pp. 214–224.

Hill, D. L., Green, S. E., Crossman, J. E., Hawkes, D. J., Robinson, G. P., Ruff, C. F., Cox, T. C., Strong, A. J., and Gleeson, M. J. (1992). Visualization of multi-modal images for the planning of skull base surgery. *In* "Proceedings of the Second Conference on Visualization in Biomedical Computing, Chapel Hill, NC," pp. 564–573.

Höhne, K. H., and Bernstein, R. (1986). Shading 3-D images from CT using grey-level gradients. *IEEE Trans. Med. Imag.* **15**, 45–47.

Höhne, K. H., Bomans, M., Pommert, A., Riemer, M., Tiede, U., *et al.* (1990). Rendering tomographic volume data: Adequacy of methods for different modalities and organs. *In* "3D Imaging in Medicine" (K. H. Höhne, H. Fuchs, and S. M. Pizer, Eds.), NATO ASI Series, Vol. 60, pp. 333–361.

Höhne, K. H., Pommert, A., Riemer, M., Schiemann, T., Schubert, R., and Tiede, U. (1992). Framework for the generation of 3D anatomical atlases. *In* "Proceedings of the Second Conference on Visualization in Biomedical Computing, Chapel Hill, NC," pp. 510–520.

Jack, C. R., Jr., Marsh, W. R., Hirschorn, K. A., Sharbrough, F. W., Cascino, G. D., *et al.*, (1990). Electrophysiologic mapping onto 3-D surface display images of the brain. *Radiology* **176**, 413–418.

Jiang, H., Robb, R. A., and Holton, K. S. (1992). A new approach to 3-D registration of multimodality images by surface matching. *In* "Proceedings of the Second Conference on Visualization in Biomedical Computing, Chapel Hill, NC," pp. 196–213.

Kamber, M., Collins, D. L., Shinghal, R., Francis, G. S., and Evans, A. C. (1992). Model-based 3D segmentation of multiple sclerosis lesions in dual-echo MRI data. *In* "Proceedings of the Second Conference on Visualization in Biomedical Computing, Chapel Hill, NC," pp. 590–600.

Kermode, A. G., Tofts, P. S., Thompson, A. J., MacManus, D. G.,

Rudge, P., *et al.* (1990). Heterogeneity of blood–brain barrier changes in multiple-sclerosis: An MRI study with gadolinium-DTPA enhancement. *Neurology* **40,** 229–235.

Kikinis, R., Cline, H., Altobelli, D., Halle, M., Lorensen, W., and Jolesz, F. A. (1992). Interactive visualization and manipulation of 3D reconstructions for the planning of surgical procedures. *In* "Proceedings of the Second Conference on Visualization in Biomedical Computing, Chapel Hill, NC," pp. 559–563.

Kübler, O., and Gerig, G. (1990). Segmentation and analysis of multidimensional data-sets in medicine. *In* "3D Imaging in Medicine" (K. H. Höhne, H. Fuchs, and S. M. Pizer, Eds.), NATO ASI Series, Vol. 60, pp. 63–81.

Levin, D., Hu, X., Tan, K. K., Galhotra, S., Pelizzari, C. A., *et al.* (1989). The brain: Integrated three-dimensional display of MR and PET images. *Radiology* **172,** 783–789.

Levoy, M. (1988). Display of surfaces from volume data. *Comput. Graphics Appl.* **8**(3), 29–37.

Mohan, R., Barest, F., Brewster, L. J., Chui, C. S., Kutcher, G. J., *et al.* (1988). A comprehensive three-dimensional radiation treatment planning system. *Int. J. Radiat. Oncol. Biol. Phys.* **15,** 481–495.

Pizer, S. M., Cullip, T. J., and Fredericksen, R. E. (1990). Toward interactive object definition in 3D scalar images. *In* "3D Imaging in Medicine" (K. H. Höhne, H. Fuchs, and S. M. Pizer, Eds.), NATO ASI Series, Vol. 60, pp. 83–105.

Robb, R. A. (1988). Multidimensional biomedical image display and analysis in the Biotechnology Computer Resource at the Mayo Clinic. *Machine Vision Appl.* **1,** 75–96.

Robb, R. A. (1990). A software system for interactive and quantitative analysis of biomedical images. *In* "3D Imaging in Medicine" (K. H. Höhne, H. Fuchs, and S. M. Pizer, Eds.), NATO ASI Series, Vol. 60, pp. 333–361.

Robb, R. A., and Barillot, C. (1989). Interactive display and analysis of 3-D medical images. *IEEE Trans. Med. Imag.* **8**(3), 217–226.

Robb, R. A., and Hanson, D. P. (1990). ANALYZE: A software system for biomedical image analysis. *In* "Proceedings of the First Conference on Visualization in Biomedical Computing, Atlanta, GA, May 22–25," pp. 507–518.

Schiemann, T., Bomans, M., Tiede, U., and Höhne, K. H. (1992). Interactive 3D-segmentation. *In* "Proceedings of the Second Conference on Visualization in Biomedical Computing, Chapel Hill, NC," pp. 376–383.

Sherouse, G. W., Bourland, J. D., Reynolds, K., McMurry, H. L., Mitchell, T. P., *et al.* (1990). Virtual simulation in the clinical setting: Some practical considerations. *Int. J. Radiat. Oncol. Biol. Phys.* **19,** 1059–1065.

van den Elsen, P. A., Antoine Maintz, J. B., Pol, E. J., and Viergever, M. A. (1992). Image fusion using geometrical features. *In* "Proceedings of the Second Conference on Visualization in Biomedical Computing, Chapel Hill, NC," pp. 172–186.

Vannier, M. W. (1992). Electronic imaging of the human body. *In* "Proceedings of the Second Conference on Visualization in Biomedical Computing, Chapel Hill, NC," pp. 478–486.

Vincken, K. L., Koster, A. S., and Viergever, M. A. (1992). Probabilistic multiscale image segmentation—Set-up and first results. *In* "Proceedings of the Second Conference on Visualization in Biomedical Computing, Chapel Hill, NC," pp. 63–77.

Waters, K. (1992). A physical model of facial tissue and muscle articulation derived from computer tomography data. *In* "Proceedings of the Second Conference on Visualization in Biomedical Computing, Chapel Hill, NC," pp. 574–583.

18

Intersubject Comparison of PET Activation Data by MRI Matching

J. D. G. Watson*

*Department of Anatomy, University College London, London, United Kingdom, WC1E 6BT;
and MRC Cyclotron Unit, Hammersmith Hospital, London, United Kingdom, W12 0HS*

I. Introduction

In this chapter I show how recent advances in technique have led to significant improvements in the study of individual subjects undergoing positron emission tomography (PET) activation experiments. The major technical advance was the advent of fully three-dimensional (3D) PET scanning, which has led to significant increases in sensitivity. The next advance was the availability of extremely detailed magnetic resonance imaging (MRI), coupled with methods of image coregistration so that individual PET results could be linked with a subject's own MR image. Recent results obtained in normal volunteers have allowed detailed investigation of the structure–function relationship of the cerebral cortex. For the particular experiment that I will describe, this has led to new insights and speculations about a part of the visual cortex previously thought to be a high-level association area.

II. Three-Dimensional PET Scanning

Conventional or 2D PET scanning is an insensitive technique, recovering only 0.5% of the radioactivity administered. International, national, and local regu-

lations on the use of radioactivity ensure that only very small doses are given to individual normal volunteers and that as few individuals as possible are used for experiments. The low sensitivity of conventional PET scanning has been such that meaningful data could not usually be obtained from single subjects, especially if the changes in regional cerebral blood flow (rCBF) were not large. This necessitated the averaging of activations from groups of subjects, in effect spreading a higher radiation dose over a number of subjects. However, the need to average across subjects then presents problems in terms of image alignment and transformation and in the use of atlases and coordinates to report results.

Conventional scanners have collimating septa, of lead or tungsten, placed in front of the detector crystals at the junctions between detector rings. These septa reduce the acceptance angle of the crystals in recording the two coincident photons emitted in opposite directions by the decay of each positron (Fig. 1). Developments in scanner design, acquisition hardware, reconstruction algorithms, and computing power were combined in the manufacture of the first commercially available 3D PET scanner (Siemens–CTI 953B; CTI, Inc., Knoxville, TN) in which the septa were fully retractable, the prototype model being installed at the MRC Cyclotron Unit in London. By increasing the acceptance angle so that all pairs of crystals were able to record coincident events, the point source sensitivity was increased some six to seven times (Bailey *et al.*, 1991). In practice, there is a three-

---

* Present address: Department of Medicine, The University of Sydney, New South Wales, Australia, 2006

FUNCTIONAL NEUROIMAGING

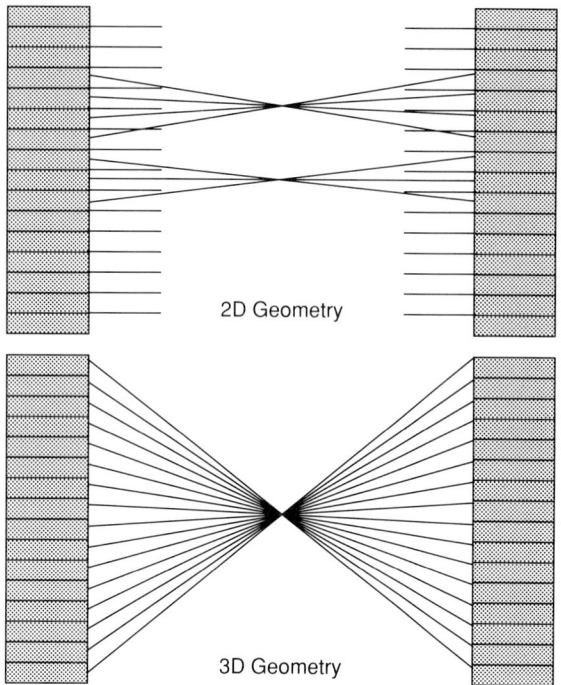

Figure 1 The planes contributing to 2D and 3D PET images are shown for the 16-ring Siemens-CTI 953B camera. In the 2D case, the image planes are built up from the detected coincident events from either three detector rings (odd-numbered planes) or four detector rings (even-numbered planes). In the 3D case, with the septa removed, any pair of rings may be in coincidence. Adapted from Bailey (1992).

fold increase in useful counts over the whole brain and a fivefold increase at the center of the field of view (Bailey *et al.*, 1991). The main drawback is an increase in scattered radiation, which results in the technique not being absolutely quantitative at the time of writing. However, the hope, ultimately borne out, was that the increase in sensitivity of 3D scanning would more than overcome such drawbacks (Townsend *et al.*, 1991). Less radiation is needed per scan and therefore more scans can be performed in each subject. By averaging more scans for each stimulus, the data quality is improved, so that the ability to detect and localize areas of activation in single subjects is enhanced greatly. In summary, it is as if five times more radiation could be given to each subject.

III. MRI Acquisition and Coregistration

PET images are low in spatial resolution and do not highlight cerebral landmarks. MRI is dramatically better at revealing the details of cerebral anatomy, achieving resolutions previously undreamed of. Other participants have discussed how such MR im-

ages may enhance lower resolution PET images. These include the coregistration of images across modalities for structure–function analysis (Chapters 23, 14, and 25) and the use of MRI to make partial volume corrections of PET images (Chapter 15). Soon it should be possible to use MR images to enhance PET images, by using a maximum likelihood approach to their reconstruction. Perhaps MR images could also be used to improve the attenuation process in PET image reconstruction.

By the end of 1991, the MRC Cyclotron Unit in London was able to obtain good quality images from the newly installed MR machine at Hammersmith Hospital (a 1-T Picker HPQ Vista system). After some trials, a sequence was developed that gave relatively spin-lattice time (T_1)-weighted images with good gray/white contrast and anatomical resolution. A radiofrequency spoiled volume acquisition was made [repeat time (T_R), 24 ms; echo time (T_E), 6 ms; nonselective excitation with a flip angle of 35°; field of view in plane, 25 × 25 cm; 192 × 256 in plane matrix with 128 secondary phase encoding steps oversampled to 256; resolution, 1.3 × 1.3 × 1.5 mm; total imaging time, 20 min].

For each subject, an average PET image was made from the 12 realigned scans obtained in the experiment. Then a rigid body coregistration with the MRI scan was performed using the Automated Image Realignment (AIR) software originally developed for PET-to-PET realignment (Woods *et al.*, 1992), adapted for MRI–PET matching (Woods *et al.*, 1993), and kindly made available by the authors. With the current sets of data, an average PET–MRI coregistration takes about 15 min to run on a SPARC 2 workstation (Sun Computers Europe, Inc., Surrey, UK); the only user interaction needed is the segmentation of the high MRI signal found particularly in the scalp, a signal that has no equivalent in the PET images. In validation studies, the mean three-dimensional error in the alignment of the two images was less than 2 mm, with maximum errors of less than 3 mm (Woods *et al.*, 1993). The reorientation parameters in terms of translations and rotations were calculated by the software and were used to coregister the PET-based images of significant rCBF change (which contain little overall anatomical information) with the subject's MR image.

IV. The PET Experiment

A. Aims

For the past four years, the collaborative group set up by Professor Semir Zeki of University College London and Professor Richard Frackowiak at the

MRC Cyclotron Unit has been studying the process of vision in normal human subjects. By using PET and visual stimuli for color or motion, the respective positions of areas V4 and V5 had been identified (Zeki *et al.*, 1991). These experiments had been done by averaging groups of subjects using a PET camera in conventional 2D mode. However, subsequent experiments that should have involved V5, an area outside the V1/V2 complex on the occipitotemporal border, suggested variability in its position. It seemed likely that the position of area V5 would vary from one individual to the next, especially as the calcarine sulcus, a major landmark in the occipital lobe, is also markedly variable in position even after stereotaxic normalization to the AC–PC line (Talairach *et al.*, 1967; Belliveau *et al.*, 1991). It was also quite possible that some of the variation merely reflected the difficulties of stereotaxic manipulation. First, the AC–PC line is a short baseline at the center of the brain and in simple geometric terms is not ideal for mapping cortical structures, particularly those lying a long way from it. Second, the occipital lobe seems more variable than the rest of the brain in terms of the relationship of its major structure, the calcarine sulcus, to the AC–PC line. Last, it seems likely that all stereotaxic methods will themselves introduce some variation to the relocation of analogous parts of different brains, which is another way of saying that stereotaxic normalization is a difficult thing to get right!

With all these caveats, there remained the most tantalizing possibility: that there might be a relationship of the functionally defined area V5 to cortical landmarks of each individual brain and that, as these landmarks varied among individuals, so would area V5. Even if such a relationship did exist, to attempt to demonstrate it was rather an exercise in speculation. No one doubts that there are functional properties related to the surface markings of the brain: the calcarine sulcus marks the horizontal border of the visual field for the striate cortex; the Rolandic sulcus marks a useful division between sensory and motor cortices. These relationships all lie in what is thought of as "primary" cortex, with deep, fairly easily recognized sulci, but V5 lies at the occipitotemporal border in areas thought of as "association" cortex and in which the sulcal pattern seemed anything but constant.

To address the issue of individual variability, a group of 12 subjects performing a visual motion task was studied, by means of 3D PET scans and high-resolution MR imaging. The experiment is described fully elsewhere (Watson *et al.*, 1993); I will concentrate on its most important aspects.

B. Methods

1. PET Scans

There were 9 male and 3 female subjects aged from 21 to 70 years (mean and SD, 43 $\pm$ 17 years). All subjects gave informed written consent. The studies were approved by the Hammersmith Hospital Medical Ethics Committee and permission to administer radioactivity was obtained from the Administration of Radioactive Substances Advisory Committee of the Department of Health, United Kingdom.

All subjects had 12 PET scans in a single 3-h session, each scan providing images of relative rCBF, which was measured by recording the distribution of cerebral radioactivity following the intravenous injection of the positron emitting ^{15}O-labeled tracer, water ($H_2{}^{15}O$). Changes in rCBF were used as a marker of the local synaptic activity in response to the visual stimuli (Raichle, 1987). Each rCBF measurement was made over the course of 3 min. There were 12 min between scans to allow for the decay of radioactivity to background levels. The integrated counts accumulated over each scan, corrected for background activity, were used as the index of relative rCBF (Mazziotta *et al.*, 1985; Fox and Mintun, 1989). On average, each subject received 1014 MBq or 27.4 mCi of $H_2{}^{15}O$ for each of the 12 scans.

The rCBF was compared in two states of stimulation, using

Stimulus A: Eyes open, with the subject viewing a high-resolution monitor, at a distance of 37 cm. The display covered the central 30° of the visual field vertically and 40° horizontally and consisted of a stationary, random array of approximately 600 small black squares each subtending 1°, displayed on a white background.

Stimulus B: Eyes open, with the same display moving in one of eight directions that changed randomly every 5 s in 45° steps from 0° to 315°. The small squares moved *en bloc* at a speed of six squares s^{-1}.

When the display was stationary, subjects were asked to fixate a target square at the center of the screen. For the moving display, the subjects fixated a stationary target square at the center. The two stimuli were alternated from scan to scan and were identical in terms of brightness and contrast.

The CTI 953B PET scanner has 16 rings of crystal detectors covering an axial field of view of 10.65 cm. A transmission scan was used to correct the emission data for the attenuating effects of the tissues of the head. The scans were then reconstructed as 31 axial planes by filtered back projection with a Hanning filter of a cutoff frequency of 0.5 cycles pixel^{-1}. The resolution of the resulting images was $8.5 \times 8.5 \times 4.3$ mm at full width, half-maximum (FWHM) (Spinks *et al.*, 1992). Each plane was displayed in a 128- $\times$ 128-pixel format, with a pixel size of 2.09×2.09 mm. The 31 original planes were transformed by interpolation to 43 planes, to produce images with approximately cubic voxels.

2. Image Transformations

All calculations and image manipulations were carried out on SPARC computers, using ANALYZE Version 5 image display software (BRU, Mayo Foundation, Rochester, MN) and PROMATLAB (MathWorks, Inc., Natick, MA). Statistical maps of significant blood flow changes were then derived using SPM software (MRC Cyclotron Unit, London, UK).

For each subject, any head movement between any 2 of the 12 scans was corrected by aligning them all with the first one, using AIR software (Woods *et al.*, 1992). Then the intercommissural (AC–PC) line, linking the anterior and posterior commissures, was identified automatically. All the images were then transformed (Friston *et al.*, 1991a) into the standard anatomical space of the stereotaxic atlas of Talairach and Tournoux (1988), which uses this line as its reference point. For the coregistration of individual PET and MR images, the PET images were not transformed into stereotaxic space.

The PET images were all filtered with a relatively small low-pass Gaussian filter (FWHM of approximately $10 \times 10 \times 10$ mm) to smooth the data in three dimensions (Friston *et al.*, 1990). This served to increase the signal-to-noise ratio by attenuating the high-frequency noise in the images and by augmenting the effects of image averaging across subjects, when performed.

3. Statistical Analysis

We used the technique of statistical parametric mapping (SPM) for data analysis (Friston and Frackowiak, 1991). The confounding effect of global flow changes was corrected by performing a pixel-based analysis of the covariance (ANCOVA) of rCBF against relative global CBF, the latter being treated as the confounding covariate (Friston *et al.*, 1990). For group analysis, the ANCOVA calculated mean values of rCBF for each experimental condition across the subjects (with the global CBF adjusted to 50 ml dl^{-1} min^{-1}) together with the associated error variance, for each pixel. Twelve means and associated variances were thus determined by pooling the data for each comparable scan across all subjects.

Finally, the difference between the mean values of rCBF obtained for each of the two visual conditions

was evaluated for each pixel by use of the t statistic. This generated a statistical parametric map (SPM[t]) of the areas of significant rCBF change associated with the difference in the tasks. On such an SPM[t], only pixels whose significance values exceeded a certain threshold were displayed. This threshold could be set to correct for the effective number of independent tests, which is less than the actual number of pixels because neighboring pixels are not truly independent. The stereotaxic coordinates of the most significant sites of change were determined and then related to the standard atlas (Talairach and Tournoux, 1988).

A similar procedure was used for analyzing the pattern of rCBF change in individual subjects. The SPM[t] was noisier than for the group as the comparison involved $\frac{1}{12}$ the data. Hence, a secondary Gaussian smoothing filter of 4 mm FWHM was applied to the SPM[t] in the x and y dimensions. The effect of this filter was a small change in the in-plane resolution, on average from 9.9 to 10.7 mm FWHM.

The average location of significant areas of change obtained from the group analysis of the 12 subjects was used to direct the search for the location of area V5 in individuals, i.e., for a bilateral prestriate area in the anterolateral parts of the occipital lobe in which cortical activation by visual motion might be expected. A search radius was set, within which activation foci could be considered as belonging to V5 in any given individual. An arbitrary radius of 15 mm was chosen, 1.5 times the FWHM of the primary smoothing filter. The distance was larger than the primary smoothing filter, otherwise an individual site of V5 far enough away from the mean to contribute little or nothing to that mean position might be excluded; but too large a distance would include areas such as the V1/V2 complex not believed to be candidates for the location of V5 in individuals. An activation was accepted as significant and belonging to V5 if it appeared on at least three contiguous axial planes. The location of the pixel with the most significant statistical score was taken to be the center of V5.

Thus, by examining a limited area of the brain, omnibus statistical testing could be used. In fact, all individual brains were tested first at the harshest threshold, $p < 0.05$, corrected for multiple nonindependent comparisons (a Z score of about 3.8). If no significant activation could be found in the searched region, the threshold was next lowered to $p < 0.001$, without a correction for multiple comparisons (a Z score of 3.09), and if necessary to a threshold of $p < 0.01$ (a Z score of 2.33).

For the coregistration of the untransformed PET and MR images obtained from individual brains, the same statistical analysis was used. The SPM[t] was then coregistered with the subject's own MRI scan, using the transformation parameters as determined above. Superimposition of the images showed the position of significant rCBF changes in relation to the gyral and sulcal pattern of that brain, thus to determine if there was any consistent relationship between the two.

C. Results

1. Group and Subgroups

I will discuss only the results for area V5, but should point out that other areas of the brain were active in this experiment (Watson *et al.*, 1993). The group of 12 subjects was analyzed as a whole, and selected subgroups of 6 were also taken. This was aimed at determining what variation there would be in the site and extent of rCBF change for area V5 with subject numbers often used for PET activation studies.

As before (Zeki *et al.*, 1991), there was an area on each lateral occipital surface associated with the perception of visual motion, felt to represent the human motion area, V5. Plate 53 shows the highly significant foci of increased rCBF induced in the 12 subjects when looking at the moving display. The average relative increase in rCBF in a 10-mm-diameter spherical region of interest centered on the pixels of most highly significant change was 4.7%. The Talairach and Tournoux coordinates show that human area V5 is located ventrolaterally at the confluence of the occipital and temporal lobes, corresponding with the inferior junction of Brodmann's areas 19 and 37.

The 12 subjects provided 72 measurements in each of the two states and thus represent a large sample size. Most studies use smaller samples. How representative would be results obtained from such smaller groups? Different subgroups of 6 subjects were taken from the whole group, and the variation in the location and extent of rCBF changes of human area V5 was determined. It was not practicable to test all 924 possible combinations of 6 from 12, but limiting cases were chosen deliberately to maximize the potential variability in position and blood flow change of V5. It was found that in a group study of only 6 subjects, drawn from a population of 12, the position of the most significant pixel of V5 in stereotaxic coordinates could vary by as much as 13 mm. Group blood flow increases recorded in response to a moving stimulus could range from 3.4 to 6.3%.

2. Individual Subjects

After stereotaxic normalization, the position of the most significant pixel corresponding to V5 in the left hemisphere varied more than that on the right, the ranges being 27 and 18 mm, respectively. There was a mean rCBF increase of 3.9 ml dl^{-1} min^{-1} in the left V5 areas (range, 1.4 to 5.4 ml dl^{-1} min^{-1}). In the right hemisphere, the mean increase was 3.7 ml dl^{-1} min^{-1} (range, 2.3 to 5.7 ml dl^{-1} min^{-1}). In relative terms the mean increases were 7.1% on the left (range, 2.6 to 9.6%) and 7.2% on the right (range, 4.2 to 11.5%).

Seventeen of the twenty-four V5 areas were significant at the harshest threshold of $p < 0.05$ (corrected for multiple comparisons), with Z scores from 3.86 to as high as 8.52. Six areas were significant in the next lower range, with Z scores of 3.09 to 3.66. In only one case did the threshold have to be lowered further in order to detect area V5 (a threshold of $0.001 < p < 0.01$, with a Z score of 2.46). As the area of search for V5 was constrained, these statistical thresholds may be considered unnecessarily harsh, but it is worth observing that the 17 V5 areas identified at the harshest level could have been reported in their own right, with no prior knowledge of their likely positions (Friston *et al.*, 1991b). Even for the single V5 result that was found at the lowest statistical threshold, no new areas appeared elsewhere in the brain that had not been identified in other subjects.

3. Coregistration of PET Results with MRI

The coregistration of PET SPM[t] images obtained from each subject's brain with the MRI scans obtained from the same brain allowed a description of the location of the activated areas in relation to the sulcal and gyral pattern of the occipital lobe within each brain, more precisely than had been previously possible (Plate 54 and Fig. 2). The pattern of the sulci in the occipital lobe was variable, and the consistency of their relationship to area V5 is discussed below.

V. Discussion

A. Group versus Individual Studies

The location of V5 in Talairach coordinates was determined in each individual using the same image realignment and stereotaxic normalization as the group analysis. For these subjects, the variation in position of V5 was 27 mm on the left and 18 mm on the right. The greater variation on the left may reflect known brain asymmetries, particularly in the region of the posterior temporal lobe (Galaburda, 1984). Subgroup analysis demonstrated that even groups of six subjects tested with an identical experimental paradigm could have mean locations for V5 that differed from each other by as much as 13 mm, close to the breadth of some cerebral gyri.

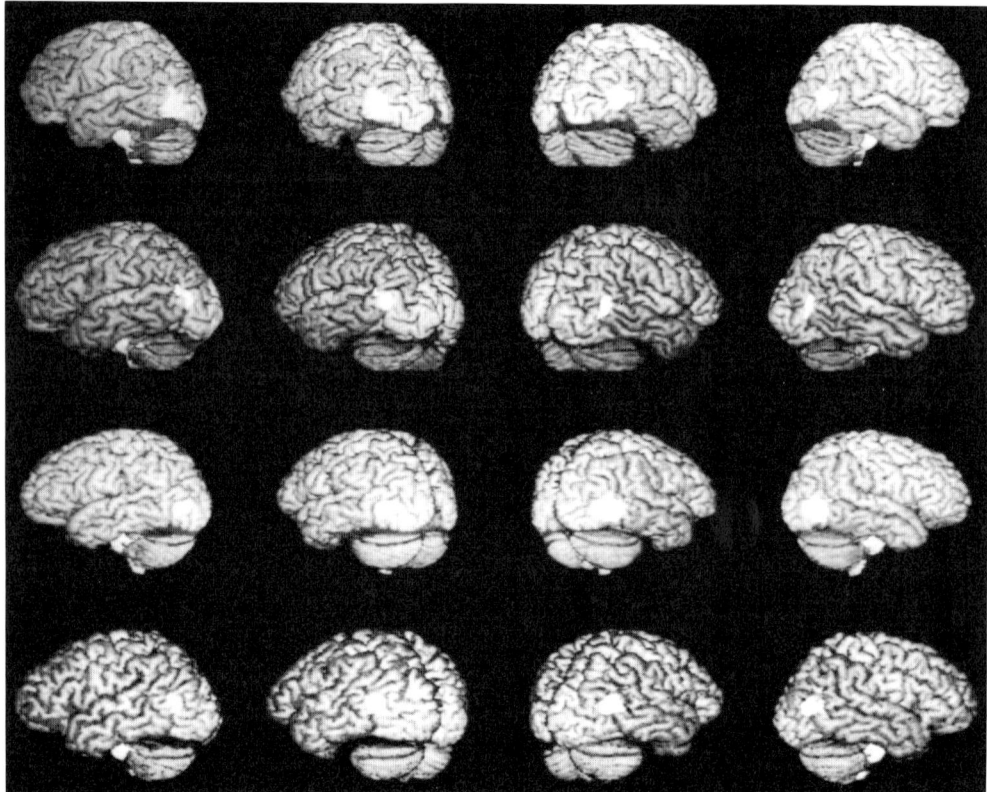

Figure 2 Data from four subjects, showing each V5 area as defined by the PET activation experiments, superimposed on the individual's own MR image. Each subject occupies a row. The images were derived from data such as those presented in Plate 54 (now shown in the top row of this figure), but are now displayed as surface-rendered objects viewed at rotations of 90° and 50° from the occipital pole, to allow the patterns of sulci and gyri to be seen. In each subject the PET SPM[*t*] image was edited to leave only V5, and the statistical threshold was lowered so that the PET image was contiguous with the cortical surface of the MRI after the PET and MR images were coregistered and superimposed, so that the process of surface rendering (to a depth of some eight pixels) correctly locates the site of V5 in terms of surface features. The PET activation sites were rendered as the bright white areas on the final images. From Watson *et al.* (1993).

In individuals, the increase in rCBF for V5 ranged from 2.6 to 11.5%, with a mean of 7.1% on the left and 7.2% on the right. When the 12 subjects were incorporated into a single group for analysis, the increase was 4.7% on each side. The subgroup analysis showed that relative increses in blood flow reported for V5 could vary from 3.4 to 6.3%. rCBF changes in averaged group data will be smaller than those recorded in individuals because of the combination of spatial filtering (which reduces the peaks of rCBF change) and the variation in the location of V5 across individuals, such that the anatomical transformation into Talairach coordinates fails to superimpose the foci from different individuals onto one another.

Should one study groups or individuals? This issue is also discussed elsewhere in this volume (Chapter 25). The answer must be to do both, as each approach provides important information, but each has limita-

tions. The very low sensitivity of conventional PET was the original rationale behind using averaged groups. Grouped data highlight the most significant and commonplace activation sites but sacrifice the individual patterns of activation and thus lose the important lessons that these patterns must contain. The referencing of grouped results to standard stereotaxic coordinates makes it easier to compare results obtained with different paradigms, in different laboratories, and with different groups of subjects (Chapter 9). However, the subgroup analysis indicated that the typically small PET subject groups must make the reporting of results in terms of standard stereotaxic coordinates uncertain. In the subgroup analysis subject selection was the only variable, and even this showed that activation sites may vary by the width of a gyrus. Thus the method of standardized coordinates is uncertain and limited, especially in relating the site of activation to the genuine anatomy of the cerebral cortex. Even if the coordinates were certain, relocating them onto the single brain used in the Talairach and Tournoux (1988) system will be valid only as far as that brain, measured in the postmortem and fixed state, reflects the actual anatomy of the individuals that made up a PET study group.

These drawbacks were addressed by the use of the increased sensitivity of 3D PET scanning to obtain results with greater statistical confidence, which were then coregistered with MR images. The sites of activation could thus be directly related to the anatomy of the cerebral cortex. But individual results alone were insufficient: for example, this study used the position of V5 defined in the analysis of the whole group as the basis on which to search for V5 in each individual. Thus both approaches have a role, the one for the screening of the cerebral areas involved in the execution of a task and the other for a more detailed study of the areas in relation to the anatomy of the brain.

B. V5 Is Related to Cortical Landmarks

Coregistration of the PET and MR images allowed an examination of the position of V5 according to individual brain structure, by using both two- and three-dimensional reconstructions (Plate 54 and Fig. 2). These images identified the pattern of sulci and gyri in the occipital lobes of each subject and demonstrated that there was a relationship of area V5 to the sulcal and gyral pattern of the occipital lobe of the human brain.

Clear structure–function relationships in the human occipital lobe have been known for many years [see Horton and Hoyt (1991a, 1991b) for new insights into some classical concepts]. Although it was plausible that such relationships could be found elsewhere in the occipital lobe, the sulcal and gyral anatomy of the lateral occipital lobe is quite varied.

The most useful landmark for identifying the position of area V5 was a sulcus present in most brains, running vertically at the border between the temporal and occipital lobes. It was identified by Cunningham (1902) as the *ascending limb of the inferior temporal sulcus* (ALITS) and is also known as the *anterior occipital sulcus*. It meets the horizontal *inferior* or *lateral occipital sulcus* almost at right angles. In 16 of the 24 hemispheres studies, the ALITS and the inferior lateral sulcus were easily identified, and in the remainder there were less well-formed sulci taking their direction. V5 lay on or posterior to the ALITS, at its junction with the inferior occipital sulcus and therefore at the confluence of the occipital and temporal lobes. This location for V5 has been previously implicated in humans in non-PET studies. Clarke and Miklossy (1990)

used two criteria: one related the position of the prestriate areas to the pattern of callosal distribution within that zone of cortex, because cortical areas have a definite relationship to strips of callosally connected cortex (Zeki, 1977a; 1977b), and the other related to the pattern of myelination within the prestriate cortex. The same region was compromised in the akinetopsic patient described by Zihl *et al.* (1983, 1991), although the lesions found were not confined to it.

C. Speculations on Why V5 Should Be Related to Particular Sulci

To me the most interesting aspect of the location for V5 is that it coincides almost exactly with *Feld 16* of Flechsig (1920), in what he calls the *gyrus subangularis* (Fig. 3). Flechsig studied the patterns of myelina-

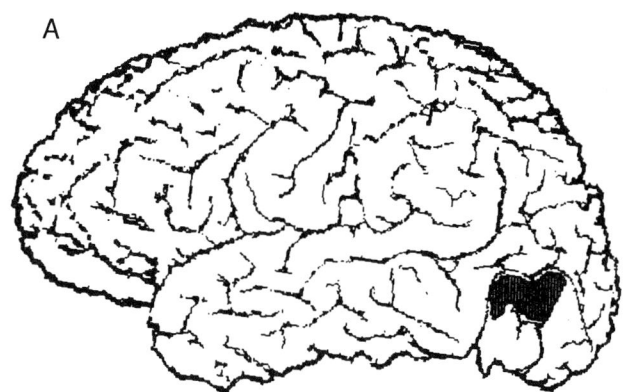

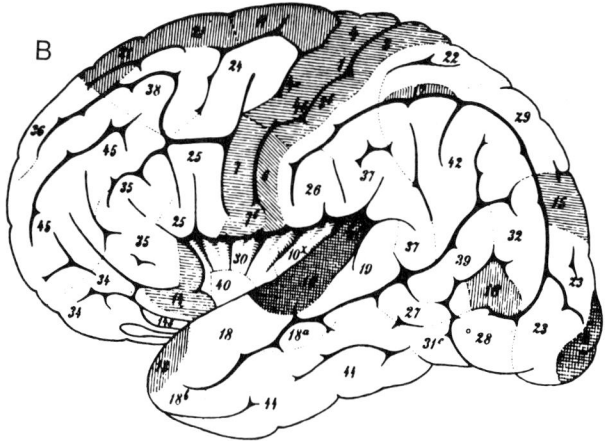

Figure 3 (A) Lateral view of the brain from one subject with a surface rendition of the position of area V5. This is the hatched area lying behind the ascending limb of the inferior temporal sulcus, also known as the anterior occipital sulcus, and above the inferior occipital sulcus. (B) Flechsig's diagram of the myeloarchitecture of the human brain. Note the position of *Feld 16*, corresponding closely with area V5 of the subject. From Watson *et al.* (1993).

tion of the cortex and is mostly responsible for the concept of primary and association areas. *Feld 16* belonged to cortex myelinated at birth, although not as heavily myelinated as certain other areas (his *Felds 1 to 10*), among which he numbers the calcarine cortex (area V1). In conjunction with the present results, which place area V5 in the same position as *Feld 16*, it seems highly likely that V5 is well demarcated in terms of its myelination, callosal connections, and functional properties from birth or before: embryological atlases often show the ALITS forming by 30 weeks [see Fig. 7 of von Bonin and Bailey (1951)]. Clarke and Miklossy (1990) showed that in V5 the heavy subcortical myelination pattern and callosal fibers lie along the superior wall of the inferior occipital sulcus. It is tempting to speculate that the microscopic features that are indicators of V5 are themselves involved in the formation of a landmark sulcus during fetal development, by the induction of differential growth patterns. This may be the link between structure and function, at least for area V5, and perhaps it was good fortune that this was the first prestriate area chosen for such detailed analysis.

In view of its early myelination, the argument can be sustained that V5 more rightfully belongs to "primary" than "association" cortex. One should always be careful in appealing to teleology but it is plausible that a motion detecting cortical area should function well in the newborn or soon thereafter. Further experiments could be designed to test these speculations, which have arisen because of advances in PET methodology and through the coregistration of PET images with high-resolution MR images.

Acknowledgment

The studies reported in this chapter were supported by the Wellcome Trust, through a grant held by Professor S. Zeki, FRS, of University College, London.

References

Bailey, D. L. (1992). 3D acquisition and reconstruction in positron emission tomography. *Ann. Nucl. Med.* **6**, 123–130.

Bailey, D. L., Jones, T., and Spinks, T. J. (1991). A method for measuring the absolute sensitivity of positron emission tomographic scanners. *Eur. J. Nucl. Med.* **18**, 374–379.

Bailey, D. L., Jones, T., Spinks, T. J., Gilardi, M.-C., and Townsend, D. W. (1991). Noise equivalent count measurements in a neuro-PET scanner with retractable septa. *IEEE Trans. Med. Imag.* **10**, 256–260.

Bailey, P., and von Bonin, G. (1951). "The Isocortex of Man." Urbana: University of Illinois Press.

Belliveau, J. W., Kennedy, D. N., McKinstry, R. C., Buchbinder, B. R., Weisskoff, R. M., Cohen, M. S., Vevea, J. M., Brady, T. J., and Rosen, B. R. (1991). Functional mapping of the human visual cortex by magnetic resonance imaging. *Science* **254**, 716–719.

Clarke, S., and Miklossy, J. (1990). Occipital cortex in man: organization of callosal connections, related myelo- and cytoarchitecture, and putative boundaries of functional visual areas. *J. Comp. Neurol.* **298**, 188–214.

Cunningham, D. J. (1902). "Text-book of Anatomy." Edinburgh, London: Y. T. Pentland.

Flechsig, P. (1920). "Anatomie des menschlichen Gehirns und Rückenmarks." Leipzig: Thieme.

Fox, P. T., and Mintun, M. A. (1989). Noninvasive functional brain mapping by change-distribution analysis of averaged PET images of $H_2^{15}O$ tissue activity. *J. Nucl. Med.* **30**, 141–149.

Friston, K. J., and Frackowiak, R. S. J. (1991). Imaging functional anatomy. In "Brain Work and Mental Activity: Quantitative Studies with Radioactive Tracers" (N. A. Lassen, D. H. Ingvar, M. E. Raichle, and L. Friberg, Eds.), pp. 267–279. Copenhagen: Munskgaard.

Friston, K. J., Frith, C. D., Liddle, P. F., Dolan, R. J., Lammertsma, A. A., and Frackowiak, R. S. J. (1990). The relationship between global and local changes in PET scans. *J. Cereb. Blood Flow Metab.* **10**, 458–466.

Friston, K. J., Frith, C. D., Liddle, P. F., and Frackowiak, R. S. J. (1991a). Plastic transformation of PET images. *J. Comput. Assist. Tomogr.* **15**, 634–639.

Friston, K. J., Frith, C. D., Liddle, P. F., and Frackowiak, R. S. J. (1991b). Comparing functional (PET) images: The assessment of significant change. *J. Cereb. Blood Flow Metab.* **11**, 690–699.

Galaburda, A. M. (1984). Anatomical asymmetries. In "Cerebral Dominance: The Biological Foundations" (N. Geschwind and A. M. Galaburda, Eds.), pp. 11–25. Cambridge, MA: Harvard University Press.

Horton, J. C., and Hoyt, W. F. (1991a). Quadrantic visual field defects: A hallmark of lesions in extrastriate cortex (V2/V3). *Brain* **114**, 1703–1718.

Horton, J. C., and Hoyt, W. F. (1991b). The representation of the visual field in human striate cortex. *Arch. Ophthalmol.* **109**, 816–824.

Mazziotta, J. C., Huang, S. C., Phelps, M. E., Carson, R. E., MacDonald, N. S., and Mahoney, K. (1985). A non-invasive positron computed tomography technique using oxygen-15 labeled water for the evaluation of neurobehavioral task batteries. *J. Cereb. Blood Flow Metab.* **5**, 70–78.

Raichle, M. E. (1987). Circulatory and metabolic correlates of brain function in normal humans. In "Handbook of Physiology: The Nervous System" (F. Plum, Ed.), Vol. 5, pp. 643–674. New York: American Physiology Society/Oxford University Press.

Spinks, T. J., Jones, T., Bailey, D. L., Townsend, D. W., Grootoonk, S., Bloomfield, P. M., Gilardi, M.-C., Casey, M. E., Sipe, B., and Reed, J. (1992). Physical performance of a positron tomograph for brain imaging with retractable septa. *Phys. Med. Biol.* **8**, 1637–1655.

Talairach, J., Szikla, G., Tournoux, P., Prossalentis, A., Bordas-Ferrer, M., Covello, L., Iacob, M., and Mempel, E. (1967). "Atlas of Stereotaxic Anatomy of the Telencephalon: Anatomo-Radiological Studies," p. 211. Paris: Masson.

Talairach, J., and Tournoux, P. (1988). "Co-Planar Stereotaxic Atlas of the Human Brain." Stuttgart/New York: Thieme.

Townsend, D. W., Geissbuhler, A., Defrise, M., Hoffman, E. J., Spinks, T. J., Bailey, D. L., Gilardi, M.-C., and Jones, T. (1991). Fully three-dimensional reconstruction for a PET camera with retractable septa. *IEEE Trans. Med. Imag.* **10**, 505–512.

Watson, J. D. G., Myers, R., Frackowiak, R. S. J., Hajnal, J. V., Woods, R. P., Mazziotta, J. C., Shipp, S., and Zeki, S. (1993).

Area V5 of the human brain: evidence from a combined study using positron emission tomography and magnetic resonance imaging. *Cereb. Cortex* **3,** 79–94.

Woods, R. P., Cherry, S. R., and Mazziotta, J. C. (1992). A rapid automated algorithm for accurately aligning and reslicing positron emission tomography images. *J. Comput. Assist. Tomogr.* **16,** 620–633.

Woods, R. P., Mazziotta, J. C., and Cherry, S. R. (1993). MRI–PET registration with automated algorithm. *J. Comput. Assist. Tomogr.,* **17,** 536–546.

Zeki, S. M. (1977a). Colour coding in the superior temporal sulcus of the rhesus monkey visual cortex. *Proc. R. Soc. London (Biol.)* **197,** 195–223.

Zeki, S. M. (1977b). Simultaneous anatomical demonstration of the vertical and horizontal meridians in areas V2 and V3 of rhesus monkey visual cortex. *Proc. R. Soc. London (Biol.)* **195,** 517–523.

Zeki, S., Watson, J. D. G., Lueck, C. J., Friston, K. J., Kennard, C., and Frackowiak, R. S. J. (1991). A direct demonstration of functional specialization in human visual cortex. *J. Neurosci.* **11,** 641–649.

Zihl, J., von Cramon, D., and Mai, N. (1983). Selective disturbance of movement vision after bilateral brain damage. *Brain* **106,** 313–340.

Zihl, J., von Cramon, D., Mai, D., and Schmid, Ch. (1991). Disturbance of movement vision after bilateral posterior brain damage: Further evidence and follow up observations. *Brain* **114,** 2235–2252.

19

MRI-Based Topographic Segmentation

David N. Kennedy,* James W. Meyer, Pauline A. Filipek, and
Verne S. Caviness, Jr.

*Center for Morphometric Analysis, Departments of Neurology and *Radiology, Massachusetts General
Hospital, Harvard Medical School, Boston, Massachusetts 02214*

I. Introduction

The brain possesses anatomically discrete processing regions. A complete understanding of brain function requires determination of *where* these sites are located, *what* operations are performed, and *how* distributed processing is organized (Zeki *et al.*, 1991). Changes in neuronal activity are accompanied by focal changes in cerebral blood flow (Fox *et al.*, 1986), blood volume (Fox and Raichle, 1986; Belliveau *et al.*, 1991), blood oxygenation (Fox and Raichle, 1986; Fox *et al.*, 1988), and metabolism (Phelps *et al.*, 1981; Prichard *et al.*, 1991). These physiological changes can be used to produce functional maps of component mental operations. By measuring these physiological changes and correlating them with behavior, we can study the relationship between anatomical structure and behavioral function.

One goal of functional cerebral imaging studies is to provide quantitative data on the location and temporal orchestration of component mental operations participating in a given cognitive or behavioral state. The analysis of location requires the understanding of brain anatomy in the individual as well as its variation across populations of individuals. As the resolving power of functional imaging methods increases, the need for precision in anatomic analysis also increases. Any method used to treat interindividual differences will yield results only as spatially accurate as the residual, unaccounted anatomic variability (Talairach and

Tournoux, 1988; Steinmetz *et al.*, 1989). Thus, it is necessary to develop new methods of anatomic analysis that can be applied repeatedly and reliably in normal subjects in order to expand the spatiotemporal window of *in vivo* brain investigation.

With this in mind, the purpose of this report is to review an anatomic analysis hierarchy that is completely supported by the information contained within high-resolution magnetic resonance imaging (MRI) and is applicable on an individual basis. It forms a fundamental groundwork for the subsequent application of increasingly advanced methods of intersubject analysis.

Over the years, the methods for making observations regarding human brain structure and function have changed dramatically. On the one hand, the most detailed method of structural assessment comes from the analysis of the postmortem brain sample. It is in this analysis only that exact identification of cyto- and myeloarchitectonic structure can be systematically assessed at a microscopic level of spatial resolution. On the other hand, *in vivo* methods are necessary for a practical approach to structural analysis that can be applied to statistically significant numbers of subjects (Caviness *et al.*, 1989).

II. Structural Description Hierarchy

The functional and structural neuroanatomist conceives of the brain in a hierarchical fashion as a function of spatial and temporal scales. Temporal analysis

FUNCTIONAL NEUROIMAGING

of brain function spans a time scale of events from that requiring an entire lifetime to the firing of a single neuron, which requires only a fraction of a millisecond (Churchland and Sejnowski, 1988). The structural scale spans the perspective from the whole brain to the single synapse. In a general sense, complete understanding of the brain requires knowledge about operations occurring across all of the spatial and temporal scales. Thus it is important to push the spatial and temporal limits of our available imaging technology toward the fastest and smallest limits.

State-of-the-art magnetic resonance imaging provides a degree of anatomic detail that provides an excellent foundation upon which to base correlative studies of structure and function. Our approach is to use this window of MRI-defined topology to establish a hierarchy of anatomic description that spans from the *whole brain* level to the *systems* level description. Anatomic segmentation and cortical localization analysis (parcellation) are important for the interpretation of functional neuroimaging data and are a precursor for intersubject comparison techniques. In the following sections, we will describe a methodology based upon high-resolution, volumetric MR images that spans anatomic segmentation to callosal-based (lobar) and cortical subparcellation methodologies.

III. Methods and Results

In this section, we will present both the general methodology and example applications of the positional normalization, structural segmentation, callosal parcellation, and cortical parcellation in use in our laboratory.

A. Image Acquisition

The following qualities are essential in image data for structural analysis: (1) the image data must faithfully represent the spatial and geometric relationships of the brain, (2) they must convey accurate anatomic information, and (3) they must be acquirable in a reasonable amount of imaging time. For the analyses to be reported here, we have acquired coronal, volumetric T_1-weighted actively spoiled gradient echo MRI scans with the following parameters: TR, 40 ms; TE, 8 ms; flip angle, 40°; field of view, 24 cm; slice thickness, 3.0 mm; matrix, 256 × 256 × 64; and averages, 1. This imaging sequence provides an acceptable basis for morphometric and structural analysis (Filipek *et al.*, 1989, 1993; Caviness *et al.*, 1989).

B. Positional Normalization

To optimize the criteria for delimiting anatomic structures across multiple scans, a technique for ensuring standardized orientation and anatomic presentation, *positional normalization*, of the MRI scans has been developed. This involves reformatting and reslicing the volumetric image data in accordance with the coronal orientation described for the Talairach atlas (Talairach and Tournoux, 1988). The standard points of reference include the midpoints of the decussations of the anterior commissure (AC) and posterior commissure (PC) and the midpoint of the genu of the corpus callosum (to define the interhemispheric plane). We choose the origin of a new coordinate system to be located at the midpoint of the AC–PC line segment. Thus, we have a Cartesian coordinate system defined as x axis increasing laterally from the subjects right to left, y axis increasing from posterior to anterior, and z axis increasing from superior to inferior (xy, transaxial; xz, coronal; and yz, sagittal orientations). By selection of these reference points and a coordinate system, we can define the image transformation (rotation and translation) necessary to create new, positionally normalized coronal images, such that the AC–PC line segment is aligned with the y axis and the plane of the interhemispheric fissure is in the yz plane. By using this postprocessing techniques, the need for any special positional protocol during the image acquisition itself is essentially eliminated (Filipek *et al.*, 1990, 1991). An example in which the same subject was scanned on two occasions, one year apart, is shown in Fig. 1. The top row shows an example slice from the original, or *native*, image datasets, selected to show the superior colliculus for both imaging sessions. Images resulting from the positional normalization procedure, also selected to demonstrate the superior colliculus, are shown in the bottom row. The anatomic detail is clearly more comparable in the normalized data.

C. Anatomic Segmentation

The first step for structural morphometry is the delineation of anatomic regions of interest, or *anatomic segmentation*. Once structural borders have been defined, subsequent morphometric analysis of volume, shape, localization, etc., can be performed on the results of the segmentation (Kennedy *et al.*, 1989; Caviness *et al.*, 1989).

On each planar MR image, anatomic segmentation is performed using *intensity contour mapping* and *differential intensity contour mapping* algorithms (Kennedy *et al.*, 1989). Anatomic structures are delineated by *primary* borders, corresponding to signal intensity

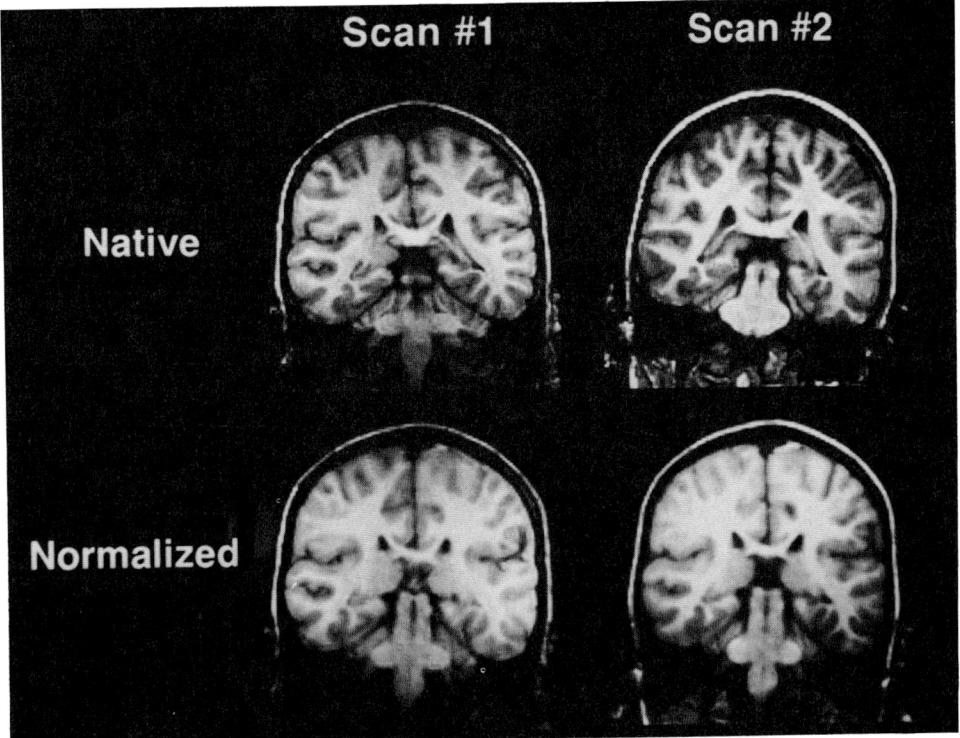

Figure 1 Example of *positional normalization* procedure. Two scans were acquired on the same individual on two occasions, one year apart. In the top row, an example image from each scan, chosen to include the superior colliculus, is shown. The bottom row shows the slice, including the superior colliculus from each scan *after* the application of the positional normalization procedure.

transitions at brain–CSF or at gray–white matter interfaces; and *secondary* borders, knowledge-based anatomic subdivisions within a gray or white matter field that are not defined by signal intensity transitions, are subsequently defined by hand by the investigator. In principle, the segmentation algorithms identify, classify, and create a continuous outline corresponding only to those voxel locations constituting the specified anatomic border. These operations have been described in greater detail elsewhere (Kennedy *et al.*, 1989; Filipek *et al.*, 1989, 1991). An example image (located at the slice of the anterior commissure) including the anatomic segmentation of cortex, white matter, caudate, lateral ventricles, putamen, and palidum is shown in Fig. 2a.

D. Callosal Parcellation

At a crude level, the functional organization of the cerebral hemispheres can be described at the lobar level. The interlobar transitions, however, are not anatomically well defined. In order to permit a subdivision of the cerebrum that maintains some of this lobar-level description and is reproducibly definable from the coronal, volumetric image data, the following procedure is used. Each positionally normalized brain is subdivided into neocortical regions as follows: *precallosal*, defined as those coronal MRI slices anterior to and not including the visualization of the genu of the corpus callosum; *pericallosal*, defined as those slices in which the corpus callosum is visualized, and further subdivided into the *anterior pericallosal*, defined as those slices anterior to and not including the anterior commissure; *posterior pericallosal*, defined as those slices posterior to and including the anterior commissure; and *retrocallosal*, defined as those slices posterior to and not including the visualization of the splenium of the corpus callosum. The anterior and posterior pericallosal regions are further subdivided into *superior* and *inferior* segments by a line drawn extending from the sylvian fissure along the superior circular insular sulcus, connecting with the superolateral tip of the lateral ventricle; and the *temporal* segment by a line drawn extending from the sylvian fissure along the inferior circular insular sulcus, connecting (by the shortest distance) with the optic trace/hippocampus–amygdala. Figure 2b shows an example image (located at the slice of the anterior commissure, which is, consequently, in the *posterior pericallosal region*) that includes the superior, inferior, and temporal callosal regions.

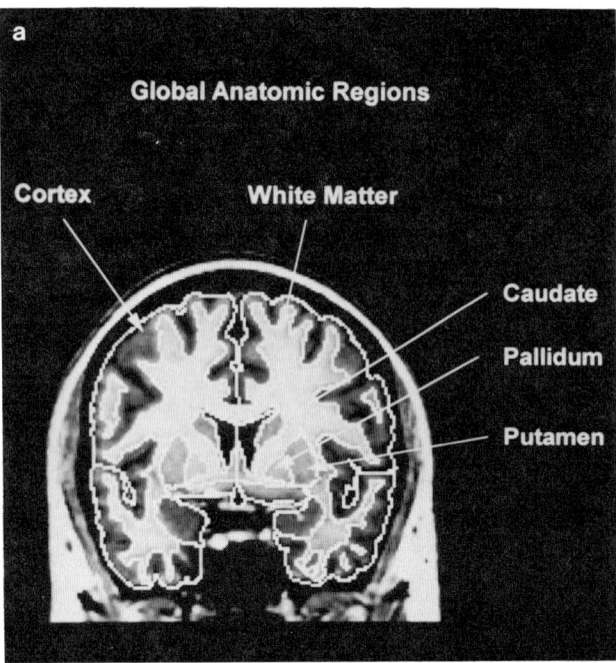

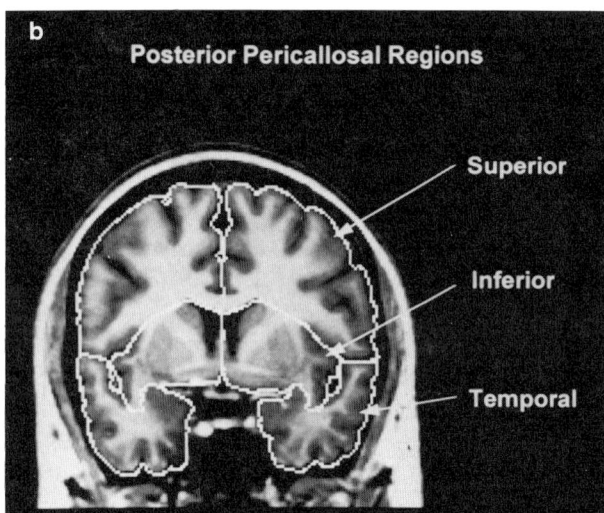

Figure 2 Examples of anatomic and callosal segmentation at the level of the anterior commissure. (a) Global anatomic structural segmentation of structures including the cerebral cortex, white matter, lateral ventricle, caudate, pallidum, and putamen. (b) Callosal segmentation showing the superior, inferior, and temporal regions. Because this slice includes the anterior commissure, it is in the posterior pericallosal region (see text for complete definitions).

E. Cortical Parcellation

Most current concepts of functional brain organization revolve around a hierarchical processing organization. This *systems level* description, reviewed by Mesulam (1985), involves unimodal primary cortical areas, surrounded by unimodal association areas, surrounded by intermodal association areas (Mesulam,

1985). The *topologies* of individual normal brains are constant, in so far as they each contain the same logical processing units. But, there is very little information within the cortex in the MRI image that would indicate the location of the borders between the functionally discrete processing areas. The primary visual cortex, with its prominent layer 4 (line of Gennari) is a possible exception in which the presence of this feature may indeed be observable by MRI (Clark *et al.*, 1992). The *topography,* and hence the spatial deployment of processing areas of individual brains, is quite variable. However, these functionally distinct regions have been shown to bear a consistent relationship to the surface features of the brain. There is lesion and post-mortem evidence that there is, to some degree, a relationship between the functional (cytoarchitectonic) regions and the surface topography of the brain (Rademacher *et al.*, 1992; Sanides, 1962; Zilles, 1990). Rademacher *et al.* (1993) demonstrated that 60% of Brodmann area 17 lies within the banks of the calcarine fissure, that Brodmann area 3b is consistently localized to the posterior bank of the central sulcus, and that Brodmann area 41 is completely contained upon Heschl's gyrus (Rademacher *et al.*, 1993).

This line of reasoning has lead to a number of methods of defining different cortical areas based upon the local cortical topography (Rademacher *et al.*, 1992; Jouandet *et al.*, 1989; Damasio and Frank, 1992). This is a level of cortical description that transcends the lobar approximations of brain regions discussed above. From an image analysis point of view, however, this presents a unique challenge. The identification of the primary and secondary fissures themselves does not provide a complete parcellation scheme for the cortex. Closure of cortical regions needs to be introduced by a set of conventions. To this end, we define *limiting planes* with respect to constant anatomic landmarks to complete the parcellation system. A complete set of operational definitions for this method is presented in Rademacher *et al.* (1992). Although these regions are not exactly analogous to actual functional or cytoarchitectonic areas, they likely correlate very strongly with specific subsets of them. A critical advantage of this method is that the definitions are unambiguously definable in a standardized fashion from the information visible in high-resolution MRI (Rademacher *et al.*, 1992).

F. Operational Implementation

After the positional normalization and anatomic segmentation procedures are performed, it is necessary to demark the location of the limiting planes and the trajectories of the limiting fissures so that their course in the coronal plane can be determined. Once this information is obtained, the cortical regions can be extracted from the results of the anatomic segmentation in the coronal plane. As with the global anatomic structures and callosal subdivisions, these cortical regions can be subsequently used for morphometric analysis.

There are several dozen sulcal trajectories and 16 limiting planes that must be identified for each hemisphere. Some of these are optimally observed within the coronal plane itself. Others, however, are optimally viewed in the axial or sagittal plane. In order to facilitate the demarcation of all of the limiting planes and sulci in their optimal plane of section and to facilitate extraction of the cortical regions, we have developed a unique interactive user interface to interact with the volumetric MRI image data. Plate 55 presents an overview of the user interface.

The main features of this user interface are as follows: (1) coronal, axial, and sagittal views of the volumetric acquisition, displayed from top to bottom, on the far right, including slice cross-referencing lines that indicate the location of the other displayed slices; (2) a zoomed version of a selected coronal, axial, or sagittal view, in the center; (3) labeling options for sulci, coronal limiting planes, or extracted cortical regions, depending on the current mode, on the left; and (4) mode selection, in the middle, on the left, for the sulci, limits, parcellation, extraction, and review modes.

1. Sulci Mode

The user is permitted to trace sulcal trajectories on the zoomed selected view. Upon completion of the trace, the user selects the desired sulcal label. The trajectory is then automatically color coded based upon the name, and the intersections of the trajectory with the other viewing planes are automatically updated. Plate 56 shows a closer look at a zoomed sagittal view. In this example, a number of trajectories have been identified in this view; the cingulate, shown in a bold line format, has been selected by the user. Colored dots (near the arrowhead, for example, the central sulcus cross-reference dot is seen) indicate where specific sulcal trajectories identified from other views intersect this view.

Figures 3 and 4 shows two explicit examples of the sulcal cross-referencing to the coronal plane. In Fig.

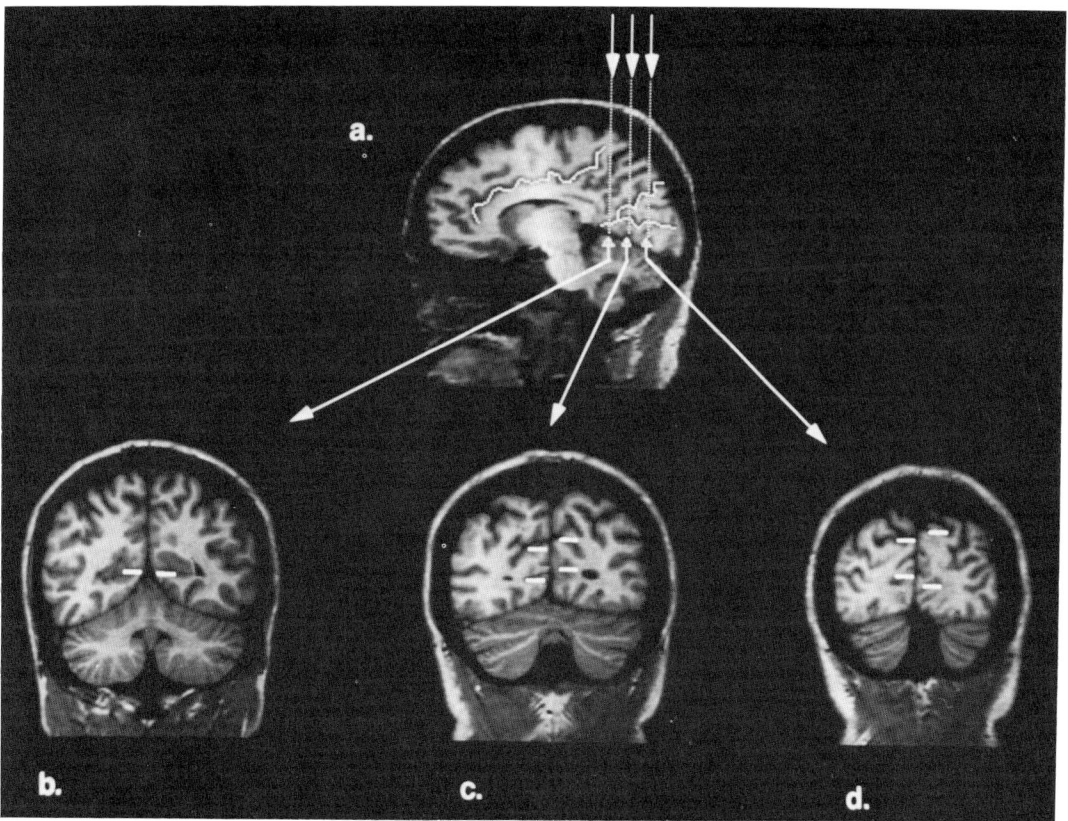

Figure 3.　Sagittal view including sulcal trajectories of the cingulate, parietooccipital, and calcarine sulci. a shows the sagittal slice with the sulcal trajectories. b–d show three coronal slices at the indicated locations and include the cross-reference marks at the intersection of the image plane and the sulci identified in the sagittal view.

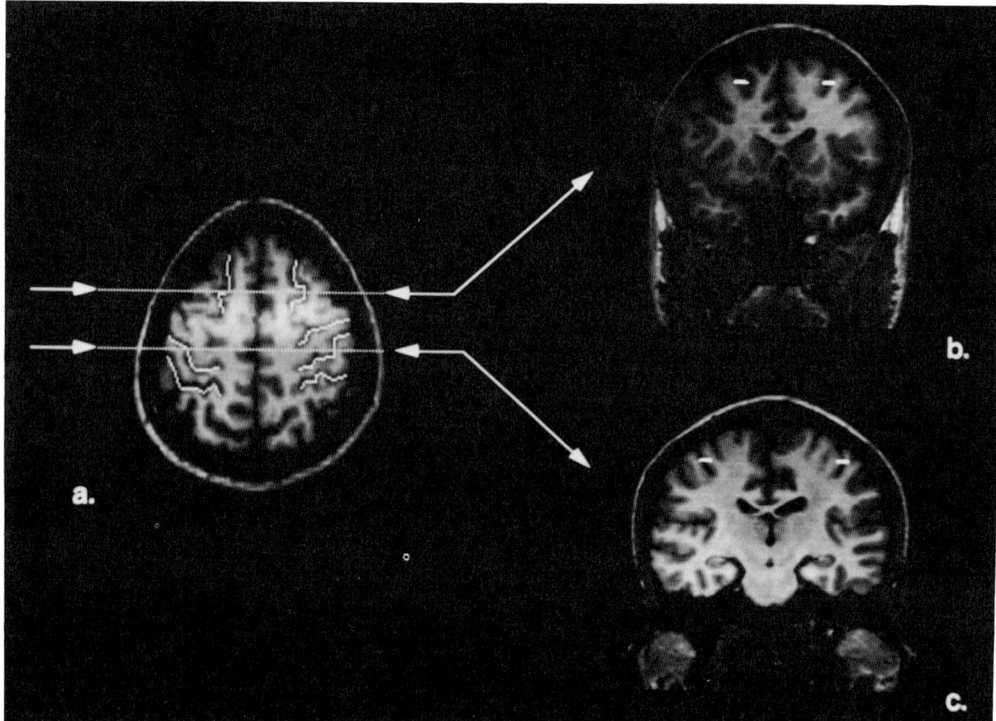

Figure 4. Axial view, including sulcal trajectories of the superior frontal, precentral, central, and postcentral fissures. a shows the axial slice with the sulcal trajectories. b–c show two coronal slices at the indicated locations and include the cross-reference marks at the intersection of the image plane and the sulci identified in the axial view.

3, the sagittal view with calcarine and parietooccipital fissures is shown, as well as three coronal planes that intersect these fissures at the location shown. Figure 4 shows an example from the axial plane in which the courses of the superior frontal, precentral, central, and postcentral fissures are demarked. In addition, there are two coronal planes, for which the intersection with the superior frontal and central sulcal trajectories is shown (as horizontal hatch marks).

2. Limits Mode

Limits mode is similar to sulci mode, except that the limiting plane choices are displayed and selected by positioning the coronal slice slider or by manual entry of the slice number in conjunction with the selection of the desired plane label. The red lines labeled A–G, shown in Plates 55 and 56, indicate the location of a subset of these plane locations. The planes can be selected separately for the right and left hemispheres, allowing for hemispheric asymmetry.

3. Parcellation Mode

Parcellation mode is the utility in which the results of the general anatomic segmentation are integrated with the results of the sulci identification mode. In this mode, the user adds the subdivision lines necessary,

based upon the sulcal identification, to subdivide the cortex into the parcellation units.

4. Extraction Mode

It is in this mode that the user selects regions of cortex, enclosed by both the original anatomic segmentation and the sulcal-based boundaries, and gives them their cortical parcellation label. Depending on the coronal location of the image, the user is permitted to select from a label menu that includes only allowable regions for that location.

5. Review Mode

Once the regions have been selected in each of the coronal slices, the user enters review mode. In this mode, the user can view all of the cortical areas defined for a given slice in a color-coded fashion (see Plate 57). We believe that this type of interface facilitates rapid evaluation of symmetry and completeness. The user can quickly and efficiently correct any labeling errors that have occurred at this point.

Plate 58 demonstrates three-dimensional visualization of the results of the cortical parcellation for the regions labeled occipital pole, precentral gyrus, superior frontal gyrus, and anterior and posterior cingulate as viewed using volume rendering from the lateral and medial views. Only the right cerebral hemisphere is shown to permit visualization of the structures on the medial surface.

IV. Discussion

We have reviewed a hierarchical method of anatomic description based upon volumetric MRI that is suitable for application to questions relating to anatomic localization (in conjunction with functional imaging methods) as well as to questions regarding fine-grained structural morphometry. As a morphometric method, this hierarchy is supported by a comprehensive set of standardized definitions relating to reproducible anatomic definition (Rademacher et al., 1992). The resulting cortical parcellation units are similar in many respects to the regions reported by Jouandet et al. (1989). Their method keys the regional transitions based upon the location of sulci in a two-dimensional flat map of the cortical surface. Consequently, the methods selected to establish closure for the creation of anatomic regions will cause significant differences in the regional details for cortical areas defined using these two methods. Also, the issues regarding the measurement of cortical surface area and its relationship to cortical volume require further study.

There are a number of other methods that allow localization of cortical areas based upon topographic information. Damasio and Frank (1992) report a topographic method of lesion localization. The described methodology for interaction with the volumetric data is similar to the interactive approach we have taken here. Their approach includes interaction directly with volumetric renderings of the image data. The method, however, provides a description of specific localities, but is not designed to form a complete parcellation system for morphometric analysis and region-of-interest selection. Evans et al. (1988) has proposed the use of an interactively deformable atlas. In this type of approach one starts with an anatomic template and interactively repositions, warps and deforms the template to conform to the anatomic topology found in the image of the brain. This method is ideal for a complete and comprehensive description of localization, but the application to a quantitative morphometric treatment would be limited based upon the precision of the complete cortical surface description.

It is intended that accurate, reproducible, fine-grained subdivision of the cerebral cortex will provide a foundation for intersubject comparison technologies. Many of the methods for intersubject comparison in use at the present time rely on the piecewise linear proportional scaling system of Talairach and Tournoux (1967, 1988). As the spatial resolution of the functional imaging methodologies increases, the limitations of this method are becoming increasingly apparent. One approach to overcome some of the limitations has been to increase the number of landmarks used in the interindividual matching problem and to allow nonlinear classes of image deformation (Bookstein, 1991; Mazziotta, et al., 1991). A cortical parcellation system, like the ones discussed here, provides a greatly enhanced set of potential landmark information (vertices of the parcellation units, intersections of sulci, etc.), which are deployed continuously over the cortical surface [as compared with the anterior and posterior commissure-based system of Talairach (1967)]. Extensions can be envisioned to expand the warping methodologies to incorporate the sulcal trajectories themselves, in addition to landmarks derived from them. Finally, the goals of intersubject analysis may not require that the entire brain of each individual be matched simultaneously. Thus warping methodologies that can act on the regional subdivisions individually may find increased utility.

Acknowledgments

This work was supported in part by Grants NS 20489, NS 24279, and NS 27950 (Drs. Filipek and Kennedy) from the National Institute of Neurological Disorders and Stroke and by HD 27802 (Drs. Filipek and Kennedy) from the National Institute of Child Health and Human Development. Dr. Kennedy also holds a Fairway Trust Fellowship.

References

Belliveau, J. W., Kennedy, D. N., McKinstry, R. C., Buchbinder, B. R., Weisskoff, R. M., Cohen, M. S., Vevea, J. M., Brady, T. J., and Rosen, B. R. (1991). Functional mapping of the human visual cortex by magnetic resonance imaging. *Science* **254,** 716–719.

Bookstein, F. L. (1991). Thin-plate splines and the atlas problem for biomedical images. *In* "Information Processing in Medical Imaging" (A. C. F. Colchester and D. J. Hawked, Eds.). Berlin: Springer-Verlag.

Caviness, V. S., Filipek, P. A., and Kennedy, D. N. (1989). Magnetic resonance technology in human brain science: Blueprint for a program based upon morphometry. *Brain Dev.* **11,** 1–13.

Churchland, P. S., and Sejnowski, T. J. (1988). Perspectives on cognitive neuroscience. *Science* **242,** 741–745.

Clark, V. P., Courchesne, E., and Grafe, M. (1992). *In vivo* myeloarchitectonic analysis of human striate and extrastriate cortex using magnetic resonance imaging. *Cereb. Cortex* **2,** 417–424.

Damasio, H., and Frank, R. (1992). Three-dimensional *in vivo* mapping of brain lesions. *Arch. Neurol.* **49,** 137–143.

Evans, A. C., Beil, C., Marrett, S., Thompson, C. J., and Hakim, A. (1988). Anatomical–functional correlation using an adjustable mri-based region-of-interest atlas with positron tomography. *J. Cereb. Blood Flow Metab.* **8,** 513–530.

Filipek, P. A., Kennedy, D. N., and Caviness, V. S. (1991). Morphometric analysis of central nervous system neoplasms. *Ped Neuro.*

Filipek, P. A., Kennedy, D. N., Caviness, V. S., Rossnick, S. L., Spraggins, T. A., and Starewicz, P. M. (1989). Magnetic resonance imaging-based brain morphometry: Development and application to normal controls. *Ann. Neurol.* **25**, 61–67.

Filipek, P. A., Kennedy, D. N., Rademacher, J., and Caviness, V. S., Jr. (1990). Error and variability incurred with MRI-based morphometry. *Ann. Neurol.* **28**.

Filipek, P. A., Richelme, C., Kennedy, D. N., and Caviness, V. S., Jr. (1994). The young adult human brain: An MRI-based morphometric analysis. *Cereb. Cortex*, in press.

Fox, P. T., and Raichle, M. E. (1986). Focal physiological uncoupling of cerebral blood flow and oxydative metabolism during somatosensory stimulation in human subjects. *Proc. Natl. Acad. Sci. USA* **83**, 1140–1144.

Fox, P. T., Mintun, M. A., Raichle, M. E., Miezin, F. M., Allman, J. M., and Van Essen, D. C. (1986). Mapping human visual cortex with positron emission tomography. *Nature* **323**, 806–809.

Fox, P. T., Raichle, M. E., Mintun, M. A., and Dence, C. (1988). Nonoxidative glucose consumption during focal physiologic neural activity. *Science* **241**, 462–464.

Jouandet, M. L., Tramo, M. J., Herron, D. M., Herrmann, A., Loftus, W. C., Bazell, J., and Gazzaniga, M. S. (1989). Brainprints: Computer-generated two-dimensional maps of the human cerebral cortex in vivo. *J. Cog. Neurosci.* **1**, 88–117.

Kennedy, D. N., Filipek, P. A., and Caviness, V. S., Jr. (1989). Anatomic segmentation and volumetric analysis in nuclear magnetic resonance imaging. *IEEE Trans. Med. Imag.* **7**, 1–7.

Mazziotta, J. C., Pelizzari, C. C., Chen, G. T., Bookstein, F. L., and Valentino, D. (1991). Region of interest issues: The relationship between structure and function in the brain. *J. Cereb. Blood Flow Metab.* **11**, 51–56.

Mesulam, M.-M. (1985). Patterns in behavioral neuroanatomy: Association areas, the limbic system, and hemispheric specialization. *In* "Principles of Behavioral Neurology," pp. 1–70. Philadelphia: F. A. Davis.

Phelps, M. E., Kuhl, D. E., and Mazziotta, J. C. (1981). Metabolic mapping of the brain's response to visual stimulation: Studies in humans. *Science* **211**, 1445–1448.

Prichard, J., Rothman, D., Novotny, E., Petroff, O., Kuwabara, T., Avison, M., Howseman, A., Hanstock, C., and Shulman, R. (1991). Lactate rise detected by 1H NMR in human visual cortex during physiologic stimulation. *Proc. Natl. Acad. Sci. USA* **88**, 5829–5831.

Rademacher, J., Galaburda, A. M., Kennedy, D. N., Filipek, P. A., and Caviness, V. S., Jr. (1992). Human cerebral cortex: Localization, parcellation and morphometry with magnetic resonance imaging. *J. Cog. Neurosci.* **4**, 352–374.

Rademacher, J., Caviness, V. S., Steinmetz, H., and Galaburda, A. M. (1993). Topographic variation of the human primary cortices: Implications for neuroimaging, brain mapping and neurobiology. *Cereb. Cortex* **3**, 313–329.

Sanides, F. (1962). "Die Architektonik des menschlichen Stirnhirns." Berlin: Springer-Verlag.

Steinmetz, H., Furst, G., and Freund, H.-J. (1989). Cerebral cortical localization: Application and validation of the proportional grid system in MR imaging. *J. Comput. Assist. Tomogr.* **13**, 10–19.

Talairach, J., Szikla, G., and Tournoux, P. (1967). "Atlas d'Anatomie Stereotaxique du Telencephale." Paris: Masson.

Talairach, J., and Tournoux, P. (1988). "Co-Planar Stereotaxic Atlas of the Human Brain." New York: Thieme Medical.

Zeki, S., Watson, J. D. G., Lueck, C. J., Friston, K. J., Kennard, C., and Frackowiak, R. S. J. (1991). A direct demonstration of functional specialization in human visual cortex. *Neuroscience* **11**, 641–649.

Zilles, K. (1990). "The Human Nervous System," pp. 575–802. San Diego: Academic Press.

20

The Role of a Computerized, Adjustable Brain Atlas for Merging of Data from Examinations Using PET, SPECT, MEG, CT, and MR Images

Martin Ingvar,§ Christian Bohm,† Lennart Thurfjell,* Lars Eriksson,‡,§ and Torgny Greitz ‡

*Centre for Image Analysis, Uppsala University, Uppsala, Sweden; †Department of Physics, University of Stockholm and Departments of ‡Neuroradiology and §Neurophysiology, Karolinska Institute/Hospital, Stockholm, Sweden

I. Introduction

In order to integrate information between and within different neuroimaging modalities, such as CT, PET, SPECT, and MRI, intra- and intersubject standardizations are required to bring the data into a compatible form. The type of standardization depends on whether the investigations are restricted to one subject or include many different subjects. This standardization can be brought about in many ways (see Chapter 11). In this chapter, however, we base our discussions and results on the CBA method (Bohm *et al.*, 1983, 1986; Greitz *et al.*, 1991a).

The CBA method uses a three-dimensional brain atlas that provides the anatomical information necessary for a correct interpretation of imaging data. It aids in identifying structures and in defining regions of interests, both in low-resolution modalities such as PET, SPECT, and MEG and in high-resolution modalities such as MRI and CT. In addition, the atlas provides the means to transform (reformat) image data into a standardized anatomy. This facilitates the analysis of intra- and intersubject data from different imaging modalities. A statistical comparison is then possible, producing average and variance images. By making an average image based on reformatted data from a group of "normal" cases, a database defining normality for each modality can be constructed. This database can then be used as a reference when interpreting data from individual cases. This is conve-

niently done by subtracting the individual formatted image from the group average image. In this way, deviations can easily be detected. The statistical significance of the deviations can also be determined since the standard deviation image corresponding to the average is known as well. We will describe the atlas and the tools it provides for merging data from the different neuroimaging modalities. Finally, some examples ar given to illustrate their use.

II. The CBA Atlas Database

The atlas is based on anatomical information derived from structures drawn onto displayed digitized photos obtained from a single cryosectioned brain and from various sources in the literature. The brain was fixated *in situ* soon after death in order to reduce systematic errors due to postmortem deformations. Basing the atlas on only one normal brain sample does not necessarily limit its usefulness as a standard because all relevant features should be present. However, if it is extreme in some structural respect, it will, of course, demand extreme transformations to adapt the atlas to most individuals. Such incidents are difficult to avoid because experience (and statistics) shows that it is difficult to find one sample that is normal in many independent ways. The probability that 10 independent parameters are within 1 SD from their mean is about 1%. This suggests that a suitably transformed brain or an average of such brains is a more convenient anatomical reference.

The definition and classification of the anatomical structures and divisions are in agreement with the standard textbooks of anatomy and the nomenclature is that of the "Nomina Anatomica" (1977). With regard to the thalamic nuclei, the nomenclature of Jones (1985) has been adapted. The boundaries of the cortical cytoarchitectonic areas ("Brodmann areas") have been determined using information from several different sources, since three-dimensional literature data on their distribution are incomplete, scarce, and partly contradictory. However, no analysis of the cytoarchitectonics of the atlas brain itself was undertaken.

The database contains at present three-dimensional representations of the brain surface, the ventricular system, and the cortical gyri and sulci, as well as the Brodmann cytoarchitectonic areas. The major basal ganglia including the thalamic nuclei, the brain stem nuclei, the lobuli of the vermis, and the cerebellar hemispheres, are also contained in the database.

The three-dimensional structures in the database representing the cortical gyri and the Brodmann areas are drawn in such a way that they include to a certain extent the underlying white matter. This is so because the marked individual variations of the cerebral cortex preclude a perfect adaptation of the atlas to the individual brain. However, the atlas program is sufficiently precise to indicate, with reasonable accuracy, the location of a cortical structure and may consequently be used as a guide to identify such structures. The construction of the cortical areas in the database thus means the inclusion of a significant portion of white matter and makes the areas unsuitable for direct use as regions of interest when quantifying data from PET and SPECT studies. When a method with high structural resolution, such as MRI, is used to adapt the atlas, the exact shape and location of the relevant cortical structure can be ascertained, drawn into a corresponding image plane, and, using a reproducible head fixation (Bergström *et al.*, 1981), transferred to a low-resolution image, such as a PET scan, to be used as a region of interest.

Even in the case of a perfect adaptation, the atlas regions are not always suitable for direct use as regions of interest (ROI). This is especially true with small structures in combination with low-resolution modalities with which the limited resolution will bring external information into the structure (partial volume effects). For these situations, the CBA program can via two-and-a-half-dimensional ROIs (Bohm *et al.*, 1992) provide "recovery coefficients" (Mazziotta *et al.*, 1981) to be used as a first-order correction. For example, a very good fit can always be obtained to basal ganglia,

such as the caudate nucleus, the putamen, or the thalamus. The CBA program can then provide a recovery coefficient for that very structure, in that very cut, and for that very instrument used.

III. Individualization of the Atlas

When used in practice, the atlas is adapted to fit the anatomy of a given individual brain as it is reproduced in a set of CT, MR, PET, or SPECT images (Plates 59–61). The general transformation is composed of a number of elementary three-dimensional transformations. These include rigid as well as nonrigid transformations. The adaptation can be made to a set of high-resolution CT or MR images, and the modified atlas is then transferred to the functional PET or SPECT images. With suitable tracers showing cortical structures, the adaptation can be made directly to the functional images with acceptable precision (Plate 60).

The adaptation process is interactively done and consists of finding suitable parameters in the transformation that affect the whole atlas volume in such a way that the selected atlas structures are brought into coincidence with the corresponding structures as presented in the images. The rigid transformation parameters include translations (TX, TY, TZ) and linear scalings (SCX, SCY, SCZ) in all three dimensions as well as in-plane and out-of-plane rotations (A, B, C). The nonrigid parameters are second-order transformations (i.e., including a higher order term such as x^2, xy, etc.) and can account for most types of individual variations in brain shape. The parameters are divided into variable scalings, skews, and scoliosis and are specified in arbitrary units in the range from -100 to 100, where 0 leaves the total transformation unaffected by the parameter.

The definition of the coordinate system used is such that the origin is located in the center of the brain, x is in the lateral direction, y is in anterior–posterior direction, and z is in the body-axis direction. The variable scalings (SCXX, SCXY, SCXZ, SCYZ, SCYY, SCYZ, SCZX, SCZY, SCZZ) will add to the first parameter (the parameter following the prefix SC) a factor (the specified value of the parameter) times the product of both parameters. SCXX will thus add to x a factor times x^2, expanding the atlas on one side. In the same way, SCXY will add to x a factor times xy, making the atlas brain thicker posteriorly or anteriorly (depending on the sign of SCXY). The geometrical effects of the remaining parameters are interpreted accordingly. The scoliosis parameters (SKXY, SKXZ, SKYX, SKYZ, SKZY, SKZX) will add to the first parameter a factor times the second parameter squared. SKXY will thus add to x a factor times y^2, displacing the anterior and posterior part of the atlas brain in the lateral direction, thus making it curved as seen from below. Curvatures in several other directions can be achieved by the remaining scoliosis parameters. The skew parameters (SWYX, SWYZ, SWZX) will add a value to the first parameter corresponding to a factor times the second parameter. SWYX will thus make y more positive for positive x and more negative for negative x (or vice versa depending on the sign of SWYX), thus deforming the atlas brain forward on one side and backward on the other. The geometrical effect of the other skew parameters are interpreted accordingly.

In practice, the adaptation is performed in a series of successive adjustments of the transformation parameters. These are normally set in a mode of the atlas software in which the parameter values can be changed under mouse control. The linear scalings and the nonrigid parameters are set only once for each individual. There will then be a separate set of examination-specific rotation and translation parameters for each subsequent investigation performed on the same individual, allowing for any differences in positioning between studies to be corrected.

IV. Reformation

Reformation is the interpolation and resampling process that results when a standardization prescription is applied to an image volume. The interpolation is necessary because the data points in the standardized volume seldom coincide with sample points in the original data volume. Different interpolation methods affect the resolution of the standardized volume differently, mainly by introducing broadening and space variability into the point spread function (PSF). However, the space variance tends to average out when a large number of standardized images is combined. A simple interpolation procedure is to use a trilinear interpolation polynomial. This gives the minimum broadening of the PSF. Higher order polynomials will cause a smoothing effect, producing a broader PSF.

The data transformation consists of a geometric deformation and a strength modifying component. The latter can be of two extreme types. It can be unity, which means that intensities are not modified even if an object is expanded or contracted. This is typical for the densities registered in CT or most parameters recorded in MR imaging. The other extreme is that the intensity is reduced with the local expansion factor

of the geometrical deformation (its Jacobian). This means that the total intensity within a given structure is not affected by the transformation. If the structure is enlarged, the intensity is reduced, keeping the total intensity constant. This case is typical for many PET and SPECT images, for example, those that record receptor densities. One can also expect situations in between these extremes. The correct choice of model is often difficult to make, but is essential for obtaining reliable quantitative results.

The errors in the reformation procedure can be considered via the point spread function. The transformed PSF is a scaled and translated version of the original PSF. The size modification is caused by the local enlargement factor, which may vary considerably over the volume. The PSF variation will thus introduce an uncontrolled element into the measuring procedure. The effect due to the positioning error is difficult to estimate. One way would be to determine this factor experimentally. However, if the deviation is small compared with the width of the PSF, it will not contribute significantly to the final result because these two effects combine quadratically. The effect due to the scale variation may in principle be corrected by applying a space variant smoothing function.

The reformation process can also be used to improve the quality of the data. By combining data from different parts of the object, it is possible to obtain a larger field of view. Resampling into a denser matrix may also be beneficial. When data from different measurements and different subjects are combined, some data point may give larger contributions to the compound systematic error (i.e., those points that in the resampling interpolation get an equal contribution from several measured points rather than from just one). Using weighted averages with which low weights given to such points may reduce systematic errors is, however, at the expense of increasing the statistical errors.

V. The Use of the CBA for Merging Neuroimaging Data

An adjustable computerized atlas may aid in several ways in the merging of data obtained from examination using various imaging modalities. The most obvious use is to correlate functional (including MEG) or histochemical data with anatomical information and also to compare the spatial distribution of functional data obtained with different methods. The atlas also serves to identify the anatomical location of differences in intra- or interindividual response to various stimuli in activation studies (Plate 63).

A. Activations Studies

Activation studies are based on the concept that the brain has limited reserves of energy. Increased brain work (activation) results in an increase of the blood flow to the region that is activated. The cerebral activation pattern can conveniently be determined by measuring the blood flow in an activated state and in a reference state (rest) and then subtracting the images. The conventional technique in PET to determine regional blood flow (rCBF) is to deliver a bolus of a freely diffusable tracer such as [^{15}O]butanol. The difference image can then be divided by the reference blood flow image to give percentage changes from the rest study. However, blood flow studies with PET are characterized by a low signal-to-noise ratio (SNR) for several reasons. With the bolus technique, most of the flow information is obtained within the first 2 min. This implies a statistical limitation. The flow model assumes constant rCBFs during the time of the measurement but may vary during this time, resulting in a systematical error. Attempts to compensate for the statistical limitation by giving higher doses result in dead time losses, counteracting the expected SNR gain. The situation with limited statistics can be improved by performing multiple low-dose injections in each individual (fractionation) (Cherry *et al.*, 1993; Ingvar *et al.*, 1994) and, in addition, by making blood flow determinations in several individuals and then averaging the blood flow information. However, interindividual averaging can be made only after a reformatting procedure in which the individual dataset is transformed into a dataset with a standard interindividual anatomy.

Repeated intra- and interindividual studies imply that the variance can be determined, for each individual and across the subjects. Images of significant changes between the two tasks may then be determined based on *t* statistics. Often descriptive *t* maps are constructed. If no correlations are assumed to exist between the voxels in the *t* maps, a large number of false-positive significances would occur, simply due to the number of comparisons made. A standard Bonferroni-type correction results in a threshold for significant differences that is too high to be of practical value (Ingvar *et al.*, 1994). However, correlations do exist between adjacent voxels. These are related to the resolution of the images, defined as the full width at half-maximum (FWHM), resulting from scanner characteristics, from the image reconstruction process, from the image data processing steps involving flow map generation, and from the atlas reformation process and the additional filtering of the individual reformatted blood flow images before subtraction. The filter usually chosen in this last filtering process is a Gaussian filter with a FWHM of around 20 mm and serves several purposes. The SNR is improved (Kanno, 1991), and the impact of any remaining individual anatomical differences is minimized.

The task to determine significant changes in statistical *t* images, considering correlations between adjacent voxels (smoothness), has been investigated by Friston *et al.* (1991). In their technique, the statistical *t* images are first transformed to a normal distribution, giving Z score images with mean zero and unit variance. A relationship can then be determined between the probability of a false positive (Q) and its Z threshold. This relationship depends on the significance level and the image smoothness. A Bonferroni correction to the threshold can be made in such a way that $Q = p/N$, *p* being the significance level, for example, $p = 0.05$. By using a look-up table of the relationship between threshold and the false-positive probability, the significance level of a selected region of interest can directly be given by comparing the ROI value with the threshold values for *p/N*, *N* being the number of pixels and $p = 0.05, 0.01$, and 0.001. This technique is attractive in that it yields a set limit for implied statistical tests. The major drawback is the necessity of filtering the images yielding not only decreased precision in the calculated size of the activated area, but also a lowered precision in the calculated point of the maximum in the activated region (Ingvar *et al.*, 1993).

An alternative approach has been tested with repeated intra- and interindividual studies of the same activation paradigms (Ingvar *et al.*, 1993). The most prominent activations for reading aloud compared with reading silently are shown in Plate 62, an exploratory significance map based on a pixel-by-pixel Student's *t* test. Reading aloud relative to reading silently activated a major part of the motor cortex and a large area of the cerebral vermis region extending to the cerebellar hemispheres, especially on the left side. The cerebral motor area activations were essentially symmetrical. Reading silently relative to reading aloud activated several discrete areas in the frontal lobes with the most prominent activation in area 46 on the left side. These activations were less symmetrical than the motor activations. These activations were also significant when evaluated by Friston's SPM technique.

Plate 63 demonstrates the result obtained in a CBF study of snake phobia, using the same method of averaging after paired subtraction. Eight phobic individuals were shown one movie with an abundance of snakes and one with more pleasant scenery. As can be seen, there is a relatively high increase in flow in the visual association areas, Brodmann 19, bilaterally with the phobic stimulation compared with the neutral stimulation.

1. Sources of Error in the Statistical Determination of Activated Regions

The overwhelming size of the dataset that each study generates creates several sources of error. Both type 1 errors, in which a correct null hypothesis is rejected, and type 2 errors, in which the null hypothesis should be rejected but was not a problem. The signal-to-noise ratio can be so low that small but true activations are not detected. The statistical approach may be too conservative in order to avoid false-positive findings, thereby rejecting true findings. In both cases, increasing the number of studies and fractionation of the rCBF procedure are possible remedies. Fractionation also has the advantage that at least the major activated areas can be detected in each case studied, allowing firm conclusions regarding the significance of an activation when all cases are averaged. Filtration of the original image is often performed in order to improve the signal-to-noise ratio. However, as was pointed out above, filtering can incur changes in both location and size of the activated region.

Another important source of error is the possibility of systematic morphological differences between groups. An anatomical reformation such as that provided by the CBA is a necessary tool for successful comparisons between groups.

2. Merging of MEG Data

The atlas may also be used in combination with CT or MRI in activation studies using MEG to identify the structural correlate to the intracerebral current sources (Fig. 1). The position information is transferred between the imaging methods and MEG using a stereotactic technique. The combination of the CT, MR, PET, SPECT, and MEG methods may become a powerful tool in the future exploration of brain functions, because full advantage may be taken of the high-time resolution of MEG, whereas the anatomical information lacking in MEG will be compensated for by the imaging methods. This integration of MEG with the methods mentioned will allow us to separate primary centers of brain function from secondary centers, secondary centers from tertiary ones, and so on, making an analysis of the complex cascade arrangement of the brain in living humans feasible (Greitz *et al.*, 1993).

B. Database Concept

1. Mean–Mean Subtraction

By subtracting average images of healthy volunteers from the mean of a group of patients or by subtracting mean images of different groups of patients within a modality, specific patient-dependent features may be identified. By combining the subtraction image with the pooled standard deviation image contained in the database, the significance of anatomical or functional differences between the two groups may be determined. As already mentioned for the activation studies, the location of areas can be interpreted by the atlas database.

2. Individual–Mean Subtraction (the Greitz Principle)

Average images from various image modalities may be used to construct databases representing mean "normal" images, from which individual images taken with the same modality can be subtracted to determine differences from the normal population (Greitz *et al.*, 1991b). Because the average image has an associated standard deviation that may be displayed in an error image, the significance of possible deviations can be determined. The subtraction can be performed as a mean–individual or as individual–mean subtraction. The technique is especially powerful in functional neuroimaging. In the diagnosis of neurological diseases it may identify functional changes in the absence of morphological changes. It could also be used to reveal anatomical anomalies and abnormalities in a given individual. The principle of this method resembles that of the diagnostic procedure in clinical practice. It is conceivable that a database of various mean images could have a meaningful purpose in that context.

This method has been used to demonstrate brain tumors, using L-methionine as a tracer, as well as a regional decrease in the cerebral metabolic rate in patients with focal epilepsy (Plate 64) and in those with dementia by subtracting the finding in the patient from the mean image displaying the metabolic rate as measured with FDG in a normal age-matched population. (Plate 65).

C. The Construction of a Functional Brain Atlas

One fascinating aspect, made feasible by intersubject standardization of CT, MRI, PET, or SPECT data into a standardized anatomy, is the possibility of creating a normalized, three-dimensional, functional brain

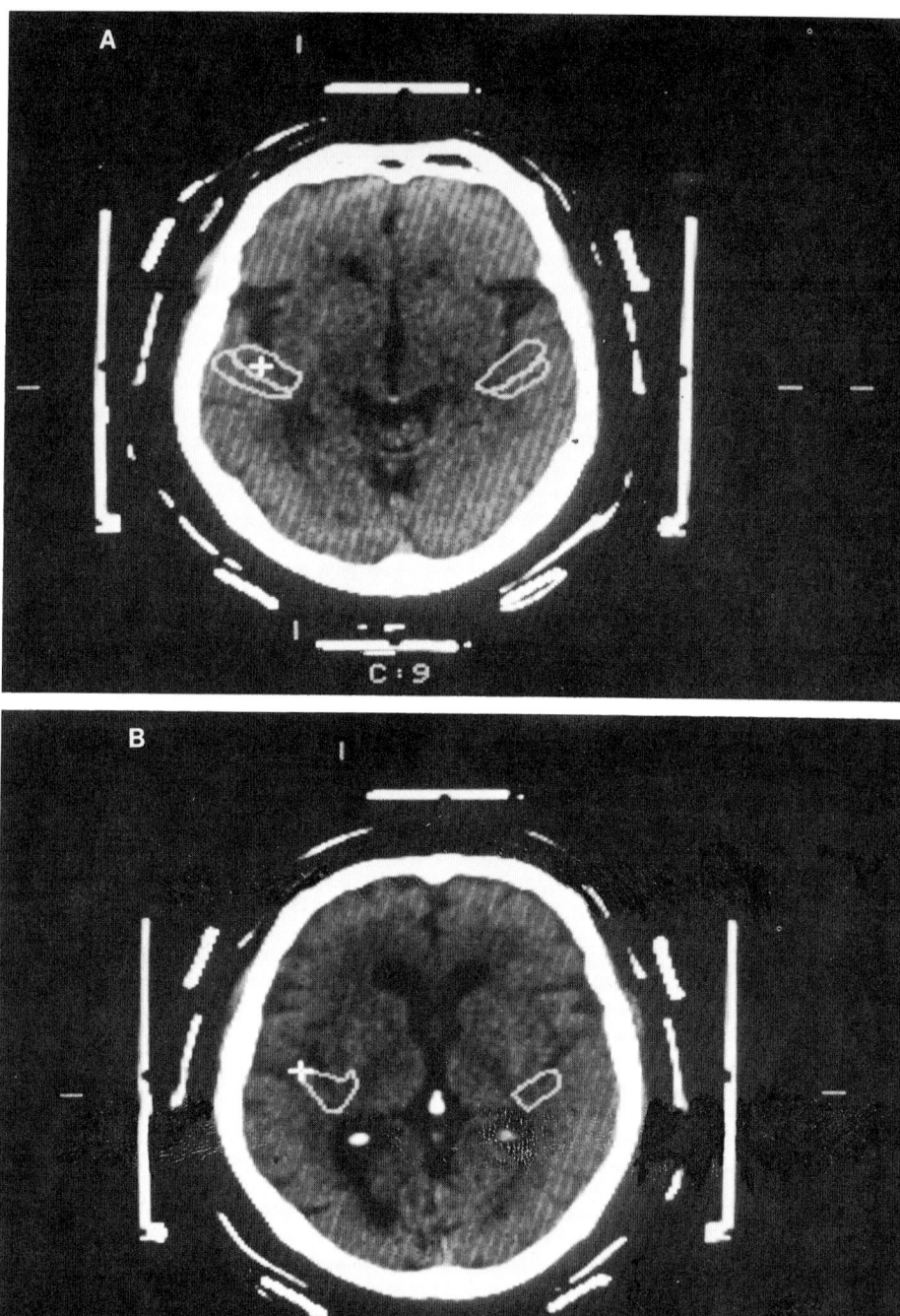

Figure 1 CT images displaying the positions (+) of two current dipoles following high and low tone stimulation, respectively, determined by stereotactic magnetoencephalography (MEG) and transferred to the CT images using a reproducible fixation. The primary and secondary auditory cortices (Brodmann's areas 41 and 42) have been drawn in automatically by the computerized atlas program. Area 42 is seen lateral and posterior to area 41 (in A). (A) Position of the dipole for low tones. (B) Position of the dipole for high tones. [Data from Greitz *et al.* (1994)].

atlas. Before the advent of nuclear medicine and the introduction of techniques to measure regional cerebral blood flow, no method was available to study brain function without interfering with the observed event. The application of image reconstruction methods allows for the first time a precise and accurate three-dimensional recording of the measured data. By reformatting images into a standardized anatomy, a variety of data from physiological experiments carried out at different centers with a standardized technique can be transferred back to a common data base (Greitz *et al.*, 1991b). Merging information in this way will serve to successfully build up a comprehensive and detailed three-dimensional functional brain atlas.

VI. Different Problems

A. Extracerebral Activations

Today, measurements of regional cerebral blood flow by PET and SPECT are used in studies of cerebral functional anatomy (e.g., Lassen *et al.*, 1991). In such studies, the anatomical correlates of the activated regions are sometimes difficult to assess, especially if subtraction image procedures are used. Such procedures yield images that contain very little anatomic information. Thus, there is a risk that, for example, paradigm-specific extracerebral blood flow changes can be interpreted as cerebral activation (Drevets *et al.*, 1992). Either a proper alignment to a case-specific morphological examination such as MRI or CT or intersubject standardization procedures will eliminate such problems. It should be pointed out that filtration procedures increases the influence of this effect.

B. Low Resolution Methods

The atlas is very helpful even with such techniques because the delimitation of larger areas sometimes is necessary for the correct diagnosis. Also, the calculation of, for example, regional CBF quantitatively requires that the choice of ROI is as independent as possible from the observer. Here, the CBA can be of great use (Plate 61). Low resolution presents a special problem in that the CBA makes it tempting to extract more detailed information than is available from the images. Knowledge of the inherent spatial resolution of the image modality should limit the smallest size of the structures used in the analysis of the images.

References

Bergström, M., Boethius, J., Eriksson, L., Greitz, T., Ribbe, T., and Widén, L. (1981). Head fixation device for reproducible position alignment in transmission CT and positron emission tomography. *J. Comput. Assist. Tomogr.* **5,** 136–141.

Bohm, C., Greitz, T., Kingsley, D., Berggren, B. M., and Olsson, L. (1983). Adjustable computerized stereotaxic brain atlas for transmission and emission tomography. *Am. J. Neuroradiol.* **4,** 731–733.

Bohm, C., Greitz, T., Blomqvist, G., Farde, L., Forsgren, P. O., Kingsley, D., Sjögren, I., Wiesel, F. A., and Wik, G. (1986). Applications of a computerized adjustable brain atlas in positron emission tomography. *Acta Radiol. Suppl.* **369,** 449–452.

Bohm, C., Greitz, T., and Thurfjell (1992). The role of anatomic information in quantifying functional neuroimaging data. *J. Neural. Transm.* **37**(Suppl.), 67–78.

Cherry, S., Woods, R. P., Hoffman, E. J., and Mazziotta, J. C. (1993). Improved detection of focal cerebral blood flow changes using 3D positron emission tomography. *J. Cereb. Blood Flow Metab.* in press.

Drevets, W., Videen, T., MacLeod, A., Haller, J., and Raichle, M. (1992). PET images of blood flow during anxiety: Correction. *Science* **256,** 1696.

Friston, K. J., Frith, C. D., Liddle, P. F., and Frackowiak, R. S. (1991). Comparing functional (PET) images: The assessment of significant change. *J. Cereb. Blood Flow Metab.* **11,** 690–699.

Greitz, T., Bohm, C., Holte, S., and Eriksson, L. (1991a). A computerized brain atlas: Construction, anatomical content and some applications. *J. Comput. Assist. Tomogr.* **15**(1), 26–38.

Greitz, T., Holte, S., Bohm, C., Eriksson, L., Seitz, R., Ericson, K., Nybäck, H., Stone-Elander, S. (1991b). A data base library as a diagnostic aid in neuroimaging. *Neuroradiology* **33**(Suppl.), 2–4.

Greitz, T., Hellstrand, E., Bohm, C., Hämäläinen, M. S., Hari, R., Ilmoniemi, R.J., Lounasmaa, O. V., and Seitz, R. (1994). The use of a computerized, adjustable brain atlas in the magnetoencephalographic localisation of intracerebral current sources activated by auditory stimulation. *Neuroreport* in press.

Ingvar, M., Eriksson, L., Greitz, T., Stone-Elander, S., Dahlbom, M., Rosenqvist, G., af Trampe, P., and von Euler, C. (1994). Methodological aspects of brain activation studies: Cerebral blood flow determined with [^{15}O]butanol and positron emission tomography. *J. Cereb. Blood Flow Metab.*, in press.

Jones, H. T. (1985). "The Thalamus." New York: Plenum.

Kanno, I. (1991). "Discussion in Brain Work and Mental Activity" (N. Lassen, D. Ingvar, M. Raichle, and L. Friberg, Eds.), pp. 433–435. Copenhagen: Munksgaard.

Lassen, N., Ingvar, D., Raichle, M., and Friberg, L. (Eds.) (1991). "Brain Work and Mental Activity," Alfred Benzon Symposium 31. Copenhagen: Munksgaard.

Mazziotta, J. C., Phelps, M. E., Plummer, D., and Kuhl, D. E. (1981). Quantitation in positron emission computed tomography. 5. Physical–anatomical effects. *J. Comput. Assist. Tomogr.* **5,** 734–743.

"Nomina Anatomica" (1977), 4th ed. Amsterdam: Exerpta Medica Foundation.

21

Modeling and Data Structure for Registration to a Brain Atlas of Multimodality Images

Michael W. Vannier*, Michael I. Miller†, and Ulf Grenander‡

*Mallinckrodt Institute of Radiology, Washington University School of Medicine, St. Louis, Missouri 63110;
†Department of Electrical Engineering, Electronic Signals and Systems Research Laboratory,
Institute for Biomedical Computing, Washington University, St. Louis, Missouri, 63110;
and ‡Division of Applied Mathematics, Brown University, Providence, Rhode Island 02912

I. Digital Electronic Atlases of the Brain

Digital electronic atlases of the brain are valuable tools for quantitative and functional neuroimaging (Pechura and Martin, 1991), especially for colocalization of volume datasets, such as those encountered with PET, SPECT, and MRI examinations (Greitz et al., 1991; Bajcsy et al., 1983; Dann et al., 1988). A suitable atlas has the utility to support neuromorphometric analyses (Shenton et al., 1992). Both activities, colocalization and neuromorphometric analysis, are based on the availability of volumetric image data with a relatively large number of uniform voxel samples as found in CT, MRI, PET, and SPECT (Jansen et al., 1989; Bohm et al., 1988; Sandor et al., 1990).

Future applications may include radiological automated diagnosis in which computer techniques are employed to interpret neuroimages (Banks et al., 1987; Lehmann et al., 1991) and radiotherapy treatment planning and evaluation (Mano et al., 1990). The use of a volume-based anatomical atlas in medical education has been explored (Höhne et al., 1992a, 1992b) and has great promise for the future—at the graduate, postgraduate, and continuing medical education levels.

Evans and associates (Evans et al., 1988, 1991; Marrett et al., 1989) described the implementation of and experience and results obtained with a 3D computerized brain atlas for topographical and functional analysis of brain subregions. A volume-of-interest (VOI) atlas was produced by manual contouring on an MRI volume dataset to yield 60 brain structures in each hemisphere, which could be adjusted, originally by global affine transformation or local interactive adjustments, to match individual MRI datasets. A nonlinear deformation (warp) capability (Bookstein, 1989) has been integrated, using a continuous 3D warp transformation derived from homologous points identified interactively in the atlas and individual MRI datasets (Evans et al., 1991).

Early efforts in the development of electronic anatomic atlases have been limited to interactive generation of orthogonal planes from a volume for display and subjective interpretation. Some of these atlases were implemented by storing precomputed planes on, for example, an analog videodisk, where an interactive control program retrieved the frame of interest. Obviously, this approach is limited to existing precomputed images and has limited utility and flexibility. The approach is most closely analogous to an electronic textbook. The registration of MR and PET imaging volumes to achieve a simultaneous display with overlap of functional areas or linear mapping of sampled volumes into a predefined stereotactic space has been applied. (Levin et al., 1989)

The components of an advanced electronic anatomic atlas consist of an image dataset, retrieval tool, matching tool, and authoring tool (Schiemann et al., 1992; Höhne et al., 1992b). The image dataset contains a voxel array with stored signal intensities, much the

FUNCTIONAL NEUROIMAGING

same as an ordinary MR, PET, or SPECT examination. In addition to intensity information at each voxel locus, information regarding the tissue type (Higer and Bielke, 1990), functional and vascular territory, anatomic nomenclature (if applicable), and related knowledge is maintained. The image dataset is linked to a hierarchical knowledge base containing textual and symbolic nonimage information.

The software tools that create, manage, and apply the atlas to user-defined needs consist of retrieval, matching, and authoring functions. The authoring function allows experts to create the hierarchical knowledge base and provides links to individual voxels or groups of voxels. The retrieval tool implements interactive exploration of atlas information, in much the same way that 3D and multiplanar reconstruction software tools allow visualization of clinical MR and PET examinations. The matching tool is intended to transform an individual MRI examination into the atlas coordinate space and achieves registration between corresponding structures, or vice versa, depending upon the application (Toga, 1990).

Electronic atlases can be characterized in terms of their voxel size (spatial resolution), information content, retrieval tools, and sample size representation (*n*, the number of individual examinations used to create the atlas). Implementation details, such as the type and speed of interaction, rendering techniques, platforms supported, and other issues, have practical but not scientific impact.

The principal limitations of electronic anatomic atlases involve the restriction to a high-*n* low-spatial-resolution space or a low-*n* (often single sample) high-spatial-resolution space. Modeling the variability among normal individuals as the ensemble average is not satisfactory. The registration of image volumes is often based on a landmark approach, with definition of homologous points (fiducials), computation of a rigid body or other affine transformations (and scaling), and resampling of one volume into the coordinate space of the other. Global matching of volumes is performed to minimize the total registration error, but this may leave significant mismatches within the volume, particularly if only point or surface features are employed.

II. The Atlas Matching Problem: Registration, Segmentation, and Labeling

The utility of an electronic brain atlas may be accessed by interactive exploration of the sampled volume using computer graphics editing and rendering tools (Vannier *et al.*, 1991). Provided that the atlas

image data volume has been labeled, structures of interest may be accessed by selecting items of interest based on their names in an associated knowledge (data) base. If the data structures and information content of the knowledge base are sufficiently rich, one may access subvolumes of interest or interrogate the atlas based on anatomic nomenclature, functional and vascular territories, tissue class, or other items of interest. Höhne and associates at the University Hospital Eppendorf in Hamburg, Germany, have designed and implemented such a system on workstations (Plate 66) (Höhne *et al.*, 1992a; Tiede *et al.*, 1992).

The process of matching a patient or normal control subject study to a predefined anatomic atlas is analogous, in many respects, to that employed in the comparison of two image volumes, from the same or different subjects. In general, the process consists of registration, segmentation, and labeling. Features are extracted from each volume and are matched to achieve a predefined degree of correspondence. This registration process is typically implemented by computing a simple global transformation matrix consisting of translation, rotation, and scaling in three orthogonal directions. The rigid transformation is applied to one volume to match another by resampling each voxel in the new coordinate system. The resampling may be done by nearest neighbor, bi- or trilinear interpolation, or cubic convolution operations, depending upon the speed and degree of accuracy required. The volumes are placed into registration so that corresponding structures occupy the same (or nearly so) coordinate locations in both (Vannier *et al.*, 1992). Segmentation of neuroimage volumes, especially from MR datasets, has been attempted using statistical image processing and pattern recognition techniques, especially supervised classification and unsupervised (cluster analysis) methods. Labeling of neuroimage volumes to identify landmarks, functional regions, and vessels or other discrete structures is performed on segmented results.

III. Pattern Theoretic Approach to Digital Anatomic Atlases

Functional neuroimaging requires digital mapping of human brain anatomy, principally for colocalization of activation sites or for neuromorphometry. Mathematical/electrical engineering researchers working in pattern theory and related fields have addressed the digital mapping of the biological structure problem and offer methods that provide important advantages over the rigid transformations or two-dimensional analyses that are commonly available. These two groups—functional neuroscientists and applied engineering mathematicians—are generally unaware of each other's existence, and we believe that all groups would benefit from the exchange of ideas, problems, and methodologies.

A major research program at Washington University in St. Louis led by Michael I. Miller and Ulf Grenander is based on construction of a realistic and precise representation of medical and biological knowledge for real-world shapes and patterns. Common to their studies of biological and natural shapes to date (hands, leaves, mitochondria, cell membranes, and amoebae) is the fact that, although the shapes being imaged may be strongly structured, they are not rigid and therefore exhibit high variability. A fundamental task in the understanding and the analysis of biomedical scenes is construction of models that incorporate both variability and structure in a mathematically precise way (Miller, 1991, 1993; Christensen *et al.*, 1992).

There is no shortage of image processing algorithms—the literature abounds with computational techniques designed to improve pictures by noise suppression or to recognize particular patterns so as to segment pictures into subpictures. Much of the greatest success to date has been in the modeling of sensor variability. For example, in CT, MR, PET, and SPECT, the physical device electronics and optical characteristics are well understood. Reconstruction algorithms that are highly tuned for accommodating sensor noise abound.

However, the variability type not in the sensor but in the shapes and biological structures themselves is much less well understood. Limitations of existing methodologies become visible for more ambitious tasks, in which the goal is to arrive at a deeper understanding of the image ensemble itself. To make this possible, more subject matter knowledge must be built into the algorithms. If the algorithm is to make sense of a biological image, with all the possible variations, normal and abnormal, it must know something about the global anatomical structures themselves and how they vary from one individual to another.

In other words, the methods must be based on a mathematical model that allows a precise representation of medical anatomical knowledge. But the enormous complexity of biological patterns, contrasted with that of synthetic objects, makes the design of the representation scheme a difficult, perhaps overwhelming endeavor. For example, in representing normal human brains, is it possible to design representations that reflect the complexity of normal human anatomy while accommodating human varia-

tion? Miller's research program rests on the belief that this can be done.

IV. Global Pattern Theory

Since the mid-1970s, researchers have built models that attempt to incorporate structure/variability at least for the simpler tasks. For example, to achieve high-quality restoration or segmentation, using probabilistic models such as Markov random fields (MRF), a good deal of success has been demonstrated. But this is not enough—what we have in mind is something more ambitious. The reason why textures can be dealt using MRF models is that most (but not all) of their variability is of a very local nature: the probabilistic dependencies extend over quite a limited range. To meet the greater challenges, global representations must be employed. Mathematical techniques for such representations began to appear in the early 1990s under the name of Grenander's global shape models (Grenander *et al.*, 1990; Grenander and Miller, 1991, 1992, 1993; Amit *et al.*, 1991; Knoerr, 1988; Srivastava *et al.*, 1991).

Grenander's global shape models attempt to represent image ensembles in terms of their typical structure via the construction of templates and their variabilities by the definition of probabilistic transformations applied to the templates. It is not appropriate for us to describe in precise mathematical detail how this is achieved or how the algorithms are implemented computationally. Simply stated, the transformations form groups (translation, scale, and rotation) and are applied so that, although a rich family of shapes may be generated from a single template, the global properties of the templates are maintained.

V. Digital Anatomical Databases

The key to the global shape models is the construction of the templates and the variations that occur around them. In all of our previous projects, the construction of the templates could be obtained with modest effort. For example, membranes, mitochondria, and amoebae are all straightforwardly defined as transformations of linear, elliptical, and spherical shapes, respectively. The corresponding templates themselves are of low complexity.

Until recently this seemed to be the major obstacle for the successful application of the global shape models. The construction of digital anatomical libraries has recently been performed at several laboratories.

In particular, the ''Visible Human'' project, undertaken by the National Library of Medicine (NLM), promises to yield results well suited to the definition of detailed anatomic templates. In the Board of Reagents report (1990), it is noted that "This Visible Human project would include digital images derived from computerized tomography, magnetic resonance imagery, and photographic images from cryosectioning of cadavers. A working group should be assembled from experts in anatomy, clinical imaging, and computer science to establish standards for recognition and computer representation of the data." Furthermore, "NLM should expand upon initial image libraries comprised of normal structure to encompass specialized image collections which represent structural information, such as embryological development, normal and abnormal variations and disease-related images."

VI. Advantages of Global Shape Models

Global shape modeling enables automatic registration, correspondence between slices, and noise suppression. This is useful in many functional neuro-imaging applications. However, more important gains will result from the ability to achieve image understanding at a deeper level. As described in the Board of Regents report (1990), the aim of the plan is not restricted to present libraries of image ensembles, in which each voxel means the observed intensity of the radiation observed by some sensor. The images will also carry symbolic values, say in the form of established names of anatomical regions, the type of tissue at a certain point, and functional or vascular territory (Board of Regents, National Laboratory of Medicine, 1990).

The global shape models will carry such symbolic values and will allow for the deformation of the coordinate system, which the template library is defined on, to be carried into the coordinate system of any given patient. If several sensors are used, fusion is automatically achieved when the global (and subsequent local) shape matching process is complete.

It appears obvious to us that a project as ambitious as the one proposed requires cooperation among medical researchers building the digital libraries and the mathematicians and engineers developing the pattern theoretic algorithms. These collaborative plans in the biomedical community are being developed simultaneously with the creation of pattern theoretic methodologies that require exactly the same empirical information that these electronic libraries will contain.

Acknowledgments

The assistance of Gary E. Christensen, Yali Amit, Marcus Raichle, Karl Heinz Höhne, and Alan C. Evans in discussions regarding these methods is gratefully appreciated.

References

Amit, Y., Grenander, U., and Piccioni, M. (1991). Structural image restoration through deformable templates. *J. Am. Stat. Assoc.* **86**(414), 376–387.
Bajcsy, R., Lieberson, R., and Reivich, M. (1983). A computerized system for the elastic matching of deformed radiographic images to idealized atlas images. *J. Comput. Assist. Tomogr.* **7**(4), 618–625.
Banks, G., Vries, J. K., and McLinden, S. (1987). Radiologic automated diagnosis (RAD). *Comput. Methods Programs Biomed.* **25**, 157–168.
Board of Regents, National Library of Medicine (1990). "Long Range Plan: Electronic Imaging."
Bohm, C., Greitz, T., Kingsley, D., Berggren, B., and Ollson, L. (1988). Adjustable computerized stereotaxic brain atlas for transmision and emission tomography. *AJNR* **4**, 731–733.
Bookstein, F. L. (1989). Principal warps: Thin-plate splines and the decomposition of deformations. *IEEE Trans. Pattern Anal. Mach. Intell.* **11**(6), 567–585.
Bookstein, F. L. (1991). "Morphometric Tools for Landmark Data." Cambridge, England. Cambridge University Press.
Christensen, G., Miller, M. I., Amit, Y., and Grenander, U. (1992). Global shape models for anatomical structures. *In* "Jour 26th Annual Conference on Information Science and Systems, Princeton University."
Dann, R., Hoford, J., Kovacic, S., Reivich, M., and Bajcsy, R. (1988). Three-dimensional computerized brain atlas for elastic matching: Creation and initial evaluation. *In* "Medical Imaging II 1988: SPIE Proceedings," Vol. 914, pp. 600–612.
Evans, A. C., Beil, C., Marrett, S., Thompson, C. J., and Hakim, A. (1988). Anatomical–functional correlation using an adjustable MRI-based region of interest atlas with positron emission tomography. *J. Cereb. Blood Flow Metab.* **8**(4), 513–530.
Evans, A. C., Dai, W., Collins, L., Neelin, P., and Marrett, S. (1991). Warping of a computerized 3-D atlas to match brain image volumes for quantitative neuroanatomical and functional analysis. *In* "Image Processing 1991: SPIE Proceedings," Vol. 1445, pp. 235–246.
Greitz, T., Bohm, C., Holte, S., and Eriksson, L. (1991). A computerized brain atlas: Construction, anatomical content, and some applications. *J. Comput. Assist. Tomogr.* **15**(1), 26–38.
Grenander, U., and Miller, M. I. (1991). "Jump-Diffusion Processes for Abduction and Recognition of Biological Shapes." Electronic Signals and Systems Research Laboratory.
Grenander, U., and Miller, M. I. (1994). Representations of knowledge in complex systems. *J. R. Stat. Soc.*, B, **56**(3).
Grenander, U., and Miller, M. I. (1993). Deformable anatomical data bases using pattern theoretic methods. *In* "Proceedings of the USAF/MIR/NLM Workshop on Electronic Imaging of the Human Body." (M. W. Vannier, R. E. Yates, and J. Whitestone, Eds.). Dayton, OH: Harry G. Armstrong Human Factors Laboratory, Wright Patterson Air Force Base.

Grenander, U., Chow, Y., and Keenan, D. (1990). "HANDS: A Pattern Theoretic Study of Biological Shapes." New York: Springer-Verlag.

Higer, H. P., and Bielke, G. (1990). (Eds.) "Tissue Characterization in Magnetic Resonance Imaging." New York: Springer-Verlag.

Höhne, K. H., Bomans, M., Riemer, M., Schubert, R., Tiede, U., and Lierse, W. (1992a). A volume-based anatomical atlas. *IEEE Comput. Graphics Appl.*, 72–78.

Höhne, K. H., Pommert, A., Riemer, M., Schiemann, Th., Schubert, R., and Tiede, U. (1992b). Framework for the generation of 3D anatomical atlases. *In* "Visualization in Biomedical Computing 1992. SPIE Proceedings," Vol. 1808, pp. 510–520.

Jansen, W., Baak, J. P., Smeulder, A. W., and van Ginneken, A. M. (1989). A computer based handbook and atlas of pathology. *Pathol. Res. Pract.* **185**(5), 652–656.

Knoerr, A. (1988). "Global Models of Natural Boundaries." Pattern Analysis Report No. 148.

Lehmann, E. D., Hawkes, D. J., Hill, D. L., Bird, C. F., Robinson, G. P., Colchester, A. C., and Maisey, M. N. (1991). Computer-aided interpretation of SPECT images of the brain using an MRI-derived 3D neuro-anatomical atlas. *Med. Inf.* **16**(2), 151–166.

Levin, D. N., Hu, X., Tan, K. K., *et al.* (1989a). The brain: Integrated three-dimensional display of MR and PET images. *Radiology* **172**, 783–789.

Levin, D. N., Hu, X., Tan, K. K., and Galhotra, S. (1989b). Surface of the brain: Three-dimensional MR images created with volume rendering. *Radiology* **171**, 277–280.

Mano, I., Suto, Y., Suzuki, M., and Iio, M. (1990). Computerized three-dimensional normal atlas. *Radiat. Med.* **8**(2), 50–54.

Marrett, S., Evans, A. C., Collins, L., and Peters, T. M. (1989). A volume of interest (VOI) atlas for the analysis of neurophysiological image data. *In* "Medical Imaging II 1989: SPIE Proceedings," pp. 467–477.

Miller, M. I. (1991). Automated segmentation of biological shapes in electron microscopic autoradiography. *In* "Proceedings of the 25th Annual Conference on Information Science and Systems, Johns Hopkins University, 1991," pp. 637–642.

Miller, M. I., Christensen, G. E., Amit, Y., and Grenander, U. (1993). "A Mathematical Textbook of Deformable Neuroanatomies." *Proc. Natl. Acad. of Sci. USA* **90**(24).

Pechura, C. M., and Martin, J. B. (Eds.) (1991). "Mapping the Brain and Its Functions." Washington, D.C.: National Academy Press.

Sandor, T., Jolesz, F., Tieman, J., Kikinis, R., LeMay, M., and Albert, M. (1991). Extraction of morphometric information from dual echo magnetic resonance brain images. *In* "Visual Communications and Image Processing '90: SPIE Proceedings," Vol. 1360, pp. 665–675.

Schiemann, T., Bomans, M., Tiede, U., and Höhne, K. H. (1992). Interactive 3D-segmentation. *In* "Visualization in Biomedical Computing 1992: SPIE Proceedings," Vol. 1808, pp. 376–383.

Shenton, M. E., Kikinis, R., Jolesz, F. A., Pollak, S. D., LeMay, M., Wible, C. G., Hokama, H., Martin, J., Metcalf, D., Coleman, M., and McCarley, R. W. (1992). Abnormalities of the left temporal lobe and thought disorder in schizophrenia. *N. Engl. J. Med.* **327**, 604–612.

Srivastava, A., Miller, M. I., and Grenander, U. (1991). Jump-diffusion processes for object tracking and direction finding. *In* "Proceedings of the 29th Annual Allerton Conference on Communication, Control and Computing, Urbana, Champaign, 1991," pp. 563–570. University of Illinois, Urbana.

Tiede, U., Höhne, K. H., Pommert, A., Riemer, M., Schiemann, T., and Schubert, R. (1993). A computerized three-dimensional atlas of the human skull and brain. *Am. J. Neuroradiol.* **14**(3), 551–559.

Toga, A. W. (Ed.) (1990). "Three-Dimensional Neuroimaging." New York: Raven Press.

Vannier, M. W., Brunsden, B. S., Hildebolt, C. F., Falk, D., Cheverud, J. M., Figiel, G. S., Perman, W. H., Kohn, L. A., Robb, R. A., Yoffie, R. L., and Bresina, S. J. (1991). Brain surface cortical lengths: Quantification with three-dimensional MR imaging. *Radiology* **180**, 479–484.

Vannier, M. W., Yates, R. E., and Whitestone, J. (1992). Electronic imaging of the human body. *In* "Visualization in Biomedical Computing 1992: SPIE Proceedings," Vol. 1808, pp. 478–486.

22

High-Resolution Evoked Potential Technology for Imaging Neural Networks of Cognition

Alan Gevins, Brian Cutillo, Don DuRousseau, Jian Le, Harrison Leong, and Michael Smith

EEG Systems Laboratory & SAM Technology, San Francisco, California 94107

I. Introduction

The functional architecture of mental processes has come to be viewed as dynamic and multifocal (e.g., Goldman-Rakic, 1988a, 1988b; Damasio, 1989; Mesulam, 1990). Especially in the case of higher cognitive functions, adequate characterization of the electrical signals generated by such distributed neural substrates requires a means for measuring moment-by-moment changes in the functional networks that are adaptively configured in response to environmental demands and in the context of purposive behavior (Eimas and Galaburda, 1989). Of all brain imaging modalities, the temporal resolution of the electroencephalogram (EEG) makes it best suited for monitoring rapid changes in brain activity. Thus, development of improved neuroelectric imaging methods addresses a central problem in cognitive neuroscience.

During the past 20 years, rapid advances have been made in such neuroimaging modalities as CT, MRI, PET, and SPECT. In contrast, although the EEG provides a subsecond temporal resolution, is completely noninvasive and harmless, and has equipment costs over an order of magnitude less than other imaging modalities, the development of a spatiotemporal electrophysiological neuroimaging modality has not been fully realized during the almost 70 years since the first EEG recording. This delay stems largely from the fact that the amount of spatial information that can be recovered from the scalp-recorded EEG has often been underestimated; hence, relatively little effort has been

made to increase its spatial resolution. Without questioning the fundamental limitations to inferences about arbitrarily complex electrical sources that may be obtained from scalp recorded brain electrical or magnetic activity, we note that the spatial information obtained from EEGs has been limited by the small number of scalp sites that are sampled during most routine recordings and by the underutilization of modern signal enhancement methods to compensate for volume conduction blurring. The former is for the most part a matter of habit, whereas the expense of computing is no longer a significant barrier. Therefore major advances in EEG technology can now be practically accomplished. The first part of this chapter reviews some of the efforts we have made to improve the capabilities of the EEG; the second part describes some of the studies in which we have applied these developing technologies.

II. High-Resolution Evoked Potential Techniques

A. Improved Sampling and Registration with MRI

1. Increased Number of Electrodes and Measurement of Electrode Positions

Adequate spatial sampling is a requirement for extracting detailed information about neurocognitive processes from scalp-recorded EPs. The 19-channel

FUNCTIONAL NEUROIMAGING

"10–20" montage commonly used in clinical and research EEG recordings has an interelectrode distance of about 6 cm on a typical adult head. This spacing may be dense enough for detecting signs of gross pathology, but is insufficient for resolving the finer topographical differences that are important in studying human perceptual and cognitive processes. To improve spatial resolution, we have increased the number of scalp electrodes to 59 and 124 (Gevins, 1988; Gevins *et al.*, 1990a), in order to provide interelectrode distances of about 3.5 and 2.25 cm, respectively. This is within the 2.5 cm range of the 3-dB point on the cortex-to-scalp point spread function, that is, the size of the scalp representation of a small, discrete neuronal source at the level of the cortex (Gevins, 1990). A reasonable goal may be to work toward increasing the number of electrodes to as many as 256, which would provide for interelectrode distances on the order of 1 cm^2. To simplify electrode application, we have been developing an EEG recording system with active electrodes that do not require preparation of the scalp (Gevins *et al.*, 1991b). Finally, in addition to increasing the number of recording electrodes, productive application of signal enhancement techniques also requires that the spatial positions of those electrodes be known. At present, we obtain this information by measuring the 3D positions of each scalp electrode with a commercial magnetic digitizer with an accuracy of about 3 mm.

2. Realistic Head Model and Alignment of Electrodes with Scalp Surface

Most attempts to increase the 3D spatial resolution of brain electrical events have relied on spherical head models that are uniform in their conductive properties. However, the head is not spherical, and its conductivity is not spatially uniform. These sources of error can be reduced by utilizing an accurate anatomical representation of a subject's brain, skull, and scalp. We have developed methods to process MRIs for accurate rendering of the scalp surface, alignment of electrode positions with this scalp surface, and construction of structured finite elements (tetrahedral volumes) to model the tissue layers of scalp, skull, and cortical surface (Gevins *et al.*, 1990a, 1991a; Le and Gevins, 1993). The structure of scalp, skull, and superficial cortex are modeled by contouring individual horizontal MRI slices and then constructing a triangular surface mesh. After the structures are outlined by an automated contour tracing algorithm, each MRI slice is viewed on a graphics screen in order to correct the outlines as necessary. The resulting series of contours are then triangularized to form a continuous 3D model. The digitized electrode positions are then aligned with the scalp surface model by translation and rotation of the *x*, *y*, and *z* axes and application of an iterative least-squares fitting algorithm that adjusts each parameter until the average distance between each electrode position and the corresponding closest scalp point is minimized. The procedure is cross-checked by comparison with the alignment of fiducial points at the nasion, inion, and preauricular notches. Plate 68 shows an example of electrode positions on reconstructed scalp surface after the alignment process.

B. Reduction of Spatial Blur Distortion

1. Laplacian Derivation

The usefulness of an increased number of electrodes is mainly limited by the distortion of neuronal potentials as they are conducted through the highly resistive skull. This distortion amounts to a spatial low-pass filtering, which causes a blurring of the potential distribution at the scalp. There are a number of methods for reducing this distortion, from the computationally simple to very intensive. The spatial Laplacian operator, usually referred to as the *Laplacian derivation* (LD), lies at the simpler and more widely accessible end. It is computed as the second derivative in space of the potential field at each electrode. The LD is proportional to the current entering and exiting the scalp at each electrode site and is independent of the location of the reference electrode used for recording. It is relatively insensitive to signals that are common to the area or local group of electrodes used to compute the LD and thus is more sensitive to cortical potentials of higher spatial frequency than to signals conducted from subcortical sources. A simple method of computing the LD assumes that electrodes are equidistant and at right angles to each other (Hjorth, 1975). This approximation is good for some electrode positions, such as midline central (Cz), but is less accurate for others such as midtemporal (T5). We have used a more accurate estimate of the LD that is based on 3D spline functions for computing the LD over the actual shape of the head (Gevins *et al.*, 1991a; Law *et al.*, 1993; Le *et al.*, submitted). One drawback to all LD methods is that it is not possible to estimate the LD at peripheral electrodes, because the set of surrounding electrodes is incomplete.

2. Finite Element Deblurring (FED)

This technique is a mathematical spatial enhancement procedure that uses an anatomically realistic model of the passive conducting properties of each subject's head and the finite element method to estimate potentials at the cortical surface from scalp potentials (Gevins et al., 1991a; Le and Gevins, 1993). Unlike other methods that estimate cortical potentials or currents (Nicholas and Deloche, 1976; Freeman, 1980; Sidman et al., 1989), FED is a true "downward continuation" method in that the cortical potential distribution is derived without prior knowledge or assumptions about the generating sources. The increase in spatial detail provided by this technique over that obtained by more traditional EP mapping methods is illustrated in Plate 70 in the case of steady-state somatosensory evoked potentials. The process is described in some detail below.

a. Finite Element Construction For the FED method described in the following section, an important first step is to represent the scalp and skull volumes by a set of finite elements with the same simple geometry. A tetrahedron was chosen as the basic finite element shape as this is the 3D object that can be formed from the fewest triangles. Horizontal contours were first generated to delineate the scalp/exterior border, the skull/scalp border, and the brain/skull border. Finite elements were then constructed from the contours in the following manner. For each point on a given contour for a given MRI slice, edges were formed between that point and (a) adjacent points on the same contour for the same slice, (b) the homologous point and the next point lying on an adjacent contour of the same slice, (c) the homologous point and the next point lying on the same contour of an adjacent slice, and (d) the homologous point and the next point lying on an adjacent contour of an adjacent slice. Triangular faces were formed from the edges and tetrahedrons were formed from the faces. These tetrahedrons, which partitioned the entire volume, constituted the finite elements (Plate 69). The cortical surface models consist of the innermost triangular faces of the original tetrahedral elements, onto which the deblurred potentials have been interpolated. The theoretical formulation and computational implementation of FED are described in Le and Gevins (1993).

b. Verification with Simulations and Subdural Grid Recording The validity of the deblurring procedure was assessed in several ways. Simulations using a spherical conducting model were performed to compare the obtainable exact solutions with the deblurring results (Le and Gevins, 1993). The scalp, skull, and brain surfaces were modeled with concentric (upper) hemispheres of radii 9, 8.5, and 8 cm, each containing 127 points that defined the vertices for a total of 432 prism-shaped finite elements. The conductivity ratio of scalp/skull and brain/skull elements was taken to

be 80. Six current dipoles within the inner hemisphere were selected which varied in depth, orientation, and horizontal location. For each dipole, the potentials at the vertices on the inner and outer surfaces were calculated as the forward solution for a three-sphere model. The potentials on the inner hemisphere were also solved for by the deblurring method, using the potentials at the outer surface. The resulting error variance ranged from 0.2 to 1.2% for the six dipoles, which shows good agreement between the deblurred potentials and the exact solutions.

As a direct verification of this method, evoked potentials recorded from a 64-channel grid over the somatosensory cortex from an epileptic patient were compared to deblurred EPs recorded at the scalp prior to surgery (Gevins et al., 1991a, 1993b in press). The patient was a 21-year-old woman with pharmacologically intractable seizures originating in the left hemisphere and with right-hemisphere dominance for handedness and speech (as determined by Wada test). Somatosensory electrical stimulation at 14.92 Hz produced EPs which were very similar for all five fingers stimulated and showed an abnormally large response known to occur for some epileptics [referred to as "giant SEP"; e.g., Shibasaki et al. (1990)]. Alignment of the cortical grid with the MRIs recorded prior to surgery was done based on information from a surgical photograph and postimplant radiograph. The deblurred potentials showed an improvement in resolution over the Laplacian derivation and were more similar to the actual recorded cortical potentials. Although this patient exhibited abnormal cortical organization and SEPs, this initial test of the deblurring method is considered valid because the method is based only on the model of head conductivity.

Additional analyses with data from this patient have shown the stability of the deblurred potentials across independent samples and for different conductivity ratios. The variability across samples was measured by finding the standard deviation of potential values at each cortical point over three independent samples of data (each 100 s of recording for five individual fingers) and then calculating the mean of these standard deviations. This number was then expressed as a percentage of the within-sample variability, which was calculated by finding the mean range in potential values for each sample. These results showed that the across-sample variability was only 4.2% of the within-sample variability, which indicates that the deblurring procedure is stable. Deblurring calculations were also performed using values of the scalp/skull and brain/skull conductivity ratio at a range of values varying +/− 50% from the standard value of 80. Results showed that different conductivity ratios produced gradual differences in the exact size of active regions and in the finer detail, but did not substantially change the pattern of activity. These preliminary findings suggest that the deblurring method merits further validation and development to remove ambiguities in interpretation of topographic maps due to tangentially oriented cortical generators.

C. Preparation of Datasets

Integrity of data is another area to which we have given particular attention, because the quality of the data is especially important when applying new and highly sensitive methods. This involves removal of instrumental and physiological artifacts and control of experimental conditions.

1. Detecting and Eliminating Artifacts

The usual practice in evoked potential studies of cognition is to automatically reject artifacted trials in which the voltage of the eye-movement measurement channels exceeds a fixed threshold or in which the EEG signals are very large due to head movements or scalp muscle activity (Barlow, 1986). Although these procedures catch large contaminants, they miss small ones. This can lead to a spurious result if there are small, consistent saccades, microblinks, or other noncerebral activities time locked to the stimulus. Although we also use an on-line artifact detection procedure to flag portions of trials and individual channels with unusually high or low amplitude, all data are examined off line using an interactive graphics program to confirm and improve the automatic detection algorithm. Improved automated artifact detection procedures using neural network pattern recognition are under continuing development (Gevins and Morgan, 1986).

2. Controlling for Spurious Between-Condition Differences

After the data have been cleared of artifacts, sets of trials are formed in order to test specific hypotheses. In forming each pair of datasets, it is imperative that the major difference between sets be related to the hypothesis being tested. It is, of course, standard practice to try to eliminate spurious differences by careful experimental design, but there is always the chance that some remaining factors differ between sets. These uncontrolled factors can include small residual eye-movement contaminants, arousal level, and response movement parameters such as response force or reaction time, all of which can affect neuroelectric signals. To ensure that the major source of

variance is actually related to the hypothesis, the sets of artifact-free trials for each condition of the hypothesis are submitted on a subject-by-subject basis to an interactive program that displays the means, *t* tests, and histogram distributions of up to 50 behavioral and physiological variables (Gevins *et al.*, 1985). These include stimulus parameters, reaction time, response magnitude and duration, error, EEG arousal index (integrated energy in the α frequency band), and eye-movement and muscle potential indices (integrated energy). The datasets are inspected for significant differences in variables not related to the hypothesis, and outlier trials are discarded until the *t* test reaches an α of 0.2 or, if this causes a severe truncation of the distribution, just over 0.05. For example, in tasks in which the force of a finger response is variable, a between-condition condition in the distribution of response forces may be present. The associated movement-related potentials could overlap the P300 EP peak and cause a spurious between-condition difference in P300 amplitude. To avoid this, the two datasets would be balanced for response force so that between-condition differences in P300 amplitudes would not be confounded by differences in movement-related potentials.

D. Integration of Spatial and Temporal Information: Evoked Potential Covariance

Topographical maps of a brain electrical event usually display the voltage over the scalp measured at a single time point, usually corresponding to an EP peak. However, the peak latency of an EP component might vary substantially between electrode sites or, as with slow potentials such as the contingent negative variation, does not exist as a discrete time point. Thus, in many cases the selection of a time point for mapping becomes somewhat arbitrary, and potentially revealing interelectrode latency differences are ignored. We have worked toward developing methods for characterizing EP components both in terms of their spatial topography and in terms of their temporal relationships between electrode locations. We refer to one such method as evoked potential covariance (EPC) analysis, and it evolved from the notion that the neural processes involved with higher cognitive functions must involve functionally related activity in widely distributed cortical and subcortical areas.

Because the EP waveform delineates the time course of event-related mass activity of a neural population, a contribution of two or more populations to task performance should be signaled by a consistent relationship between the morphology of their EP waveforms and consistent time delay (Adey *et al.*,

1961; Callaway and Harris, 1974; Livanov, 1977; Gevins and Bressler, 1988). If the relationships are linear, as they often appear to be, this coordinated activity might be statistically characterized by the lagged covariance between the EPs, or segments of EPs, from different regions. Of course, this simple idea becomes more complicated when EPs are measured at the scalp, in which case the genesis of any specific covariance of this type is unknown and a consistent statistical relationship between two regions might be due to direct or indirect neurotransmission between cortical regions, to imposed synchronization from one or more areas, or to common volume conduction from remote sources. As a result of this ambiguity, interpretations of EPCs in terms of the underlying neural processes that generate them must be made very cautiously. Ongoing investigations are studying the neurogenesis of EPCs using a primate preparation (Bressler and Nakamura, 1992; Bressler et al., in press) and subdural grid recordings in epileptic patients (Gevins et al., 1993a in press). In the meanwhile, we have found this method to be a useful analytic tool for quantitatively characterizing the spatiotemporal changes in brain electrical activity that occur in conjunction with adaptive cognitive functions; it is worthwhile to note that results with this method to date have been highly consistent with the known large-scale functional neuroanatomy of the cerebral cortex (Gevins et al., 1987, 1989a, 1989b, 1990b).

Our current EPC procedure is described in Gevins et al. (1989a), and an example of an EPC display is provided in Plate 71. There are two main concerns with the interpretation of the EPC measure, both of which are the subject of ongoing research. The first is the extent to which the covariance measure actually reflects the coordinated activity of a functional neural network. We merely note here that statistical interdependency between channels (not necessarily linear) is a necessary but not sufficient feature of functional neural networks. The second is the degree to which it is possible to measure the activity of cortical networks immediately underlying each electrode. There is no general solution to this latter issue, but the ambiguity can be mitigated to some extent by careful experimental design and by the use of spatial filters such as the Laplacian derivation which tends to be more sensitive to superficial (i.e. cortical) sources. Ongoing work on disambiguating deblurred evoked potentials due to tangentially oriented cortical sources should also greatly simplify the interpretation of EPCs (see above). Until these issues are settled any interpretations of EPCs in terms of the underlying neural processes that generate them must be made very cautiously.

III. Applying the Tools

In this section, we review some results of recent studies of basic neurocognitive functions. These studies suggest that each basic neurocognitive process may be characterized by a sequence of spatiotemporal patterns of distributed, coordinated processing, signs of which are evident in evoked potential covariance measures. The findings support the concept that the formation and regulation of such distributed networks involve the integrative activity of areas of prefrontal cortex.

A. Deblurring of Language-Related EPs

In addition to its utility for increasing the spatial resolution of sensory EPs, the FED method promises to be a useful tool in the analysis of higher-order functions. For example, it has been used to increase the spatial resolution of EPs related to component processes in reading that were elicited during a simple cued matching task that required one of four types of matching judgments (Gevins et al., manuscript in preparation): graphic (visual identity of unfamiliar nonletter character strings), phonemic (homophonic pseudowords), semantic (antonymy), and grammatic (noun–verb agreement). Each trial of this task began with a cue that indicated which one of the four conditions to expect. One second later this cue was followed by the first stimulus, which in turn was followed one second later with the comparison stimulus. Fifteen percent of the trials were "mismatch" trials to which subjects responded by pressing a button with their left index finger. Eighty-five percent of the trials were "match" trials to which no response was to be made. The four conditions were presented in random order, as were the occurrence of match and mismatch trials. EEGs were recorded from nine right-handed subjects using a 59-electrode montage. Application of a 3D spline Laplacian derivation resulted in a set of 43 nonperipheral electrodes, which were analyzed. The FED method was performed for two subjects for whom MRI-based head models had been constructed. Several striking between-condition differences were evident in highly localized EP patterns. For example, larger amplitude EP peaks occurred in the grammatic condition (relative to the other language tasks) at 442 ms after the first stimulus and about 300 ms after the second stimulus. These potentials were most prominent in the regoin of Broca's language area of the left hemisphere (e.g., Plate 72), and their task correlates are consistent with the postulated functional neuroanatomy of this region.

B. EPCs Related to Preparatory Processes

Even in the highly controlled conditions of the laboratory, a stimulus does not fall upon a blank brain state. There is always some degree of expectation based on what has occurred during preceding trials, because the perceptual interaction between one's self and one's environment always occurs in the context of prior experience. One way to study the effects of expectation in the controlled conditions of the laboratory is to deliberately manipulate preparatory activity by means of a get-ready cue. Higher resolution evoked potentials have proven particularly fruitful in this area. An example suggesting the modulation of neural networks associated with preparatory processes was found during the cued prestimulus interval of a visuomotor judgment task. EPC patterns were computed in an interval from 500 to 875 ms after subjects had been visually cued to prepare to make a graded pressure response with the index finger of either the right or the left hand when the next numeric stimulus was presented (Gevins *et al.*, 1987, 1989b). (The numeric stimulus was always presented 1 s after the get-ready cue.) Plate 73 shows the preparatory interval for the right hand for those trials for which the response was subsequently either accurate or inaccurate. (Accurate response trials were defined as those trials whose response error was less than the mean error over the whole session comprising several hundred trials.) The "network" pattern for those trials with subsequently accurate responses have covariances of the left prefrontal electrode with electrodes overlying the same motor, somatosensory, and parietal areas that were involved in actual response execution. The preparatory pattern preceding inaccurate responses differed markedly from that preceding accurate responses in that it had fewer and weaker covariances. Thus, it is possible that inaccurate performance of this task was due in part to a failure of prefrontal regions to initially prepare and coordinate the activity of cortical areas used in subsequent production of the response.

Functional network patterns have also been measured during a task involving working memory, that is, the process of holding a small amount of information in awareness while it is used in some mental operation (Gevins and Cutillo, 1993). We used a task in which a graded pressure response was made with the right-hand index finger according to the magnitude of the visual stimulus number (from 1 to 9) presented two trials previously (Gevins *et al.*, 1990b). In a random 20% of trials, the current stimulus number was the same as the number presented two trials previously, and no response was to be made to these match trials. For comparison purposes, a control task was also included in which the graded pressure response was made according to the number of the current trial, rather than the number presented two trials previously. During the period before onset of the number stimulus, EPCs for both working memory and control tasks were focused on electrodes over midline and bilateral premotor and right posterior areas. However, dramatic preparatory EPC differences were also observed, with the working memory condition being distinguished by stronger EPCs overall and strong left-sided EPCs between precentral and anterior parietal and anterior occipital sites. Thus, as with the prestimulus differences related to subsequent response accuracy, these results also suggest that the prefrontal regions of the brain tend to be involved in the anticipatory activation of those specialized brain regions that will participate in an upcoming cognitive event.

Degradation of this anticipatory activation appears to accompany states of fatigue, a fact that may be important for understanding and predicting the performance failures that tend to occur in fatigued individuals. For example, the working memory task described above was used to determine predictive, leading indicator neuroelectric signs of operational fatigue due to extended sessions of task performance (Gevins *et al.*, 1990b). This experiment was conducted with the participation of five highly skilled Air Force test pilots who practiced the tasks extensively prior to the EEG recording session. The main object was to study changes in EPC patterns in a long recording session, in particular, to search for EEG changes that preceded significant behavioral signs of operational fatigue. Twenty-seven EEG channels were used to determine 18 channels of nonperipheral Laplacian derivation evoked potentials. EPC patterns between all pairwise combinations of these 18 channels were computed. Changes in the EPCs during the prestimulus interval were observed over the course of a recording session that lasted from 10 to 14 h. The changes appeared after 7–8 h of performance, but before behavioral signs of fatigue became significant. The overall magnitude of the covariances was reduced with fatigue, and the topographic pattern was altered. Specifically, the pattern changed from one strongly focused on midline central and precentral sites, to one focused primarily on right-sided precentral and parietal electrodes. It appeared that fatigue may have affected the transient allocation of attentional resources to processes associated with maintaining the two numbers and possibly also the preparatory processes involving the contents of working memory.

Finally, we have also seen evidence of preparatory networks related to the nature of the feature extraction process to be performed on an expected stimulus. In the study of language processing mentioned above, the graphic task required the matching of two strings of Japanese Katakana characters. Because Katakana characters have about the same degree of complexity as letters, but were highly unfamiliar to our subjects, it was expected that their encoding would involve a greater amount of neural activity compared with the encoding of letters. This expectation was supported by the observation that the amplitude of an evoked potential peak at about 340 ms in the graphic condition was larger over occipital regions in the cued prestimulus interval, suggesting that extrastriate cortical regions were being activated in preparation for processing the expected unfamiliar stimulus.

IV. Conclusions

Recent advances in recording and analysis technology promise to increase the sensitivity and specificity of measurements of the neurophysiological basis of perception, cognition, and action. More detailed evoked potential measurements have been achieved by increasing the number of electrodes and using a means of spatial signal enhancement, such as Laplacian derivation or the finite element deblurring (FED) method. Information about distributed processing and its temporal relationships is provided by the evoked potential covariance (EPC) measure. The signs of rapidly shifting patterns of statistical interdependency between sites that are reviewed above are particularly intriguing in light of their consistency with historical and contemporary findings about brain–behavior relationships from clinical and experimental sources. The development of neurophysiological measurement technology is by no means complete. The next step is concerned with removing ambiguities in interpretation of topographic maps in terms of cortical generators. This will require development of better methods of "source analysis," which is underway at several laboratories. With these developments, high-resolution evoked potentials, both by themselves and in combination with other functional neuroimaging modalities, will likely play an increasingly important role both in cognitive neuroscience and in clinical neurology.

Finally, the ability to accurately characterize the subsecond spatiotemporal dynamics of neurocognitive processes will likely promote the development of more realistic biological conceptions of mental func-

tions. Because of the stimulus–response format inherent in most experimental designs, many models of cognitive functioning have a passive tone. The brain is conceived of as reacting to a given stimulus, and the stages leading to an elicited response are inferred from measures of reaction time, EP peak latencies, and so on. However, experience, observation, and inference all suggest that cognitive processes are highly interactive and proactive. Perception is a synthesis of sensation, current brain state, and past cognitive experience. This synthesis relies on a continuously updated, dynamic internal representation of what one imagines one's self and one's environment to be like at any given moment. Moreover, effector and sensory systems are used to actively probe the environment for information relevant to maintaining and updating the self/world model. Each perception, each action, is incorporated into the internal model, and new perceptions and actions are in turn influenced through the model's role in directing attentional and conceptual processes. It is challenging, but fruitful, to design experimental situations that emphasize this dynamic and interactive nature of cognition. Areas of particular interest include preparatory processes, which precede the stimulus and are directed by the internal model; retrieval and self-reflection, in which past experience and self-concerns are consciously compared with current events; and assessment of feedback, which governs the updating of the model. Although it seems that the frontal cortex plays a pivotal role in all of these processes (Fuster, 1989; Stuss and Benson, 1986; Stuss, 1991), it is simplistic to consider the frontal lobes as only executive in nature. Rather, it is likely that many areas are involved in a constellation of rapidly changing functional networks that provide the delicate balance between stimulus-locked behavior and purely imaginary ideation. With even further advances in brain imaging technology in the 1990s, it is realistic to hope to achieve increasingly detailed and direct measurements of the organization and interrelationships of sensory and higher cognitive behaviors in health and in disease.

Acknowledgments

This research has been supported by competitive grants from The National Institute of Mental Health, The National Institute of Neurological Diseases and Stroke, The Air Force Office of Scientific Research, The Office of Naval Research, The National Science Foundation, and The National Institute of Alcohol Abuse and Alcoholism of the United States federal government. Thanks to all members of the EEG Systems Laboratory and SAM Technology, past and present, for their vital contributions to the work presented here.

References

Adey, W., Walter, D. and Hendrix, C. (1961). Computer techniques in correlation and spectral analysis of cerebral slow waves during discriminative behavior. *Exp. Neurol.* **3**, 501–524.

Ary, J. B., Klein, S. A., and Fender, D. H. (1981). Location of sources of evoked scalp potentials: Corrections for skull and scalp thicknesses. *IEEE Trans. Biomed. Eng.* **28**, 447–452.

Barlow, J. S. (1986). Artifact processing (rejection and minimization) in EEG data processing. In "Handbook of Electroencephalography and Clinical Neurophysiology" (F. H. Lopes da Silva, W. Storm van Leeuwen, and A. Remond, Eds.), Vol. 2, pp. 15–65. Amsterdam: Elsevier.

Bressler, S. L., and Nakamura, R. C. (1992). "Inter-Area Synchronization in Macaque Neocortex during a Visual Pattern Discrimination Task." Presented at the Conference on Computational and Neural Systems, July 1992, San Francisco, CA.

Bressler, S. L., Coppola, R., and Nakamura, R. (1993). Cortical interactions in the macaque cortex. *Nature (London)*, in press.

Callaway, E., and Harris, P. (1974). Coupling between cortical potentials from different areas. *Science* **183**, 873–875.

Damasio, A. R. (1989). Time-locked multi-regional retroactivation: A systems-level proposal for the neural substrates of recall and recognition. *Cognition* **33**, 25–62.

Efron, B. (1982). "The Jackknife, the Bootstrap, and Other Resampling Plans." Philadelphia: Society for Industrial and Applied Mathematics.

Eimas, P. D., and Galaburda, A. M. (1989). Some agenda items for a neurobiology of cognition: An introduction. *Cognition* **33**, 1–23.

Freeman, W. J. (1980). Use of spatial deconvolution to compensate for distortion of EEG by volume conduction. *IEEE Trans. Biomed. Eng.* **27**, 421–429.

Fuster, J. M. (1989). "The Prefrontal Cortex: Anatomy, Physiology, and Neuropsychology of the Frontal Lobe." New York: Raven Press.

Gevins, A. S. (1990). Analysis of multiple lead data. In "Event-Related Potentials of the Brain" (J. Rohrbaugh, R. Johnson, and R. Parasuraman, Eds.), pp. 44–56. New York: Oxford University Press.

Gevins, A. S. (1988). Recent advances in neurocognitive pattern analysis. In "Dynamics of Sensory and Cognitive Processing of the Brain" (E. Basar, Ed.), pp. 88–102. Heidelberg: Springer-Verlag.

Gevins, A. S., and Bressler, S. L. (1988). Functional topography of the human brain. In "Functional Brain Imaging" (G. Pfurtscheller, Ed.), pp. 99–116. Bern: Hans Huber Publishers.

Gevins, A., and Cutillo, B. (1986). Signals of cognition. In "Handbook of Encephalography and Clinical Neurophysiology," Vol. 2, "Clinical Applications of Computer Analysis of EEG and Other Neurophysiological Signals" (F. Lopez da Silva and A. Remond, Eds.), pp. 335–381. Amsterdam: Elsevier.

Gevins, A., and Cutillo, B. (1993). Neuroelectric evidence for distributed processing in human working memory. *Electroenceph. Clin. Neurophysiol.* **87**, 128–143.

Gevins, A. S., and Morgan, N. H. (1986). Classifier-directed signal processing in brain research. *IEEE Trans. Biomed. Eng.* **33**, 1058–1064.

Gevins, A. S., Doyle, J. C., Cutillo, B. A., Shaffer, R. E., Tannehill, R. S., Bressler, S. L., and Zeitlin, J. (1985). Neurocognitive pattern analysis of a visuomotor task: Low-frequency evoked correlation. *Psychophysiology* **22**, 32–43.

Gevins, A. S., Morgan, N. H., Bressler, S. L., Cutillo, B. A., White, R. M., Illes, J., Greer, D. S., Doyle, J. C., and Zeitlin, G. M.

(1987). Human neuroelectric patterns predict performance accuracy. *Science* **235**, 580–585.

Gevins, A. S., Cutillo, B. A., Bressler, S. L., Morgan, N. H., White, R. M., Illes, J., and Greer, D. S. (1989a). Event-related covariances during a bimanual visuomotor task. I. Methods and analysis of stimulus- and response-locked data. *EEG Clin. Neurophysiol.* **74**(1), 58–75.

Gevins, A. S., Cutillo, B. A., Bressler, S. L., Morgan, N. H., White, R. M., Illes, J., and Greer, D. S. (1989b). Event-related covariances during a bimanual visuomotor task. II. Preparation and feedback. *EEG Clin. Neurophysiol.* **74**(2), 147–160.

Gevins, A. S., Brickett, P., Costales, B., Le, J., and Reutter, B. (1990a). Beyond topographic mapping: Towards functional-anatomical imaging with 124-channel EEGs and MRIs. *Brain Topogr.* **3**(1), 53–64.

Gevins, A. S., Bressler, S. L., Cutillo, B. A., Illes, J., and Fowler-White, R. M. (1990b). Effects of prolonged mental work on functional brain topography. *EEG Clin. Neurophysiol.* **76**, 339–350.

Gevins, A. S., Le, J., Brickett, P., Reutter, B., and Desmond, J. (1991a). Seeing through the skull: Advanced EEGs use MRIs to accurately measure cortical activity from the scalp. *Brain Topogr.* **4**(2), 125–131.

Gevins, A. S., DuRousseau, D., and Libove, J. (1991b). "Electrode System for Brain Wave Detection." U.S. Patent No. 5,038,782.

Gevins, A., Cutillo, B., Bressler, S., Barbero, N., and Laxer, K. (1993a). Distributed cortical networks during a somatosensory discrimination task. *Electroenceph. Clin. Neurophysiol.*, in press.

Gevins, A., Cutillo, B., and Smith, M. E. Neurocognitive decomposition of reading with high resolution evoked potentials. Manuscript in preparation.

Gevins, A. S., Le, J., Martin, N., Desmond, J., McLaughlin, J., and Brickett, P. (1993b). High resolution EEG: 124-channel recording, spatial enhancement and MRI integration methods. *Electroenceph. Clin. Neurophysiol.*, in press.

Goldman-Rakic, P. S. (1988a). Topography of cognition: Parallel distributed networks in primate association cortex. *Annu. Rev. Neurosci.*, **11**, 137–156.

Goldman-Rakic, P. S. (1988b). Changing concepts of cortical connectivity: Parallel distributed cortical networks. In "Neurobiology of Neocortex" (P. Rakic and W. Singer, Eds.), pp. 177–202. New York: Wiley.

Hjorth, B. (1975). An on-line transformation of EEG scalp potentials into orthogonal source derivations. *Electroenceph. Clin. Neurophysiol.* **39**, 526–530.

Law, S. K., Nunez, P. L., and Wijesinghe, R. S. (1993). High resolution EEG using spline generated surface Laplacians on spherical and ellipsoidal surfaces. *IEEE Trans. Biomed. Eng.* **40**(2), 145–153.

Le, J., and Gevins, A. (1993). Method to reduce blur distortion from EEGs using a realistic head model. *IEEE Trans. Biomed. Eng.* **40**(6), 517–528.

Le, J., Menon, V., and Gevins, A. Local estimate of surface Laplacian derivation on a realistically shaped scalp surface. *Electroenceph. Clin. Neurophysiol.*, submitted for publication.

Livanov, M. N. (1977). "Spatial Organization of Cerebral Processes." New York: Wiley.

Mesulam, M. (1990). Large-scale neurocognitive networks and distributed processing for attention, language, and memory. *Ann. Neurol.* **28**(5), 597–613.

Nicholas, P., and Deloche, G. (1976). Convolution computer processing of the brain electrical image transmission. *Int. J. Bio-Med. Comput.* **7**, 143–159.

Rush, S., and Driscoll, D. (1968). Current distribution in the brain from surface electrodes. *Anesthesia Analgesia* **47**, 717–723.

Rush, S., and Driscoll, D. (1969). EEG electrode sensitivity—An application of reciprocity. *IEEE Trans. Biomed. Eng.* **16,** 15–22.

Shibasaki, H., Nakamura, M., Nishida, S., Kakigi, R., and Ikeda, A. (1990). Wave form decomposition of "giant SEP" and its computer model for scalp topography. *Electroenceph. Clin. Neurophysiol.* **77,** 286–294.

Sidman, R. D., Kearfott, R. B., Major, D. J., Hill, D. C., Ford, M. R., Smith, D. B., Lee, L., and Kramer, R. (1989). Development and application of mathematical techniques for the noninvasive localization of the sources of scalp-recorded electric potentials. *In* "IMACS Transcripts on Scientific Computing" (J. Eisenfield and D. S. Levine, Eds.), Vol. 5, pp. 133–157. Basel: J. C. Baltzer.

Stuss, D. T. (1991). Self, awareness, and the frontal lobes: A neuropsychological perspective. *In* "The Self: Interdisciplinary Approaches" (J. Strauss and G. R. Goethals, Eds.), pp. 255–278. New York: Springer-Verlag.

Stuss, D., and Benson, D. F. (1986). "The Frontal Lobes." New York: Raven Press.

23

Registration of PET and SPECT with MRI by Anatomical Surface Matching

**Charles A. Pelizzari,* David N. Levin,† Chin-Tu Chen,†
and George T. Y. Chen***

*Departments of *Radiation and Cellular Oncology and †Radiology, The University of Chicago,
Chicago, Illinois 60637*

I. Introduction

Functional information from nuclear medicine images is critical in many research, diagnostic, and therapy planning applications. In particular, 3D functional image sets from emission computed tomography (ECT) modalities provide a unique source of detailed information concerning both normal function and abnormalities of the brain. Analysis of functional information from positron (PET) or single photon (SPECT) emission computed tomography is frequently complicated by the lack of direct visualization in nuclear medicine images of relevant neuroanatomy. In many cases a set of anatomical images from magnetic resonance imaging (MRI) would constitute a useful anatomical template for analysis of ECT data, were it possible to establish a correspondence between the anatomical and the functional image spaces at an appropriate level of accuracy. Use of such an anatomical template may be of particular interest in planning procedures such as neurosurgery or radiation therapy in which a lesion is manifested by some functional abnormality visualized in the nuclear medicine images, but spatial localization with the required accuracy directly from the functional images is impossible. In some research applications, in which patterns of response in groups of subjects rather than in a single individual are of interest, relating a particular subject's functional image dataset to an anatomical scan may provide a means of effecting a transformation into a homogeneous coordinate system within which individual results may be averaged or otherwise analyzed. In situations in which functional information concerning a single individual is to be analyzed, the use of that individual's neuroanatomy as visualized in MRI as a template for interpretation of the functional image data is of direct interest. This latter class of single-subject analysis includes essentially all clinical applications, in addition to a large number of research situations. In this chapter, we review a number of techniques for registration of a set of functional images with an anatomical image scan of the same subject, with particular attention paid to methods that utilize global shape properties of the subject's anatomy to effect the image registration.

II. Overview of Image Registration Methods

A number of methods have been developed for registration of an anatomical scan with a set of functional images of the same subject, which we denote *intrasubject* image registration. Several types of anatomical and functional datasets may be relevant to a particular problem, some of which are listed in Table 1. In this chapter we discuss registration of 3D datasets from tomographic modalities, i.e., anatomical images from MRI or CT and functional images from PET or SPECT. Depending on the particular application at hand, the manner in which registered data are dis-

FUNCTIONAL NEUROIMAGING

Table 1 Types of Image Data to Be Considered

	Anatomic	Functional
Tomographic	CT and MRI	PET and SPECT
Single projection	Diagnostic radiograph and reconstructed radiograph	Planar scintigraph
Multiple projection	Biplane, stereo angiography	

played or analyzed may vary. For example, for a given slice of a PET scan, a corresponding MRI slice may be desired for use as an anatomical template for regional function analysis (Mazziotta, 1991; Maguire, 1986; Chen, 1988). For surgical planning, a 3D display of MRI-defined brain anatomy with added functional information from PET or SPECT may be useful (Levin, 1989; Valentino, 1991). In the former case, anatomical information must be transformed into the space of the functional images; in the latter, functional information must be transformed into the MRI space.

In each case, the transfer of information from one image space to the other requires the knowledge of a coordinate transformation relating the position of voxels in one study to those in the other. If this coordinate transformation is known, information may be moved freely from one study to the other in either direction—functional to anatomic or anatomic to functional. The essence of any image registration procedure is to define this *interscan coordinate transformation*. For intrasubject registration of brain scans, the interscan coordinate transformation may be taken to be a rigid-body transformation, i.e., consisting only of 3D translation and rotation, apart from known image magnification factors. For intersubject registration, for transformation of an individual subject's image dataset into a canonical coordinate system such as an atlas, and for registration of image data in parts of the body where anatomy is not rigid, more complicated transformations are required. The various methods that have been developed differ in their approach to defining this transformation, as shown in Table 2. In this chapter, we address methods belonging to only one subclass of registration methods, namely retrospective methods using anatomical surface matching. Before describing any method in detail, we briefly discuss the differences in the classes of methods listed in Table 2.

The initial distinction made in Table 2 is between methods in which the subject is or is not positioned reproducibly with respect to the planes of the various imaging devices, thus imposing a single coordinate system on all scans. We refer to this as *a priori* defini-

tion of the interscan coordinate transformation, and it may be accomplished by immobilization of the subject within a mask or other device with which the imaging planes are then carefully aligned. Alignment of a scan plane with some well-defined anatomical feature such as the canthomeatal plane, as is commonly done for PET brain studies, also falls into this category. A method of this class will produce registration accuracy dependent on the care taken in immobilization and alignment. Because different scanners may vary considerably in the slice thickness, separation, and magnification of imaging planes, alignment of a single plane in each of two modalities may not ensure that any other planes are aligned. However, if the alignment is done with sufficient care and the geometry of the imaging devices is well known, coordinates in different modalities can be related to each other (Vogl, 1989; Meltzer, 1990). For repeated imaging of a subject

Table 2 Classification of Image Registration Techniques

A priori control of scanning geometry
    Immobilization; markers for repositioning

A posteriori recovery of interscan transformation
    Prospective: impose coordinate system on patient
        Stereotactic frame
            Rigidly fixed
            Carried on mask
        Applied fiducial marks
            Attached to anatomical landmarks
            On mask
    Retrospective: attempt to use patient-intrinsic coordinate system
        Point landmarks
        Curves on 2D radiographs
        Three-dimensional shape properties
            Matching spatial moments of 3D volume
            Correlation of voxel density distribution
            Matching of anatomical surfaces
    Indirect: relate scans to intermediate coordinate system
        Anatomically defined atlas; transform to "standard" anatomy
        Mathematically defined coordinate system, e.g.
            Talairach

in the same scanner, this is a natural technique.

If the interscan coordinate transformation is calculated from information in the images, rather than controlled during the scans, we refer to the image registration method as depending on *a posteriori* determination of the transformation. One example of such a method is the use of a stereotactic localizer frame rigidly fixed to the patient's skull, as is commonly done for implantation of depth electrodes, stereotactic biopsy, interstitial brachytherapy, radiosurgery, and other procedures. The localizer frame typically consists of radiopaque rods in a well-known geometric arrangement that produce a characteristic pattern of bright spots in the image slices. From measured coordinates of the rod images, a coordinate transformation from the localizer frame to the images may be calculated. As long as the mounting hardware remains attached to the patient, physical positions known relative to the frame may be transformed into the image coordinate system and vice versa. By use of localizer rods visible in multiple modalities (Bergström, 1981; Olivier, 1984), for example, water-filled tubes in MRI and activated copper wires or tubes filled with ^{68}Gd-doped solution in PET, it is possible to calculate transformations from each modality to the common frame coordinate system. This allows information to be transferred from one modality to another; thus the studies are registered. Stereotactic frames carried on a mask custom-fitted to the patient (Schad, 1987) or a system of fiducial points applied either to the patient surface or to a mask (Kessler, 1991) may be used in the same way without the inconvenience of bony fixation of the frame, but at the expense of some decrease in accuracy of registration. Image registration methods that rely on the use of a stereotactic or fiducial-based coordinate system attached to the subject prior to imaging have the virtue that the identification of the features in the images that are used to define the interscan coordinate transformation is not subject to error. In addition, the well-known geometry of the frame or fiducial system allows such methods to be self-calibrating; that is, once the interscan coordinate transformation has been calculated, it can be checked by transforming the positions of the markers from one scan to the other, and an objective estimate of registration error thus can be generated (when fiducial marks that must be removed and replaced between scans are utilized, additional uncertainty in the coordinate transformation may result due to variation in the mark positions). This is an important advantage, because verification of correct registration is otherwise quite difficult.

Registration using a stereotactic frame or placed fiducial markers is limited to prospective use, in the sense that only scans made with the system of markers in place may be utilized. Data without the marker system, for example, diagnostic images acquired in normal clinical practice, cannot be incorporated using these methods. *Retrospective* image registration methods are those that recover the interscan coordinate transformation from information intrinsic to images of the subject, without either control of the scanning geometry (for example, by careful alignment of the scan planes as described above) or the imposition of an extrinsic coordinate system (by fiducial or frame placement). Such methods rely on the identification of corresponding features in the scans to be registered and the calculation of a coordinate transformation that optimally matches these features. A number of such techniques that utilize different types of features in the image datasets to supply constraints in the calculation of the interscan coordinate transformation have been developed. Methods based on the matching of homologous 3D point landmarks have been applied successfully in matching PET and SPECT with MRI (Evans, 1989) as well as in relating image datasets of individuals to the canonical coordinate system of an atlas (Evans, 1991; Bookstein, 1991), using nonlinear transformations that permit local and global anatomical distortions. Below we discuss several methods that utilize global 3D shape properties of anatomical and functional datasets in order to calculate the required interscan coordinate transformation for intrasubject image registration.

III. Registration by Surface Matching

Due to differences in imaging principles, a given anatomical object may or may not appear in multiple imaging modalities. However, it may be possible to segment 3D models of one or more anatomical objects that are visualized in each of two or more modalities. If these anatomical objects may be assumed not to have changed their shape from one scan to another, which is a reasonable assumption for intracranial structures, and if the scanners are geometrically accurate (or their distortions are well enough known to be corrected for), then the 3D image-based models should have the same shape. Under the assumption that all objects in the 3D "scene" translate and rotate together without relative motion as the subject moves from one scanner to another, it should be possible to find a single global transformation that optimally matches one or more pairs of 3D objects visualized in each of two modalities. This transformation essentially defines the difference in position of the imaged volume of the subject in the two scanners; it is precisely the interscan coordinate transformation described earlier.

A number of methods that attempt to match 3D shape properties of visualized objects to effect *a posteriori* recovery of the interscan coordinate transformation have been developed. If the imaged volume of a given object in each of two scans is the same, then it should be possible to calculate the interscan coordinate transformation simply by evaluating the spatial moments of the volume and then finding the transformation that aligns the first (centroid) and second (moments of inertia, principal axes of inertia) moments to define the translational and rotational part of the transformation, respectively. This method has been applied to matching of multiple anatomical scans (Gamboa-Aldeco, 1986) and to registration of anatomical and functional images (Bajcsy, 1989; Kovacic, 1989; Alpert, 1990). The underlying assumption that the moments should match, i.e., that the 3D objects are identical, may be violated in practical situations, in which the anatomical object being matched may not be completely covered by the scan. This may lead to errors in the calculated transformation, because missing data can modify the moments of the object being considered in the two scans differently. Holupka (1992) has modified the moments technique by analytically representing the surface as an expansion in a set of orthogonal functions such as spherical harmonics. This analytic representation can then be used to "complete" the surface in regions of missing data, reducing the sensitivity of the calculated transformation to nonidentical scan volumes. Because the analytic representation is simply an interpolating function, however, it does not necessarily fill in missing regions correctly, so this method cannot be expected to perform well for very large or complex missing regions. Bajcsy *et al.* (1989) have also used principal-axis matching as the first step in a more complex registration procedure, which includes local elastic distortion, for matching to an atlas or for use in areas of the body where anatomy is deformable. Rusinek *et al.* (1993) have compared principal axis matching with direct surface fitting for registration of brain images using extensive computer stimulations. Their results "suggest that [surface fitting] is the method of choice for registering brain images" and "confirm the feasibility of registration of multimodality scans with accuracy better than 2 mm using [surface fitting]."

An interactive method developed by Kapouleas (1991) uses shape properties of the brain to match PET with MRI in a two-step process. First, the midline of the brain is identified on PET and on axial MRI slices by positioning a line on each slice. A plane is fitted to the midlines in each modality separately and then a transformation that matches the two planes is calculated. This determines the left–right translation and the rotations about the anterior–posterior and inferior–superior axes of the patient. Using this partial transformation, the PET image data are reformatted along a set of sagittal MRI planes that were acquired at the same time as the axial MRI; thus they are in a known relation to the planes on which the midline was defined. The user then interactively adjusts the remaining degrees of freedom (rotation about the left–right axis, translation in the sagittal plane) to match the reformatted sagittal PET slices with the sagittal MRI. Consistency of registration between 2 and 4 mm was reported in tests on patient image data using a nonparametric statistical analysis. The accuracy achieved was somewhat operator dependent, as might be expected for a purely interactive method.

Several methods that search through a space of possible interscan transformations and attempt to maximize the congruence of 3D surface models of one or more pairs of anatomical objects from each of two scans have been developed. The essential features of all such methods are illustrated schematically in Fig. 1. A transformation that matches one of the models (model "B") to the other (model "A") is to be found. Model A may be thought of as being a stationary surface onto which model B, represented as a set of 3D points, is to be placed. The transformation that, when applied to model B, fits it best onto model A is to be found. Given a starting estimate of the transformation, the points constituting model B are transformed. A figure of merit for congruence is calculated, which is typically the mean or mean square distance of points on model B from the surface of model A. One or more of the parameters (three translations,

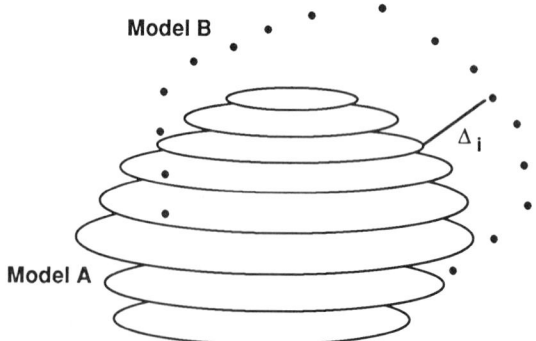

Figure 1 Schematic representation of surface matching. A transformation that matches the points that constitute model B most closely with model A is to be found. The average distance from the points on model B to the surface of model A, such as Δ_i, is a common figure of merit for congruence of the surfaces.

Plate 77 Head surface sampled with a 3D digitizer from subject 2. Each blue + represents one of the 479 points sampled. Four views are presented: (A) left view, (B) left lateral view, (C) left posterior oblique view, and (D) anterior–posterior view. Superimposed on the digitized head are the locations of 29 electrodes (small pink spheres) used to record EEG during self-paced, voluntary movements of the right index finger. The electrodes were about 3 mm thick and were placed according to the international 10-20 system. The head surface was digitized on an occasion prior to the EEG recording, so the electrode positions were registered onto the digitized head using the least-mean-squares registration algorithm described in the text. In this case, the RMS and maximum errors of the registration were 5.0 and 6.5 mm, respectively. Also shown is the sphere that was fitted to the scalp portion of the head (all points above the eyebrows, ears, and inion), using the modified least-mean-square-error function proposed by Lükenhüner *et al.* (1990). This sphere had a radius of 92.4 mm and the mean and maximum distances of the scalp points from the sphere surface were 8.1 and 17.5 mm, respectively.

Plate 78 Three EEG equivalent dipole locations mapped into the respective digitized head (subject 2). The dipoles were computed from the EEG recordings made with the electrodes shown in Plate 77, using the BESA program (Toro *et al.*, 1993a, 1993b). Instead of assuming that the electrodes were in the ideal 10-20 system locations, the actual electrode positions were computed by projecting them onto the sphere that best fitted the scalp (Plate 77). The spherical coordinates of the dipole locations and directions calculated by BESA were transformed into rectangular coordinates by scaling the "eccentricities" with the radius of the best-fitting sphere and converting the angles into lengths along the rectangular system that has its origin at the center of the best-fitting sphere, its z axis through Cz, and its x axis in the plane defined by those two points and Fpz. The dipole directions are not shown here but could be easily added. The four views, A, B, C, and D, are the same as those in Plate 77.

Plate 79 Five MEG equivalent dipole locations mapped into the respective digitized head (subject 2). The dipoles were computed from the MEG recordings made with the seven-channel BTI magnetometer (model 607) at nine probe locations. One dipole was computed for each of the following time instants: -128, 0, 51, 126, and 243 ms with respect to the onset of the finger movement. Each time instant corresponds to a peak in the magnetic field waveform. The dipole locations were mapped into the digitized head using a set of coordinate transformation equations that converted the locations from the system defined by the nasion and left and right preauricular points to the system defined by the source of the magnetic digitizer. The four views, A, B, C, and D, are the same as those in Plate 77.

Plate 80 Transcranial magnetic stimulation (TMS) grid (green +) superimposed on the respective digitized head (subject 5). The head surface (404 points represented by blue +s) was digitized on an occasion prior to the TMS session, so the scalp grid was registered onto the digitized head using the least-mean-squares registration algorithm described in the text. The red dot represents the reference point on the grid during TMS. Also shown is the center of gravity (COG) of TMS (yellow sphere) computed from the EMG recorded at the finger abductor muscle (Wassermann *et al.*, 1992a). From the COG, a line perpendicular to the scalp was drawn (in yellow) to visualize the projection of the magnetic field into the head. This line was computed by fitting a sphere to the grid points, using the modified least-mean-square-error function proposed by Lükenhüner *et al.* (1990). The four views, A, B, C, and D, are the same as those in Plate 77.

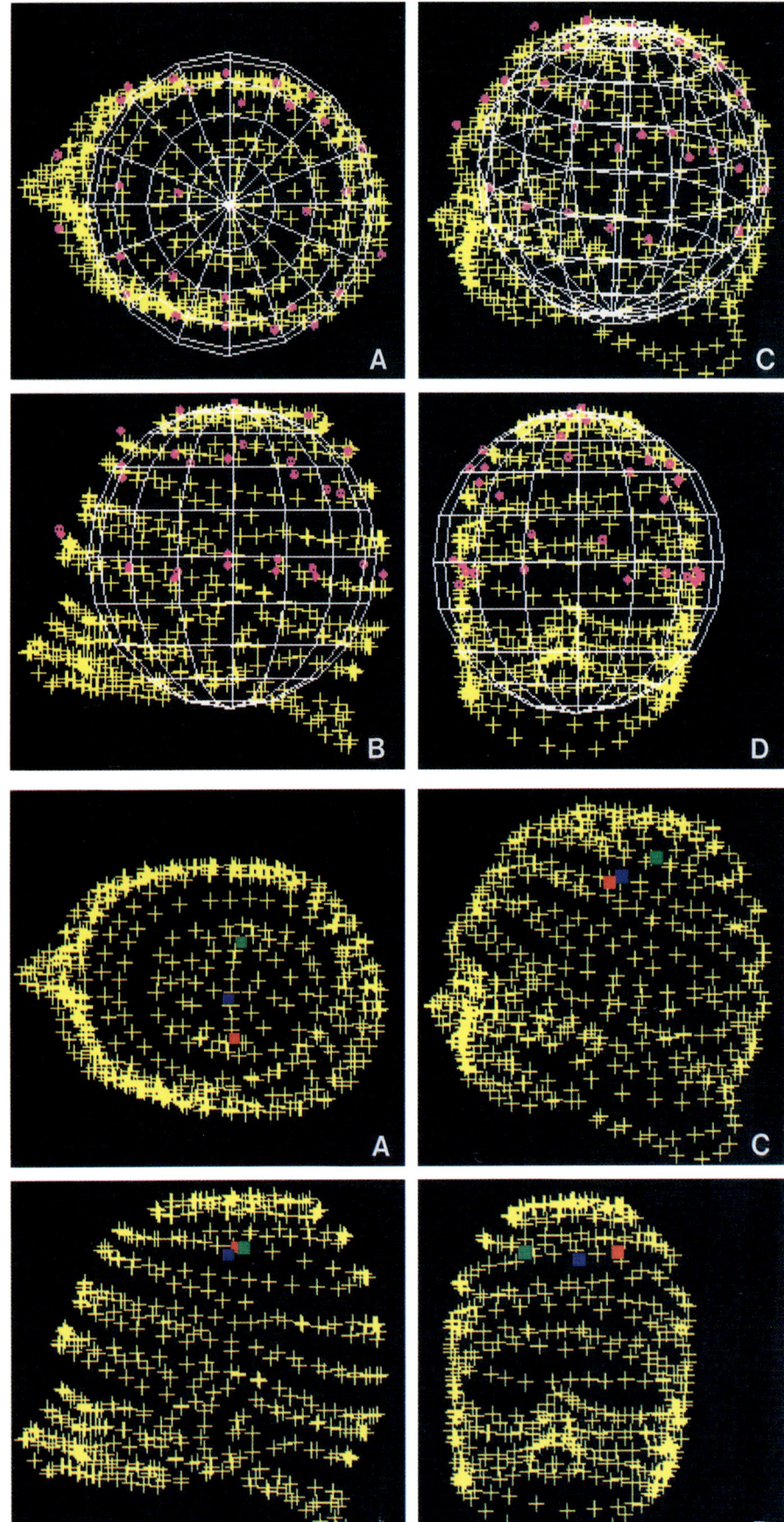

Plate 77

Plate 78

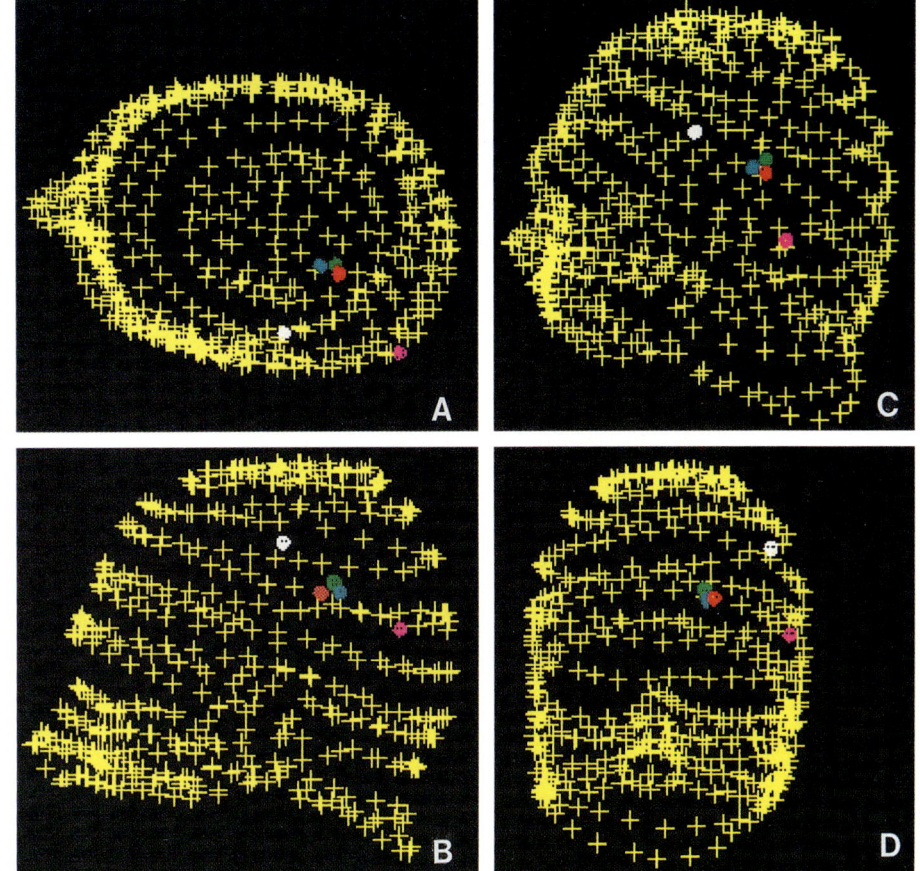

Plate 79

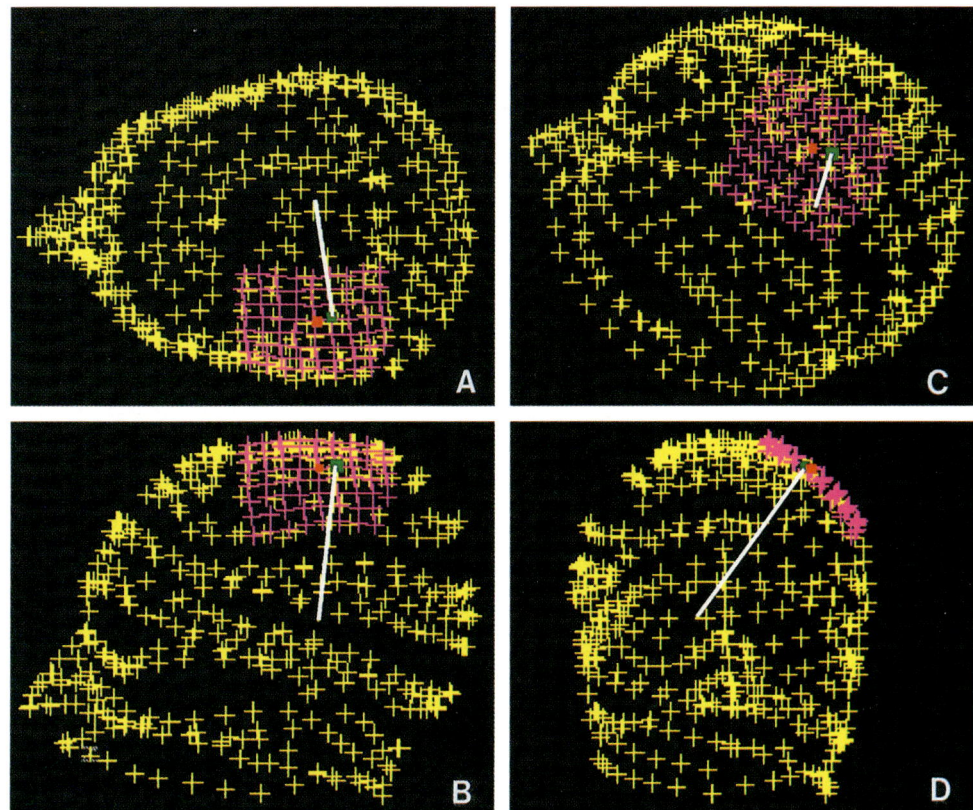

Plate 80

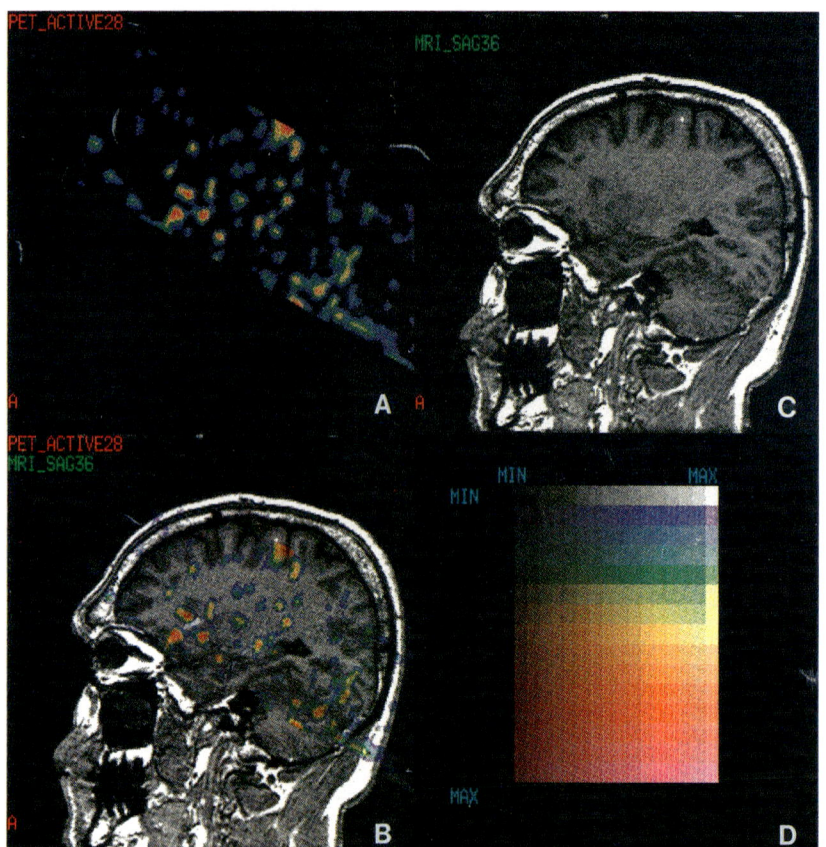

Plate 81 Location of the contralateral EEG dipole (white cross) mapped into MR and compared with the subtraction PET (subject 2). This dipole is the same as that shown in the left hemisphere of Plate 78 and was mapped into this MR slice using the registration and mapping technique described in the text. The PET image was obtained after registering the PET brain contours with MR brain contours, subtracting the mean rest set from the mean active set, and reslicing the PET images along the sagittal plane coplanar with MR slices. The threshold of the subtraction PET images thus obtained was adjusted so as to show the most active regions in red and the least active ones in blue, whereas the MR is shown in gray scale. In this case, there were two discernible peaks in the subtraction PET active region, both in slices left to the dipole location. The distances from these two PET peaks to the dipole were 13 and 25 mm. The four views, A, B, C, and D, are the same as those in Plate 77.

Plate 82 Location of one of the five MEG dipoles (white circle) mapped into MR and compared with the subtraction PET (subject 2). This dipole is the same as that shown in yellow in the left hemisphere of Plate 79 and was mapped into this MR slice using the registration and mapping technique described in the text. The PET image was processed in the same manner as that described in Plate 81 and was superimposed on the MR.

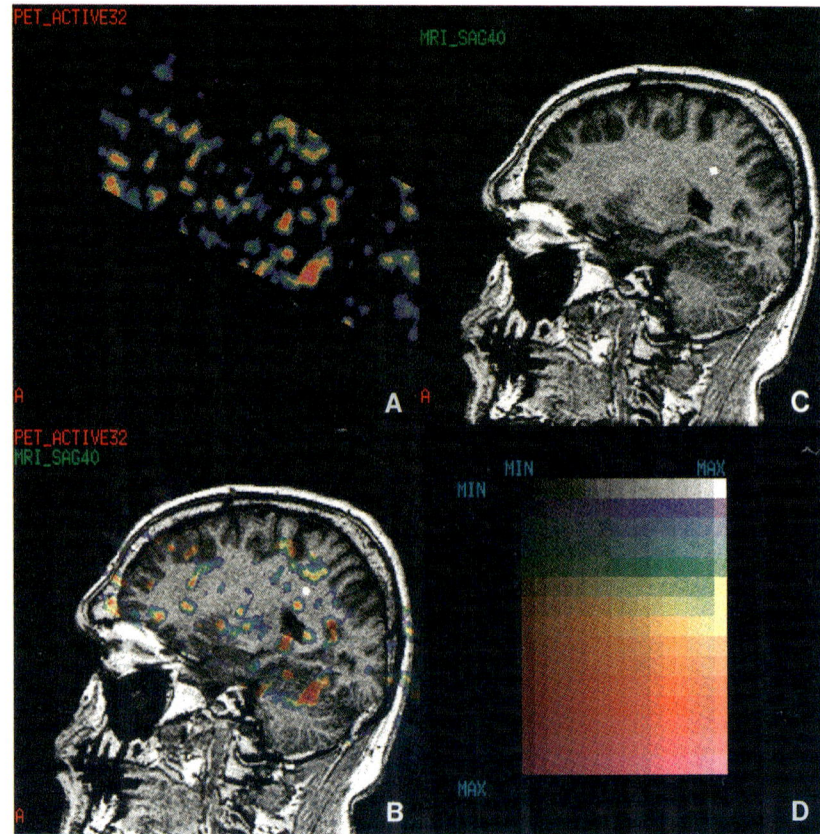

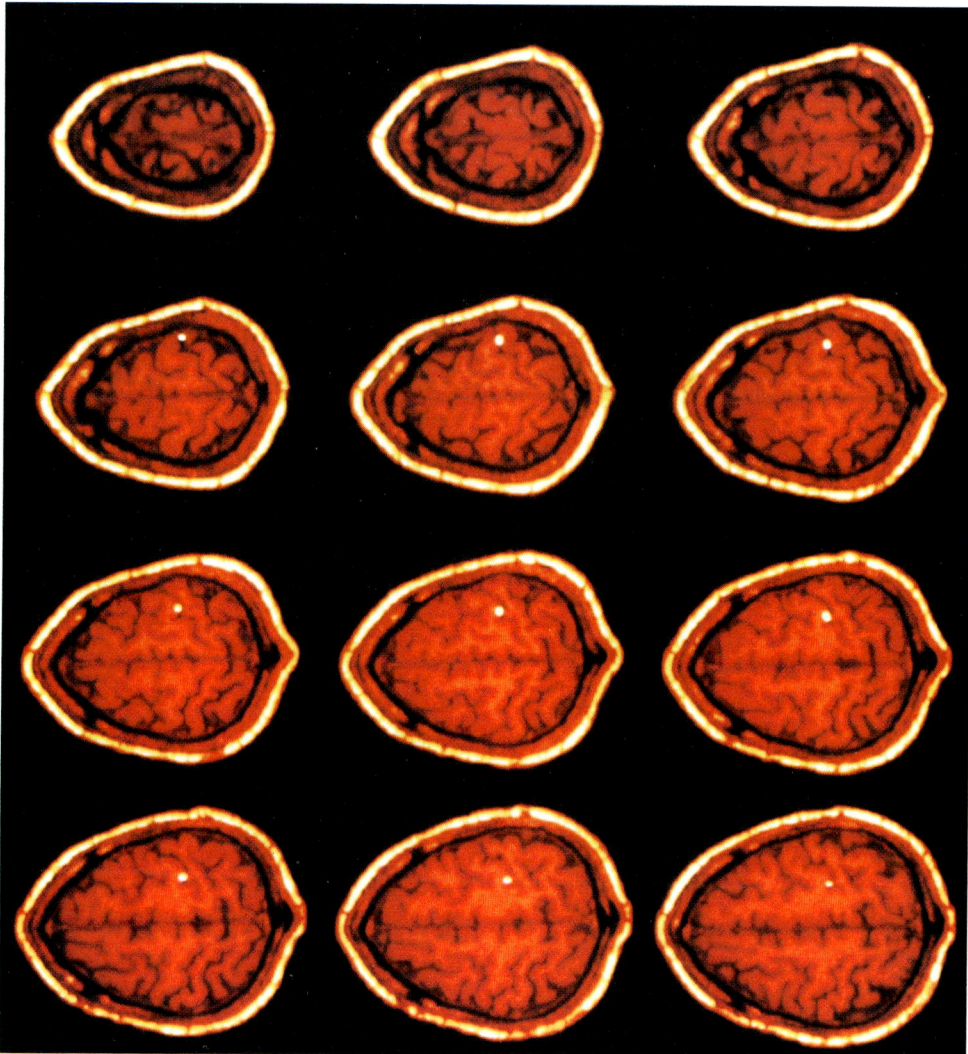

Plate 83 Intersection of the TMS COG projection with sequential axial MR slices (subject 5). The parameters of the yellow line shown in Plate 80 were mapped into MR using the registration and mapping technique described in the text. The intersection of this line with each sagittal MR slice was computed, and the area surrounding the corresponding pixel was masked in white. The entire volumetric MR was then resliced axially to yield the slices shown. Whenever necessary, the intersections on the axial slice were slightly enlarged to make them more visible.

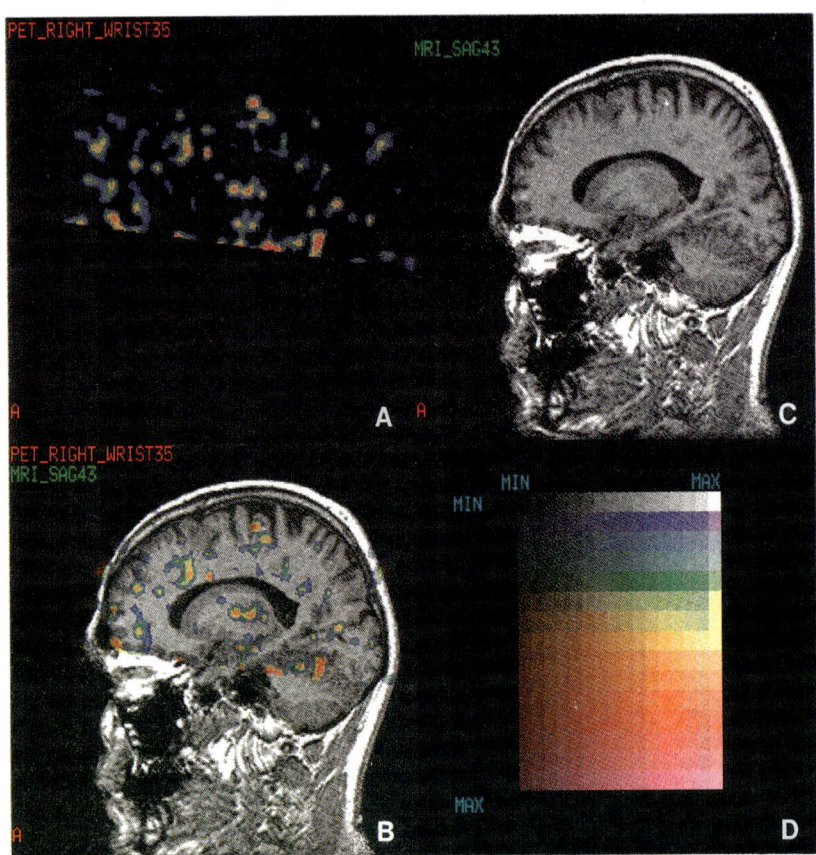

Plate 84 One of the intersections of the TMS COG projection with sagittal MR slices (white square) compared with the subtraction PET (subject 5). The intersection of the yellow line shown in Plate 80 with each sagittal MR slice was computed after the line parameters were mapped into MR using the registration and mapping technique described in the text. The PET image was processed in the same manner as that described in Plate 81 and was superimposed on the MR slices. This particular slice was selected because it contains one of the two discernible peaks in the subtraction PET's active region. In this case, the intersection was 6 mm away from the PET peak.

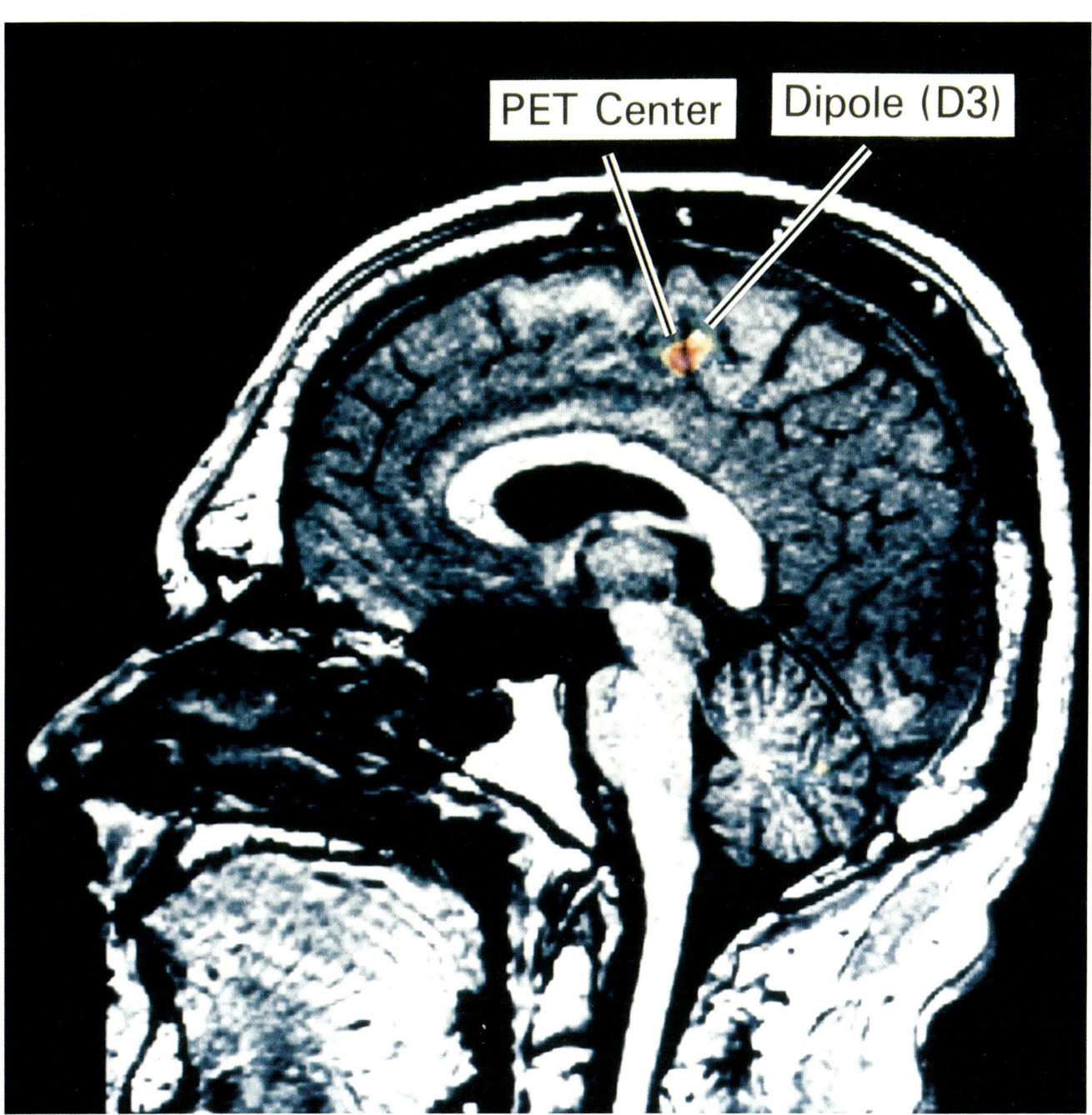

Plate 87 Multimodal sagittal image of the contralateral left hemisphere (sagittal slice No. 51). The rCBF PET image registered with the corresponding sagittal MRI was obtained after averaging three images obtained during the execution of self-paced right index finger movements after the injection of H_2O^{15} and subtraction from averaged rest scans. The location of source 3 (i.e., D3; see Fig. 2) in the spherical head model, in the same subject executing the same task, has been projected into the PET and MRI images (open cross) after the appropriate coordinate transformations and rotations. See Chapter 25 for more details of the technique. Both the dipole source and the active PET region are located in the anterior bank of the supplemental motor cortical region. The distance between the dipole source location (left arrow) and the center of the active PET region (right arrow) is approximately 6 mm. The Talairach and Tournoux (1988) atlas coordinates of the registered PET and dipole source 3 are approximately a, 3-4, and E_1 in the left hemisphere. (Coordinates x, y, z are +0.4 cm horizontal, +0.5 cm medial-lateral, and +4.6 cm top to bottom.)

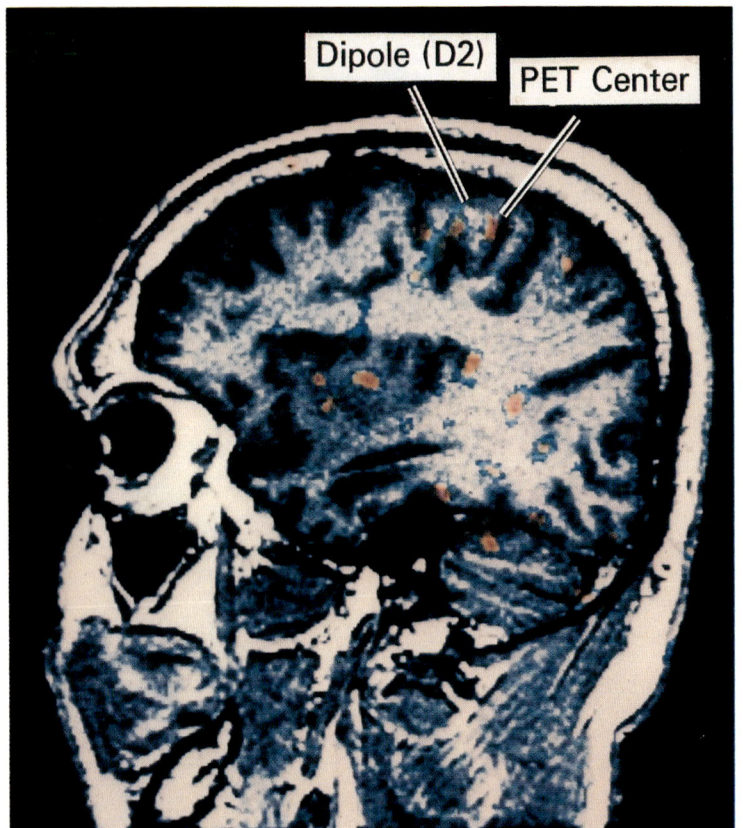

Plate 85 Multimodal sagittal image of the ipsilateral right hemisphere (sagittal slice No. 74). The rCBF PET image registered with the corresponding sagittal MRI was obtained after averaging three images obtained during the execution of self-paced right index finger movements after the injection of H_2O^{15} and subtraction from averaged rest scans. The location of source 2 (i.e., D2; see Fig. 2) in the spherical head model, in the same subject executing the same task, has been projected into the PET and MRI images (open cross) after the appropriate coordinate transformations and rotations. See Wang *et al.* (1993a) for more details of the technique. Both the dipole source and the active PET region are located near the ipsilateral hand region in the anterior bank of the central sulcus. The distance between the dipole source location (left arrow) and the center of the active PET region (right arrow) is approximately 10 mm. The Talairach and Tournoux (1988) atlas coordinates of the registered PET and dipole source 2 are approximately c, 3, and E_2 in the right hemisphere. (Coordinates x, y, z are +1.4 cm horizontal, +4.1 cm medial-lateral, and +5.0 cm top to bottom.)

Plate 86 Multimodal sagittal image of the contralateral left hemisphere (sagittal slice No. 36). The rCBF PET image registered with the corresponding sagittal MRI was obtained after averaging three images obtained during the execution of self-paced right index finger movements after the injection of H_2O^{15} and subtraction from averaged rest scans. The location of source 1 (i.e., D1; see Fig. 2) in the spherical head model, in the same subject executing the same task, has been projected into the PET and MRI images (open cross) after the appropriate coordinate transformations and rotations. See Chapter 25 for more details of the technique. Both the dipole source and the active PET region are located near the hand region in the anterior bank of the central sulcus. The distance between the dipole source location (left arrow) and the center of the active PET region (right arrow) is less than 3 mm. The Talairach and Tournoux (1988) atlas coordinates of the registered PET and dipole source 1 are approximately c, 3, and E_2 in the left hemisphere. (Coordinates x, y, z are +1.4 cm horizontal, +4.1 cm medial-lateral, and +5.0 cm top to bottom.)

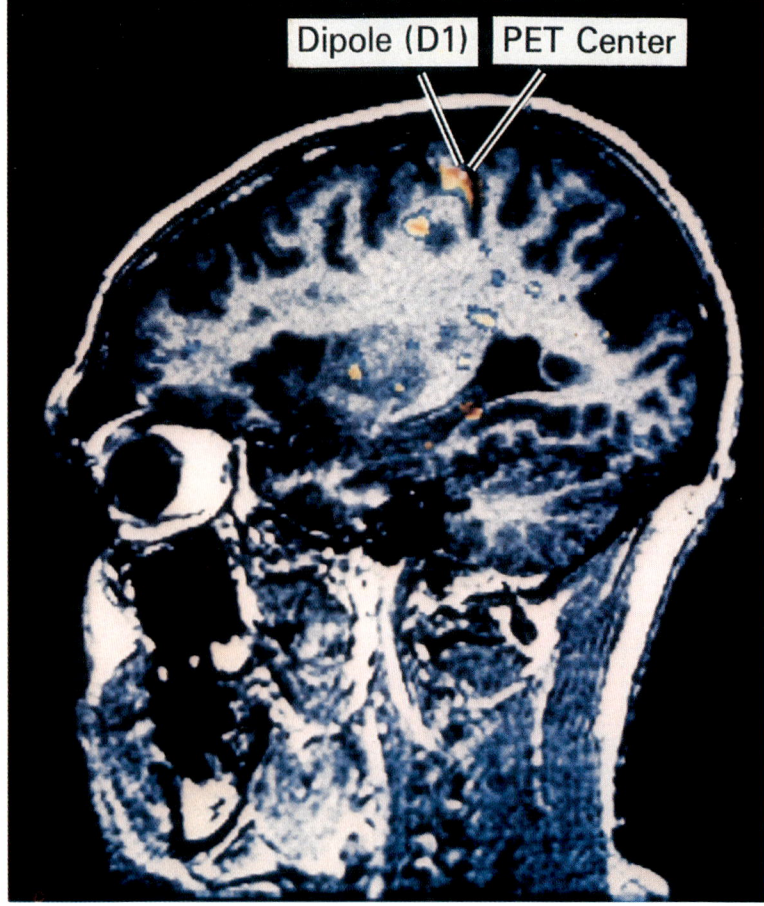

three rotations) of the transformation are varied, model B is transformed according to the new transformation, and the change in the congruence measure is evaluated. Parameter variation is continued until satisfactory congruence is achieved.

Individual methods differ in their approaches to searching the space of allowed transformations and in their calculations of the figure of merit by which surface congruence is judged. van Herk (1992) and Jiang (1992) use a distance transformation or "chamfer matching" algorithm to evaluate the mean distance of a set of points from one 3D model to the surface of the other model. Each uses some combination of grid search and gradient-based nonlinear parameter search within an allowed region of the space of possible translations and rotations to find the transformation that minimizes the mean distance between the two models. Each also uses a coarse initial search to identify the most promising regions of the parameter space, followed by a finer final search. Oghabian and Todd-Pokropek (1991) use the mean of a distance calculated at each point as the figure of merit and incorporate a multiresolution search of the parameter space. The space is first searched at a coarse scale, with the figure of merit calculated from a low-resolution representation of the surface models so local shape details do not constrain the search. Starting from the minimum found in the coarse search, the space is searched at a finer scale using a somewhat higher resolution representation of the surfaces. Resolution is increased and the scale of the parameter search reduced until satisfactory convergence is achieved.

The method developed at the University of Chicago (Pelizzari, 1989) has been used by a number of investigators for registration of PET (Pelizzari, 1987; Levin, 1988; Valentino, 1991; Mazziotta, 1991; Turkington, 1991b) and SPECT (Holman, 1991; Turkington, 1991a, 1991b) with MRI. Early work on registration of PET with MRI relied on matching external surface models (Pelizzari, 1987, 1989). This required the availability of PET transmission scans, which are routinely made in some institutions but not in others. An additional difficulty with the use of transmission scans is the possibility of patient motion between the transmission and the emission scans. The assumption in using a head surface model from transmission scans is that the emission images are registered with the transmission images; thus, if the transmission scan is registered with MRI, then the emission scan is also. If the patient moves between the transmission and the emission studies, the external surface model from the transmission study is not registered correctly with the emission data; thus the registration of emission images to MRI based on the external surface is also incorrect. In re-

cent work (Levin, 1989; Turkington, 1991a, 1991b; Holman, 1991), brain surface models from MRI and from PET or SPECT have been directly matched, eliminating the need for transmission images. In the case of tracers that exhibit only focal uptake, the brain surface is not visualized in PET or SPECT, and external surface matching based on transmission images may still be required. The difficulty of reliably segmenting anatomical surfaces from nuclear medicine images was originally perceived to be a source of uncertainty in registration. Early work (Pelizzari, 1987, 1989) used a simple binary thresholding method for surface segmentation, which due to poor resolution in PET led to suboptimal identification of external and brain surfaces. To compensate for this uncertainty in surface location on PET, scale factors were introduced into the interscan transformation in addition to the rigid body translations and rotations. When the scale factors in the in-plane directions were found to differ significantly from unity, the PET surfaces were resegmented with a different threshold and the fitting procedure was repeated. Recent results (Turkington, 1991b; T. G. Turkington, private communication, June 1992) have shown that improved segmentation schemes incorporating gradient information can reliably segment brain and external surfaces from PET and SPECT, obviating the need for scaling in the interscan transformation.

Estimates of registration accuracy for this method that have been published include <2 mm in translation and <2° in rotation based on PET and MRI brain phantom studies with attached fiducial markers (Turkington, 1991b); 2–3 mm in plane and 1-mm axial translation based on the positions of thalami in merged MRI and SPECT (Holman, 1991); 3–4 mm in 3D based on linear fiducials in head phantom in PET, CT, and MRI (Pelizzari 1989); and 2–4 mm in 3D based on misregistration of anatomical landmarks in MRI, ^{15}O, and ^{18}FDG PET (Pelizzari, 1991). A significant negative aspect of this technique, shared by other retrospective techniques, is that it does not provide a direct estimate of registration accuracy for a given case. The figure of merit for matching of surfaces cannot be interpreted simply in terms of registration accuracy and in fact may be quite large for a good fit of the surfaces due to noise in one or the other image dataset. Accuracy must be evaluated by the user in each case by measurement of deviations between visible 3D landmarks or examination of reformatted slices for congruence of anatomical structures.

A problem common to nonlinear parameter search techniques is the possibility of the search terminating in a local minimum of the residual, rather than finding the global minimum as desired. Holman (1991) has published contour plots showing local minima in the parameter space for SPECT/MRI brain surface registration located 5–10° away from the global minimum. Several methods for dealing with this problem have been developed. As mentioned above, several authors have used an initial coarse search of the parameter space to find favorable regions, followed by detailed searching in the regions thus identified (van Herk, 1992; Jiang, 1992). The Chicago image registration program addresses this problem by allowing the operator to interactively adjust all the transformation parameters and to prealign the two surface models (Fig. 2). This process, which typically takes less than 30 s, provides the parameter search algorithm with a reasonable starting point. The nonlinear parameter search used (Powell's method) then reliably locates the global minimum. Some users of the Chicago program have reported that no prealignment has been found to be necessary for registration of SPECT with

MRI using the brain surface (T. G. Turkington, private communication, June 1992). The current version of the program also allows the simultaneous matching of two or more structures from each image study when this is desirable.

IV. Results

An application of surface-based image registration that has been of considerable interest in our institution is the planning of neurosurgery for focal epilepsies and brain tumors. In many instances, an area of hypometabolism on interictal [18]FDG PET is associated with epileptic foci, which cannot be anatomically localized from PET alone with sufficient precision to aid in surgery planning. Ictal PET may show foci of hypermetabolism. These foci are typically not demonstrated on MRI. We have developed methods for producing

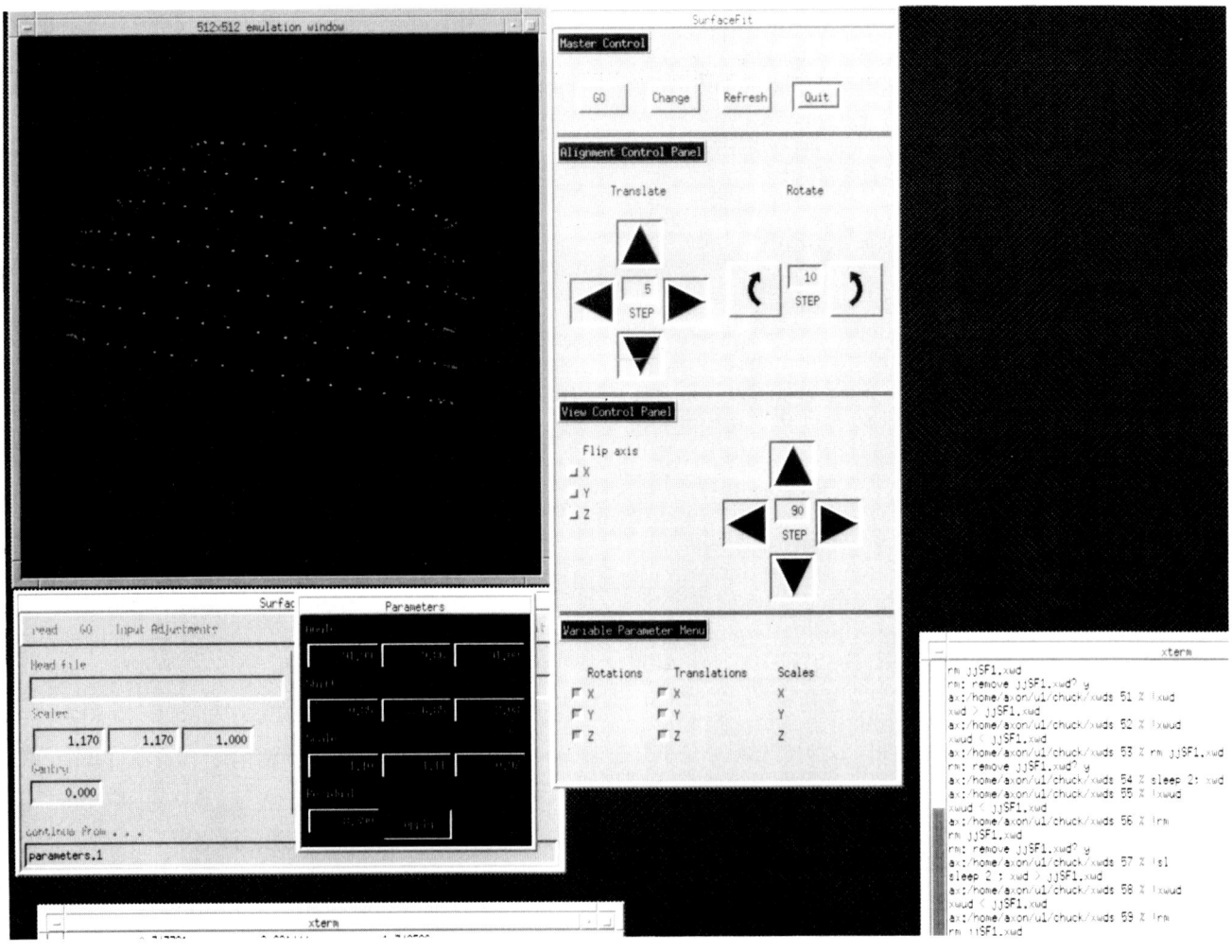

Figure 2 User interface of the Chicago image registration program, SurfaceFit. Panel at right is used to interactively prealign the two surface models before beginning the parameter search.

3D volume-rendered MRI brain models that incorporate functional information from PET (Levin, 1989), allowing neurologists and neurosurgeons to view the functional image data in the context of an accurate and realistic 3D cortical map. This has proven quite valuable in planning surgical approaches and in anticipating complications due to juxtaposition of critical cortical regions to the lesion. The process by which such models are produced is outlined in Fig. 3. A set of sagittal MRI slices covering the entire brain is acquired, and the brain is segmented from these slices to improve the quality of the final volume renderings. Transverse PET slices, taken parallel to the base of the skull, are registered with the sagittal MRI using the surface fitting procedure described above. As mentioned previously, the brain surface is used for this registration step. Transmission PET images are thus not needed for the image registration, although they are made and used in the reconstruction of the PET emission images. The brain surface is segmented from the emission images by thresholding at a level

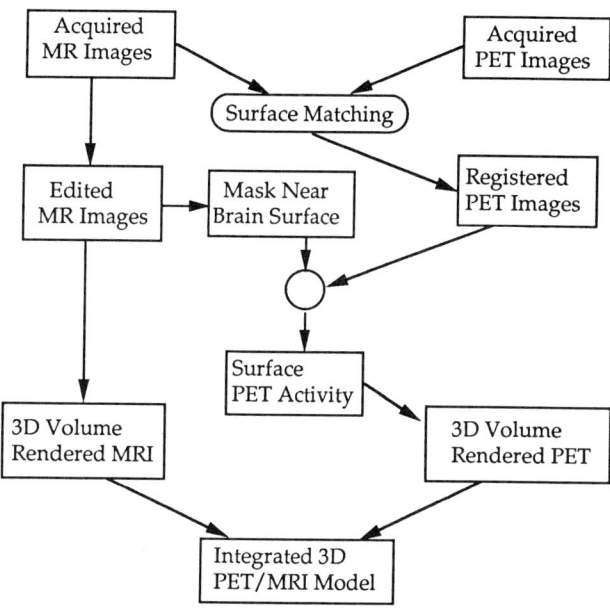

Figure 3 Procedure for producing integrated 3D MRI/PET brain models.

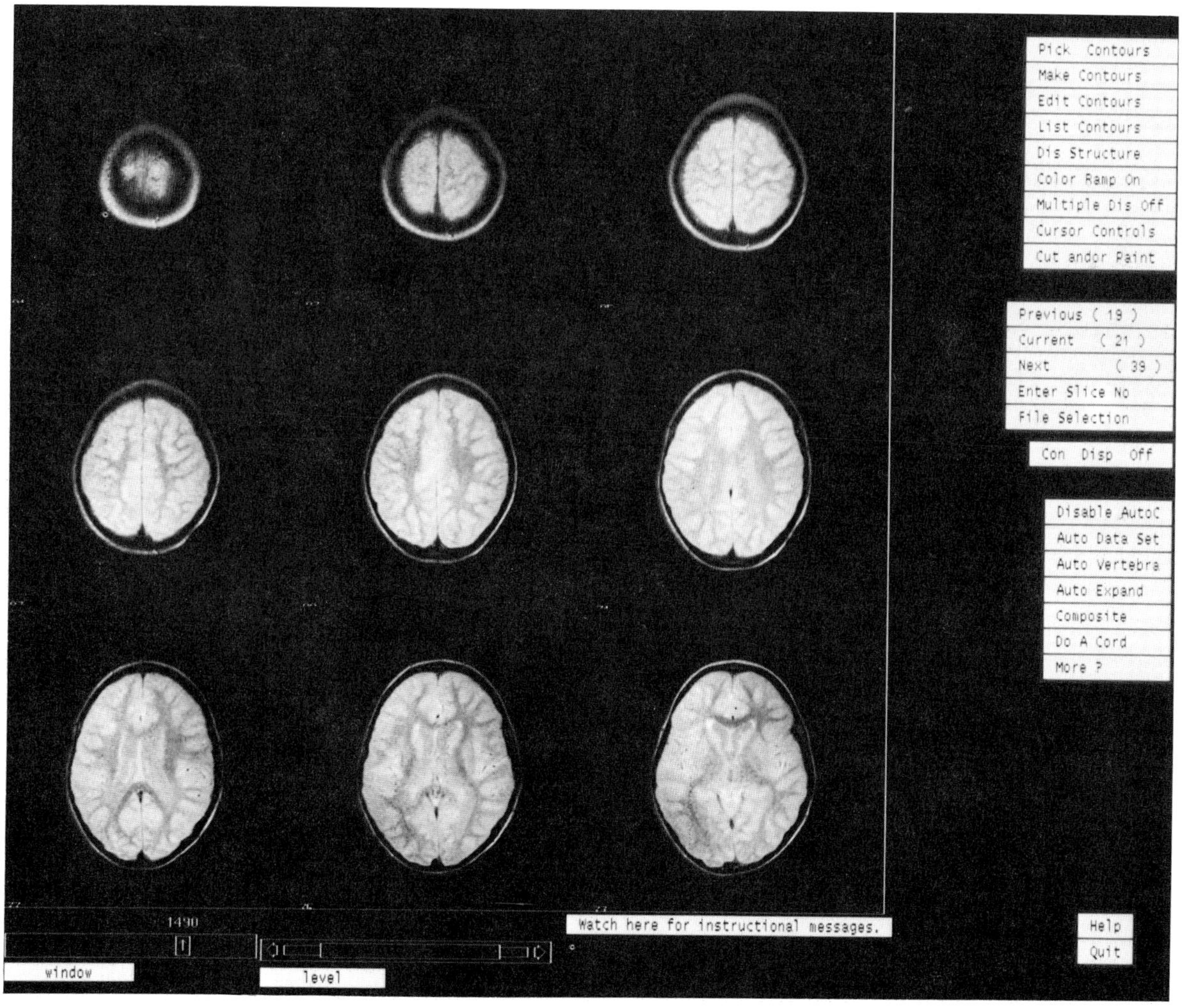

Figure 4 Axial MRI slices from a patient with acute focal encephalitis, during seizure.

of 30–40% of the study maximum. For each slice in the sagittal MRI study, a reformatted registered PET slice is produced. This produces exactly corresponding volumes of PET and MRI image data. To produce a 3D image optimized to show cortical surface metabolic activity, the registered PET slices are masked to zero beyond a depth of 1 or 2 cm inside the MRI-defined brain surface. The two image volumes are rendered separately using a Pixar Image computer with ChapVolumes software. Typically 64 azimuthal views of the brain are produced, allowing later viewing of a rotating brain "movie." The separately rendered MRI and PET volumes are combined, the MRI in gray scale and the PET in color, to produce a final 3D brain model with anatomy from MRI coded with function from PET. Figure 4 illustrates unremarkable proton-density weighted axial MRI slices from a 9-year-old patient experiencing continuous electrical seizure activity due to a focal encephalitis. Figure 5 shows [18]FDG PET metabolic rate images of the same patient, demonstrating an intense focus of hypermetabolism. Plate 74 shows the PET study reformatted along the planes of both axial and coronal MRI studies. The registered PET data have been encoded in color and added to the gray-scale MRI slices. The surface fitting program display in Fig. 2 shows a brain surface model from the axial PET study being fitted to the brain surface from a sagittal MRI used to produce a 3D volume rendering. In Plate 75, the registered PET data have been reformatted along the sagittal MRI planes, and the PET and MRI have been volume rendered separately and finally added together, the PET again in color and the MRI in gray. In this model, the location of the hypermetabolic focus astride the motor and sensory areas is clearly demonstrated. This type of presentation has been found quite useful in planning cortical resections in cases of focal epilepsy.

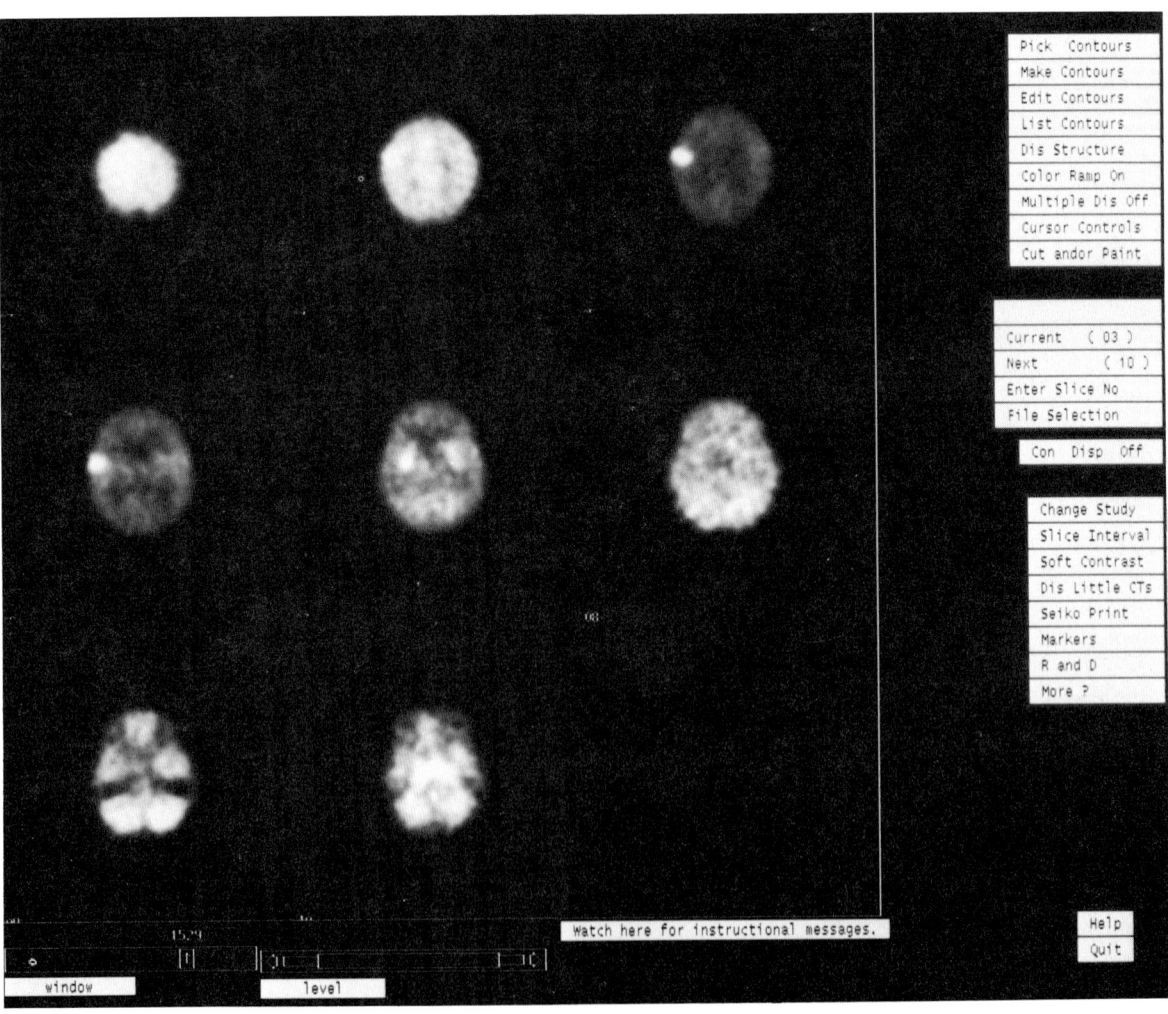

Figure 5   [18]FDG PET scan of the same patient as that in Fig. 4, during seizure.

V. Discussion

Anatomical and functional images of the same subject may be registered by matching 3D models of a surface that can be visualized in both modalities. Several surface matching methods have been published, all of which are retrospective techniques in that they require no preparation of the patient or scanner prior to image acquisition in order to allow registration. Retrospective techniques, including those based on matching of intrinsic anatomical landmarks, share the property of not providing a well-defined measure of registration accuracy for a given case. Phantom and patient studies with markers have shown accuracy on the order of 2–4 mm to be achievable by surface matching for registration of PET or SPECT with MRI, largely limited by image quality in the nuclear medicine images. This level of accuracy is adequate for many clinical and research applications. Improved parameter search methods, more reliable segmentation of structures from PET and SPECT, improvements in nuclear medicine image quality, and the ability to simultaneously match multiple pairs of objects should result in further improvements in the registration accuracy attainable.

References

Alpert, N. M., Bradshaw, J. F., Kennedy, D., and Correia, J. A. (1990). The principal axis transformation—A method for image registration. *J. Nucl. Med.* **31**(10), 1717–1722.

Bajcsy, R., and Kovacic, S. (1989). Multiresolution elastic matching. *Comput. Vision Graphics Image Process.* **46**(1), 1–21.

Bergström, M., Boëthius, J., Eriksson, L., Greitz, T., Ribbe, T., and Widén, L. (1981). Head fixation device for reproducible position alignment in transmission CT and positron emission tomography. *J. Comput. Assist. Tomogr.* **5**(1), 136–141.

Bookstein, F. L. (1991). Thin-plate splines and the atlas problem for biomedical images. *In* "Information Processing in Medical Imaging," pp. 326–342. Berlin: Springer-Verlag.

Chen, C.-T., Pelizzari, C. A., Chen, G. T. Y., Cooper, M. D., and Levin, D. N. (1988). Image analysis of PET data with the aid of CT and MR images. *In* "Information Processing in Medical Imaging," pp. 601–611. New York: Plenum.

Evans, A. C., Marrett, S., Collins, L., and Peters, T. M. (1989). Anatomical–functional correlative analysis of the human brain using three dimensional imaging systems. *In* "SPIE Vol. 1092: Medical Imaging III—Image Processing," pp. 264–274.

Evans, A. C., Marrett, S., Torrescorzo, J., Ku, S., and Collins, L. (1991). MRI–PET correlation in three dimensions using a volume-of-interest (VOI) atlas. *J. Cereb. Blood Flow Metab.* **11**, A69–A78.

Gamboa-Aldeco, A., Fellingham, L. L., and Chen, G. T. Y. (1986). Correlation of 3D surfaces from multiple modalities in medical imaging. *In* "Medicine XIV/PACS IV SPIE Meeting," Newport Beach, CA.

Holman, B. L., Zimmerman, R. E., Carvalho, P. A., Schwartz, R. B., Loeffler, J. S., Alexander, E., Pelizzari, C. A., and Chen, G. T. Y. (1991). Computer-assisted superimposition of magnetic resonance and high resolution Tc-99m HMPAO and Tl-201 SPECT images of the brain. *J. Nucl. Med.* **32**, 1478–1484.

Holupka, E. J., and Kooy, H. M. (1992). A geometric algorithm for medical image correlations. *Med. Phys.* **19**(2), 433–438.

Jiang, H., Holton, K., and Robb, R. (1992). Image registration of multimodality 3-D medical images by chamfer matching. *In* "SPIE Vol. 1660: Biomedical Image Processing and Three-Dimensional Microscopy," pp. 356–366.

Kapouleas, I., Alavi, A., Alves, W. A., Gur, R. E., and Weiss, D. W. (1991). Registration of three-dimensional MR and PET images of the human brain without markers. *Radiology* **181**(2), 731–739.

Kessler, M. L., Pitluck, S., Petti, P., and Castro, J. R. (1991). Integration of multimodality imaging data for radiotherapy treatment planning. *Int. J. Rad. Oncol. Biol. Phys.* **21**, 1653–1667.

Kovacic, S., Gee, J. C., Ching, S. L., Reivich, M., and Bajcsy, R. (1989). Three-dimensional registration of PET and CT images. *In* "IEEE Engineering in Medicine and Biology Society 11th International Conference," pp. 548–549.

Levin, D. N., Hu, X., Tan, K. K., Galhotra, S., Pelizzari, C. A., Chen, G. T. Y., Beck, R. N., Chen, C. T., Cooper, M. D., Mullan, J. F., Hekmatpanah, J., and Spire, J. P. (1989). The brain: Integrated three-dimensional display of MR and PET images. *Radiology* **172**, 783–789.

Levin, D. N., Pelizzari, C. A., Chen, G. T. Y., Chen, C. T., and Cooper, M. D. (1988). Retrospective geometric correlation of MR, CT and PET images. *Radiology* **169**, 817–823.

Maguire, G. Q. J., Noz, M. E., Lee, E. M., and Schimpf, J. H. (1986). Correlation methods for tomographic images using two and three dimensional techniques. *In* "Information Processing in Medical Imaging," pp. 267–279. Boston: Martinus Nijhoff.

Mazziotta, J. C., Pelizzari, C. A., Chen, G. T. Y., Bookstein, F. L., and Valentino, D. (1991). Region of interest issues: The relationship between structure and function in the brain. *J. Cereb. Blood Flow Metab.* **11**, A51–A56.

Meltzer, C. C., Bryan, R. N., Holcomb, H. H., Kimball, A. W., Mayberg, H. S., Sadzot, B., Leal, J. P., Wagner, H. N., and Frost, J. J. (1990). Anatomical localization for PET using MR imaging. *J. Comput. Assist. Tomogr.* **14**(3), 418–426.

Oghabian, M. A., and Todd-Pokropek, A. (1991). Registration of brain images by a multi-resolution sequential method. *In* "Information Processing in Medical Imaging," pp. 165–174. Berlin: Springer-Verlag.

Olivier, A., Peters, T. M., and Bertrand, G. (1984). New stereotactic instrument for use with CT, DSA, MR and PET scan. *Can. J. Neurol. Sci.* **11**, 336.

Pelizzari, C. A., Chen, G. T. Y., Spelbring, D. R., Weichselbaum, R. R., and Chen, C. T. (1989). Accurate three-dimensional registration of PET, CT and MR images of the brain. *J. Comput. Assist. Tomogr.* **13**, 20–27.

Pelizzari, C. A., Chen, G. T. Y., Halpern, H., Chen, C. T., and Cooper, M. D. (1987). Three dimensional correlation of PET, CT and MRI images. *J. Nucl. Med.* **28**(4), 683.

Pelizzari, C. A., Evans, A. C., Neelin, P., Chen, C. T., and Chen, G. T. Y. (1991). Comparison of two methods for 3D registration of PET and MRI images. *In* "IEEE Engineering in Medicine and Biology Society 13th International Conference," pp. 221–223.

Rusinek, H., Tsui, W. H., Levy, A. V., Noz, M. E., de Leon, M. J. (1993). Principal axes and surface fitting methods for three-dimensional image registration. *J. Nucl. Med.* **34**, 2019.

Schad, L. R., Boesecke, R., Schlegel, W., Hartmann, G. H., Sturm, V., Strauss, L., and Lorenz, W. J. (1987). Three dimensional image correlation of CT, MR, and PET studies in radiotherapy treatment planning of brain tumors. *J. Comput. Assist. Tomogr.* **11**(6), 948–954.

Tan, K. K., Levin, D. N., Pelizzari, C. A., and Ghen, G. T. Y. (1990). Interactive stereotaxic localization of brain anatomy. *Radiology* **177**(P), 217.

Turkington, T. G., Jaszczak, R. J., Greer, K. L., Coleman, R. E., and Pelizzari, C. A. (1991a). Correlation of SPECT images of a 3D brain phantom using a surface fitting technique. *In* "IEEE Nuclear Science Symposium and Medical Imaging Conference," pp. 2154–2157.

Turkington, T. G., Jaszczak, R. J., Pelizzari, C. A., Harris, C. C., MacFall, J. R., and Hoffman, J. M. (1991b). Measurement of accuracy in registration of PET and SPECT brain images. *Radiology* **181**(P), 186.

Valentino, D. J., Mazziotta, J. C., and Huang, H. K. (1991). Volume rendering of multimodal images: Application to MRI and PET imaging of the human brain. *IEEE Trans. Med. Imag.* **10**(4), 554–562.

van Herk, M., Gilhuis, K., Holupka, E., and Kooy, H. (1992). A new method for automatic three-dimensional image correlation. *Med. Phys.* **19**(4), 1134.

Vogl, G., Schwer, G., Jauch, M., Wiethölter, H., Kindermann, U., and Müller-Schauenberg, W. (1989). A simple superposition method for anatomical adjustments of CT and SPECT images. *J. Comput. Assist. Tomogr.* **13**(5), 929–931.

24

Locating Evoked Potential Dipoles in Magnetic Resonance Images

Vernon L. Towle, Raif Cakmur,‡ David N. Levin,* Charles Pelizzari,†
Mitchell Brigell,§ Gastone Celesia,§ Jeffrey A. Steck,
Robert Grzeszczuk,* and Jean-Paul Spire

Departments of Neurology, Radiology, and Radiation Oncology,† The University of Chicago, Chicago,
Illinois 60637; ‡Department of Neurology, Dokuz Eylul University, Izmir, Turkey; and §Department of
Neurology, Loyola University Medical Center, Chicago, Illinois 60611*

I. Introduction

The ability to merge MR and CT images of brain structure with PET and SPECT images of brain function has allowed more comprehensive and informative images of the intact human brain. MEG dipoles have also been displayed on MRI brain slices (Papanicolaou *et al.*, 1990; Suk *et al.*, 1991), and, using computationally intensive, but realistically shaped dipole models, electrophysiologic dipoles have been superimposed on MR images (Nakajima *et al.*, 1990). Sensory evoked potentials complement PET and SPECT, but have a temporal resolution of about four orders of magnitude better than the temporal resolution of those techniques. Evoked potentials are more functionally limited, however, because they require synchronization with an external stimulus. Their spatial resolution has not yet been determined. Recently, techniques that make it possible to determine the location of electrophysiologic recording electrodes in MR images have been developed (Myslobodsky and Bar-Ziv, 1989; Myslobodsky *et al.*, 1990; Jack *et al.*, 1990; Grzeszczuk *et al.*, 1990; Tan *et al.*, 1991; Gevins and Illes, 1991; Towle *et al.*, 1993). Van den Elsen and Viergever (1991) have superimposed scalp-recorded epileptic spikes on an MR image using a spherical dipole model, but noted some difficulty with the spherical fitting process. We have developed a strategy for determining the location of cerebral evoked potentials within 3D MR images of the brain. With this technique it may be possible to associate sensory, motor, and cognitive cerebral potentials with their anatomical generators.

II. Methods

A. Subjects

Three normal volunteers aged 33–45 years with no neurologic complaints were tested.

B. Stimulation

Somatosensory evoked potentials (SEPs) and pattern visual evoked potentials (VEPs) were obtained using standard stimulating techniques. For somatosensory stimulation, brief electrical pulses were applied to the surface of the skin over the median nerve at the wrist and the posterior tibial nerve at the medial ankle. Stimulus intensity was adjusted to cause a small twitch of the thumb or toes at a stimulus rate of 6 Hz. Two to five replications of 1000 stimuli were presented to each limb. To obtain pattern reversal VEPs, subjects viewed a B/W monitor containing 1° checks that reversed position at 2 alternations/s. The subjects fixated either the center or the left or right edges of the display to activate one or both of the occipital poles.

C. Electrophysiologic Recordings

The evoked potentials were recorded from scalp electrodes placed according to the International 10–20 System (Jasper, 1958). Twenty-one channels of EEG were recorded with a bandpass of 1–3 kHz. Averaged waveforms were digitally filtered with a bandpass of 30–500 Hz to remove any stimulus artifact for SEPs and with a bandpass of 1–100 Hz for VEPs. A linked ear reference was used, with the baseline portion of the waveforms being set to zero volts.

D. Dipole Localization

A spatiotemporal dipole model (Scherg and von Cramon, 1985) was used to analyze the waveforms as fixed dipoles with overlapping activation functions. A gradient descent algorithm (Neuroscan, Inc.) was used to minimize the variance between the empirically obtained recordings and the equivalent dipole solutions. Each dipole was initially placed at the center of the isotropic spherical head model, and its location and temporal activation function was allowed to vary until a model that best fit the recorded waveforms was identified. A single dipole was used to model the P100 component of the pattern VEPs and the P40 component of tibial nerve SEPs. Three dipoles were used to model the P14, N20, and P25 components of median nerve responses.

E. MRIs

MRIs were obtained from a Siemens magnetom 1.5-T using a T_1 weighting function. Sixty-four 1.17-mm slices were obtained during a single 11-min scan. The surfaces of the skin and brain were manually edited and rendered as 3D images after the manner of Levin *et al.* (1988).

F. Electrode Locations

The locations of the recording electrodes were obtained using an RF localizer (Polhemus Corp., Colcester, VT), which returns the Cartesian coordinates of the electrodes relative to a sensor attached to the forehead. It has a 1.4-mm accuracy in our hands (Towle *et al.*, 1993). During the same measurement session, the locations of 150 arbitrary points on the scalp were obtained, forming a patient-specific coordinate system encoding the electrode locations and scalp.

G. Merging Coordinate Systems

Three sets of Cartesian coordinates must be related to each other in order to register the equivalent dipoles of the electrophysiologic recordings within MR im-

ages of the brain anatomy (Fig. 1). The electrodes exist within physical space, the anatomical structures exist within MR images, and the dipoles are mapped within the isotropic spherical model of the head.

Because the electrode locations and the surface of the scalp were encoded in the same coordinate system, the electrodes were translated and rotated to the surface of the head in the MR image by fitting the edited skin of the MR image with the digitized scalp (Fig. 2), using the surface correlation algorithm developed by Pelizzari *et al.* (1989). This procedure allows the electrode locations to be superimposed on the MR image with a two- to three-pixel resolution. Individual electrodes can be located with a 2- to 3-mm average accuracy. One advantage of this retroactive fitting technique is that radioopaque markers need not be placed on the scalp to indicate the electrode positions at the time of the MR scan. Alternatively, if all of the electrode locations can be located in the MR image, separate digitization of the electrode locations is unnecessary.

The center of the spherical dipole model is located within the image containing the electrodes by determining the best-fitting sphere, i.e., the sphere that minimizes the distance between the surface of the sphere and the scalp electrodes (Fig. 3). We have found that scalp electrode positions are well approximated by a sphere, with an average error of 6% of the radius of the sphere. The center of the best-fitting sphere, which we call Descartes' point, is located near the floor of the third ventricle about 6 mm anterior to the posterior commissure on the midline (Towle *et al.*, 1993).

In order to minimize the discrepancy between the spherical model and the dolichocephalic head, we have warped the spherical model (Fig. 4) by applying an elliptical transformation based on the distances between the anterior–posterior electrodes ($F_{pz}–O_z$) and the lateral electrodes ($T_3–T_4$). This process will reduce the eccentricity of dipoles in the lateral regions and increase the eccentricity of dipoles located in anterior and posterior regions. No adjustment is made in the vertical direction. After the center of the spherical model is placed at Descartes' point and the axes are scaled to the size and shape of the head, the horizontal axes of the dipole model are rotated to be parallel to the plane determined by a line between the frontal F_{pz} electrode position and the occipital O_z electrode position and by the lateral electrode positions, $T_3–T_4$. These axes can deviate from the horizontal MR coordinates by as much as 30°, depending on the position of the head within the scanner (Fig. 5). This alignment strategy has the advantage of not requiring the digitization of fiducial points and not assuming perfect

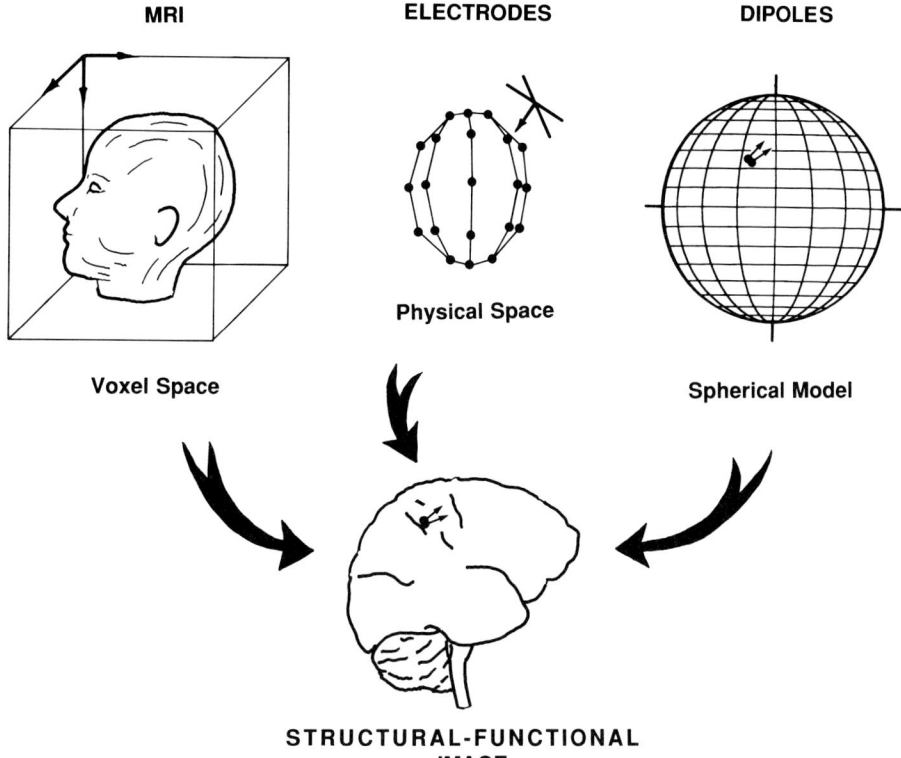

Figure 1   Diagram of the three types of information and coordinate systems that must be merged in order to register evoked potential dipoles within MR images. Brain structure is addressed using the MRI video display coordinates; the electrode locations are measured in patient-specific Cartesian coordinates produced by the localizer; and the dipoles are initially defined using the coordinates of the spherical model.

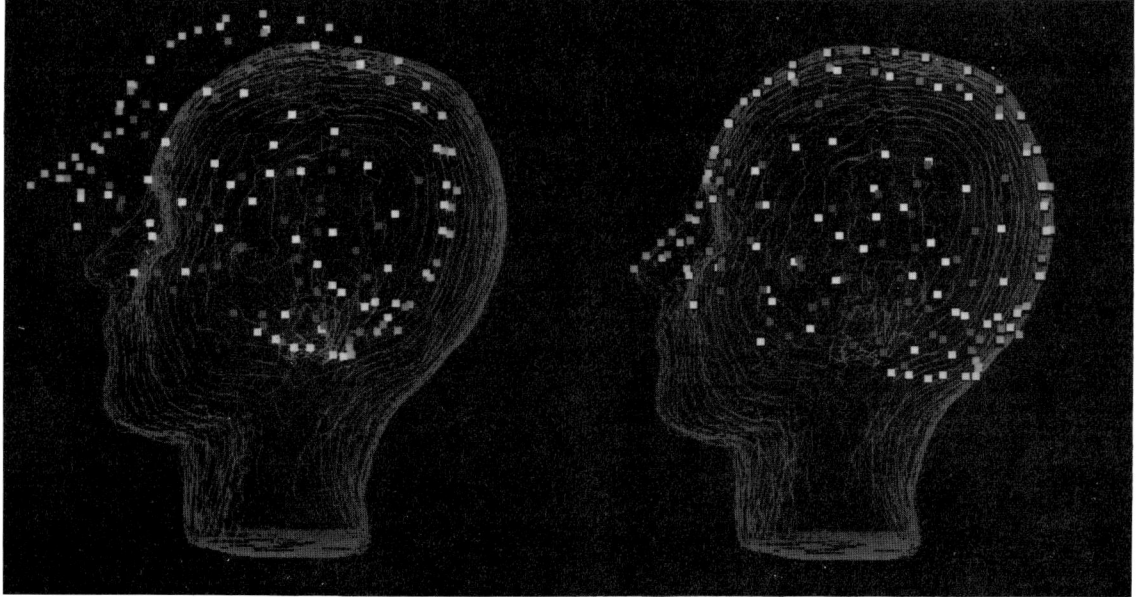

Figure 2   The electrodes are located in the MR image through a surface matching algorithm that fits 150 points digitized from the scalp with an edited MRI surface of the head. This transformation matrix is then applied to the electrode coordinates.

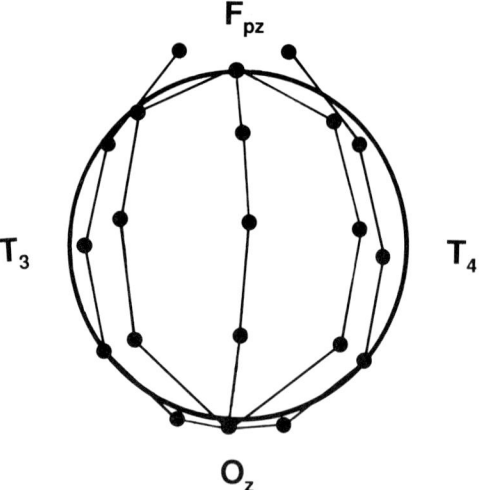

Figure 3 The spherical model is located such that its center coincides with the center of a sphere which minimizes the distance between the electrode locations and the sphere. The frontal and occipital electrodes lay outside of the sphere and the temporal electrodes lay within the sphere.

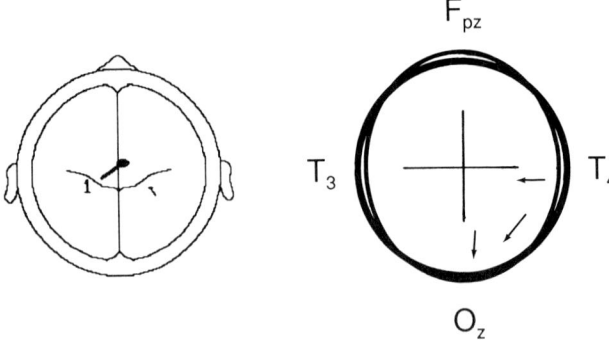

Figure 4 To correct for the nonspherical shape of the head, the dipole coordinates are scaled using an elliptical transformation based on the distance between the F_{pz}–O_z and the T_3–T_4 electrode locations.

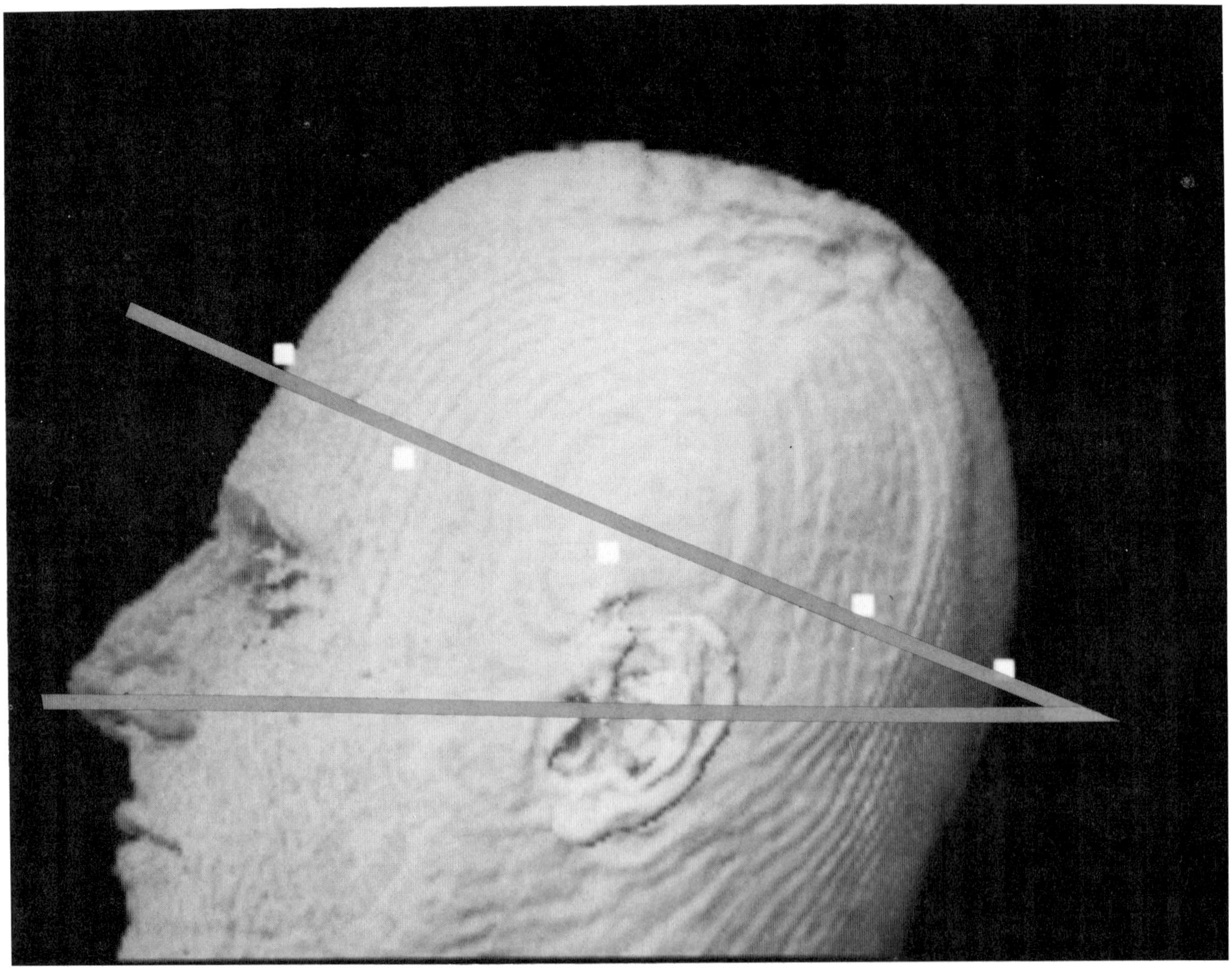

Figure 5 The orientation of the axes of the spherical model is based on a plane defined by the orientation of a line passing through the F_{pz} and O_z electrodes and the T_3 and T_4 electrodes. This plane is rotated to match the horizontal plane of the MR coordinates.

symmetry of the head. If the individual subject's electrode locations are not taken into consideration when the dipole parameters are calculated, it is advisable to base these rotations on all of the electrodes, rather than these four. The coordinate transformation procedures are described in more detail in the Appendix.

III. Results

An example of the averaged scalp waveforms resulting from left median nerve stimulation at the wrist of one subject is shown in Plate 76, along with the scalp distribution of the response 20 ms after the stimulus. The dipole model predicted 94% of the variance of the empirical waveforms. The location and orientation of dipoles associated with the N20 component from five replications of the median nerve SEP from this subject are displayed both within the spatiotemporal dipole model and within the MR image in Fig. 6. The dipoles were located in or over the right hemisphere in the approximate hand area of the postcentral gyrus. The average deviation of each replication from the mean was 4 mm.

Figure 7 displays the mean dipole location resulting from stimulation of the left median nerve, left tibial nerve, and left visual field of a different subject. The locations of all three dipoles within the right hemisphere are generally consistent with the organization

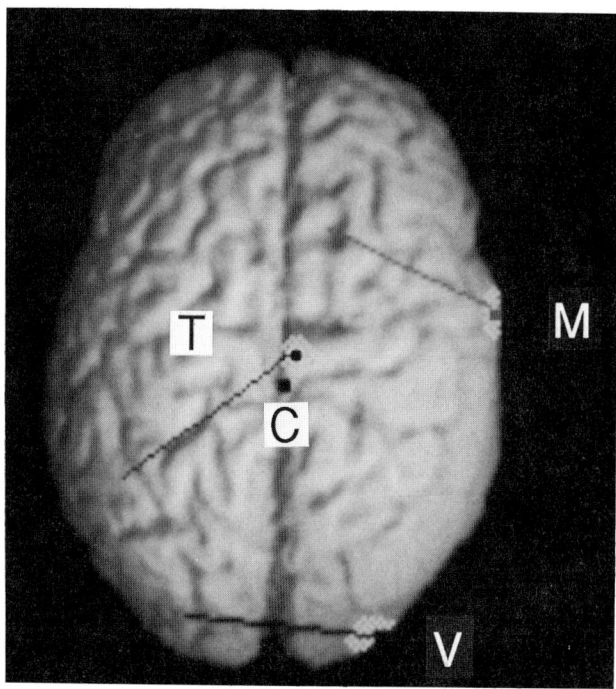

Figure 7 Vectors indicating the location and orientation of the initial cortical responses to stimulation of the left wrist (M), left ankle (T), and left visual field (V) of a different subject.

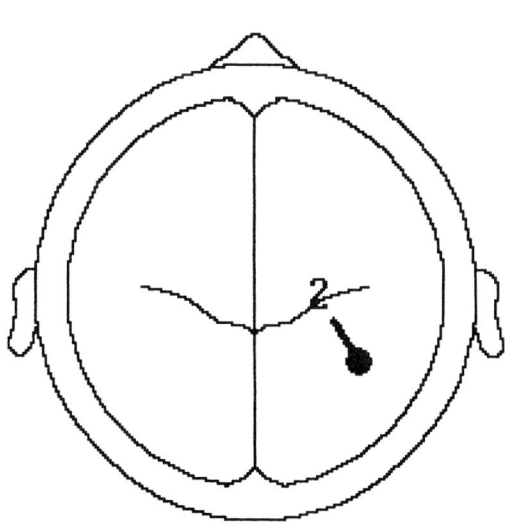
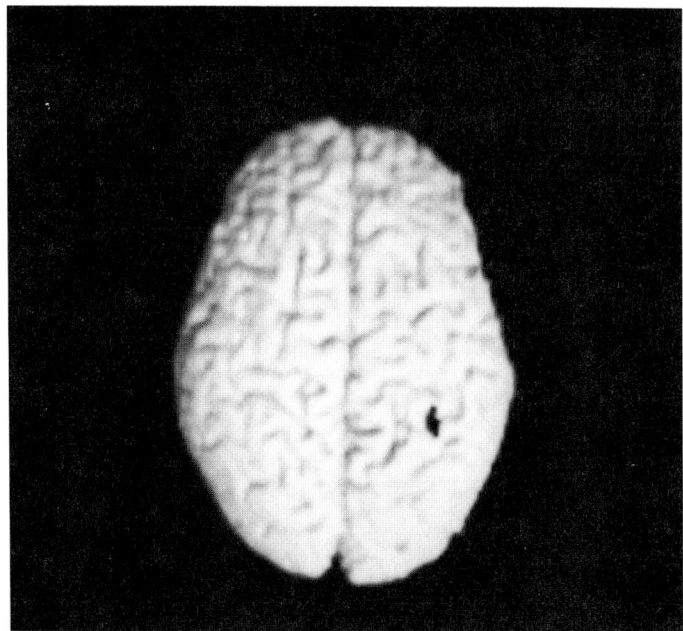

Figure 6 The location of the dipole associated with the N20 component of the left median nerve somatosensory evoked potential (SEP) from the subject whose data appear in Fig. 5 and Plate 76. Five replications of the dipole deviated from their mean location by 4 mm.

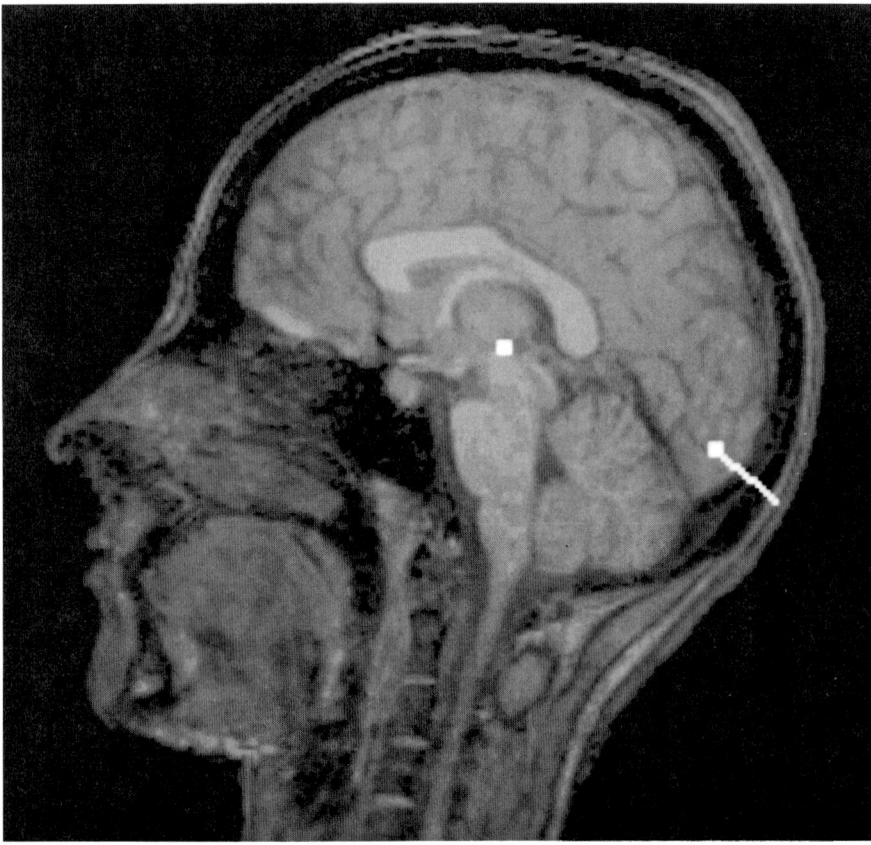

Figure 8 The location and orientation of the cortical response (P100) to full-field checkerboard pattern stimulation displayed on a midsagittal MR slice of the subject appearing in Fig. 2.

of the sensory and visual cortices of humans. In some cases it is more appropriate to display the location of the dipoles by viewing them in standard 2D MRI slices of the brain. Figure 8 shows the location of a full-field pattern VEP from a third subject displayed on a midsagittal slice. The dipole is located near the midline at the level of the calcarine fissure, consistent with a cortical generator. This relationship with cortical anatomy cannot necessarily be appreciated by viewing the distribution of the VEP on the scalp.

IV. Discussion

Using the procedure described above, it is possible to register evoked potentials in MR images, allowing the creation of functional cortical maps based on electrophysiologic recordings. The technique is amenable to various types of electrophysiologic recordings, including visual (Mehta *et al.*, 1990), somatosensory (Buchner and Scherg, 1990) and auditory evoked potentials (Scherg and von Cramon, 1990), movement-related potentials (Toro *et al.*, 1991), and perhaps, to

a lesser extent, cognitive event-related potentials (Starr *et al.*, 1991) and epileptic spikes (Ebersole, 1991; Rose *et al.*, 1987), which involve large areas of the brain. Crucial for the interpretation of dipole models, which yield hypothetical points of zero volume as solutions, is the ability to selectively activate specific brain areas (van Essen *et al.*, 1992; Desmedt and Ozaki 1991). Unlike PET and SPECT, this technique cannot define volumes of interest.

A second difficulty with this technique is that very high quality recordings are necessary, in order to obtain dipole stability. Because the solutions are primarily based on the distribution of response amplitude over the scalp, they are very sensitive to noise in the electrophysiologic recordings. Many patients may not be able to relax well enough to obtain adequate records. Dipole reliability is a necessary, but not sufficient condition for obtaining valid dipoles. Reporting some index of spatial variability across replications or displaying multiple dipoles, as we have done in Fig. 6, should be a necessary requirement for credible recordings. A set of requirements for assessing the validity of dipole solutions has not yet been widely accepted, but will likely involve low dipole variability, adequate spatial sampling by the electrode montage, biologically realistic dipole activation functions, and low residual variances.

The validity of the technique also depends on the adequacy of the spherical model to accurately reflect the volume currents within the brain and skull (Fender, 1991). We have employed post hoc corrections to compensate for the obvious differences between a sphere and the human head, but more promising results may be obtained with realistic head-shaped models (Nakajima *et al.*, 1990; He *et al.*, 1987). When advances are made in these areas, we can expect more useful images that communicate both the spatial and the functional aspects of the intact human brain.

Appendix

The coordinate system used to describe locations within the spherical volume conduction model of the head is based on the locations of four 10–20 system electrodes, F_{pz}, O_z, T_3, T_4, and the center of the best-fit sphere as they appear in the MR image. Consider the MRI coordinates of these locations to be vectors:

$$F_{pz} \rightarrow \mathcal{A}$$
$$O_z \rightarrow \mathcal{P}$$
$$T_3 \rightarrow \mathcal{L}$$
$$T_4 \rightarrow \mathcal{R}$$
$$\text{center} \rightarrow \mathcal{C}.$$

The origin of the spatiotemporal dipole model coordinate system is defined as point C. Vectors of unit length in the direction of the axes are signified by $\hat{x}$, $\hat{y}$, and $\hat{z}$. The y axis is parallel to the line between F_{pz} and O_z, with $+y$ anterior:

$$\hat{y} = \frac{\mathcal{A} - \mathcal{P}}{|\mathcal{A} - \mathcal{P}|}.$$

The z axis is perpendicular to the y axis and to the line between T_3 and T_4, with $+z$ superior:

$$\hat{z} = \frac{(\mathcal{R} - \mathcal{L}) \times \hat{y}}{|(\mathcal{R} - \mathcal{L}) \times \hat{y}|}.$$

The x axis is perpendicular to the y and z axes, with $+x$ to the right:

$$\hat{x} = \hat{y} \times \hat{z}.$$

If the MRI coordinates are left handed (i.e., $\hat{x} \times \hat{y} = -\hat{z}$), it is important when calculating the above cross-products to use right-hand conventions to keep the axes pointed in the proper directions.

Once the unit vectors $\hat{x}$, $\hat{y}$, and $\hat{z}$ are known, MRI coordinate $\mathcal{D}$ can be transformed into dipole model coordinates x_s, y_s, and z_s, by taking the dot products:

$$x_s = (\mathcal{D} - \mathcal{C}) \cdot \hat{x}$$
$$y_s = (\mathcal{D} - \mathcal{C}) \cdot \hat{y}$$
$$z_s = (\mathcal{D} - \mathcal{C}) \cdot \hat{z}.$$

Electrode locations in the spherical dipole model may then be scaled to more precisely fit the surface of the sphere:

$$x_s' = \frac{x_s |\mathcal{R} - \mathcal{L}|}{2r} \quad y_s' = \frac{y_s |\mathcal{A} - \mathcal{P}|}{2r} \quad z_s' = z_s,$$

where r is the radius of the best-fit sphere.

To transform the dipole model coordinates into MRI coordinates, the scaling is inversed to return to the actual head shape:

$$x_s = \frac{2x_s' r}{|\mathcal{R} - \mathcal{L}|} \quad y_s = \frac{2y_s' r}{|\mathcal{A} - \mathcal{P}|}.$$

The location vector $\mathcal{D}$ in MRI coordinates is then

$$\mathcal{D} = \mathcal{C} + x_s \hat{x} + y_s \hat{y} + z_s \hat{z}.$$

Acknowledgments

We are grateful to Halina Wilczek, Samuel Frank, and Drs. Yue Cao and Lucio Parmeggiani for their contributions to this study.

References

Buchner, H., and Scherg, M. (1990). "Multiple Sources of Median Nerve Somatosensory Evoked Potentials Revealed by Brain Electric Source Analysis." Paper presented at the Fourth International Evoked Potentials Symposium, Toronto, 1990.

Desmedt, J. E., and Ozaki, I. (1991). SEPs to finger joint input lack the N20-P20 response that is evoked by tactile inputs: Contrast between cortical generators in areas 3b and 2 in humans. *Electroenceph. Clin. Neurophysiol.* **80**, 513–521.

Ebersole, J. S. (1991). EEG dipole modeling in complex partial epilepsy. *Brain Topogr.* **4**, 113–123.

Fender, D. H. (1991). Models of the human brain and the surrounding media: Their influence on the realiability of source localization. *J. Clin. Neurophysiol.* **8**, 381–390.

Gevins, A. S., and Illes, J. (1991). Neurocognitive networks of the human brain. *Ann. N.Y. Acad. Sci.* **620**, 22–44.

Grzeszczuk, R., Tan, K. K., Levin, D. N., Pelizzari, C. A., Chen, G. T. Y., Milton, J., Spire, J.-P., and Towle, V. L. (1990). Radiographic localization of cortical electrodes with respect to MR-derived 3-D brain models. *Radiology* **177**(P), 290.

He, B., Musha, T., Okamoto, Y., Homma, S., Nakajima, Y., and Sato, T. (1987). Electric dipole tracing in the brain by means of the boundary element method and its accuracy. *IEEE Trans. Biomed. Eng.* **34**, 406–414.

Jack, C. R., Jr., Marsh, W. R., Hirschorn, K. A., Sharbrough, F. W., Cascino, G. D., Karwoski, R. A., and Robb, R. A. (1990). EEG scalp electrode projection onto three-dimensional surface rendered images of the brain. *Radiology* **176,** 413–418.

Jasper, H. H. (1958). The ten twenty electrode system of the international federation. *Electroenceph. Clin. Neurophysiol.* **10,** 370–375.

Levin, D. N., Hu, X., Tan, K. K., and Galhotra, S. (1989). Surface of the brain: Three-dimensional MR images created with volume-rendering. *Radiology* **171,** 277–280.

Mehta, A. D., Simpson, G. V., Scherg, M., Vaughan, H. G., Jr., and Weiss, K. (1990). "Spatiotemporal Analysis of Visual Activity in Primates. I. Retinotopic Activation of Human Visual Cortex." Paper presented at the 20th annual meeting of the Society for Neuroscience, St. Louis.

Myslobodsky, M. S., and Bar-Ziv, J. (1989). Locations of occipital EEG electrodes verified by computed tomography. *Electroenceph. Clin. Neurophysiol.* **72,** 362–366.

Myslobodsky, M. S., Coppola, R., Bar-Ziv, J., and Weinberger, D. R. (1990). Adequacy of the international 10-20 electrode system for computed neurophysiologic topography. *J. Clin. Neurophysiol.* **7,** 507–518.

Nakajima, Y., Homma, S., Musha, T., Okamoto, Y., Ackerman, R. H., Correia, J. A., and Alpert, N. M. (1990). Dipole-tracing of abnormal slow brain potentials after cerebral stroke—EEG, PET, MRI correlations. *Neurosci. Lett.* **112,** 59–64.

Papanicolaou, A. C., Baumann, S., Rogers, R. L., Saydjari, C., Amparo, E. G., and Eisenberg, H. M. (1990). Localization of auditory response sources using magnetoencephalography and magnetic resonance imaging. *Arch. Neurol.* **47,** 33–37.

Pelizzari, C. A., Chen, G. T. Y., Spelbring, D. R., Weichselbaum, R. R., and Chen, C-T. (1989). Accurate three-dimensional registration of CT, PET, and/or MR images of the brain. *J. Comput. Assist. Tomogr.* **13,** 20–26.

Rose, D. F., Sato, S., Smith, P. D., Porter, R. J., Theodore, W. H., Friauf, W., Bonner, R., and Jabbari, B. (1987). Localization of magnetic interictal discharges in temporal lobe epilepsy. *Ann. Neurol.* **22,** 348–354.

Scherg, M., and von Cramon, D. (1985). Two bilateral sources of the late AEP as identified by a spatio-temporal dipole model. *Electroenceph. Clin. Neurophysiol.* **62,** 32–44.

Scherg, M., and von Cramon, D. (1990). Dipole source potentials of the auditory cortex in normal subjects and in patients with temporal lobe lesions. "Advances in Audiology" *In* (F. Grandori, M. Hoke, and G. L. Romani (Eds.), Vol. 6, pp. 165–193.

Starr, A., Kristeva, R., Cheyne, D., Lindinger, G., and Deecke, L. (1991). Localization of brain activity during auditory verbal short-term memory derived from magnetic recordings. *Brain Res.* **558,** 181–190.

Suk, J., Ribary, U., Cappell, J., Yamamoto, T., and Llinas, R. (1991). Anatomical localization revealed by MEG recordings of the human somatosensory system. *Electroenceph. Clin. Neurophysiol.* **78,** 185–196.

Tan, K. K., Levin, D. N., Pelizzari, C. A., Grzeszcuk, R., Chen, G. T. Y., Erikson, R. K., Milton, J., Spire, J.-P., and Towle, V. L. (1991). Interactive device for performing image-guided cranial procedures. *J. Magn. Reson. Imag.* **1,** 198.

Toro, C., Matsumoto, J., Roth, B. J., and Hallet, M. (1991). "Dipole Source Analysis of Movement Related Cortical Potentials." Paper presented at the annual meeting of the American EEG Society, Philadelphia.

Towle, V. L., Bolanos, J., Suarez, D., Tan, K., Grzeszczuk, R., Levin, D. N., Cakmurk, R., Frank, S., and Spire, J.-P. (1993). The spatial location of EEG electrodes: Locating the best-fitting sphere relative to cortical anatomy. *Electroenceph. Clin. Neurophysiol.* **86,** 1–6.

van den Elsen, P. A., and Viergever, M. A. (1991). Marker guided registration of electromagnetic dipole data with tomographic images. *In* "Information Processing in Medical Imaging" (A. C. F. Colchester and D. J. Hawkes, Eds.) Berlin: Springer-Verlag.

van Essen, D. C., Anderson, C. H., and Felleman, D. J. (1992). Information processing in the primate visual system: An integrated systems perspective. *Science* **255,** 419–423.

25

Multimodal Integration of Electrophysiological Data and Brain Images: EEG, MEG, TMS, MRI, and PET

Binseng Wang,* Camilo Toro, Eric M. Wassermann, Thomas A. Zeffiro, Robert W. Thatcher, and Mark Hallett

Biomedical Engineering and Instrumentation Program, National Center for Research Resources; and Human Motor Control Section, Medical Neurology Branch, National Institute of Neurological Disorders and Stroke, National Institutes of Health, Bethesda, Maryland 20892

I. Introduction

Although there are several imaging technologies that offer high spatial resolution to study the brain, none can provide the temporal resolution of electrophysiological techniques (Thatcher *et al.*, 1994). Conversely, the latter cannot compete with the former in terms of anatomical detail. Therefore, there is a natural desire to integrate different modalities of data and images for the research and diagnosis of brain disorders (Pechura and Martin, 1991). For example, Gevins *et al.* (1990, 1991) have mapped the spatial distribution of the scalp-recorded electroencephalogram (EEG) onto the cortical surface, as well as EEG dipole sources into magnetic resonance (MR) images of the brain. Kuriki *et al.* (1987), Reite *et al.* (1988), Yamamoto *et al.* (1988), and Papanicolaou *et al.* (1990) have mapped magnetoencephalogram (MEG) dipole sources onto MR images.

Often it is sufficient to integrate electrophysiological data with only one modality of three-dimensional (3D) images. Sometimes, however, other image modalities are needed to provide a more complete understanding. In particular, positron emission tomography (PET) images, properly registered and overlaid with MR, can provide an additional, independent means to identify the physiologically active brain regions (e.g., Grafton *et al.*, 1991).

We report here a method to integrate EEG and MEG dipole sources and transcranial magnetic stimulation (TMS) scalp maps with MR and PET images. Instead of using fiduciary markers visible to MR or PET for mapping the 3D data into the images (e.g., Papanicolaou *et al.*, 1990), each subject's head surface was sampled by a digitizer and used as an intermediary framework to hold all electrophysiological data. Each digitized head was registered with the respective MR head surface using a surface registration algorithm (Pelizzari *et al.*, 1989). The transformation parameters obtained from the registration were used to map the electrophysiological data into MR. Finally, the mapped MR was registered and overlaid with the PET image using again the surface registration technique. This report concentrates on the methodological issues of multimodality integration. The physiological significance of the results are addressed by other chapters of this volume.

II. Methods

A. Data and Image Acquisition

Six healthy adult volunteers, four men and two women, participated in this study. The research protocols (one for each modality) were approved by the clinical research subpanel of the National Institute of Neurological Disorders and Stroke, and all subjects gave their written informed consent for the studies. In

---

* On leave from the State University of Campinas, Brazil.

addition, a plastic adult skull model (Model 24-6981T, Carolina Biological Supply, Burlington, NC) was used to test the methods and evaluate precision at each step.

EEG recordings were obtained from four subjects while conducting self-paced right-index-finger abduction/adduction, at a rate of about 0.25 Hz. MEG recordings were obtained from two subjects doing the same task. TMS scalp maps were made on four subjects using the EMG recorded from the right-finger abductor muscle while stimulating the contralateral motor cortex. The details of EEG and MEG recordings and TMS mapping have been reported previously by Toro *et al.* (1993, 1994) and Wassermann *et al.* (1992a), respectively and, thus, will not be repeated here. The Brain Electric Source Analysis (BESA) program (Neuroscan, Inc.) was used to compute three equivalent dipole sources from each set of EEG recordings (Scherg and Berg, 1990), using the strategy described by Toro *et al.* (1993a). Five equivalent dipole sources were computed from each set of MEG recordings, one for each main peak, using a software supplied by the manufacturer of the magnetometer, Biomagnetic Technology, Inc. (San Diego, CA).

MR images were obtained with a 1.5-T GE Signa system. From each subject, 124 contiguous sagittal volumetric MR slices were obtained. The pixels were 0.98×0.98 mm, whereas the slice thickness was 1.5 mm. Regional cerebral blood flow (CBF) images were obtained with a Scanditronix 2048-15 PET scanner using $H_2^{15}O$ as the radioactive tracer, injected intravenously in 33-mCi boluses. Measurements of changes in CBF were obtained using a modified autoradiographic technique (Herscovitch *et al.*, 1983; Raichle *et al.*, 1983). From each subject 15 transaxial slices, 6.5 mm thick, with an in-plane pixel size of 2 mm were obtained in each one of three different states: rest, active, and passive. In the rest state, the subject was instructed to lay quietly with eyes closed. In the active state, the subject moved his or her right index finger in the manner described above. In the passive state, the finger was moved by the examiner with about the same rate and range of movement. Each subject underwent eight scans, three at rest, three in an active state, and two in a passive state. The data of each state were averaged and globally normalized to a mean of 100. The mean rest set was subtracted from the mean active set, thus providing a set of subtraction images that are presumably linearly related to tissue activity due to active movement of the index finger (Fox *et al.*, 1988; Fox and Mintun, 1989).

We used a plastic skull model to calibrate the registration of MR and surface digitization. To scan the plastic skull model with MR, the upper portion of the skull was removed, and 12 2- $\times$ 2-mm holes were drilled into, but not through, its inner surface. This shell was placed upside down, filled with about 500 ml of saline (0.9% NaCl), and placed inside a MR head coil on top of two 500-ml saline bags. This arrangement provided a good picture of the skull model's inner surface, which was also digitized with the magnetic digitizer. After registration of the two surfaces, the coordinates of the 12 holes determined by the digitizer were mapped into the MR and compared with the actual positions in the image.

B. Data and Image Integration

Electrophysiological data and 3D images were integrated using the head surface as the common reference framework (Fig. 1). This method assumed that two different representations of each subject's head surface can be obtained, one using a 3D digitizer and another from the individual's MR slices, and these two representations can be registered using a mathe-

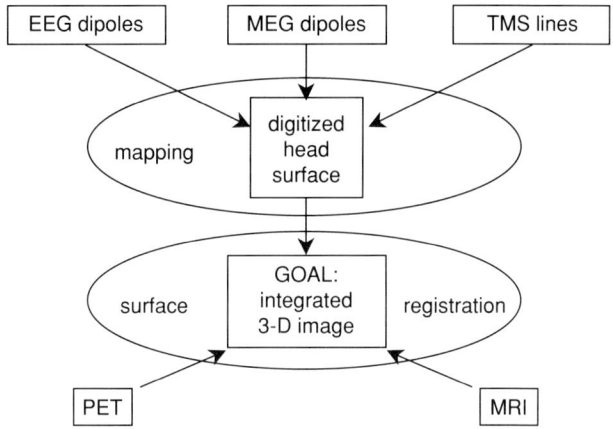

Figure 1 Schematic diagram showing how the digitized head surface can be used as a common framework for storing three-dimensional (3D) electrophysiological data and for integrating them with 3D images. The coordinates of 3D objects, such as equivalent-dipole-source locations and directions computed from EEG and MEG recordings and projections of transcranial magnetic stimulation (TMS) sites on the scalp, were first mapped into the digitized head through coordinate transformations. The digitized head surface was then aligned with the head surface contours obtained from MR scans using a surface registration algorithm. This allowed the mapping of 3D objects from the digitized head into MR slices. The PET images were integrated by registering the brain surface contours obtained from PET and MR slices. The registered PET was then resliced along the sagittal plane, coplanar with the MR slices. The resliced PET images were then overlaid on the corresponding MR slices, which were previously mapped with the 3D electrophysiological data, thus achieving the goal of an integrated multimodality 3D image.

matical algorithm. The transformation parameters that make one surface representation aligned with the other provided a means to map 3D coordinates from one coordinate system to the other. The entire integration method can be divided into six steps. The first one was head surface digitization. Next, each type of electrophysiological data had to be transferred from its original coordinate system into the digitized-head coordinate system. The third step was the registration of the digitized head with the head contours obtained from the MR images. The parameters obtained from the registration were then used to map data from the digitized heads into MR images. The fifth step was the registration of PET and MR images. Finally, the MR images with electrophysiological data already mapped on were overlaid onto the PET images, thus completing the integration process.

1. Head Surface Digitization

A magnetic-field digitizer (Polhemus, Colchester, VT) was used to sample the head surface and to measure the 3D coordinates of markings or electrode positions on the scalp. The digitizer's magnetic source was fixed on the top of a plastic frame, which was mounted on the top of the head with self-adhesive wraps (Wang et al., 1994). This method is preferable to holding the subject's head still by using either a chin rest (Gevins et al., 1990) or a bite bar (Law and Nunez, 1991). Although the sessions sometimes lasted more than an hour, the volunteers reported no discomfort because they were able to move their heads whenever they wished.

From each subject, 350–450 points were obtained. The points were about 2–3 cm apart from each other, spiraling down from the top of the head. Two to three readings were made at each point. The mean values (for each of the three coordinates) were accepted as the coordinates of that point if the difference between each reading and the mean was less than 1 mm; otherwise, the data were discarded. This procedure avoided including erroneous readings whenever the digitizer probe was not held steadily against the head surface. The average localization uncertainty has been estimated to be 3.2 ± 0.4 mm (Wang et al., 1994).

Positions on the head, such as electrode locations and stimulation sites, were digitized from each subject whenever an experiment was carried out, but each head surface needed to be digitized only once. Data obtained in different sessions from the same subject were registered through an algorithm that minimizes the mean-square-root distance (error) between the transformed and the measured coordinates of a set of 10 points. This least-mean-square error (LMSE) regis-

tration technique have an estimated precision of 5.7 mm (Wang et al., 1994).

2. Mapping into Digitized Heads

a. Mapping EEG Sources into Digitized Heads
The BESA program assumes that the head can be modeled by a sphere with three concentric layers, with its center approximately at the middle of the posterior commissure and a radius of 85 mm (Scherg and Berg, 1990). In an attempt to achieve a more precise mapping for each individual, we fitted a sphere to the scalp portion of the digitized head surface, i.e., the points above the eyebrows, ears, and inion, using the modified least-mean-square error function proposed by Lükenhüner et al. (1990). The radius of this best-fitting sphere was used to scale the dipole "eccentricities" provided by BESA. The best-fitting-sphere center, together with C_z and F_{pz}, defined for each subject a rectangular coordinate system, from which the dipole source locations and orientations calculated with BESA were mapped into the digitized head.

b. Mapping MEG Sources into Digitized Heads
The software used for the computation of MEG sources also assumes a spherical head model. However, the computed source locations were in rectangular coordinates with respect to a system defined by the nasion and left and right preauricular points. Thus the mapping of MEG sources into the digitized head was achieved by determining a set of equations for coordinate transformation between the MEG coordinate system and the digitized-head coordinate system.

c. Mapping TMS Scalp Maps into Digitized Heads
The grid of scalp positions used in TMS was digitized for each subject. Whenever the TMS grid was not acquired in the same session as the head surface, the grid coordinates were mapped into the digitized head using the LMSE registration algorithm mentioned previously. After the center of gravity of the TMS map has been computed, its coordinates are linearly interpolated from the coordinates of the nearest points on the grid. The grid points were also used to determine the perpendicular line to the scalp at the center of gravity, by fitting a sphere to the grid points. Again, the error function proposed by Lükenhüner et al. (1990) was used.

3. Registration of the Digitized Heads with MR Images

The surface registration algorithm developed by Pelizzari et al. (1989) was used to align each digitized head with the respective MR head surface. For this purpose, the head contour of each MR slice was outlined manually with a trackball. A few points were removed from each digitized head prior to the registration to reduce possible misalignments caused by sagging of soft tissue on the face and difficulties in reliably identifying scalp surfaces in the most lateral MR slices (Wang *et al.*, 1994). The RMS misfits of the registrations ranged between 1.8 and 3.0 mm, with an average of 2.4 mm.

4. Mapping Data from Digitized Heads into MR Images

From each registration, a set of rotation and translation parameters was obtained. These parameters were used to deduce four sequential coordinate transformations that converted the coordinates of any point from the digitized-head coordinate system into the MR's coordinate system. Four transformations were needed because the registration algorithm devised by Pelizzari *et al.* (1989) uses the centroids of each surface as an intermediate coordinate system.

BESA source locations were mapped into MR by masking a plus-shaped region of interest with white color. BESA orientations could not be mapped because they are usually not coplanar with the parasagittal slices. Instead, a point 1 cm away in that direction was computed and mapped onto the respective MR slice, so the direction could be visualized if desired. MEG source locations were represented by white circles. To visualize the projection of the TMS center of gravity into the brain of each subject, we computed the intersection of the perpendicular line with each sagittal slice and masked a square of 3 × 3 pixels around the intersection.

5. Registration of MR and PET Images

Instead of head contours, brain contours were used to register PET and MR images because it is easier to discern the brain in PET images. Head surface would be available if transmission images were acquired with the PET scanner. The PET brain contours were obtained from the global average of all eight rest, active, and passive image sets, using an edge detection algorithm. Often manual editing of the contours was necessary to remove sharp edges. As the brain contours obtained from each image set overlaid well on the contour obtained from the global average, we assumed that there was no head motion during the PET scan.

The MR brain contours were outlined manually with a trackball and required training and the proficiency of the operator. The PET and MR brain contours were registered using the algorithm developed by Pelizzari *et al.* (1989). After each registration, the global averaged PET was resliced along the sagittal

plane and overlaid on the corresponding MR slices. Proper alignment of the two sets of images was considered to be achieved whenever the higher activity areas were confined to gray matter areas along the brain sulci. Otherwise the brain contours were revised and the registration procedure was repeated.

6. Superposition of PET Images

Once a satisfactory registration was achieved, the mean rest PET set was subtracted from the mean active set. This set of images was then resliced into 124 slices along the sagittal plane, coplanar with the MR slices, using the registration parameters. The resliced PET subtraction images were then overlaid on the corresponding MR slices, which were previously mapped with dipole locations or TMS line intersections. Now the electrophysiological data can be compared to active PET regions, having in the background the neuroanatomic substrate provided by MR.

III. Results

Although it is only an intermediate step of the integration method, it is instructive to visualize electrophysiological data within the framework provided by the digitized head. Plate 77 shows a typical digitized head with the positions of the electrodes used for recording EEG. Also shown is the sphere that best fit the scalp surface with the least-mean-square error. This sphere was used to map BESA sources into the digitized head. Plate 78 shows three EEG-source locations and Plate 79 shows five MEG-source locations mapped into the respective digitized heads. Plate 80 shows a digitized head with a line perpendicular to the scalp surface projecting into the brain from the TMS center of gravity. This line provides a means to visualize the trajectory of the magnetic field created by the coil on the scalp.

EEG and MEG dipoles and TMS lines integrated with MR and PET images were visualized on 2D slices as there were no means to render integrated 3D objects together with images. Plate 81 compares, on a single sagittal MR slice, the location of the main contralateral dipole source of cortical EEG potentials with the increased regional CBF detected by PET. Both sets of data were obtained from the same subject executing self-paced right-index-finger voluntary movements. The orientation of the dipole could not be shown as it was not coplanar with this slice. A notion of the proximity of each dipole to the respective increased regional CBF region was obtained by measuring the distance between the dipole location and the peak of the nearest activated PET region. This distance varied in four subjects from 9 to 25 mm, with the mean at 17 mm, for the main contralateral dipole. The mean distances for the ipsilateral and middle dipoles were 32 and 36 mm, respectively. However, often there were multiple increased regional CBF regions around these dipoles, and these regions were not as strongly activated as those near the contralateral motor cortex (Wang *et al.*, 1992).

The location of one of the five MEG sources is compared with the increased regional CBF detected by PET on Plate 82. As suggested by this figure, none of the five magnetic dipoles came close to the activated PET regions, nor even to the central sulcus. However, as will be discussed later, this result may due to the fact that the model and assumptions used to compute these dipole sources were inadequate.

Plate 83 shows the intersections of the projection of the TMS center of gravity with nine sequential axial MR slices. These intersections were consistently just anterior to the central sulcus in every subject. Data obtained from four subjects also suggest that each projection line runs parallel to the respective sulcus for about 10 mm right after penetrating the brain (Wassermann *et al.*, 1992b). Plate 84 shows how close one of the intersections came to the peak of the increased regional CBF region within PET. The distance between the TMS projection and the peak of the activated PET region varied in four subjects from 5 to 22 mm, with the mean at 13 mm.

IV. Discussion

The results show that the digitized head surface provides a simple and inexpensive way to integrate different types of electrophysiological data and images. Compared with the mapping technique based on the alignment of anatomical landmarks (Boesecke *et al.*, 1990), this new method has the advantage of not requiring *a priori* knowledge of anatomical structures nor experience in identifying them, except when registering PET brain images. On the other hand, when compared with the mapping methods based on markers (Berström *et al.*, 1981) or frames visible to MR (Kuriki *et al.*, 1987; Reite *et al.*, 1988; Yamamoto *et al.*, 1988; Papanicolaou *et al.*, 1990), our method does not require a special or new MR scan each time new electrophysiological data are acquired. In fact, one can use previously acquired MR images, thus saving time and expense.

In spite of being effective and useful, the integration method developed is still primitive. Even though each subject's head surface needs to be digitized only once, the digitization process is slow and laborious.

This disadvantage can be overcome by designing a cap with many magnetic sensors that can digitize the entire head surface within a few minutes. Naturally head surface digitization and registration can be replaced altogether in the future when MR labels more accurate than the vitamin E pills presently used become available. However, one still must face the need of a new scan each time new electrophysiological data are acquired. MR head contour drawings are also slow and tedious, as are the surface registration programs available presently. Both issues are being addressed by other researchers [see, for example, Hall *et al.* (1992) and Jiang *et al.* (1992), respectively]. Finally, powerful 3D image and object visualization and manipulation programs are needed to display the dipole locations and directions within the merged MR and PET image. Alternatively, one would like to be able to reslice the merged MR and PET image in the planes defined by the dipoles directions or the TMS lines.

The precision of the mapping process itself, i.e., of points digitized from the head surface into MR images, has been estimated to be 3–6 mm (Wang *et al.*, 1993). This value is greater than the 2 mm of mean error distance reported by Gevins *et al.* (1990), but seems adequate for the integration of electrophysiological data with 3D brain images due to the intrinsic resolution of the data and images. The equivalent dipole sources computed from MEG and EEG recordings have spatial uncertainties of 8–10 mm (Cohen and Cuffin, 1991), whereas the resolution of TMS scalp maps is about 5–10 mm (Wassermann *et al.*, 1992a). Only direct cortical recordings or stimulation has higher spatial resoution. On the other hand, PET images have an inherent resolution limitation imposed by the 2- $\times$ 2- $\times$ 6.5-mm pixel size, and the MR–PET registration probably adds at least 5 mm of additional uncertainty.

That MEG dipole locations were found to be quite far from the increased regional CBF detected by PET is most likely due to the fact that the model used to compute the dipoles assumes only a single dipole can be active at a time. As demonstrated by the EEG dipoles computed with BESA, at least two main dipoles were active simultaneously, one in the contralateral cortex and another in the ipsilateral side (Toro *et al.*, 1993). Thus the MEG dipole computed by BTI's program was actually the geometric mean of all the active dipoles at each one of the five time instants. Another factor that might have contributed further to the inaccuracy of the MEG dipole locations was the extremely low signal-to-noise ratio (SNR) of fields generated by a single finger movement. Low SNR significantly increases uncertainty of the dipole computations.

The head surface digitization and registration technique described can also be useful for a variety of other purposes, due to its ability to correlate positions within the head with locations and directions on the head surface. For example, Lufkin *et al.* (1990) and Fishman *et al.* (1991) have already shown that 3D multimodal image integration techniques can be useful for radiation therapy, craniofacial surgeries, neurosurgical planning, and transcranial biopsies. New applications are likely to emerge as the technique is improved in terms of speed and precision. Extension to other parts of the body, such as the chest, the knee, and elbow joints, also seems promising.

Acknowledgments

The authors are grateful to J. Trettau, W. Groves, R. Hill, and L. Johnson for technical assistance; to B. J. Hessie for skillful editorial assistance; and to Drs. S. Bookheimer, B. J. Roth, A. Pascual-Leone, J. Valls-Solé, C. N. Chen, R. Levin, and C. A. Pelizzari for their cooperation. The support of Dr. M. Eden, Director of BEIP–NIH, is appreciated, as well as that provided by UNICAMP, CNPq, and FAPESP, Brazil, to the first author.

References

Berström, M., Boëthius, J., Eriksson, L., Greitz, T., Ribbe, T., and Widén, L. (1981). Head fixation device for reproducible position alignment in transmission CT and positron emission tomography. *J. Comput. Assist. Tomogr.* **5,** 136–141.

Boesecke, R., Bruckner, T., and Ende, G. (1990). Landmark based correlation of medical images. *Phys. Med. Biol.* **35,** 121–126.

Cohen, D., and Cuffin, B. N. EEG versus MEG localization accuracy: Theory and experiment. (1991). *Brain Topogr.* **4,** 95–104.

Fishman, E. K., Magid, D., Ney, D. R., Chaney, E. L., Pizer, S. M., Rosenman, J. G., Levin, D. N., Vannier, M. W., Kuhlman, J. E., and Robertson, D. D. (1991). Three dimensional imaging. *Radiology* **181,** 321–337.

Fox, P., Mintun, M. A., Reiman, E. M., and Raichle, M. E. (1988). Enhanced detection of focal brain responses using inter-subject averaging and change-distribution analysis of subtracted PET images. *J. Cereb. Blood Flow Metab.* **8,** 642–653.

Fox, P., and Mintun, M. A. (1989). Noninvasive functional brain mapping by change-distribution analysis of averaged PET images of $H_2^{15}O$ tissue activity. *J. Nucl. Med.* **30,** 141–149.

Gevins, A. S., Brickett, P., Costales, B., Le, J., and Reutter, B. (1990). Beyond topographic mapping: Towards functional-anatomical imaging with 124-channel EEGs and 3-D MRIs. *Brain Topogr.* **3,** 53–64.

Gevins, A. S., Le, J., Brickett, P. Reutter, B., and Desmond, J. (1991). Seeing through the skull: Advanced EEGs use MRIs to accurately measure cortical activity from the scalp. *Brain Topogr.* **4,** 125–131.

Grafton, S. T., Woods, R. P., Mazziotta, J. C., and Phelps, M. E. (1991). Somatotopic mapping of the primary motor cortex in humans: activation studies with cerebral blood flow and positron emission tomography. *J. Neurophysiol.* **66,** 735–743.

Hall, L. O., Bensaid, A. M., Clarke, L. P., Velthuizen, R. P., Sil-biger, M. L., and Bezdeck, J. C. (1992). A comparison of neural network and fuzzy clustering techniques in segmenting magnetic resonance images of the brain. *IEEE Trans. Neural Networks* **3,** 672–682.

Herscovitch, P., Markham, J., and Raichle, M. E. (1983). Brain oxygen utilization measured with oxygen-15 radiotracers and positron emission tomography: Generation of metabolic images. *J. Nuc. Med.* **26,** 416–417.

Jiang, H., Holton, K., and Robb, R. (1992). Image registration of multimodality 3-D medical images by chamfer matching. *Proc. SPIE Biomed. Image Process. Three-Dimensional Microsc.* **1660,** 356–366.

Kuriki, S., Isobe, Y., Mizutani, Y., and Murase, M. (1988). Magnetic responses evoked by verbal and nonverbal stimuli. *In* "Biomagnetism '87" (K. Atsumi, M. Kotani, S. Ueno, T. Katila, and S. J. Williamson, Eds.), pp. 262–265. Tokyo: Tokyo Denki University Press.

Law, S. K., and Nunez, P. L. (1991). Quantitative representation of the upper surface of the human head. *Brain Topogr.* **3,** 365–371.

Lufkin, R. B., Robinson, J. D., Castro, D. J., Jabour, B. A., Duckwiler, G., Layfield, L. J., and Hanafee, W. N. (1990). Interventional magnetic resonance imaging in the head and neck. *Topogr. Magn. Reson. Imag.* **2,** 76–80.

Lükenhüner, B., Pantev, C., and Hoke, M. (1990). Comparison between different methods to approximate an area of the human head by a sphere. *In* "Auditory Evoked Magnetic Fields and Electric Potentials," Vol. 6, "Advances in Audiology" (F. Grandori, M. Hoke, and G. L. Romani, Eds.), pp. 103–118. Basel: Karger.

Papanicolaou, A. C., Baumann, S., Rogers, R. L., Saydjari, C., Amparo, E. G., and Eisenberg, H. M. (1990). Localization of auditory response sources using magnetoencephalography and magnetic resonance imaging. *Arch. Neurol.* **47,** 33–37.

Pechura, C. M., and Martin, J. B. (Eds.) (1991). "Mapping the Brain and Its Functions." Washington, D.C.: National Academy Press.

Pelizzari, C. A., Chen, G. T. Y., Spelbring, D. R., Weichselbaum, R. R., and Chen, C. T. (1989). Accurate three-dimensional registration of CT, PET, and/or MR images of the brain. *J. Comput. Assist. Tomogr.* **13,** 20–26.

Raichle, M. E., Martin, W. R. W., Herscovitch, P., Mintun, M. A., and Markham, J. (1983). Brain blood flow measured with intravenous $H_2^{15}O$. II. Implementation and validation. *J. Nucl. Med.* **24,** 790–798.

Reite, M., Teale, P., Zimmerman, J., David, K., and Whalen, J. (1988). Source location of a 50 msec latency auditory evoked field component. *Electroenceph. Clin. Neurophysiol.* **70,** 490–498.

Scherg, M., and Berg, P. (1990). "BESA—Brain Electric Source Analysis Handbook," Version 1.7. McLean, VA: Neuroscan.

Thatcher, R. W., Toro, C., Pflieger, M., and Hallett, M. (1994). Human neural network dynamics using multimodal registration of EEG, PET and MRI. *In* "Functional Neuroimaging: Technical Foundations" (R. W. Thatcher, M. Hallett, T. Zeffiro, E. R. John, and M. Huerta, Eds.). Orlando, FL: Academic Press.

Toro, C., Matsumoto, J., Deuschl, G., Roth, B., and Hallett, M. (1993). Source analysis of scalp-recorded movement-related electrical potentials. *Electroenceph. Clin. Neurophysiol.* **86,** 167–175.

Toro, C., Wang, B., Zeffiro, T. A., Thatcher, R. W., and Hallett, M. (1994). Movement related cortical potentials: Source analysis and PET/MRI correlation. *In* "Functional Neuroimaging: Technical Foundations" (R. W. Thatcher, M. Hallett, T. Zeffiro, E. R. John, and M. Huerta, Eds.). Orlando, FL: Academic Press.

Wang, B., Toro, C., Zeffiro, T. A., Nagamine, T., and Hallett, M. (1992). Method for mapping electrophysiological sources into brain images. *In* ''Science Innovation '92 Program,'' p. 89.

Wang, B., Toro, C., Zeffiro, T. A., and Hallett, M. (1994). Head surface digitization and registration: A method for mapping positions on the head onto magnetic resonance images. *Brain Topogr.*, in press.

Wassermann, E. M., McShane, L. M., Hallett, M., and Cohen, L. G. (1992a). Noninvasive mapping of muscle representations in human motor cortex. *Electroenceph. Clin. Neurophysiol.* **85,** 1–8.

Wassermann, E. M., Wang, B., Toro, C., Zeffiro, T. A., Valls-Solë, J., Pascual-Leone, A., and Hallett, M. (1992b). Projecting transcranial magnetic stimulation (TMS) maps into brain MRI. *Soc. Neurosci. Abstr.* **18,** 939.

Yamamoto, T., Williamson, S. J., Kaufman, L. Nicholson, C., and Llinas, R. (1988). Neuromagnetic localization of neuronal activity in the human brain. *Proc. Natl. Acad. Sci. USA* **85,** 8732–8736.

26

Movement-Related Cortical Potentials: Source Analysis and PET/MRI Correlation

Camilo Toro, Binseng Wang, Thomas Zeffiro, Robert W. Thatcher, and Mark Hallett

Human Motor Control Section, Medical Neurology Branch, National Institute of Neurological Disorders and Stroke; and Biomedical Engineering and Instrumentation Program, National Center for Research Resources, National Institutes of Health, Bethesda, Maryland 20892

I. Introduction

Understanding of the processes involved in the preparation, initiation, and completion of willful motor activity in humans has been the focus of intense neurophysiological research. The sequence of activation and the contribution of various cortical and subcortical structures to the initiation and execution of voluntary movements are important issues in human motor physiology. Knowledge of these mechanisms may provide insights into processes such as the pathophysiology of movement disorders, the recovery of function after brain injury, the acquisition of motor skills, and motor development in the immature brain. Much of our current understanding of these mechanisms has originated from single unit studies in primates and from studies of motor deficits as a result of local brain lesions in patients. More recently, with the development of positron emission tomography (PET) and the improvement of electrophysiological instrumentation and analysis techniques, it has become possible to study the intact human brain as it prepares and executes voluntary motor activity. Although PET activation related to voluntary motor activity provides an unambiguous spatial localization of brain areas involved in the execution of voluntary movements, these images are devoid of any temporal resolution. Electrophysiologic studies from scalp EEG and MEG recordings, on the other hand, provide a

high temporal resolution, but localization of their source generators is elusive. An ideal scenario would be one in which strengths from PET, MRI, and electrophysiological studies could be exploited in the generation of functional images with information in both the space and the time domains. The convergence of these independent pieces of functional and anatomical information would aid the understanding the dynamic network interaction that ultimately underlies the processes in effect during voluntary motor behavior.

In this chapter, we review the current understanding of motor cortex activation in the setting of voluntary movements from the perspective of movement-related cortical potentials (MRCPs) and regional cerebral blood flow (rCBF) activation measured by PET. We review a source analysis model of the MRCPs (Toro *et al.*, 1993) implemented in a three-layer spherical head model using the brain electrical source analysis (BESA) method (Scherg *et al.*, 1989), and we describe the use of multimodal registration techniques as a tool to test the physiological relevance of proposed source analysis models. Finally, we demonstrate the potential use of PET and MRI images in the development of physiologically valid constraints that simplify some of the ambiguities inherent to the solution of the "inverse problem" and contribute to the understanding of the fine temporal structure of cortical activation during voluntary movements.

II. Results

A. Cortical Activation during Voluntary Movements

1. Movement-Related Cortical Potentials (MRCPs)

a. Scalp Recordings Simple repetitive self-paced voluntary movements are accompanied by a series of well-defined and localized scalp electrical slow field potentials. These potentials are referred to as MRCPs (Kornhuber and Deecke, 1965; Vaughn *et al.*, 1968; Deecke *et al.*, 1976; Shibasaki *et al.*, 1980; Tarkka and Hallett, 1991). As local field potentials result from synchronous shifts in the membrane properties of neuronal aggregates sufficiently large to generate an equivalent dipole measurable at the scalp surface (Mitzhorf, 1991), the location strength and the orientation of the sources underlying the generation of the MRCPs are thought to reflect the magnitude, timing, and location of the cortical regions (dipole layers) active during the motor task.

The earliest component of the MRCPs is known as the Bereitschaftspotential (BP) (Kornhuber and Deecke, 1965; Deecke *et al.*, 1976; Shibasaki *et al.*, 1980). This component develops as early as 1.5 s prior to EMG onset, and it is felt to relate to an earlier aspect of motor intention and preparation (Kutas and Donchin, 1980; Libet *et al.*, 1982). The BP has a bilateral distribution over the central and midline regions. A sharper rise of the BP surface negativity at approximately 500 ms before EMG onset constitutes the onset of the negative slope (NS') component. This component becomes progressively more lateralized to the central regions and in particular over the contralateral hemisphere as movement onset approaches, reaching its peak amplitude at approximately 100 ms before EMG onset over the contralateral central and midline electrodes (Shibasaki *et al.*, 1980; Tarkka and Hallett, 1991). The motor potential (MP) is the best defined waveform component of the MRCPs. The MP begins some 30 ms before EMG onset and has two distinct peaks. The onset of the MP is associated with a very sharp focalization of the surface scalp negativity, which has been called the initial slope of the MP (isMP) (Tarkka and Hallett, 1991). The first peak of surface negativity is seen over the central and parietal areas at 30 to 40 ms after EMG onset. This peak is referred to as the parietal peak of the MP (ppMP) (Tarkka and Hallett, 1991). A later large amplitude peak with frontocentral negativity and parietal positivity takes place at about 100 ms after EMG onset. This component has been labeled the frontal peak of the MP (fpMP) (Tarkka and Hallett, 1991). Additional

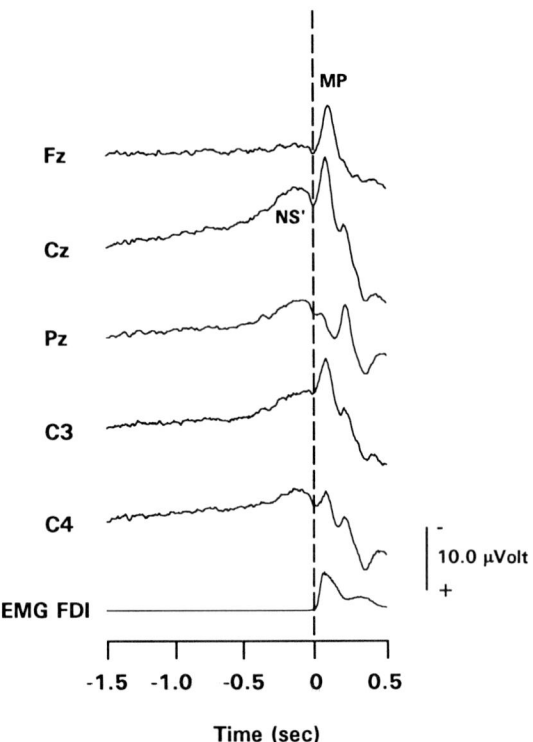

Figure 1 Waveform morphology of MRCPs elicited by self-paced index finger abduction movements in one normal volunteer. The negative slope (NS') and the motor potential (MP) components are indicated.

peaks follow the fpMP, those components that have been labeled under the general term of "reafferent response" and are likely to represent different aspects of sensory feedback and evaluation of motor performance.

b. Direct Cortical Recordings of MRCPs Direct cortical recordings of MRCPs in epileptic patients (Lee *et al.*, 1986; Neshige *et al.*, 1988; Toro *et al.*, 1989; Ikeda *et al.*, 1992) and nonhuman primates (Sasaki and Gemba, 1991; Johnson *et al.*, 1980) with implanted subdural electrodes suggest that both sensorimotor cortices undergo activation during the premovement period, with a bias for a much larger activation contralaterally as movement onset approaches. A large somatotopically organized contribution of the contralateral sensorimotor cortex develops at the time of the MP. Despite the fact that an important role of SMA in the genesis of scalp-recorded MRCPs and MREFs has been suggested (Deecke and Kornhuber, 1978; Lang *et al.*, 1991), direct cortical recordings in humans (Ikeda *et al.*, 1992; Allison *et al.*, 1991) and primates

(Sasaki and Gemba, 1991) show only a modest amplitude cortical potential over the SMA during the premotor period in comparison with the activation in the contralateral primary sensorimotor cortex.

c. MEG Recordings and Their Relation to MRCPs

Self-paced voluntary movements in humans are also associated with the development of discrete magnetic fields, which are referred to as movement-related magnetic fields (MRMF). These magnetic fields have been divided into a series of waveform components (Kristeva *et al.*, 1991). The readiness field (RF) corresponds to the slowly increasing magnetic field strength preceding the movement onset. This component peaks at about 100 ms before movement onset and is known as the motor field (MF). A peak that occurs following movement onset and that has a current flow direction opposite that of the MF has been labeled the movement-evoked field I (MEFI). Additional magnetic peaks in the postmovement period have been labeled movement-evoked field II (MEFII) and movement-evoked field III (MEFIII). Although MEG recordings capture only the cortical sources oriented tangentially to the scalp surface, similarities in the timing and topography of the generators for MRMFs and MRCPs can be drawn, especially the timing of the peak activity of the MF and the peak of NS' (pNS') and the timing of the MEFI and the fpMP, respectively. Cheyne *et*

al. (1989) and Kristeva *et al.* (1991) reported on the satisfactory modeling of this magnetic activity at about the time of the MF with two homologous sources located in the vicinity of the hand sensorimotor regions. The MEFI, which can be considered the magnetic counterpart to the fpMP, was also well modeled by a single generator in the contralateral sensorimotor cortex. MEG studies, however, have not shown clear evidence of SMA participation in the magnetic responses to self-paced voluntary movements (Cheyne *et al.*, 1989; Kristeva *et al.*, 1991). An explanation given for the lack of SMA activation on MEG recordings is the presence of bilateral SMA generators with exactly opposite orientation, resulting in field cancellation (Kristeva *et al.*, 1991). Superimposition of the location of MRMF sources in response to foot, tongue, and finger movements onto activated PET images and MRI indicates a close intermodal concordance in the localization of the activated brain regions (Walter *et al.*, 1992).

2. rCBF Changes during Voluntary Motor Activity

PET imaging is based on the assumption of functional coupling of neuronal activity, energy metabolism, and regional cerebral blood flow (rCBF) (Yorowsky *et al.*, 1981; Herscovitch *et al.*, 1993). rCBF measurements with PET during voluntary repetitive hand movements have shown activation of the contra-

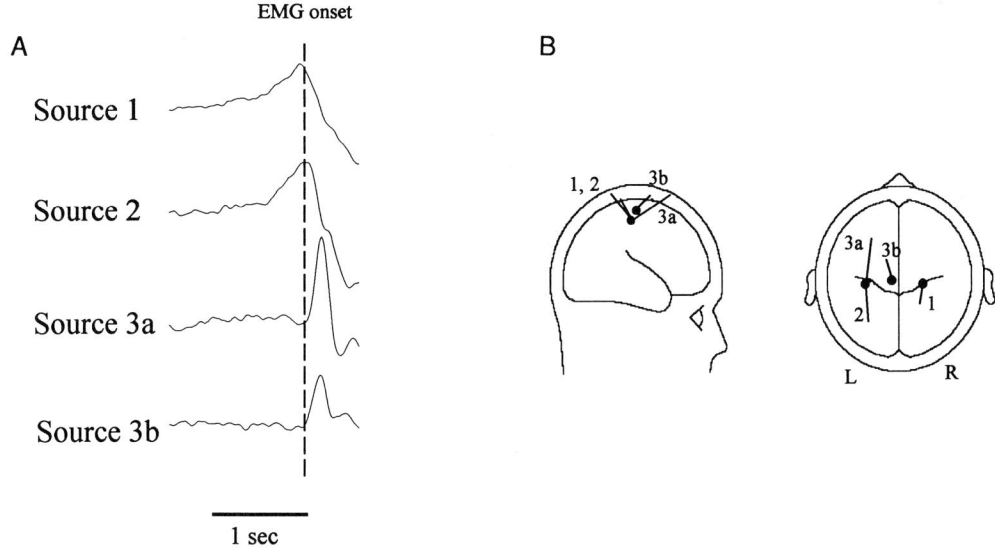

Figure 2 Source analysis model of the MRCPs calculated on the grand-averaged MRCP waveforms from 10 normal individuals. (A) Time history of the relative output of each one of the proposed sources. (B) The solution at the pNS' is calculated with two sources (sources 1 and 2), located on each side of the sphere. The solution at the fpMP is also calculated with two sources: source 3a, located in the same vicinity as source 2, and source 3b, free of any location or orientation constraints. These four sources account for over 92% (SD, 1.81) of the signal in the period from 200 ms before movement onset to 200 ms after movement onset. For further details on the model, see Toro *et al.* (1993).

lateral and ipsilateral sensorimotor regions, premotor cortex, and SMA (Roland *et al.*, 1985; Fox and Applegate, 1989; Colebatch *et al.*, 1991). Variation in the task demands, including cognitive aspects and other technical factors, may account for the qualitative and quantitative differences in these studies. Homuncular organization of the primary sensorimotor cortex in humans has been demonstrated using simple repetitive movements (Colebatch *et al.*, 1991; Grafton *et al.*, 1991), indicating that this technique can be used as a reliable noninvasive method for identification of the various motor cortical regions.

B. Source Analysis Model of the MRCPs

Based on the evidence collected from MRCPs recorded from subdural and scalp electrodes in human and nonhuman primates, as well as results from activated PET studies during voluntary movements, we have proposed a source model of the MRCPs (Toro *et al.*, 1993). In this model, the activity at the instant of the pNS' was modeled with two homologous sources (sources 1 and 2) over each side of the spherical head, which were assumed to represent the activation of both central regions during the premovement period. The imposition of the constraint to remain in homologous areas of each hemisphere was justified by evidence from PET (Roland, 1985; Fox and Applegate, 1989; Grafton *et al.*, 1991; Colebatch, 1991) and electrophysiological studies indicating bilateral activation of the precentral regions during voluntary movements (Neshige *et al.*, 1988; Sasaki and Gemba, 1991). The fpMP was also modeled with two sources (sources 3a and 3b). Source 3a was constrained in location to remain in the same vicinity as the location of the contralateral source derived at the pNS' (source 2) but free of orientation constraints. Source 3b was free of any orientation or location constraints. The constraints for source 3a were physiologically justified by the fact that subdural recording over the central regions have shown that sites displaying the maximum amplitude NS' are the same as those with the largest amplitude MP (Neshige *et al.*, 1988). The addition of source 3b with no added constraints to the model was introduced with the assumption that it would improve the solution by representing the source activity generated by other areas distant from the location of source 3a, in particular activity originating from the ipsilateral hemisphere or the midline structures (Ikeda *et al.*, 1992). This strategy offered a satisfactory solution for both the instant of the pNS' and that of the fpMP as well as the entire time window from −200 ms before to 200 ms after movement onset in a group of 10 normal volunteers. Projection of the averaged coordinates of sources 1, 2, and 3a obtained

in these 10 subjects to a Talairach atlas (Talairach and Tournoux, 1988) indicated a location about 2.0 cm anterior to the central sulcus.

C. Use of Multimodal Registration Techniques and Validation of Source Analysis Models

Due to the functional coupling between neuronal activity and rCBF, the cortical areas showing increases in rCBF in response to simple self-paced movements are likely to overlap spatially with those cortical areas giving rise to the dipoles of the MRCPs elicited in a similar motor paradigm. We exploited this situation in order to test other assumptions made in the formulation of the MRCPs dipole model. With the use of multimodal registration techniques, we projected the location of the MRCPs source generators calculated in a spherical three-layer head model into each subject's activated H_2O^{15} PET (Toro *et al.*, manuscript in preparation), which had been properly registered into corresponding MR images. A detailed three-dimensional characterization of the scalp surface allowed the definition of the best-fitted sphere to each subject's real head shape. The location of the recording electrodes with respect to the center of this sphere were used in the calculation of the source location in the spherical head model. A surface registration between the digitized scalp surface and the skull surface obtained from MRI images permitted the rotations and coordinate transformations necessary to project the source locations in the spherical head onto MRI images with the overlaid activated PET (Wang *et al.*, 1994a, 1994b). Because the sources in our model are always positioned in relatively close proximity to the vertex, which is the portion of the skull that best approximates a sphere, the theoretical foundations for source modeling using a three-shell spherical model are generally valid (Fender, 1991; Nunez, 1981; Van Oosterom, 1991). The localization accuracy of spherical head models for sources close to the vertex is as satisfactory as that of models based in real head shapes (Roth *et al.*, 1993).

Once PET, MRI, and electrophysiological data are in registration, the dipole sources can be projected into the PET and MR images and the relation in space among the source location, anatomical landmarks, and areas of rCBF activation can be estimated.

In this pilot study, four subjects underwent H_2O^{15} PET scanning during conditions of rest and self-paced movements. The MRCPs were also recorded during a similar motor paradigm. The source locations were derived with the same model strategy previously defined (Toro *et al.*, 1993). The PET scans after proper registration with high-resolution MRI images showed

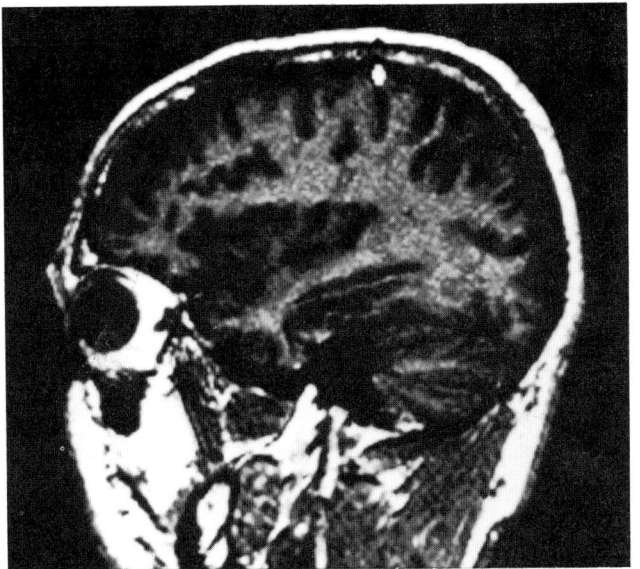

Figure 3 Multimodal saggital image across the left hemisphere. The rCBF PET image registered with the corresponding saggital MRI slice was obtained after averaging of three images obtained during the execution of self-paced right index finger movements after the injection of H_2O^{15} and subtraction from averaged rest scans. The location of sources 2 and 3a in the spherical head model in the same subject executing the same task have been projected into the PET and MRI images (open square) after the appropriate coordinate transformations and rotations. See Wang *et al.* (1994a, 1994b) for further details of the technique.

discrete increases in rCBF over the precentral and to a lesser extent the postcentral gyrus. The activation was bilateral but much more well defined over the contralateral hemisphere. Activation of the medial cortical regions (SMA and cingulate gyrus) was prominent in only one of the subjects (Thatcher *et al.*, 1994). The location of the contralateral sources (sources 2 and 3a) in the MRCPs model fell in close proximity (4.0 to 20.0 mm) to the location of the peak rCBF activation over the hand sensorimotor cortex in PET in favor of the physiological validity of our source analysis model. Estimation of the relation of the ipsilateral source (source 1) and midline source (source 3b) were more difficult to establish as the PET activation in these areas was weaker and variable across subjects.

D. Use of PET and MRI Information in the Development of Physiologic and Anatomic Constraints in Source Analysis Models

The use of PET imaging and its registration with electrophysiologic data represent a powerful tool for the validation of the physiological relevance of the proposed source analysis model. This method, in theory, can be applied to any form of evoked potential data elicited under a variety of motor, sensory,

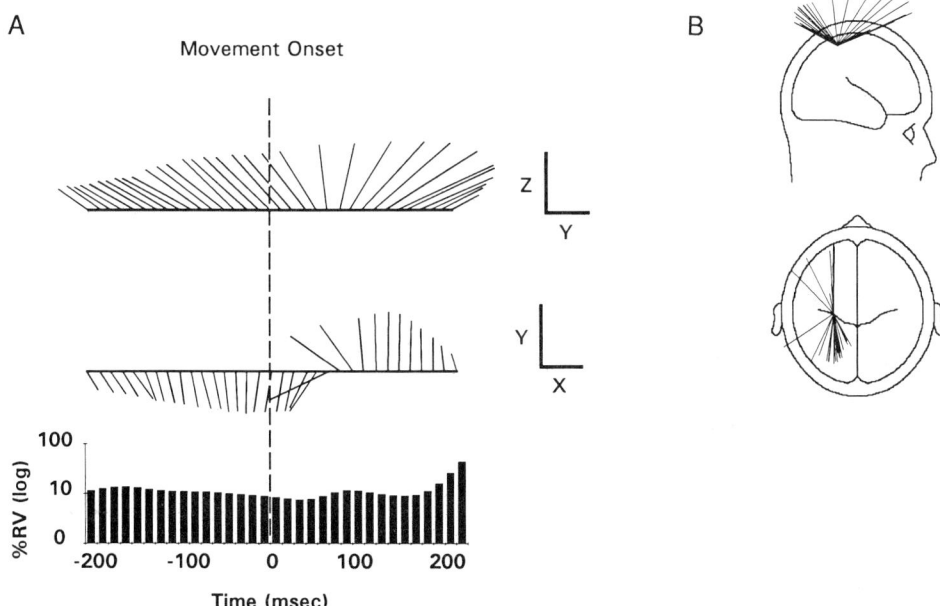

Figure 4 (A) Time history in two different planes for source orientation, strength, and residual variance, using a single dipole model of the MRCPs during the time period of 200 ms before to 200 ms after EMG onset computed at 12-ms time intervals. The source location has been constrained to a region corresponding to the location of the central sulcus as defined from PET and MRI images. (B) Same as in A but orientation and strengths of the instantaneous solutions have been projected over the constrained source locations within the spherical head model.

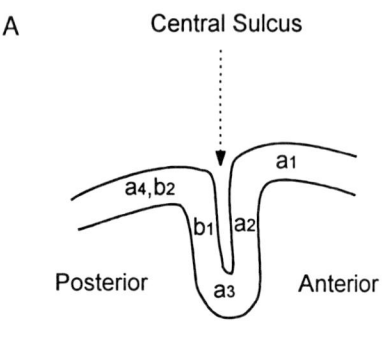

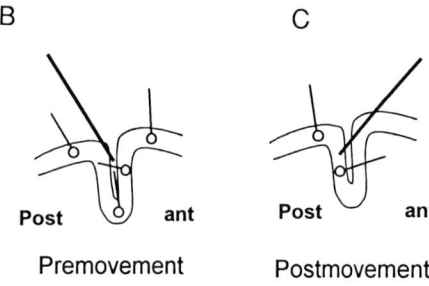

Figure 5 (A) Schematic diagram of the cortical mantle regions in the vicinity of the contralateral central sulcus, showing activation in PET (a1, crest of the precentral gyrus; a2, anterior bank of the central sulcus; a3, floor of the central sulcus; a4, crest of the postcentral gyrus; b1, posterior bank of the central sulcus; b2, crest of the postcentral gyrus). (B) Diagram of the suggested relative orientation of the resulting dipoles from the activated cortical areas (thin lines) during the premovement period and the resulting source orientations from the vectorial sum of the output of these regions (thick line). (C) Similar to B but during the postmovement period.

and cognitive tasks. This approach, however, is aimed at validating the localization accuracy of a given model but does not permit making any direct inferences on the timing of activation of the cortical structures revealed by PET. Independent knowledge of the general source localization gives the solid foundations to exploit further the high temporal resolution strengths inherent in electrophysiologic recordings (Scherg and Berg, 1991; Thatcher *et al.*, 1994). Activated PET images can guide the implementation of simpler source analysis models in which both the location and orientation of a single generator or multiple-source generators could be constrained by the location and three-dimensional orientation of the activated cortical mantle as revealed by activated PET and MR images. The formulation of these unambiguous and physiologically valid constraints permits the study of the relative contribution of defined cortical regions to the scalp electrical fields with a high degree of temporal accuracy.

Following this rationale we have conducted some

initial simulations on the MRCP sources using PET and MRI results to guide the formulation of location constraints. A single dipole solution was investigated using only the source in the contralateral sensorimotor area. After determining the three-dimensional localization of the contralateral central sulcus, a set of coordinate rotations and transformations permitted the projection of this position back into the spherical head model. Using this single dipole model, we have explored the instantaneous dipole orientation and strength solutions at closely spaced time intervals during the period from 200 ms before to 200 ms after EMG onset. The results of these simulations are repre-

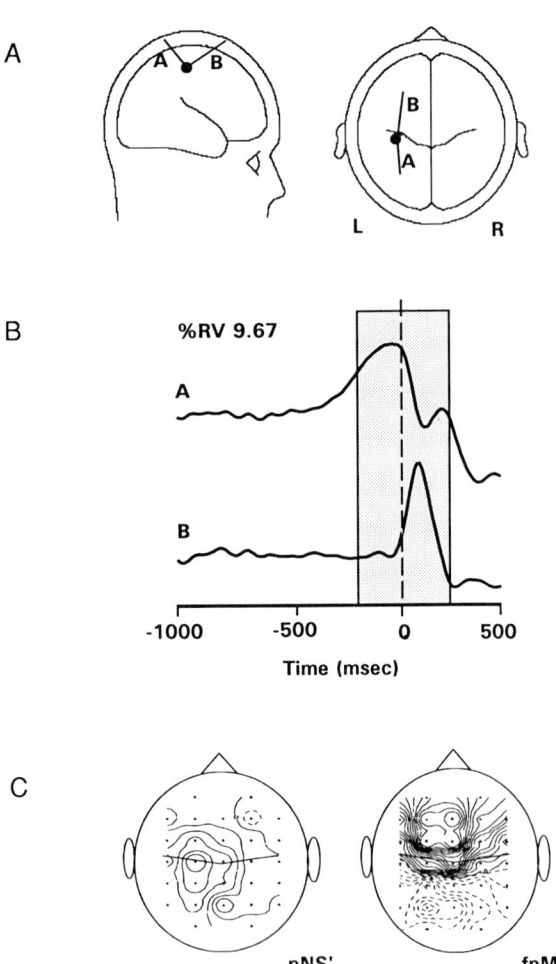

Figure 6 (A) Diagram of the location and orientation in space of the sources in the contralateral central region active in proximity to movement onset. (B) Time history of the activity of these two sources during the period of −200 to 200 ms (dotted area). Source A is active mostly during the premovement period, and the timing of its peak activity corresponds to the latency of the pNS'. Source B is active during the postmovement period, and its peak output corresponds to the timing of the fpMP. (C) The timing and orientation features of the dipole model agree with observed topographic features of the pNS and fpMP components of the MRCPs.

sented in Fig. 4. The dipole analysis revealed a source of fairly constant strength during the 200-ms period before movement with an orientation that can be proposed to result from the contribution of the dipole layers in the crown of the pre- and postcentral gyrus and the anterior bank and floor of the central sulcus as diagramed in Fig. 5. Vectorial summation of these would likely result in an equivalent source of predominantly radial and slightly posterior orientation. Following movement onset, the dipole solution undergoes a reorganization in its orientation, after which the source achieves a new orientation that can be proposed to result predominantly from the activity of tangential oriented sources presumably in the posterior bank of the central sulcus. These data are in favor of our dipole model interpretation for sources 2 and 3a by providing evidence of two distinct events in the contralateral central sulcus during the time period close to EMG initiation, as summarized in Fig. 6. This single dipole solution explains close to 90% of the residual variance of the MRCPs during this 400-ms interval centered at movement onset.

A similar simulation with no location constraints results in a slightly better fit (residual variance of approximately 5–8%), but the source location is quite unstable and often nonphysiological (such as locating the source outside of the skull) as shown in Fig. 7. The instability in source location is likely to result from the simultaneous activity of multiple sources at

defined time instants as proposed in our model of the MRCPs (Toro *et al.*, 1993) and from the overall sensitivity of the source analysis model to background signal noise.

III. Conclusions

Source modeling of the MRCPs and MRMF in response to simple self-paced finger movements suggests that contralateral and to a lesser extent ipsilateral and midline cortical activation of the sensorimotor cortex constitute the source generators of the MRCPs. The overall localization strategy of the MRCP source model has been validated with the use of activated rCBF PET images obtained in response to a similar motor paradigm. The localization congruency of these two independent methods suggest that activated PET images registered into high-resolution MRI can be used for the design of anatomically valid location and orientation constraints to be used in dipole source solutions of electrophysiologic recordings. Extension of this preliminary work includes the use of multiple sources constrained in location to the active cortical areas on activated PET scans. Orientation constraints guided by detailed three-dimensional analysis of the geometry of the activated cortical mantle can be implemented as further refinement to the models. This approach removes localization ambiguities inherent to

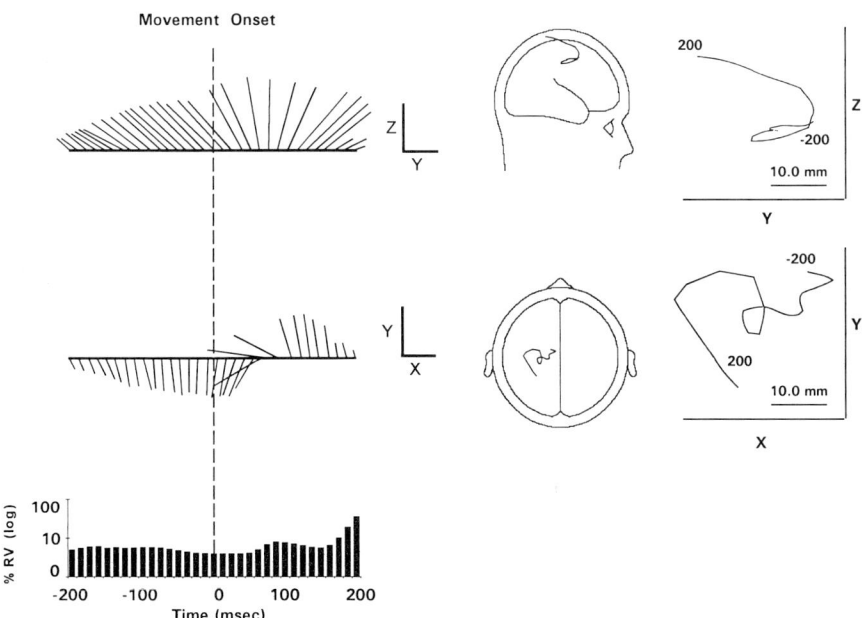

Figure 7 Simulation of the instantaneous source location, orientation, strength, and residual variance, using a single dipole model of the MRCPs in the interval of 200 ms before to 200 ms after EMG onset calculated at 12-ms time intervals. The source location, as opposed to the example in Fig. 4, has not been constrained to the central sulcus. Note that the source location is quite unstable and often nonphysiologically placed outside the skull.

the "inverse problem" and shifts the emphasis of the dipole modeling more toward the understanding of the fine temporal dynamics of cortical activation.

References

Allison, T., McCarthy, G., Jasiorkowski, J., Roessler, E., and Spencer, D. (1991a). "Functional Localization of Structures in the Mesial Wall of the Human Cortex." Presented at the annual meeting of the American Electroencephalographic Society, Philadelphia, Pa.

Cheyne, D., and Weinberg, H. (1989). Neuromagnetic fields accompanying unilateral finger movements: Pre-movement and movement-evoked fields. *Exp. Brain Res.* **78,** 604–612.

Colebatch, J. G., Deiber, M. P., Passingham, R. E., Friston, K. J., and Frackowiak, S. J. (1991). Regional cerebral blood flow during voluntary arm and hand movements in humans. *J. Neurophysiol.* **65,** 1392–1401.

Deecke, L., Grozinger, B., and Kornhuber, H. H. (1976). Voluntary finger movements in man: Cerebral potentials and theory. *Biol. Cybernetics* **23,** 99–119.

Deecke L., and Kornhuber, H. H. (1978). An electrical signal of participation of the "supplementary" motor cortex in human voluntary finger movement. *Brain Res.* **159,** 473–476.

Fender, D. H. (1991). Models of the human brain and the surrounding media: Their influence on the reliability of source localization. *J. Clin. Neurophysiol.* **8,** 381–390.

Fox, P. T., and Applegate, C. N. (1989). Simple hierarchy of motor regions in cerebral cortex suggested by positron emission tomography. *In* "XXXI International Congress of Physiological Sciences, Helsinki, Finland," Addendum 3. [Abstr.]

Grafton, S. T., Woods, R. P., Mazziota, J. C., and Phelps, M. E. (1991). Somatotopic mapping of the primary motor cortex in humans: Activation studies with cerebral blood flow and positron emission tomography. *J. Neurophysiol.* **66,** 735–743.

Herscovitch, P. (1994). Radiotracer techniques for functional neuroimaging with positron emission tomography. *In* "Functional Neuroimaging: Technical Foundations" (R. W. Thatcher, M. Hallett, T. Zeffiro, E. R. John, and M. Huerta, Eds.). Orlando, FL: Academic Press.

Ikeda, A., Liiders, H. O., Burges, R. C., and Shibasaki, H. (1992). Movement-related potentials recorded from supplementary motor area and primary area. *Brain* **115,** 1017–1043.

Johnson, R., Jr. (1980). Event related potentials accompanying voluntary movements in the rhesus monkey. *Prog. Brain Res.* **54,** 70–76.

Kornhuber, H. H., and Deecke, L. (1965). Hirnpotentialänderungen bei Willkürbewegungen und passiven Bewegungen des Menschen: Bereitschaftspotential und reafferente Potentiale. *Pflügers Arch.* **284,** 1–17.

Kristeva, R., Cheyne, D., and Deecke, L. (1991). Neuromagnetic fields accompanying unilateral and bilateral voluntary movements: Topography and source analysis. *Electroenceph. Clin. Neurophysiol.* **81,** 284–298.

Kutas, M., and Donchin, E. (1980). Preparation to respond as manifested by movement-related brain potentials. *Brain Res.* **202,** 95–115.

Lee, B. I., Liiders, H., Lesser, R. P., Dinner, D. S., and Morris, H. H. (1986). Cortical potentials related to voluntary and passive finger movements recorded from subdural electrodes in humans. *Ann. Neurol.* **20,** 32–37.

Lang, W., Cheyne, D., Kristeva, R., Lindinger, G., and Deecke, L. (1991). Functional localization of motor processes in the human cortex. *In* "Event-Related Brain Research" (C. H. M. Brunia, G. Mulder, and M. N. Verbaten, Eds.), EEG Suppl. 42, pp. 97–115. Amsterdam: Elsevier.

Libet, B., Wright, E. W., Jr., and Gleason, C. A. (1982). Readiness potentials preceding unrestricted "spontaneous" vs. planned voluntary acts. *Electroenceph. Clin. Neurophysiol.* **52,** 322–335.

Mitzdorf, U. (1991). Physiological sources of evoked potentials. *In* "Event-Related Brain Research" (C. H. M. Brunia, G. Mulder, and M. N. Verbaten, Eds.), EEG Suppl. 42, pp. 47–57. Amsterdam: Elsevier.

Neshige, R., Lüders, H., and Shibasaki, H. (1988). Recording of the movement-related potentials from scalp and cortex in man. *Brain* **111,** 719–736.

Nunez, P. (1981). "Electric Fields of the Brain." Oxford: Oxford University Press.

Raichle, M. E. (1987). Circulatory and metabolic correlates of brain function in normal humans. *In* "The Handbook of Physiology," Vol. 5, "The Nervous System," Part 2, "Higher Functions of the Brain" (V. B. Mountcastle, F. Plum, and S. R. Giger, Eds.), pp. 643–674. The American Physiology Society.

Roland, P. E. (1985). Cortical organization of voluntary behavior in man. *Hum. Neurobiol.* **4,** 155–167.

Roth, B., Balish, M., Gorbach, A., and Sato, S. (1993). How well does a three-sphere model predict positions of dipoles in a realistically shaped head? *Electroenceph. Clin. Neurophysiol.* **87,** 175–184.

Sasaki, K., and Gemba, H. (1991). Cortical potentials associated with voluntary movements in monkeys. *In* "Event-Related Brain Research" (C. H. M. Brunia, G. Mulder, and M. N. Verbaten, Eds.), EEG Suppl. 42, pp. 80–96. Amsterdam: Elsevier.

Scherg, M., Vajsar, J. J., and Picton, T. W. (1989). A source analysis of the human auditory evoked potentials. *J. Cog. Neurosci.* **1,** 336–355.

Scherg, M., and Berg, P. (1991). Use of prior knowledge in brain electromagnetic source analysis. *Brain Topogr.* **4,** 143–150.

Shibasaki, H., Barrett, G., Halliday, E., and Halliday, A. M. (1980). Components of the movement-related cortical potentials and their scalp topography. *Electroenceph. Clin. Neurophysiol.* **49,** 213–226.

Talairach, J., and Tournoux, P. (1988). "Coplannar Stereotaxic Atlas of the Human Brain." Stuttgart: Thieme.

Tarkka, I. M., and Hallett, M. (1991). Topography of the scalp recorded motor potentials in human finger movements. *J. Clin. Neurophysiol.* **8,** 331–341.

Thatcher, R. W., Toro, C., Pflieger, M., and Hallett, M. (1993). Human neural network dynamics using multimodal registration of EEG, PET and MRI. *In* "Functional Neuroimaging: Technical Foundations" (R. W. Thatcher, M. Hallett, T. Zeffiro, E. R. John, and M. Huerta, Eds.). Orlando, FL: Academic Press.

Toro, C., Cruz, R., and Gates, R. (1989). Cortical movement related potentials associated with simple hand and face movements. *Neurology* **39,** 414. [Abstr.]

Toro, C., Matsumoto, J., Deuschl, G., Roth, B., and Hallett, M. (1993). Source analysis of the scalp-recorded movement-related cortical potentials. *Electroenceph. Clin. Neurophysiol.* **86,** 167–175.

Toro, C., Wang, B., Zeffiro, T., Thatcher, R., and Hallett, M. (1993). Cortical activation accompanying self-paced movements: Integration of equivalent dipole sources with MR and PET images. Manuscript in preparation.

Van Oosterom, A. (1991). History and evolution of methods for solving the inverse problem. *J. Clin. Neurophysiol.* **8,** 371–380.

Vaughn, H. G., Costa, L. D., and Ritter, W. (1968). Topography of the human motor potential. *Electroenceph. Clin. Neurophysiol.* **25,** 1–10.

Walter, H., Kristeva, R., Knorr, U., Schlaug, G., Huang, Y., Steinmetz, H., Nebeling, B., Herzog, H., and Seitz, R. (1992). Individual somatotopy of primary somatosensory cortex revealed by intermodal matching of MEG, PET and MRI. *Brain Topogr.* **5,** 183–187.

Wang, B., Toro, C., Zeffiro, T., and Hallett, M. (1994a). Head surface registration: A method for mapping positions on the head onto magnetic resonance images. *Brain Topogr.,* in press.

Wang, B., Toro, C., Wassermann, E. M., Zeffiro, T. A., Thatcher, R. W., and Hallett, M. (1994b). Multimodal integration of electrophysiological data and brain images: EEG, MEG, TMS, MRI and PET. *In* "Functional Neuroimaging: Technical Foundations" (R. W. Thatcher, M. Hallett, T. Zeffiro, E. R. John, and M. Huerta, Eds.), Orlando, FL: Academic Press.

Yarowsky, P. J., and Ingvar, D. H. (1980). Neuronal activity and energy metabolism. *Fed. Proc.* **40,** 2353–2362.

27

Human Neural Network Dynamics Using Multimodal Registration of EEG, PET, and MRI

Robert W. Thatcher, *,† Camilo Toro,* Mark E. Pflieger,‡ and Mark Hallett*

*Medical Neurology Branch, Clinical Neuroscience Program, National Institutes of Neurological Disorders and Stroke, National Institutes of Health, Bethesda, Maryland 20892; and ‡Neuroscan, Inc., El Paso, Texas 79902

I. Introduction

Recent studies report zero phase locking of coherent multiunit activity during perceptual and motor tasks (Gray et al., 1989; Eckhorn et al., 1988; Murthy and Fetz, 1992). These studies and others (Atiya and Baldi, 1989; John, 1963; Thatcher and John, 1977) have hypothesized that the temporal characteristics of pools of oscillating neurons are used to encode information and to label various features of an object by phase-locked and coherent activity of the corresponding feature extracting neurons. Specifically, phase locking serves to link associated features in different neural systems to form a coherency of spatially organized phase and frequency relationships within and between neural networks (Grossberg, 1976; Grossberg and Somers, 1991; von der Malsburg and Schneider, 1986; Baldi and Meir, 1990).

Similar properties of phase locking and coherency between distributed neural networks have been reported by Gevins and colleagues in visual–spatial tasks using scalp-recorded EEG and evoked potential analyses in humans (Gevins et al., 1989a, 1989b; Gevins and Bressler, 1988). Phase locking and coherency between scalp-recorded EEG was also recently observed in a human voluntary motor movement task using measures of instantaneous EEG coher-

ence and phase (Thatcher et al., 1993a, 1993b). The latter study showed rapid increases and decreases in the magnitude of EEG coherence during different stages of motor movement. One of the important hypotheses that emerged from these studies is that phase locking and coherency may represent necessary and critical properties that are generalizable between multiunit animal studies and noninvasive human EEG studies. However, before this hypothesis can be properly tested, improved spatial and temporal resolution of human scalp-derived electrophysiological measurements is necessary.

The purpose of the present paper is to present, for the first time, a method to improve the spatial and temporal resolution of human neural network dynamics using multimodal registration of PET, MRI, and EEG. The crux of the method is the computation of "instantaneous dipole coherence" to measure the dynamics of neural network coupling that precedes and follows a motor movement. Our approach is made up of three steps: (1) anatomically register MRI-referenced electrophysiological dipoles obtained during a movement task to MRI-referenced PET activation obtained during the performance of the same task (Toro et al., 1994; Wang et al., 1994); (2) analytically compute an EEG-derived time series for each of the MRI- and PET-validated dipoles using a pseudoinverse method (Penrose, 1955; Ben-Israel and Greville, 1974; Mosher et al., 1992); and (3) compute instantaneous EEG coherence and phase from the derived

† Present address: Veterans Affairs Medical Center, Neurology Service, Bay Pines, Florida 33504.

FUNCTIONAL NEUROIMAGING

time series in order to study the time history of the MRI- and PET-registered dipoles (Thatcher *et al.*, 1986). A specific goal of this approach is to exploit the advantages of multimodal registration of independent modalities. For example, multimodal registration of PET, MRI, and EEG allows for the anatomical localization of functional measures and, specifically, the physiological validation of dipole source activation. This conclusion is based on the assumption that the superimposition of independently derived dipole sources onto regions of PET activation is strong evidence in support of the physiological validity of the dipole sources (Toro *et al.*, 1994; Wang *et al.*, 1994). Once the anatomical locations of dipole sources are independently validated, one can apply analytical solutions to the inverse dipole source problem (Scherg, 1992; Wang *et al.*, 1992, 1993). This is a significant advantage because, without *a priori* knowledge of the location of the dipole sources, numerical analyses in which the risk of becoming trapped in local minima will always be present. Further, without *a priori* knowledge, the inverse solution of the dipole source is indeterminate; i.e., many different source locations can give rise to identical voltage distributions on the scalp (Scherg and Berg, 1991). Finally, it is hoped that this technique may yield subcentimeter spatial resolution as well as subsecond temporal resolution of the neural network switching that occurs before and after self-paced voluntary movement.

II. Materials and Methods

A. Subjects

A healthy right-handed 30-year-old male volunteer participated in the study.[1] The PET, MRI, and EEG protocol was approved by the clinical research subpanel of the National Institute of Neurological Disorders and Stroke, and the subject gave his written informed consent to participate in the study.

B. Finger Movement Paradigm

The subject was comfortably seated in a recliner chair with his arms resting on the arm rests of the chair while he performed self-paced right hand index

---

[1] A total of four subjects in which MRI, PET, and EEG were co-registered have been studied. Because of space limitations the results of only one subject are presented in this chapter. It should be noted that the one subject is unique in the strength or magnitude of the SMA dipole. However, the temporal dynamics of dipole coherence (i.e., the latency of dipole switch onset and offset and slope values) were consistent and similar across the four subjects (Thatcher *et al.*, 1993b).

finger abductions at a rate of approximately one abduction every 4 to 5 s. The subject was asked to keep his eyes open during the task and to fixate his gaze on a target 3 m away. A total of 240 movement trials were divided into blocks of 30 movements each. A 2- to 5-min rest period occurred between each block of movements. For purposes of this study, only the first 134 trials were analyzed.

C. EEG Recording Techniques

EEG data were recorded using 29 gold-plated electrodes applied to the scalp with collodion. The electrodes were applied to the scalp at the conventional 10–20 locations in addition to intermediate positions. Two extra channels were used to monitor EOG, and one extra bipolar channel was used to monitor EMG. The 29 scalp and 2 EOG recordings were made against a linked-ears reference. Interelectrode impedances were kept below 5 kΩ. The data were filtered using a bandpass of 0.1 to 30 Hz and digitally sampled at a rate of 100 Hz with 12-bit analog-to-digital resolution. The EMG activity from the right first dorsal interosseous (FDI) muscle was filtered with a bandpass of 100 to 1000 Hz, full wave rectified, and fed into a Schmidt trigger set to fire at EMG burst onset (Barrett *et al.*, 1985). The EEG data were collected from 3.0 s before EMG onset to 1 s after EMG onset.

D. Dipole Source Analyses

Dipole locations were computed using the Brain Electric Source Analysis (BESA) program (Sherg and Berg, 1991) and by adjusting the spherical coordinates based on the sphere that best fit the subject's scalp (Wang *et al.*, 1993). The coordinates of the best fit dipoles were computed for a three-shell head model of 85 mm radius. Values for scalp thickness and skull thickness were assumed to be 7 and 8 mm, respectively. The cortical surface was approximated at 70 mm and the dura, at 72 mm eccentricity. The dipole moments were computed from the averaged cortical motor movement potentials in the interval of -212 to $+200$ ms (at which movement onset is defined at $t = 0$). Three equivalent dipole sources accounted for 95.96% of the variance of the averaged motor movement potentials. Two of the equivalent dipole sources were constrained to be bilaterally located over the motor cortical region corresponding to the hand region, and the third equivalent dipole source was unconstrained and located medially and deeper, corresponding to the supplemental motor area (SMA). The two bilateral motor cortex equivalent dipoles were derived at a latency corresponding to the peaks of the premovement MRCPs (i.e., pNS'), and the third, supplemental motor area (SMA) dipole was derived from the peak of the frontal postmovement potential (i.e., fpMp) (Toro *et al.*, 1993). The dipoles were labeled as dipole 1 for the ipsilateral motor cortex dipole, dipole 2 for the contralateral motor cortex dipole, and dipole 3 for the contralateral supplemental motor area, or SMA dipole. Details of the source analysis are given in TORO *et al.* (1993, 1994).

E. Multimodal Registration Procedures

The subject's head surface was used as a common framework to integrate the three types of data (i.e., EEG, MRI, and PET). The multimodal registration procedure was a four-step process. First, the scalp surface and the location of each of the 29 electrodes were determined with a three-dimensional magnetic digitizer. Second, the digitized head surface was registered with the head contour obtained from the same subject's MRI. Third, the three equivalent dipole sources determined by the BESA program were mapped into the MRI coordinate system defined by the registered MRI and digitized head. Fourth, positron emission tomography (PET) images obtained from the same subject undergoing the same motor movements were then superimposed on mapped MRIs by registering the brain contours obtained from both the MRI and the PET [see Wang *et al.* (1993) for further details].

F. Analytical Dipole Time Series Derivation

As described previously, the locations and orientations for three equivalent dipoles were obtained using the BESA spatiotemporal fitting procedure (Sherg and Berg, 1991) with respect to the movement-locked average EEG potentials. Keeping these locations and orientations fixed, time series of each dipole were analytically derived with respect to raw EEG movement-related epochs using a pseudoinverse procedure (Mosher *et al.*, 1990; Penrose, 1955).

For each time sample, the analytical pseudoinverse procedure computes the fixed-orientation dipole moments that minimize the sum (across electrodes) of squared differences between (a) the potential actually measured at an electrode and (b) the sum of theoretical dipole potentials computed for that electrode. The theoretical potential for a single dipole equals the fixed-orientation moment times a volume conduction weight, which is defined as the potential at an electrode produced by a unit dipole moment. For M dipoles and N scalp electrodes, an M-by-N matrix, W, represents all of the volume conduction weights. That

is, W_{ij} represents the theoretical attenuation of unit dipole i as observed at scalp location j for a three-shell spherical head model (Ary *et al.*, 1981). An M-by-M symmetric matrix, V, can be formed from the volume conduction weights matrix W by forming the sum of cross-products across electrodes:

$$V_{ij} = \sum_{k}^{N} W_{ik}W_{jk}.$$

For each N-dimensional time sample, z, of measured potentials across scalp electrodes, an M-dimensional weighted vector, y, can be formed such that

$$y_i = \sum_{k}^{N} W_{ik}z_k.$$

Then the M-dimensional dipole moment time series vector x is computed from the matrix equation $x = V^{-1}y$.

In actual practice, the measured scalp potentials are referenced in some fashion, whereas the theoretically computed dipole potentials are absolute values (i.e., referenced to infinity). To take this into account, it is necessary only to reference each volume conduction weight in the same way that the measured potentials are referenced. For our case of a linked A1–A2 reference, the average of the A1 and A2 volume conduction weights was subtracted from the other volume conduction weights for each dipole. This referenced weights matrix played the role of W in the above computations.

G. Instantaneous Dipole Coherence and Phase

The method of complex demodulation was used to compute instantaneous (or event-related) EEG coherence and phase for each pairing of the three derived dipole time series described above. Complex demodulation, which is characterized by a center frequency, f, and a half-bandwidth, b, produces a complex time series from a real time series, $z(t)$, in two stages (Otnes and Enochson, 1978). The first stage consists of shifting the center frequency down to zero, which results in a complex time series. The real part of this frequency-shifted time series is obtained by multiplying $z(t)$ by $\cos(2\pi ft)$, and the imaginary part is obtained by multiplying $z(t)$ by $\sin(2\pi ft)$. The second stage consists of a low-pass filter with a half-power cutoff, b, that is applied to both the real and the imaginary time series. The net result of this two-stage process is a complex bandpass-filtered time series having a bandpass from $f - b$ to $f + b$.

Instantaneous coherence and phase are derived from the correlation of two sets of complex time series obtained via complex demodulation. Let $x_i(t)$ and $y_i(t)$ represent the complex values of the first and second time series, respectively, for trial epoch number i and time t. The complex correlation of x and y at time t is given by

$$\rho_{xy}(t) = \frac{\sum_i [X_i(t) - \langle x \rangle(t)][Y_i(t) - \langle y \rangle(t)]^*}{\sqrt{\sum_i |X_i(t) - \langle x \rangle(t)|^2 \sum_i |Y_i(t) - \langle y \rangle(t)|^2}},$$

where the asterisk denotes complex conjugation, the vertical bars denote the magnitude of a complex number, and the angular brackets denote averaging across epochs. Note that $\langle x \rangle$ and $\langle y \rangle$ are complex average potentials (i.e., event related) that are removed prior to forming the cross-products. Because the original time series were obtained by complex demodulation, the complex correlation time series is implicitly specific to the particular center frequency f and bandwidth b. The instantaneous coherence $\gamma^2 xy$ and phase delay τ_{xy} are given by

$$\gamma^2 xy(t, f, b) = |\rho_{xy}(t)|^2$$

and

$$\tau_{xy}(t, f, b) = \frac{1}{2\pi f} \tan^{-1}\left(\frac{\text{Im}[\rho_{xy}(t)]}{\text{Re}[\rho_{xy}(t)]}\right),$$

where Re and Im denote the real and imaginary parts of a complex number.

Instantaneous coherence and phase for each band of interest were computed for successive 10-ms samples from −600 ms premovement to +500 ms postmovement (i.e., 60 premovement samples + 50 postmovement samples) across 134 movement-related epochs for all possible pairings of the three dipole time series. The DC offset was removed from each trial by computing a mean value for the first 200 sample points and then subtracting the mean from each sample point. The filter was initialized at the beginning of each trial and then the sample points between −3000 ms and −600 ms were used as an extended warmup period for the filter.

III. Results

A. Source Locations of Equivalent Dipoles

Figure 1 shows some of the waveforms elicited during the self-paced voluntary finger movement task. The Bereitschaftpotential (BP), the negative slope (NS'), the peak of the NS' (pNS'), and the frontal peak of the motor potential (fpMP) are indicated. Figure 2B shows the dipole source moments for the three equivalent sources obtained from the waveforms elic-

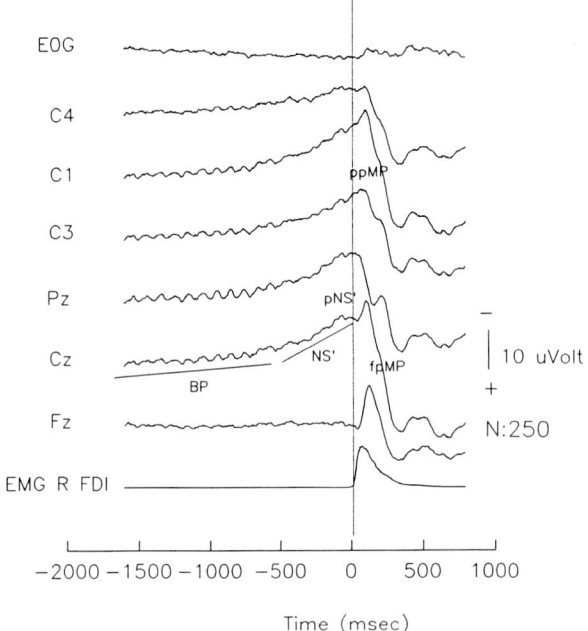

Figure 1 Waveform morphology of the movement response cortical potential (MRCP) elicited by self-paced voluntary finger abductions in the subject of this study ($N = 250$). The BP' (Bereitschaftpotential), the negative slope (NS'), the peak of the NS' (pNS'), the parietal peak of the motor potential (ppMP), the frontal peak of the motor potential (fpMP), and the FDI EMG are shown.

ited during the task. The arrows show the latency interval over which the dipole source localizations were computed. Figure 2A consists of head diagrams showing the locations of the three sources.

B. Multimodal Registration of Equivalent Dipoles, PET, and MRI

Plate 85 shows the location of ipsilateral motor cortex dipole 2 with respect to the registered MRI and PET. This equivalent dipole source registered within approximately 10 mm of the center of the active PET region located in the anterior bank of the ipsilateral central sulcus, near to the hand region. Plate 86 shows the location of contralateral motor cortex dipole 1. This equivalent dipole source registered within less than 3 mm of the center of the active PET region located in the anterior bank of the contralateral central sulcus, near to the hand region. Plate 87 shows the location of contralateral supplemental motor area (SMA) dipole 3. This equivalent dipole source registered within approximately 6 mm of the center of the active PET region located in the contralateral supplemental motor area.

These analyses show that there was relatively good coregistration between the location of the three equivalent dipoles and the independently obtained PET activation regions.

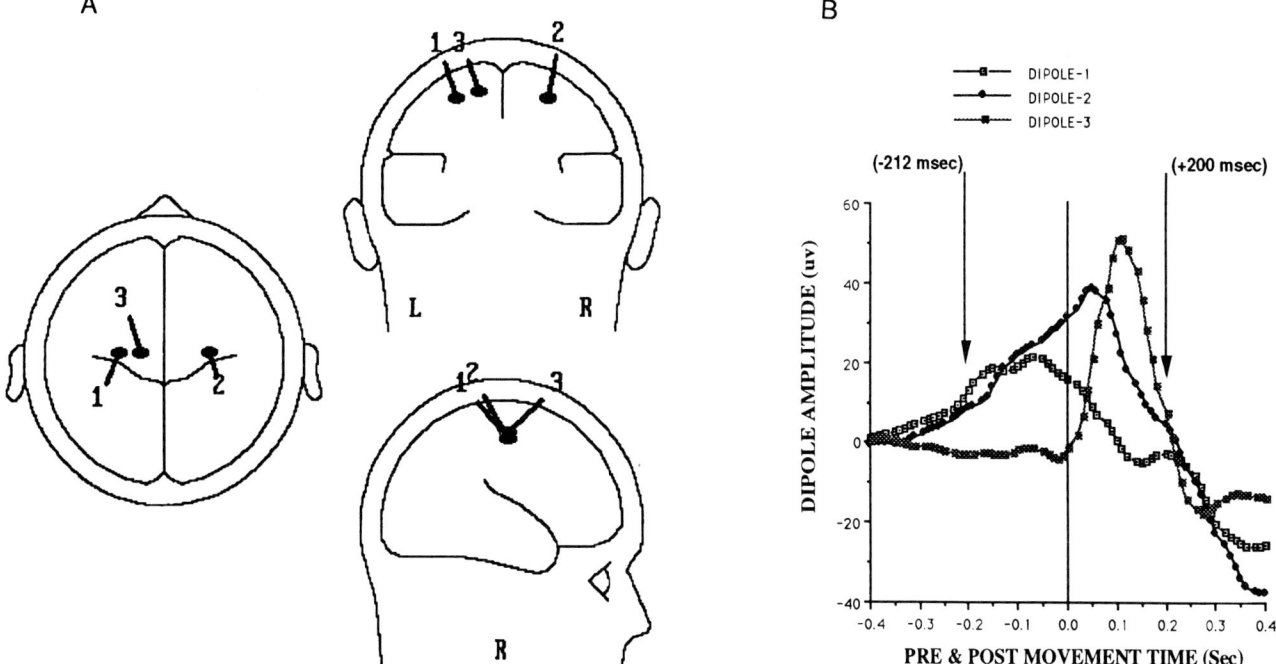

Figure 2 Dipole source analyses of the MRCPs shown in Fig. 1. (A) The three dipole solutions over the latencies between −212 and +200 ms were calculated with two sources located on each side of the best fitting sphere (D1, ipsilateral; D2, contralateral) and one source (i.e., D3) located near the SMA. These three sources accounted for approximately 96% of the variance of the MRCP. (B) The time history of the moment magnitude of each of the three equivalent dipole sources. For further details on the methods and model, see Toro *et al.* (1993a).

C. Instantaneous Coherence between the Pseudoinverse Derived Dipole Time Series

Figure 3 shows the results of the instantaneous coherence analyses among the time series computed for the various combinations of the three dipoles. Although changes in coherence as a function of time were noted in the center frequency range from 3 to 25 Hz, the strongest effects were seen in the θ frequency band (i.e., 4 to 7 Hz). As seen in Fig. 3A, for dipoles 1 and 2 there was a bimodal change in θ coherence between −600 and −300 ms, involving first a decline and then an increase in the magnitude of coherence. This was followed by a relatively steady-state level of coherence from −300 to 0 ms, after which there was an abrupt decrease in coherence between 0 and +50 ms postmovement. A slow recovery or increase in coherence was noted between +50 and 500 ms postmovement. In Fig. 3B, the coherence analyses for dipoles 1 and 3 were different than the analyses for dipoles 1 and 2. For example, there was a slow increase in coherence beginning at approximately −600 ms and reaching a peak at approximately −50 ms, after which there was a sudden drop in coherence just prior to movement (i.e., approximately −25 ms). During the postmovement period, coher-

ence between dipoles 1 and 3 showed a marked increase, reaching a peak at approximately +200 ms and then declining sharply.

An inverse relationship was evident between the coherence trajectories from dipoles 1 and 3 and those from dipoles 2 and 3, as shown in Fig. 6C. That is, dipoles 2 and 3 exhibited a decrease in coherence between approximately −300 and −50 ms, after which there was a sudden increase in coherence just prior to movement (i.e., approximately −25 ms). During the postmovement period, coherence between dipoles 2 and 3 exhibited a decline followed by a marked increase at approximately +200 ms.

D. Instantaneous Phase between the Pseudoinverse Derived Dipole Time Series

Figures 4A and 4B show an 180° phase reversal between the pseudoinverse derived time series from dipoles 1 and 2 and that from dipoles 1 and 3 during the premovement period. A rapid shift in phase from 180° to approximately 90° between dipoles 1 and 2 occurred at approximately +50 ms postmovement. Rapid shifts in phase between dipoles 1 and 3 were noted in the premovement period as well as during

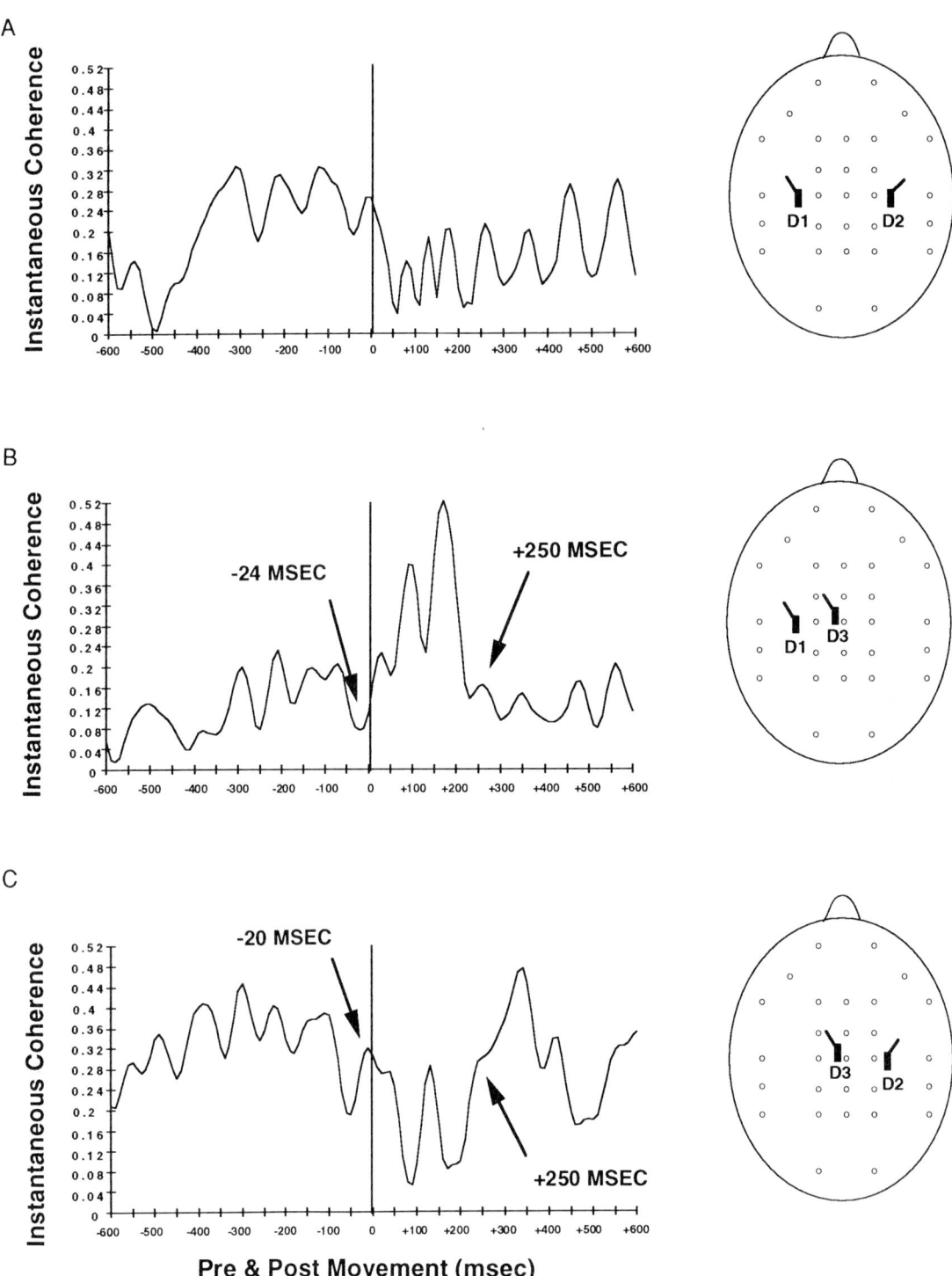

Figure 3 Instantaneous coherence (10-ms resolution) among the pseudoinverse derived dipole time series, using a center frequency of 4.25 Hz and a bandwidth of 3.5 Hz. Instantaneous coherence on the *y* axis is plotted against pre- and postmovement time (milliseconds) on the *x* axis. On the right side of the figure are diagramatic representations of the location of the dipoles (see Plates 85 to 87 for exact locations). (A) Instantaneous coherence between the ipsilateral motor cortex (D2) and the contralateral motor cortex (D1). (B) Instantaneous coherence between the ipsilateral motor cortex (D2) and the contralateral supplemental motor area (SMA) (D3). (C) Instantaneous coherence between the contralateral motor cortex (D2) and the SMA (D3).

A   B

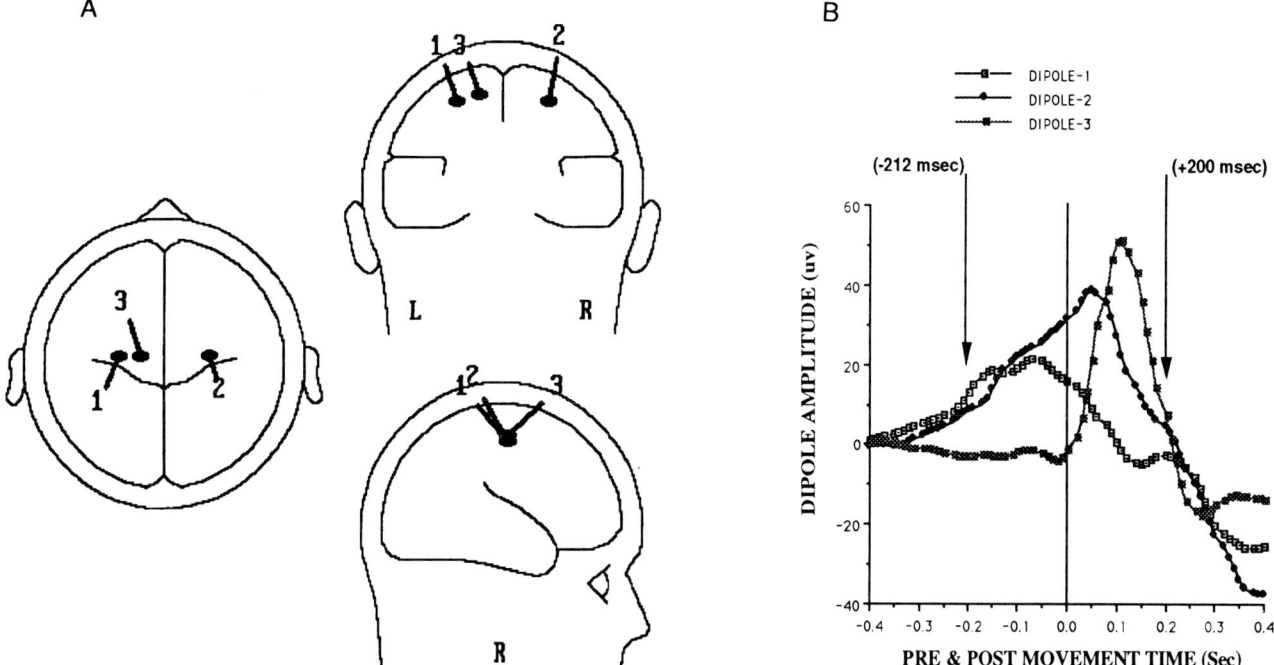

Figure 2 Dipole source analyses of the MRCPs shown in Fig. 1. (A) The three dipole solutions over the latencies between −212 and +200 ms were calculated with two sources located on each side of the best fitting sphere (D1, ipsilateral; D2, contralateral) and one source (i.e., D3) located near the SMA. These three sources accounted for approximately 96% of the variance of the MRCP. (B) The time history of the moment magnitude of each of the three equivalent dipole sources. For further details on the methods and model, see Toro *et al.* (1993a).

C. Instantaneous Coherence between the Pseudoinverse Derived Dipole Time Series

Figure 3 shows the results of the instantaneous coherence analyses among the time series computed for the various combinations of the three dipoles. Although changes in coherence as a function of time were noted in the center frequency range from 3 to 25 Hz, the strongest effects were seen in the θ frequency band (i.e., 4 to 7 Hz). As seen in Fig. 3A, for dipoles 1 and 2 there was a bimodal change in θ coherence between −600 and −300 ms, involving first a decline and then an increase in the magnitude of coherence. This was followed by a relatively steady-state level of coherence from −300 to 0 ms, after which there was an abrupt decrease in coherence between 0 and +50 ms postmovement. A slow recovery or increase in coherence was noted between +50 and 500 ms postmovement. In Fig. 3B, the coherence analyses for dipoles 1 and 3 were different than the analyses for dipoles 1 and 2. For example, there was a slow increase in coherence beginning at approximately −600 ms and reaching a peak at approximately −50 ms, after which there was a sudden drop in coherence just prior to movement (i.e., approximately −25 ms). During the postmovement period, coher-

ence between dipoles 1 and 3 showed a marked increase, reaching a peak at approximately +200 ms and then declining sharply.

An inverse relationship was evident between the coherence trajectories from dipoles 1 and 3 and those from dipoles 2 and 3, as shown in Fig. 6C. That is, dipoles 2 and 3 exhibited a decrease in coherence between approximately −300 and −50 ms, after which there was a sudden increase in coherence just prior to movement (i.e., approximately −25 ms). During the postmovement period, coherence between dipoles 2 and 3 exhibited a decline followed by a marked increase at approximately +200 ms.

D. Instantaneous Phase between the Pseudoinverse Derived Dipole Time Series

Figures 4A and 4B show an 180° phase reversal between the pseudoinverse derived time series from dipoles 1 and 2 and that from dipoles 1 and 3 during the premovement period. A rapid shift in phase from 180° to approximately 90° between dipoles 1 and 2 occurred at approximately +50 ms postmovement. Rapid shifts in phase between dipoles 1 and 3 were noted in the premovement period as well as during

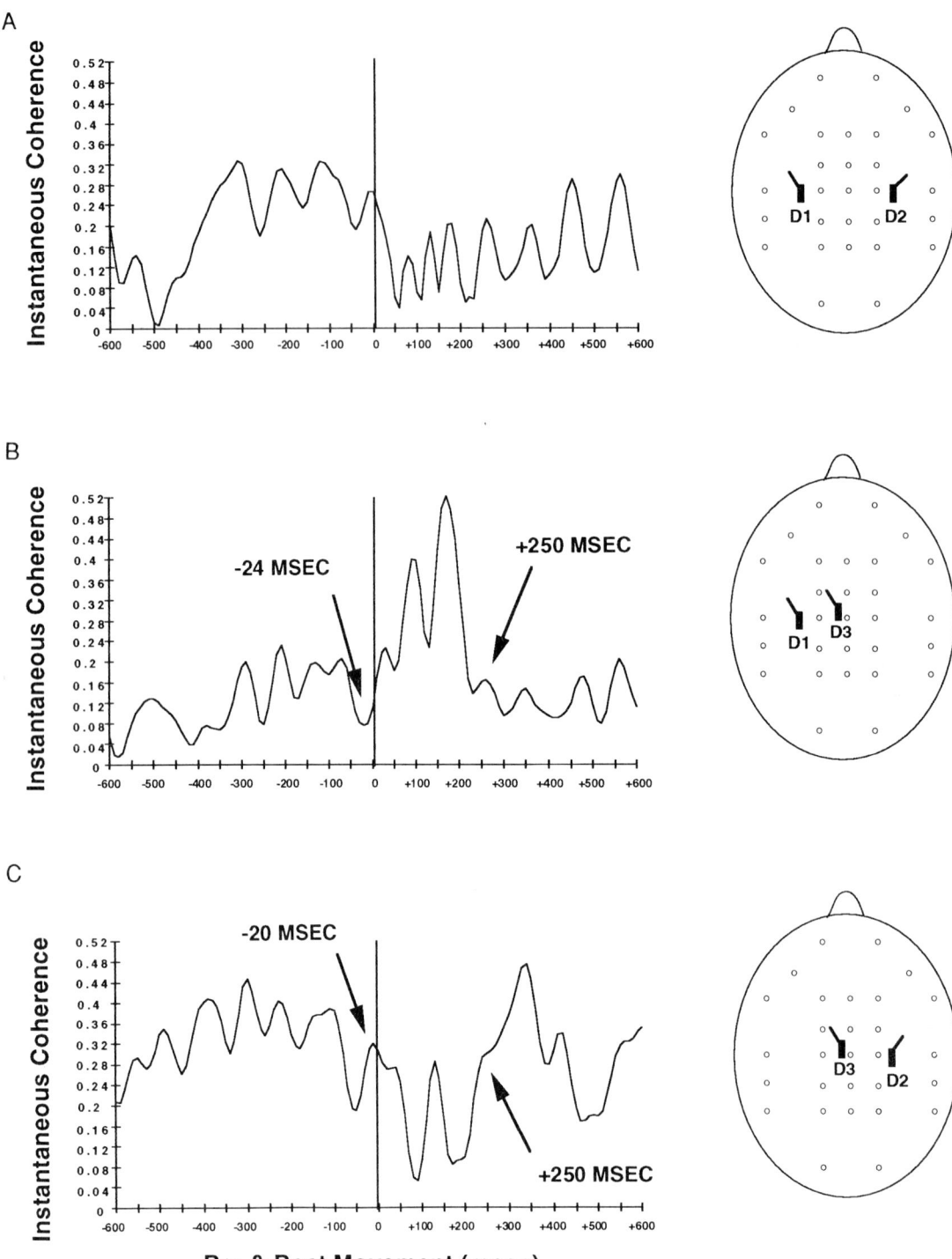

Figure 3 Instantaneous coherence (10-ms resolution) among the pseudoinverse derived dipole time series, using a center frequency of 4.25 Hz and a bandwidth of 3.5 Hz. Instantaneous coherence on the *y* axis is plotted against pre- and postmovement time (milliseconds) on the *x* axis. On the right side of the figure are diagramatic representations of the location of the dipoles (see Plates 85 to 87 for exact locations). (A) Instantaneous coherence between the ipsilateral motor cortex (D2) and the contralateral motor cortex (D1). (B) Instantaneous coherence between the ipsilateral motor cortex (D2) and the contralateral supplemental motor area (SMA) (D3). (C) Instantaneous coherence between the contralateral motor cortex (D2) and the SMA (D3).

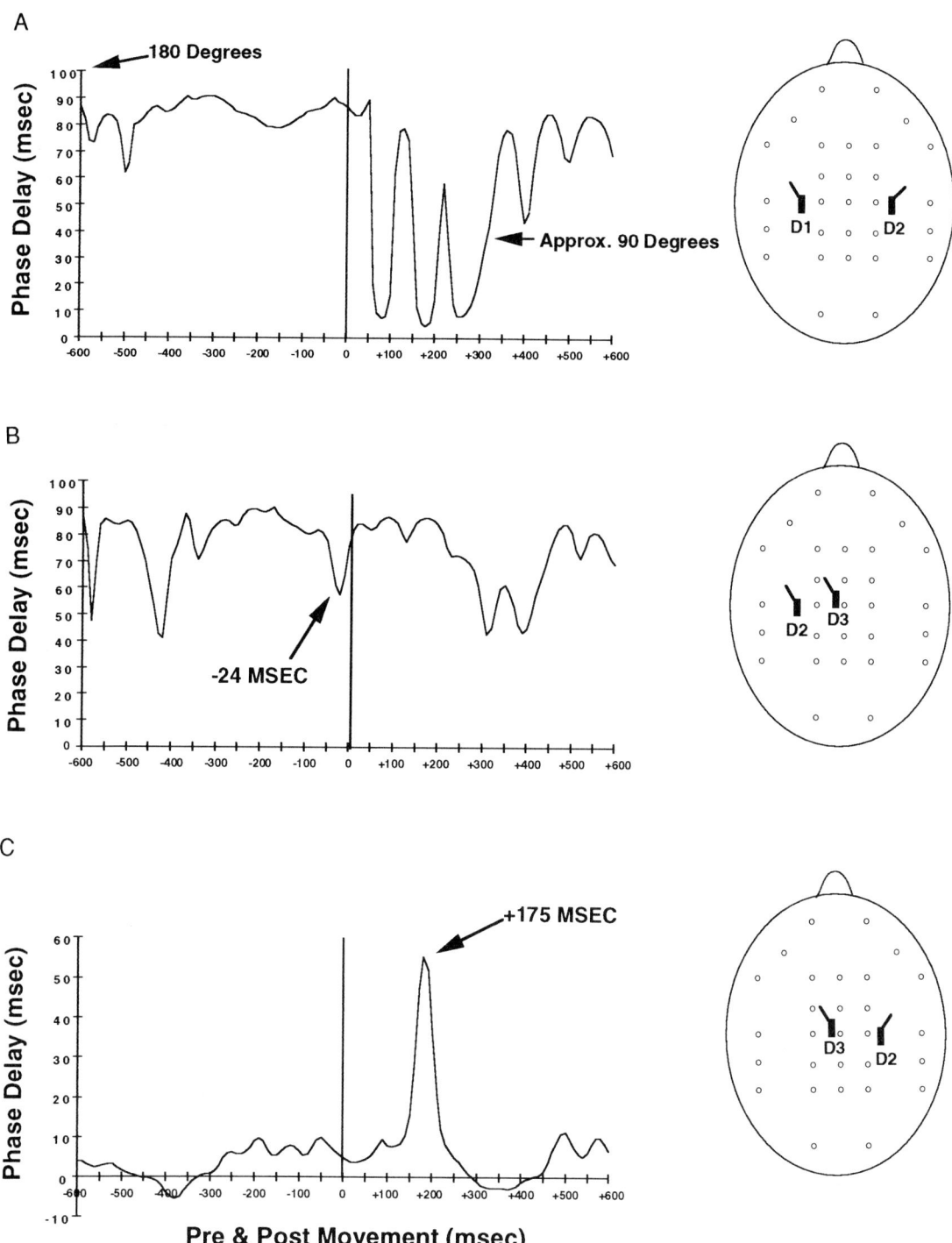

Figure 4   Instantaneous phase delay among the pseudoinverse derived dipole time series, using a center frequency of 4.25 Hz and a bandwidth of 3.5 Hz. Phase delay (milliseconds) on the y axis is plotted against pre- and postmovement time (milliseconds) on the x axis. On the right side of the figure are diagramatic representations of the location of the dipoles (see Plates 85 to 87 for exact locations). (A) Instantaneous phase delay between the ipsilateral motor cortex (D2) and the contralateral motor cortex (D1). (B) Instantaneous phase delay between the ipsilateral motor cortex (D2) and the contralateral SMA (D3). (C) Instantaneous phase delay between the contralateral motor cortex (D1) and the contralateral SMA (D3).

the postmovement period. As seen in Fig. 4C, a distinctly different phase trajectory was observed between dipoles 2 and 3. For example, the phase relationship was near 0° during the entire premovement period with a rapid increase in phase at approximately +150 ms postmovement.

IV. Discussion

A. Assumptions and Limitations

In this technique, the original dipole locations and orientations were determined using averaged time-domain data. The averaging procedure in effect throws away the "background EEG" activity that was not synchronized with the motor movement. The coherence analysis, on the other hand, is a frequency domain analysis of precisely this background EEG activity (i.e., with the average removed). Thus, the two forms of analysis are complementary approaches to the same data. Because the coherence analysis was not sensitive to the time-locked average activity used to estimate the set of dipole sources, the results of this analysis are of potential physiological interest because they are not dependent upon a signal-to-noise averaging process. Instead, the analysis focuses on the magnitude and timing of "coupling" relations that precede and follow the timing of evoked potential peaks. To this extent, the "dipole coherence" analysis may be of value in the study of the subsecond neural network dynamics involved in the mediation of perception and cognition. A further advantage of this technique is that it involves an analytic and not a numeric solution to the inverse problem and thus avoids many of the pitfalls of the latter process. This stems from the use of *a priori* knowledge from multiregistration with MRI and PET (Wang *et al.*, 1993).

At the same time, the reader should be aware of the preliminary nature of this study and the assumptions relied upon. First, it is assumed that the location and orientation of the dipoles remained fixed during the analysis period. Second, it is assumed that the analytically derived dipole moments are causally related to the distribution of scalp voltages recorded at each instant of time. Third, it is assumed that the coherence and phase measures reflect the magnitude of coupling or "phase coherency" shared between the dipole moments.

B. Face Validity of the Technique

In spite of the above noted limitations, there was considerable evidence to validate the physiological foundations of the technique. First, the anatomical

accuracy of the registration of the electrophysiological dipoles with the center of the PET-activated regions varied from approximately 3 to 10 mm (see Plates 85 to 87). Second, the dipoles were located in cortical regions that are known to subserve finger movements (i.e., the anterior bank of the central sulcus and the SMA). Third, the time course of the dipole coherence events corresponded well with the time course of evoked potential (Toro *et al.*, 1993, 1994) and event-related desynchronization events (Pfurtsheller *et al.*, 1988) obtained in similar if not identical motor movement tasks. Finally, the observed rapid changes in electrophysiological coupling between distributed brain regions was similar to that observed by Gevins *et al.* (1989a, 1989b) in subjects performing a motor movement task.

C. Competition between Dipoles

As described elsewhere, inverse relationships and 180° phase reversals in EEG coherence are believed to reflect competition between connected neural assemblies (Thatcher *et al.*, 1986, 1987, 1992). For example, for three interconnected neural assemblies, A, B, and C, increased coupling between A and B may be at the expense of coupling between A and C, B and C, or both. In the present study, increased coupling between the ipsilateral motor cortex dipole and the contralateral SMA dipole was inversely related to the magnitude of coupling between the contralateral motor cortex dipole and the contralateral SMA dipole (see Fig. 3). This is indicative of dynamic competition between the ipsilateral and contralateral motor cortex and the SMA. Another example of possible competition was seen in the coherence relationships between the ipsilateral and the contralateral motor cortex dipoles. In this case, there was a rapid decrease in coupling between the ipsilateral motor cortex (D2) and SMA (D3) immediately after motor movement (i.e., between 0 and 50 ms), which occurred simultaneously with an increase in coupling between the contralateral motor cortex dipole (D1) and the SMA dipole (D3).

D. SMA as a Neural Network Switch Element

The SMA dipole was strongly coupled to the ipsilateral motor cortex dipole during the premovement period because these regions exhibited relatively high coherence and a zero phase lag (see Figs. 3C and 4C). In contrast, during the premovement period, the SMA dipole was weakly coupled to the contralateral motor cortex dipole with variable but near 180° phase relationships (see Fig. 3B). Evidence for an SMA role as a neural network switching element was seen by the

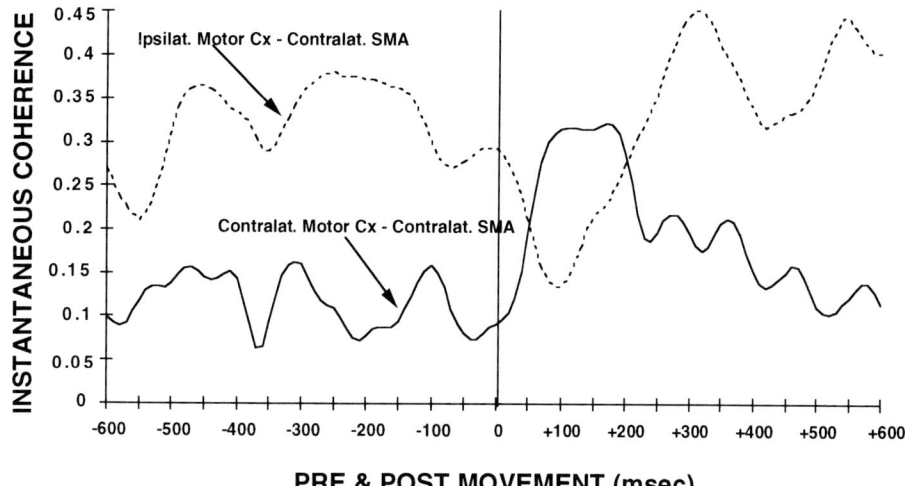

Figure 5 Instantaneous coherence (10-ms resolution) among the pseudoinverse derived dipole time series, using a center frequency of 7 Hz and a bandwidth of 4 Hz. Coherence on the y axis is plotted against pre- and postmovement time (milliseconds) on the x axis. The dashed line is instantaneous coherence between the time series from the ipsilateral motor cortex and that from the contralateral SMA. The solid line is instantaneous coherence between the time series from the contralateral motor cortex and that from the contralateral SMA.

rapid (i.e., 20 to 50 ms) reversal in coherence values immediately after the motor movement (see Fig. 3). The label of the SMA dipole as a switching element is based upon the speed at which the coupling dynamics changed and the primary relationship that the SMA dipole held with respect to the other dipoles, especially the contralateral motor cortex dipole (see Figs. 3 and 5). A more detailed analysis of the dynamics of the SMA changes in coupling with respect to the ipsilateral and contralateral cortex is shown in Fig. 5. In this figure, the center frequency of the filter was set to 7 Hz and the bandwidth was limited to 4 Hz. These filter settings provided a smoother picture of the time course of coherence changes.

E. Human Neural Network Dynamics and Zero Phase Coupling

The instantaneous coherence and phase analyses used in the present study may provide new information about the dynamics of neural interaction that occurred during the finger movement task. Three of the most significant dynamical features were (1) the presence of oscillations in coherence and phase, (2) the duration and rate of large changes in coherence and phase, and (3) the presence of zero phase locking. The presence of oscillations in dipole coherence is a function of the bandwidth of the filter; i.e., oscillations diminish as the bandwidth narrows. This suggests that the oscillations are due to periodic shifts in fre-

quency in one or both channels. The amplitude and frequency of these oscillations may be of relevance in dynamical modeling of the coupling phenomena. We are currently conducting simulation analyses to learn more about the basis of the oscillations in the dipole coherence. The duration of the large changes in dipole coherence refers to the interval over which a relatively stable level of coherence suddenly changes to a new stable level. In the present study, this interval was approximately 50 to 100 ms (see Figs. 3 and 5). The rate of change in coherence between the pre- and the postmovement periods was estimated by derivatives to be from approximately 0.001 to 0.003 ms. Finally, zero phase locking was present only between the SMA dipole and the contralateral motor cortex dipole. As mentioned previously, this is suggestive of strong coupling between these regions, which persists even though coherence may radically change (see Figs. 3 and 4). Although more analyses must be performed on a larger number of subjects, these findings tentatively suggest that the dynamics of neural network coupling observed in multiunit studies in animals (e.g., Gray *et al.*, 1989; Eckhorn *et al.*, 1988; Murthy and Fetz, 1992) may be similar to those observed in noninvasive human EEG studies.[2]

---

[2] Although the PET scan is not "noninvasive," we believe that truly noninvasive techniques, such as functional MRI, provide adequate spatial resolution of regional blood flow to replace the PET [see Turner *et al.* (1993) and Turner and Jezzard (1993)].

Acknowledgment

We acknowledge Dr. Brad Roth for his critical and constructive comments.

References

Ary, J. P., Klein, S. A., and Fender, D. H. (1981). Location of sources of evoked scalp potentials: Corrections for skull and scalp thicknesses. *IEEE Trans. Biomed. Eng.* **37,** 447–452.

Atiya, A., and Baldi, P. (1989). Oscillations and synchronizations in neural networks: An exploration of the labeling hypothesis. *Int. J. Neural Syst.* **1**(2), 103–124.

Baldi, P., and Meir, R. (1990). Computing with arrays of coupled oscillators: An application to preattentive texture discrimination. *Neural Comput.* **2,** 458–471.

Barrett, G., Shibasaki, H., and Neshige, R. (1985). A computer-assisted method for averaging movement-related cortical potentials with respect to EMG onset. *Electroenceph. Clin. Neurophysiol.* **60,** 276–281.

Ben-Israel, A., and Greville, T. N. E. (1974). "Generalized Inverses Theory and Applications." New York: Wiley.

Bendat, J. S., and Piersol, A. G. (1980). "Engineering Applications of Correlation and Spectral Analysis." New York: Wiley.

Eckhorn, R., Bauer, R., Jordan, W., Brosch, M., Kruse, W., Munk, M., and Reitboek, H. J. (1988). Coherent oscillations: A mechanism of feature linking in the visual cortex? *Biol. Cybernetics* **60,** 121–130.

Gevins, A. S., and Bressler, S. L. (1988). Functional topography of the human brain. *In* "Functional Brain Imaging" (G. Pfurtscheller, Ed.), pp. 99–116. Berlin: Hans Huber.

Gevins, A. S., Cutillo, S. L., Bressler, S. L., Morgan, N. H., White, R. M., Illes, J., and Greer, D. S. (1989). Event-related covariances during a bimanual visuomotor task. I. Methods and analysis of stimulus- and response-locked data. *Electroenceph. Clin. Neurophysiol.* **74**(1), 58–75.

Gevins, A. S., Cutillo, S. L., Bressler, S. L., Morgan, N. H., White, R. M., Illes, J., and Greer, D. S. (1989). Event-related covariances during a bimanual visuomotor task. II. Preparation and feedback. *Electroenceph. Clin. Neurophysiol.* **74**(2), 147–160.

Gray, C. M., Konig, P., Engel, A. K., and Singer, W. (1989). Oscillatory responses in cat visual cortex exhibit inter-columnar synchronization which reflects global stimulus properties. *Nature (London)* **338,** 334–337.

Grossberg, S. (1976). Adaptive pattern classification and universal recoding. I. Parallel development and coding of neural feature detectors. *Biol. Cybernetics* **23,** 187–202.

Grossberg, S., and Somers, D. (1991). Synchronized oscillations during cooperative feature linking in a cortical model of visual perception. *Neural Networks* **4,** 453–466.

John, E. R. (1963). "Mechanisms of Memory." New York: Academic Press.

Mosher, J. C., Lewis, P. S., and Leahy, R. M. (1992). Multiple dipole modeling and localization from spatio-temporal MEG data. *IEEE Trans. Biomed. Eng.* **39**(6), 541–557.

Murthy, V. N., and Fetz, E. E. (1992). Coherent 25- to 35Hz oscillations in the sensorimotor cortex of awake behaving monkeys. *Proc. Natl. Acad. Sci. USA* **89,** 5670–5674.

Otnes, R. K., and Enochson, L. (1978). "Applied Time Series Analysis," pp. 212–215. New York: Wiley.

Penrose, R. (1955). A generalized inverse for matrices. *Proc. Cambridge Phil. Soc.* **51,** 406–413.

Pfurtscheller, G., Steffan, J., and Maresch, H. (1988). ERD mapping and functional topography: Temporal and spatial aspects. *In* "Functional Brain Imaging" (G. Pfurtscheller, Ed.), pp. 117–130. Berlin: Hans Huber.

Scherg, M., and Berg, P. (1991). Use of prior knowledge in brain electromagnetic source analysis. *Brain Topogr.* **4,** 143–150.

Scherg, M. (1992). Functional imaging and localization of electromagnetic brain activity. *Brain Topogr.* **5**(2), 103–111.

Talairach, J., and Tournoux, P. (1988). "Co-Planar Stereotaxic Atlas of the Human Brain." New York: Thieme Medical.

Thatcher, R. W., and John, E. R. (1977). "Functional Neuroscience: Foundations of Cognitive Processes." New Jersey: Erlbaum.

Thatcher, R W., Krause, P., and Hrybyk, M. (1986). Corticocortical association fibers and EEG coherence: A two compartmental model. *Electroenceph. Clin. Neurophysiol.* **64,** 123–143.

Thatcher, R. W., Walker, R. A., and Giudice, S. (1987). Human cerebral hemispheres develop at different rates and ages. *Science* **236,** 1110–1113.

Thatcher, R. W. (1992). Cyclic cortical reorganization during early childhood. *Brain Cog.* **20,** 24–50.

Thatcher, R. W., Toro, C., and Hallett, M. (1993a). Neural network switching during voluntary finger movements. *In* "International Federation of Clinical Electroencephalography, Vancouver, B.C." [Abstr.]

Thatcher, R. W., Toro, C., Pflieger, M. E., and Hallett, M. (1993b). Multimodal registration of EEG, PET and MRI: Analyses of Neural Network Switching. *Proceedings of Society of Magnetic Resonance in Medicine: Functional MRI of the Brain.* Arlington, VA, June 17–19, pp. 171–181.

Toro, C., Matsumoto, J., Deuschl, G., Roth, B. J., and Hallett, M. (1993a). Source analysis of scalp-recorded movement-related electrical potentials. *Electroenceph. Clin. Neurophysiol.* **86,** 167–175.

Toro, C., Wang, B., Zeffiro, T. A., Thatcher, R. W., and Hallett, M. (1994). Movement related cortical potentials: Source analysis and PET/MRI correlation. *In* "Functional Neuroimaging: Technical Foundations" (R. W. Thatcher, M. Hallett, T. Zeffiro, E. R. John, and M. Huerta, Eds.). Orlando, FL: Academic Press.

Turner, R., Jezzard, P., Wen, H., Kwong, K. K., Le Bihan, D., Zeffiro, T., and Balaban, R. S. (1993). Functional mapping of the human visual cortex at 4 and 1.5 tesla using deoxygenation contrast EPI. *Magn. Reson. Magazine* **29,** 277–279.

Turner, R., and Jezzard, P. (1993). MR studies of brain functional activation using echo-planar imaging. *In* "Functional Neuroimaging: Technical Foundations" (R. W. Thatcher, M. Hallett, T. Zeffiro, E. R. John, and M. Huerta, Eds.). Orlando, FL: Academic Press.

von der Malsburg, C., and Schneider, W. (1986). A neural cocktail-party processor. *Biol. Cybernetics* **54,** 29–40.

Wang, B., Toro, C., Wasserman, E. M., Zeffiro, T. A., Thatcher, R. W., and Hallett, M. (1994). Multimodal integration of electrophysiological data and brain images: EEG, MEG, TMS, MRI, and PET. *In* "Functional Neuroimaging: Technical Foundations" (R. W. Thatcher, M. Hallett, T. Zeffiro, E. R. John, and M. Huerta, Eds.). Orlando, FL: Academic Press.

Wang, J., Williamson, S. J., and Kaufman, L. (1992). Magnetic source images determined by a lead-field analysis: The unique minimum-norm least-squares estimation. *IEEE. Trans. Biol. Med.* **39**(7), 665–675.

Wang, J., Kaufman, L, and Williamson, S. J. (1993b). Imaging regional changes in the spontaneous activity of the brain: An extension of the minimum-norm least-squares estimate. *Electroenceph. Clin. Neurophysiol.* **86,** 36–50.

28

Integration of MEG, EEG, and MRI

H. J. Wieringa,* M. J. Peters,* and F. H. Lopes da Silva†

*Department of Applied Physics, Low Temperature Division, University of Twente, Enschede, The Netherlands; and †Graduate School of Neurosciences, Institute of Neurobiology, Faculty of Biology, University of Amsterdam, 1098 SM Amsterdam, The Netherlands

I. Introduction

The simultaneous recording of EEG and MEG data can be used to estimate the sources of activity within the human brain. In this way, the strength of a source can be used to estimate the size of the active cortical layer. By depicting the estimated patch of activity in an MR image, the relevance of the calculated results can be evaluated.

The estimation of the sources from the measured EEGs or MEGs is called the solution of the inverse problem. In order to solve this problem, one has to make assumptions, namely, to model both the volume conductor and the sources. With respect to the former, the head is customarily described by four compartments with homogeneous conductivity representing, respectively, the brain, the cerebrospinal fluid (CSF), the skull, and the scalp. These compartments can be described, in a first approximation, by concentric best fitting spheres (see Fig. 1) or, preferably, by an approximation to their realistic shape. The best fitting spheres or the realistically shaped compartments can be obtained using the magnetic resonance imaging (MRI) data of a subject. With respect to the model of the source, a patch of active cortex is described usually by an equivalent current dipole (ED). The inverse problem for a single ED is a six-parameter estimation problem, in which three parameters determine the dipole's position and three, its components. The estimation procedure is limited commonly to the localiza-

tion of the source. Accordingly only half of the parameters are calculated due to the fact that the influence of the volume conductor does not allow a precise estimation of the strength of ED, based on EEG data, whereas MEG data give only the possibility of estimating the tangential components. However, a more powerful estimation procedure can be followed by using both EEG and MEG data. Here we show how all six parameters can be determined more accurately if both EEG and MEG data are used.

A further problem is that in most practical cases one does not know how many sources are active at the same time. Here again the use of both MEG and EEG data can help us to decide if a single ED is enough to describe the measurements or if more sources have to be discriminated. Another advantage of combining MEG and EEG data is that both types of signals contain information that is partly independent. The noise in the measurements is also to a large extent uncorrelated, and thus simultaneous electric and magnetic measurements have the highest information content (Pascual-Marqui and Biscay-Lirio, 1991).

The functional localization of brain sources of activity based on MEG and EEG should preferably be carried out in combination with the MRI of the same subject. First, the MRI can be used to derive a model of the head, which is necessary for the calculation of the location of electric activity. Second, the MRI can be used to indicate the location of the sources within the head, thereby combining functional with structural in-

FUNCTIONAL NEUROIMAGING

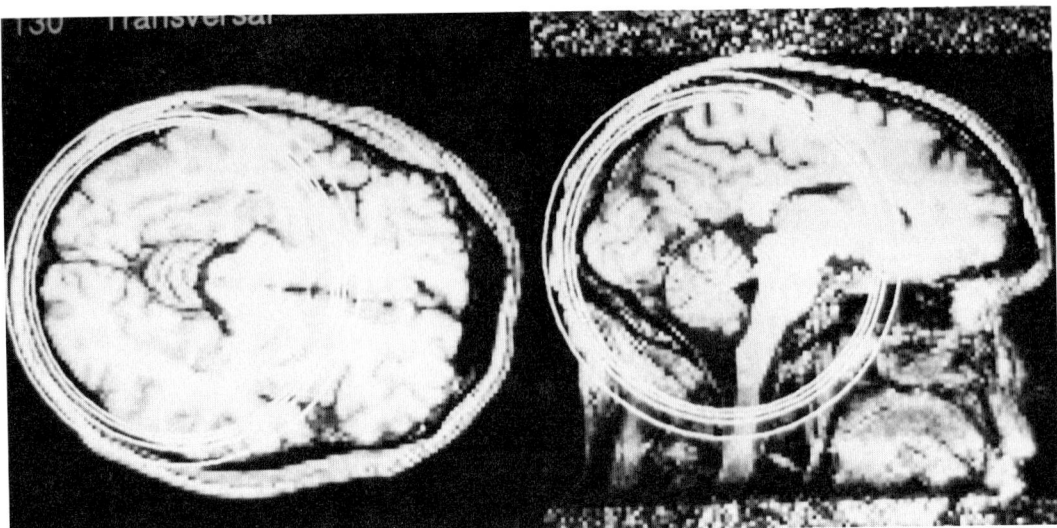

Figure 1 A model of the head as a volume conductor consisting of four concentric spheres, describing the brain, the CSF, the skull, and the scalp, superimposed on an MRI scan. The outer sphere was obtained from the MRI by fitting it locally to the outer surface of the head. The ratios between the radii are, respectively, 1.0, 0.92, 0.88, and 0.85.

formation. Finally, the position of the source depicted in the MRI enables us to validate the physiological significance of the result and, if necessary, to correct the estimated position within the error estimate.

II. Integration of MEG and EEG

Our knowledge of the conductivity distribution within the head is rather limited. The dependency of the potential distribution of an equivalent dipole on head model parameters has been investigated systematically by Stok (1987). In his study, the head was described by concentric spheres and the sources were radial or tangential dipoles. The conductivities were allowed to change by a total of 30% in steps of 5% and the radii by 2.5% in steps of 0.5%. From all possible combinations, the "worst-case" maximum and worst-case minimum potential were selected. The influence of changes in the conductivity and radii on the dipole parameters was computed for the worst-case combinations of both the conductivities and the radii, for sources at various depths. The inverse procedure was based on a reference model. The conductivities used in the reference model for the scalp, skull, fluid, and brain compartments were, respectively, 0.33, 0.0042, 1.0, and 0.33 S/m. Values of the radii were 75, 69, 66, and 64 mm, respectively. It was found that both the sphere radii and the conductivities greatly influence the strength of the EEG dipole and much less so its location. We repeated these simulations in order to investigate the influence of the model parameters on the orientation of the EEG dipole. Although both the

strength and the position of the EDs were influenced by changes in the conductivities, we found that the ratio between the radial and the tangential components of the EEG–EDs was hardly influenced by the model parameters. Furthermore, we were able to show that, when the influence of the actual shape of the four compartments (brain, fluid, skull, and scalp) is taken into account, the variation in the direction of the MEG–ED is smaller than 4° (Meijs *et al.*, 1988). The fact that the orientation of the dipole was preserved agrees with the findings of Cuffin *et al.* (1991), who studied the influence of the real head on the potential distribution over the scalp by means of activated implanted electrodes. When the head is described by a set of concentric spheres, the MEG is not influenced by the radii, nor by the conductivities. Thus, the location and the tangential components of the dipole can be derived from the MEG (i.e., five parameters describing the ED), and the orientation can be reliably derived from EEG data (i.e., the sixth parameter describing the ED). In other words, using both EEG and MEG, all six parameters describing the dipole can be found more reliably than when using EEG or MEG data alone. Once the strength and the orientation of the dipole are known, this dipole can be depicted in an MRI dataset.

III. The MRI Data

An MRI scanner has the possibility of making different types of scans, thereby varying the output numbers for different types of tissue. The two most important scanning methods are the so-called T_1-weighted and the T_2-weighted scans. In a T_1-weighted scan, the CSF is hardly distinguishable from the skull. In a T_2-weighted scan, the CSF is highlighted, whereas no difference can be observed between the gray and the white matter of the brain.

The output of the scanner consists of a number of slices, each of which is made of a (square) plane of volume elements, called voxels. Each voxel can be given a certain value. The spatial resolution, the number, and the thickness of the slices can vary. Slices can have gaps in between, they can be contiguous, or they can overlap. By translating the value of each voxel into a color or gray value, the slices can easily be visualized.

One of the difficulties in quantifying and analyzing magnetic resonance images is that a certain tissue type does not have a specific voxel value. Even within one scan, the value of voxels from the same tissue can vary over the different slices of that scan. The relative positions of the voxel values of the different tissue types remain intact. In practice, we used MRI data obtained from a Philips Gyroscan S15/ACS 1.5-T system. A 3D-volume T_1-weighted scan was performed, which gave 256 transversal slices, each of 256 × 256 voxels. Each voxel represents a volume of 1 × 1 mm.

A. Segmentation

Both for generating models and for 3D displays, the MRI scans have to be analyzed. In each slice, the head has to be discriminated from the background. Within the head, various structures have to be discriminated visually, such as the brain, the eyes, the ventricles, part of the skull, and the CSF. However, being able to discriminate them visually is not enough. A computer has to be instructed in order to make quantitative analysis of the images possible. To do this, information about the nature of the different tissue types has to be provided. In principle, an operator could mark the different tissue types on each slice, with the help of various image-processing techniques. Nevertheless, this is time consuming and has to be avoided when one is dealing with a large number of patients. Therefore, we have to resort to algorithms for automatic segmentation of MRI scans (Bomans et al., 1990). Because of the high resolutoin of the scans that are being used, these techniques can be quite successful. Nevertheless, it is difficult to get hold of the exact form of the skull from an MRI scan; for instance, it is difficult to discriminate between skull and the frontal sinus. Furthermore, the same type of tissue may have voxels with different values within the same scan. To obtain a reliable segmentation of

an MRI scan, we have first to compute a histogram of a slice representing the distribution of the number of pixels having given gray values. In this way, a peak in the histogram indicates gray values that are present more often in the image than others. The histogram of an MRI slice usually shows two or three peaks. One of the peaks comes from the background pixels with low gray values. Another peak represents the pixels corresponding to the brain and skin compartments. This peak is sometimes divided into two subpeaks, one representing the gray matter and the second representing the white matter and skin. Smoothing the histograms and taking the gradient, the computer can automatically locate the peaks. These locations are used for the actual segmentation by a method called "region growing." According to this technique, one or more points of a picture are taken as starting points. These are called seed points and are assumed to be included in the region of interest. From these points, the growing operation is started by determining if the neighbors of the seed points satisfy certain criteria. If they do, these points are added to the region of interest. This process is repeated by examining all the neighbors of these new region points and checking if they satisfy the same criterion. The process stops when no more points can be added to the region. Using region growing, the head can be easily separated from the background, thereby eliminating the noise outside the head, which is certainly present in the MRI.

The threshold used for discrimination of the head from the background is derived from the analysis of the histograms (Figs. 2a and 2b). After the growing process is completed, a check has to be made to ascertain if there are points that are not yet defined as being part of the head, but are completely enclosed by points that are. These points are then also to be marked as part of the head.

Separating the brain compartment is more difficult, because the skin and the brain partly have the same gray values. Any growing operation would therefore probably lead to large parts of the skin also being included in the brain compartment. To avoid this, a "mask" is used. A mask defines the points that are allowed to be added to the region of interest during the growing operation. A mask can be generated by selecting all points in the slice with gray values that correspond clearly to the brain compartment. These values belong to the peak(s) in the histogram; hence, the range of the values of voxels of interest is already known. However, as point out earlier, large parts of the skin can have the same gray values. To avoid extending the growing operation beyond the borders of the brain compartment and into the skin, an "eroa

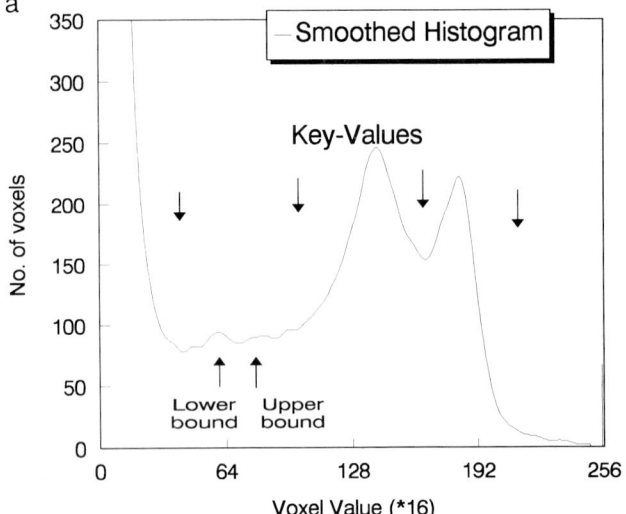

b

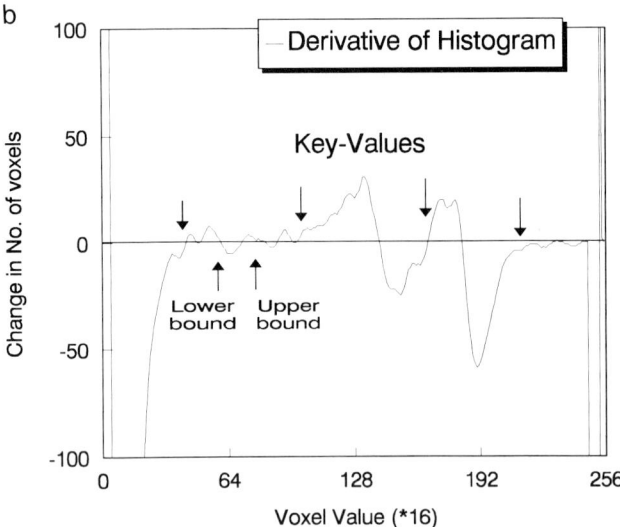

Figure 2 The smoothed histogram obtained from an MRI scan of a slice (a) and its derivative (b), with key values.

sion operation'' is performed. This means that, from a set of points, all those points that are neighbors of a point that is not part of the set are removed. If necessary, this process can be repeated a number of times.

The resulting set of points is the mask. As the brain has its center around the middle of the head, the seed points are selected from a small region in the middle of the head, and of course they belong to the mask. Then region growing is performed with the condition that the points that are added have to be part of the mask. The region found in this way will correspond to brain tissue, but in this way the complete brain compartment will not be defined. By doing a ''dilation,'' the reverse process of an ''erosion,'' the result-

ing set will practically consist of all brain matter. Isolated points inside the brain have to be added to the brain compartment.

The area that has been derived from these operations is the brain, but its outer contour does not align with the gyri and sulci of the brain. To construct mathematical models of the volume conductor, this is not inconvenient because the detailed surface of the brain is not relevant for these type of models. After the determination of the contours of the brain (including CSF) compartment has been completed, subdivisions can be made based on the gray values of subcompartments. In this way, for example, the regions corresponding to the ventricles can be estimated.

Finally, the skull compartment is extracted, using very low gray values that lie within the head and are not part of the brain as seed points. Then, again through a growing operation, points below a certain gray value are added followed by a closing operation.

B. Generation of the Model

Once the segmentation process is completed, the points at the surface of the regions of interest can be identified. This is done by tracing lines from the center of the slice toward the edge. When a given region ends, the tracing is stopped, and the corresponding coordinates represent a point on the surface of the region. By repeating this process at various angles until a full circle has been covered, a description of the contour points is obtained. To avoid points lying very close together on small contours, the distance between points along the contour is kept approximately the same. The aim is to obtain the desired number of points on the largest slice, which lies about the middle of the complete scan. These points can be used for solving the forward problem using a realistically shaped head model following a collocation method (Kemppainen and Peters, 1991). To increase the accuracy of this method the normal vector on the surface is also generated. The normal vector can easily be derived from the original MRI data, by determining the (3D) gradient of the gray values at the contour point.

Another way to solve the forward problem is to use the boundary-element method. This is examplified in Fig. 3. From the points generated according to the method described above, a triangulated surface can automatically be generated. The procedure uses points lying on two contours. Usually it starts with two points close together at the back of the head, for example, points A1 and A(*i* + 1) in Fig. 3. These two points form the start of a triangle. The procedure follows the contour in one given direction. The third

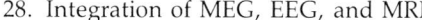
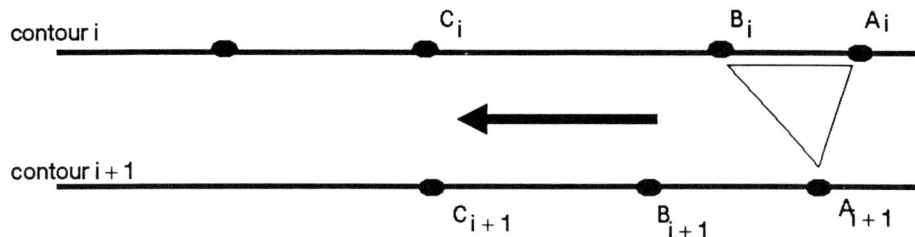

Figure 3 Graphic representation of the application of the principle of triangularization, as explained in the text.

point of the triangle lies on one of the two contours; we chose the point that lies closest to the point on the contour as the third point. For example, in the example in Fig. 3, B1–A$(i + 1)$ is shorter than A1–B$(i + 1)$. The procedure is continued by checking if this third point lies closer to the next point on the other contour B$(i + 1)$ than to the point on the contour that was part of the last triangle A$(i + 1)$. If this is so, the points Bi and B$(i + 1)$ form the start of a new triangle, and the part of the surface that is skipped forms another triangle. If not, then Bi and A$(i + 1)$ form the start of a new triangle. This process is repeated until all points on the contours are connected by triangles. Then the next contour is handled, until all contours are done. As a criterion for the distance between points, the planar angle between two points is taken instead of the Euclidean distance. This avoids initially skipping points that lie on, for instance, the nose. An example of an automatically triangulated head, using the procedure described above, is shown in Fig. 4.

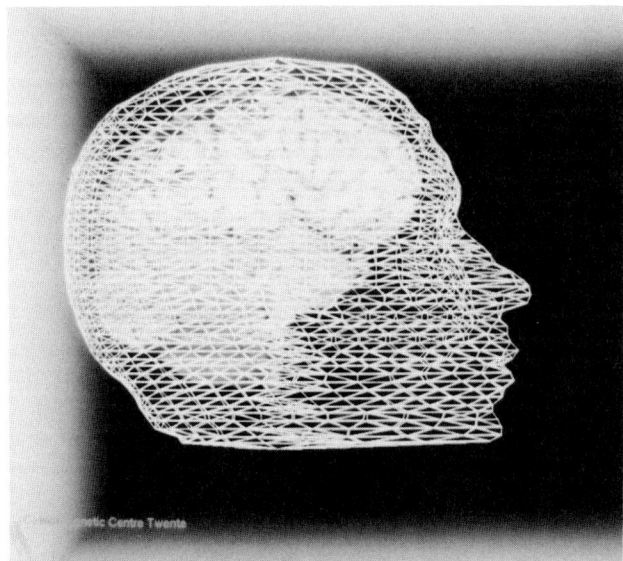

Figure 4 A fully automatic triangulated head model.

C. Three-Dimensional Display

The slices obtained by the MRI scanner provide data on the scanned volume, in our case, the head. This gives us the opportunity to display these data in various ways. The simplest method is to display each slice separately, converting the MRI values to gray values. This does not, however, give a good insight into the shape and location of the various anatomical objects. It is possible to depict the MRI data in a 3D-data space. An observer may obtain a view of this space from any angle. By using the previously described segmentation procedure, certain tissue types can be made visible or invisible, or the corresponding image parameters may be changed in any other way. By tracing rays from the screen into this virtual 3D space, a 3D view can be generated on the screen. Where the ray hits a surface, which has been chosen to be visible, one can calculate the normal to that surface by calculating the gradient of the original MRI data. Based on this surface normal, combined with the viewing direction and with the direction of an imaginary light source, we may code any pixel on the screen with a color or gray value. The color coding can be calculated from basic mathematical principles that hold for the reflection of light on surfaces. This process of "ray tracing" or volume rendering has been well described in the literature (Robb and Barillot, 1989; Tiede *et al.*, 1990).

The segmentation of the brain, derived using the method described above, will result in a rather smooth surface. The segmentation does not follow the detailed contours of the gyri and sulci, but yields only a more or less smooth outer surface. A 3D image of the brain with more details may be obtained by using another rendering method, namely, that of transparent rendering. This means that not only is the surface of the object important, but also the volume elements below the surface.

All these 3D rendering techniques show the surface of an object. However, the information inside the object is also available. By making "cut-away" views, this information can be made visible. The fastest way is to start with an existing 3D view of a surface and to define the cutting plane. The interception point from the ray into the object and the cutting plane is calculated. If this point lies within the object, the original MRI data are displayed at that point. If the point is outside the object, the original information either remains on screen or is cleared from the screen, depending on which side of the cutting plane the original information was present. The illusion of a transparent surface can be created. When the original (surface) color is not replaced by the MRI data, a new color is calculated as the sum of a small fraction of the original color and a large fraction of the original MRI data. There is not yet much experience with 3D views of clinical data in a hospital environment. It is therefore by no means clear what the most convenient way to present in practice the 3D data is. It is known that the 3D effect can be enhanced by drawing supporting objects, like a cube around the 3D object, using shades and even using motion. The suggestion of motion can be created by showing different views quickly one after the other. The subsequent frames can best be generated with the light source at a constant position relative to the observer. Current computer power is not yet sufficient to generate the frames in real time. Normally, the necessary frames are generated at an earlier time and stored on disk.

IV. Markers and Coordinate Systems

The goal of the 3D displays is not just to present MRI data, but to be able to indicate the position of an active area of the brain, most of the time represented by a current equivalent dipole, in such a way that its position is unambiguous. One of the practical problems in this respect is the fact that three different coordinate systems generally have to be used. The first is the MRI-coordinate system. The MRI data are presented in a simple cube, in which the coordinates are integers, running in our case from 0 to 255, in all three orthogonal directions. If the voxels are not isotropic, however, the coordinate system is orthogonal, but not orthonormal. If the slices are not contiguous, interpolation of the data may be necessary.

The second coordinate system is the real world coordinate system. A magnetometer system picks up the magnetic brain activity of a subject under it. The source of the magnetic field can be calculated only with respect to the position of the sensors that measured the magnetic field. If one wants to know the position of this source in the brain, one has at least to know the distance and orientation of the head with respect to the sensors. Various solutions exist for this problem, all of which consist of placing some sort of markers on the head of the test person, at known locations (Ahlfors and Ilmoniemi, 1989). These locations have to be described with respect to a coordinate system. A convenient coordinate system has been described by de Munck (1989). In this coordinate system, the origin O is located at the middle of the line segment connecting the ear canals. The (positive) y axis runs from the origin to the right ear canal, and the (positive) x axis runs from O to the inion. The positive z axis starts from the origin and has its orientation normal to the xy plane. The position of any point on the head with respect to this coordinate system can easily be found, by measuring the distances from this point to the inion and to the ear points. Its position can then be calculated from these distances. Other points can be used instead of the ones mentioned above. The inion could very well be replaced with the nasion. The principle remains the same.

The third coordinate system is necessary to account for the use of spheres as models for the head in the inverse solution. The coordinates of the current equivalent dipole are relative to the origin of the sphere(s). Usually, a vectorial addition is sufficient to transform these coordinates into the head-coordinate system. To be able to display the location of the equivalent dipole in the MRI data, the two coordinate systems have to be matched. To be able to match them, at least three points have to be known in both coordinate systems. From these three points, a coordinate transformation can be constructed, consisting of scaling, rotation, and translation.

These three points can be found in the MRI scans by using markers. The fluid gadolinium shows up very well on (T_1-weighted) MRI scans, but also Vaseline and vitamin C tablets can be used. Small Plexiglas holders are attached to the test person's head before the scanning starts. Afterwards, the MRI coordinates from these markers can be found in the slices. Their real-world or head coordinates can be measured after they are placed on the head. If a large slice thickness is used, or a large gap between slices exists, it may not be possible to find the position of the markers in the scan accurately, if at all. To increase the accuracy of the position of the markers and to be able to match both CT and MRI data, a wedge-shaped marker can be used. An alternative approach could be to match the surface of the head derived from the MRI scans with a large number of surface points measured from the test person. These points could be at the locations of the electrodes, or just random points, generated with the help of a 3D digitizer (Gevins, 1989). A least-squares routine should be able to handle this problem.

V. Evaluation by Means of MR Images

In the cortex, the pyramidal neurons form the main source of electric activity. Due to the axial alignment of their apical dendrites and to the lamellar organization of the synaptic inputs, the population of pyramidal neurons generates dipole fields (Lopes da Silva and van Rotterdam, 1993). It is interesting to establish a quantitative relationship between the strength of the estimated ED and the dimensions of the cortical dipole layer generated by the local pyramidal cells. In order to realize this objective, we have to make some assumptions about the quantitative characteristics of the cortical dipole layer. While recording electrocorticograms, Freeman found the largest transcortical potential differences to be 1 mV over a distance of 1.5 mm. Assuming the specific resistance of the cortical tissue to be, on average, 25 Ωmm, one can estimate the transcortical dipole current density to be about 270 nAmm^{-2} (Freeman, 1975). In a very simplified way, one can calculate the strength of the ED caused by the activity of such a cortical dipole layer having a given surface (S) and distance between the poles (d). In the case of visually evoked EDs, Stok (1986) calculated for the largest components measured, having a strength of 100 nAm, that the area of the cortical layer activated should be about 400 mm^2, assuming for simplicity that the poles were separated by a distance of 1 mm and that the dipole current density was 250 nA/mm^{-2}. Thus, taking into account these basic quantities, we can estimate the active cortical area corresponding to a given ED and depict this area in an MR image. As indicated above, in practice, both the localization and the tangential component are obtained from MEG data. The angle between the tangential and the radial component is deduced from EEG data. In this way, not only the localization but also the strength and the orientation of the ED are estimated. The direction of a current dipole corresponds to the direction of the intracellular current. However, the direction of this current can be known only if the pattern of synaptic activation underlying a given field is also known from basic electrophysiological studies. For example, if we assume that an evoked field component is primarily caused by excitatory synapses in middle or deep layers of the cortex, the main intracellular current is oriented toward the cortical surface.

In order to have a measurable potential or magnetic field, a population of neurons has to be activated. One activated neuron can be described by a current dipole (if the observation point is not nearby), and a population can be described by a dipole layer. We assume that the current dipoles are continuously distributed over the layer. The electric potential and the magnetic field for any such a homogeneous dipole layer are determined by the shape of the layer's rim and corresponding curvature.

Consequently, a curved homogeneous dipole layer is equivalent to a planar one having the same rim and the same current dipole density. The field and potential distribution due to the latter can, at distances comparable to the dimensions of the layer, be approximated by a single current dipole situated in the center of the planer dipole layer. In other words, a curved dipole layer can be described by an ED that is orientated perpendicular to the plane with the same rim as that of the true activated area. A schematic illustration is shown in Fig. 5. Knowledge of the direction of the dipole and the extension of the activated patch of neurons can be used to reposition the dipole within the error estimate in order to obtain the correct solution. Only a dipole layer, where all the conditions mentioned above are met within the error estimate, can be a solution. An illustration is shown in Fig. 6.

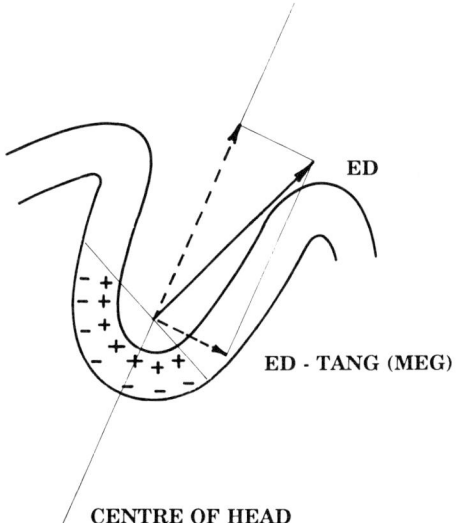

Figure 5 The location, orientation, and strength of the tangential component of the ED (ED-TANG) was obtained using the MEG. The orientation of the ED was based on EEG data. The radial direction can be estimated in the MRI by fitting a sphere. Combining the results gives an estimation of the position, strength, and orientation of the ED. ED = $\tau \times S$, where τ is the current dipole density and S is the area of the surface of the dipole layer.

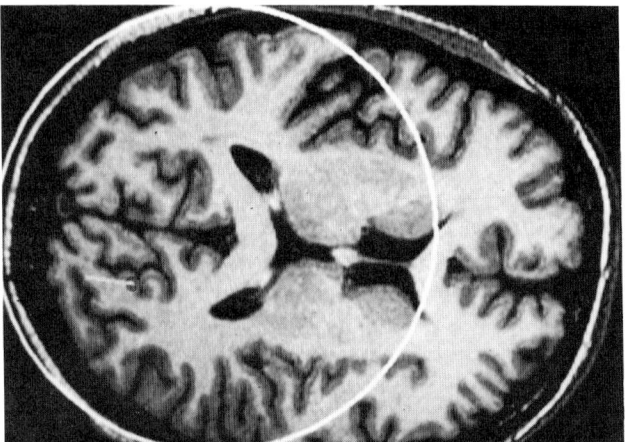

Figure 6 The VEF measured is part of a study of spatial attention on electric and magnetic responses of the brain to visual stimuli. These consisted of checkerboard patterns presented randomly to the left and right side. The target stimuli contained an extra dot in the otherwise black part of the checkerboard. The stimuli were presented on a liquid-crystal display. The checkerboard patterns were presented for a duration of 300 ms, with an interstimulus interval of 500, 600, or 700 ms. Subjects were instructed to maintain fixation at the fixation dot while attending to one visual field and counting the number of targets presented in that field. The MEG was recorded at 57 different locations over the posterior and temporal regions of the head. For each position of the magnetometer, the subjects received a series of stimuli, over 2 min, in which they attended the right or the left visual field, respectively. Very similar equivalent dipole sources locations (within 2 mm) at a latency of about 170 ms were computed for attended and unattended stimuli. In both cases, a dipole was localized in the lateral posterior cortex, contralateral to the visual field of stimulus presentation.

As discussed by Williamson *et al.* (1991), it is in principle possible to derive both the strength and the location of an ED from combined MEG and MRI data only. The tangential component of a dipole is recorded magnetically. If the local normal to the cortical surface is known from MRI, the direction of the total dipole is known. Combination of these findings gives the total current dipole moment. However, if there is still an error in the location of the dipole, then the strength obtained in this way can have a large error. This is illustrated for a dipole calculated from visual evoked fields. For the inverse procedure, two different models of the head were used. The first one consisted of a sphere, fitted to the inner surface of the skull at the back of the head. The second one was a triangulated surface description of the inside of the skull, derived from MR images of the subject. The inverse solution was in the latter case calculated using the boundary element method. The results are shown in Fig. 7. A difference of 1 cm is found in the locations of

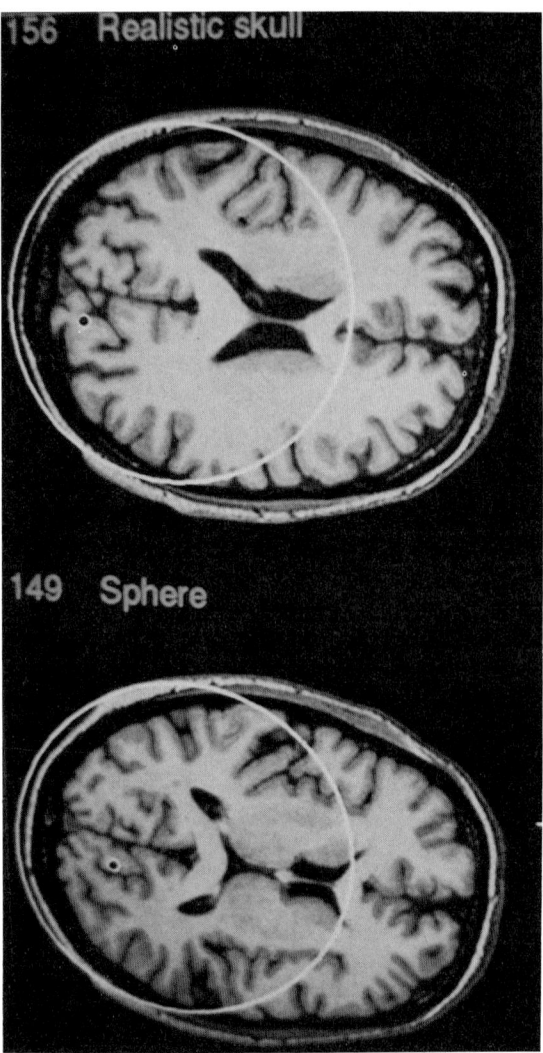

Figure 7 Localization of a source obtained using two different models of the head. In both cases, the model consists of a homogeneous compartment, either bordered by the inner surface of the skull using boundary elements (top) or by a sphere fitting the outer surface of the head, in which case the inverse problem was solved analytically (bottom). Both images show the fitted sphere. Note the difference in localization of the EDs of about 1 cm.

the dipoles, which could be explained by the difference in volume conduction. Both results are acceptable from an electrophysiological point of view, and it is the common opinion that both models are adequate as models for the head to localize activity from MEG measurements. Because the local normal to the cortical surface is totally different and there is an uncertainty about the center of the sphere, especially when a realistically shaped model of the head is used, it is obvious that the strengths of the ED obtained from these two solutions will differ.

VI. Conclusion

The fairly new and still improving MRI technique gives a host of possibilities for rendering structural information, displaying it, and providing a method to evaluate the results. The integration of MRI with EEG and MEG provides a functional imaging technique. Of course, at this moment, this technique can be used only for those cases in which the electrical activity of the brain can be described by just a few equivalent current dipoles.

Acknowledgments

The secretarial assistance of Trúc Ngô-Hà and Cristine Knaap-Cabi is gratefully acknowledged.

References

Ahlfors, S., and Ilmoniemi, R. J. (1989). Magnetometer position indicator for multichannel MEG. *In* "Advanced in Biomagnetism" (S. J. Williamson, M. Hoke, G. Stroink, and M. Kotani, Eds.), pp. 693–696. New York: Plenum.

Bomans, M., Höhne, K. H., Tiede, U., and Riemer, M. (1990). 3-D segmentation of MR images of the head for 3-D display. *IEEE Trans. Med. Imag.* **2**, 177–183.

Cuffin, B. N., Cohen, D., Yunokuchi, K., Maniewski, R., Purcell, C., Cosgrove, G. R., Ives, J., Kennedy, J., and Schoner, D. (1991). Tests of EEG localization accuracy using implanted sources in the human brain. *Ann. Neurol.* **29**(2), 132–138.

Freeman, W. J. (1975). "Mass Action in the Nervous System," p. 454. New York: Academic Press.

Gevins, A. (1989). Dynamic functional topography of cognitive tasks. *Brain Topogr.* **1/2**, 37–56.

Kemppainen, P. K., and Peters, M. J. (1991). On the forward solution of electroencephalography and magnetoencephalography. *Clin. Phys. Physiol. Meas.* **12**(Suppl. A), 95–99.

Lopes da Silva, F., and van Rotterdam, A. (1993). Biophysical aspects of EEG and magnetoencephalogram generation. *In* "Electroencephalography: Basic Principles, Clinical Applications and Related Fields," (E. Niedermeyer and F. H. Lopes da Silva, Eds.), Third ed., Baltimore/Munich: Urban & Schwarzenberg.

Meijs, J. W. H., ten Voorde, B. J., Peters, M. J., Stok, C. J., and Lopes da Silva, F. H. (1988). On the influence of various head models on the EEGs and MEGs. *In* "Functional Brain Imaging" (G. Pfurtscheller and F. H. Lopes da Silva, Eds.), pp. 31–47. Berlin: Hans Huber.

de Munck, J. C. (1989). "A Mathematical and Physical Interpretation of the Electromagnetic Field of the Brain." Ph. D. thesis. The Netherlands: University of Amsterdam.

Pascual-Maqui, R. D., and Biscay-Lirio, R. (1991). "Proceedings, 8th International Conference on Biomagnetism, Munster."

Robb, R. A., and Barillot, C. (1989). Interactive display and analysis of 3-D medical images. *IEEE Trans. Med. Imag.* **3**, 217–226.

Stok, C. J. (1986). "The Inverse Problem in EEG and MEG with Application to Visual Evoked Responses." Ph.D. thesis. The Netherlands: University of Twente.

Stok, C. J. (1987). The influence of model parameters on EEG/MEG single dipole source estimation. *IEEE Trans. Biomed. Eng.* **34**, 289–296.

Tiede, U., Hoehne, K. H., Bomans, M., Pommert, H., Riemer, M., and Wieneke, G. (1990). Investigation of medical 3-D rendering algorithms. *IEEE Trans. Comput. Graphics*, 41–53.

Williamson, S. J., Lu, Z., Karron, D., and Kaufman, L. (1991). Advantages and limitations of magnetic source imaging. *Brain Topogr.* **4**, 169–180.

29

Magnetoencephalographic Imaging of Cognitive Processes

Robert L. Rogers

Neuromagnetism Laboratory, Epilepsy and Brain Mapping Center, Hospital of the Good Samaritan,
Los Angeles, California 90017

I. Introduction

All ionic current flow is accompanied by a predictable and measurable magnetic flux that surrounds the current perpendicular to the direction of the flow of electrons. Until recently, technology that could accurately measure the small magnetic fields associated with ionic currents in the human brain, which are on the magnitude of one billionth the strength of the Earth's magnetic field, was not available. Superconductive quantum interference devices (SQUIDs) are now being used to detect the magnetic fields around the outer surface of the brain, which result from the activity of large ensembles of neurons. It has been estimated that approximately 10,000 neurons need to be simultaneously active in order to produce a magnetic field large enough to be measured using available technology (Williamson and Kaufmann, 1987).

Electric potentials and magnetic fields of the brain share many common traits, but differences in the way in which currents and magnetic fields behave in the cranium allow them to provide complementary information. Brain parenchyma and the various fluids of the brain readily conduct electric currents that can be detected as differences in potentials at the outer surface of the scalp. Magnetic fields are not conductive and therefore circle the source in which they are produced. Also, whereas electric currents are greatly influenced by the boundaries of different tissue layers, such as the skull, cerebral fluids, and cerebral tissues,

which differ vastly in their conductivity and have a profound effect on the direction of flow, magnetic fields are relatively unaffected by such layers (Barth *et al.*, 1986). Therefore, magnetic fields recorded noninvasively are primarily due to intracellular, dendritic currents, that is, the primary or impressed current source with relatively little contribution from secondary or volume conducted currents. These differences make the inverse solution, estimating the location of sources from externally measured potentials or fields, more straightforward and less information dependent with regard to these brain structures in order to provide viable solutions.

Present methods of localization of sources using magnetic field measurements rely upon dipole models in which a current flows between positive and negative poles and can be readily defined by the Biot–Savart law. If the dipole is located tangential to the outer surface of the head, the accompanying radial magnetic fields will enter and exit the outer surface of the head and can be picked up by the sensors. The strongest point at which the flux exits the head is referred to as the maximum, and the corresponding point of reentry is called the minimum. The amplitude of the signal will diminish in all directions from these two extrema, forming the distinctive dipolar pattern demonstrated in Fig. 1c, which was constructed from the waveforms to the right (Fig. 1b) at a latency of 120 ms. The source is then determined using a least-squares iteration method in which the dipole is moved around until the best possible solution is obtained. The inverse fields are then correlated with the forward solution in order to provide an estimate of the reliability of the fit to the model.

Magnetoencephalography (MEG) is able to locate sources within a few millimeters (Barth *et al.*, 1986). One recent study using surgically implanted electrodes concluded that electrical measurements were able to provide accuracy using EEG measurements that were close to those made using MEG (Cohen *et al.*, 1990). However, several aspects of this study rendered this conclusion misleading. For instance, the signal-to-noise ratio in the study was typically over 40:1 for electrical signals and in most instances was less than 10:1 for their magnetic counterparts. These discrepancies in no way reflect any real measurements made using actual sources produced in the human brain. Indeed, in their own analysis Cohen *et al.* (1990) reported high correlations between the accuracy of localization and the signal-to-noise ratio for both types of data. Although there is a slightly better signal-to-noise ratio for EEG measurements compared with that for MEG signals found in human subject evoked response studies, these differences are comparatively small and can be overcome by using a greater number of trials. The low signal-to-noise ratios reported by Cohen *et al.* (1990) are likely due to several reasons. The equipment used in the study is quite antiquated and does not reflect the noise levels of newer SQUID-based sensors. Also the placement and orientation of the dipoles will greatly influence the magnitude of signals seen on the outer surface of the brain. Cohen *et al.* (1990) place a majority of the implanted electrodes in such a way as to produce primarily tangential fields that are essentially invisible to the detectors, which apparently picked up a small radial component thus, producing diminutive amplitudes in the signal strength. Considering the fact that so many factors were stacked in favor of the EEG procedure, it is quite remarkable that the MEG still provided slightly more accurate overall results.

There is no doubt that some signals will be more readily measured using EEG, whereas others will be more amenable to MEG measurements, depending on a number of factors, including depth, orientation, and the strength of the source. Models that can simultaneously utilize EEG and MEG signals are now being developed and hopefully will provide the most accurate results and render any arguments as to which is better for localization of sources a moot point.

II. Early Contributions of MEG

Much of the earliest work in MEG was aimed at validating the procedures and concentrated on localizing signals whose origins were well established. Several of these studies used phantoms, skulls from cadavers, and implanted electrodes in humans in order to establish the accuracy of MEG localization (e.g., Barth *et al.*, 1986), which indicated that under these controlled conditions accuracies within a few millimeters were obtainable, but that deeper sources were associated with increases in variability. Romani *et al.* (1982) used a single-channel MEG system in a couple of subjects in auditory evoked response (ER) and steady-state evoked response paradigms to show that N100 emanated from the superior plane of the temporal lobe and that the response reflected the well-established tonotopic representation in the lateral–medial plane.

Some of the first investigations in our laboratory were undertaken to extend these findings to the auditory ERs. One study utilized our seven-channel neuromagnetometer and a randomly selected group of 10 subjects to validate earlier studies, to localize N100 and P200 under standardized conditions, registered onto each subject's MRI, and thus to further establish the efficacy of MEG for routine localization of ERs

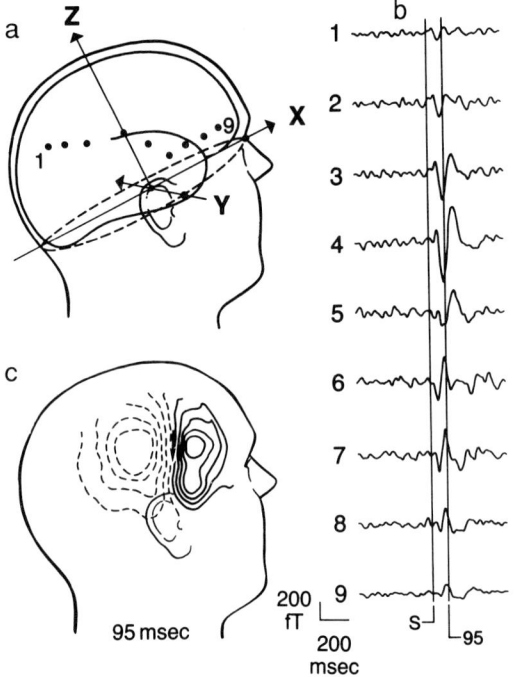

Figure 1 Construction of contour maps for dipole localization. (a) Sample for which waveforms were recorded in relation to the subject's head. (b) Waveforms from each location and changes in the amplitude of N100. (c) Isocontour map constructed from these data.

(Papanicolaou *et al.*, 1990a, 1990b). This study indicated that auditory N100 and P200 could be localized within a few millimeters of the primary auditory cortex on the superior plane of the temporal lobe. Another study used a similar paradigm to explicate the test–retest reliability of multiple procedures performed at different times (Baumann *et al.*, 1991). This study indicated that relatively high reliability was obtained.

Another interesting finding of our auditory ER investigations was that during the time course of N100 there was a highly significant and reliable movement of the dipole in an anterior direction along the superior plane of the temporal lobe (Rogers *et al.*, 1990b). Figure 2 illustrates this effect in one of our subjects. Note how the location of the dipole mirrors the contours on the temporal lobes created by the transverse sulci in both hemispheres. This effect likely represents the sequential activation of adjacent cortical columns during the time course of N100. Another study (Rogers *et al.*, 1990a) comparing the time-dependent movement of N100 to ipsilateral versus contralateral stimulation demonstrated that ipsilateral stimulation also resulted in an anterior time-dependent movement of the activation along the superior plane of the temporal

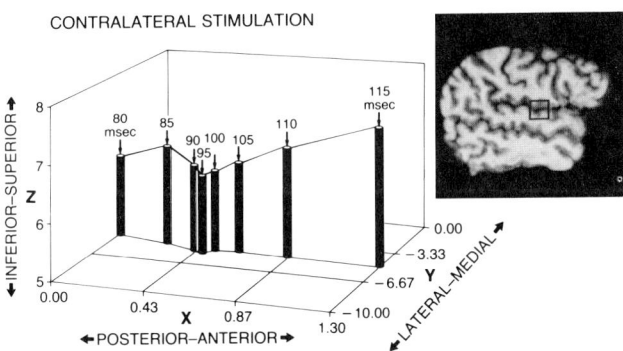

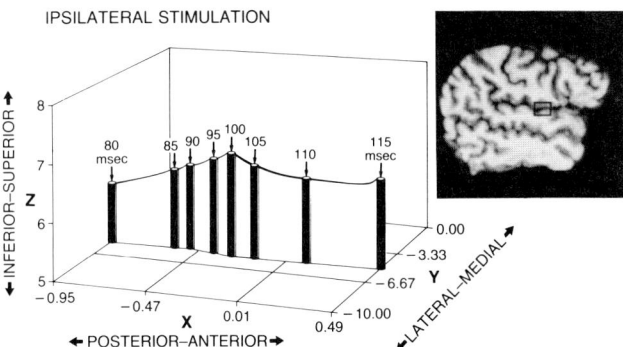

Figure 2 Time-dependent changes in dipole localization during the course of the N100 evoked response.

lobe but that it was slightly posterior to that seen during contralateral stimulation at any given latency. This appears at first to be in conflict with previous studies (Reite *et al.*, 1981; Hari and Makela, 1988), which reported that ipsilateral stimulation resulted in activity that was somewhat anterior to contralateral activity when the two were compared at their peak latencies. However, this is due to the fact that ipsilateral activity peaks at a later latency, in which the neuronal activation has progressed.

III. MEG Studies of P300

The consensus among a majority of researchers is that P300, the late positive component of ERs to aberrant, rare, and meaningful stimuli, reflects cognitive processes. This has resulted in a large volume of P300 literature over the past three decades as well as numerous attempts to establish its clinical relevance. Most studies on the nature and significance of P300 can be arranged into two broad categories. In the first are studies aimed at identification of the cognitive operations reflected by P300, which usually involve manipulation of task demands and observation of the resulting variations in amplitude, latency, and morphology.

One of the most relevant findings that has emerged from such efforts is the distinction between two varieties of P300: an early one with an average peak latency of about 240 ms and a later one with a peak latency of approximately 350 ms, called P3a and P3b, respectively (Squires *et al.*, 1975). P3a is obtained with aberrant, unexpected, nontarget stimuli that occur while the subject is engaged in a different task (Roth, 1973). It is interpreted as an index of a preattentive, basic sensory mechanism, sensitive to changes in environmental background stimulation (Squires *et al.*, 1975). In contrast, P3b obtained with task-relevant, attended stimuli is considered an index of higher order cognitive operations (Ritter and Vaughan, 1969).

The second category includes studies whose main purpose is the identification of the brain structures generating P300. The majority of MEG studies to date have concentrated on the anatomy and physiology of P300. One of the first studies in our laboratory that fall into this category used an oddball auditory stimulation in which a deviant tone was presented on 10% of the stimulus presentations (Rogers *et al.*, 1991). Figure 3 shows the electrical and magnetic waveforms in response to the frequent and rare stimuli. In the top portion of the figure, it can be seen that typical electrical evoked responses were obtained using this paradigm. That is, for frequent presentations clear

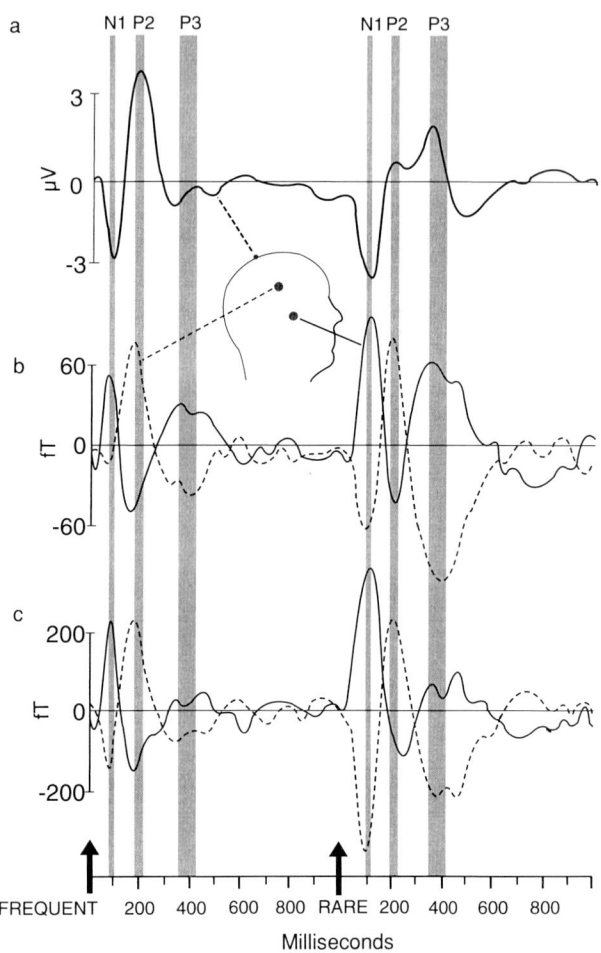

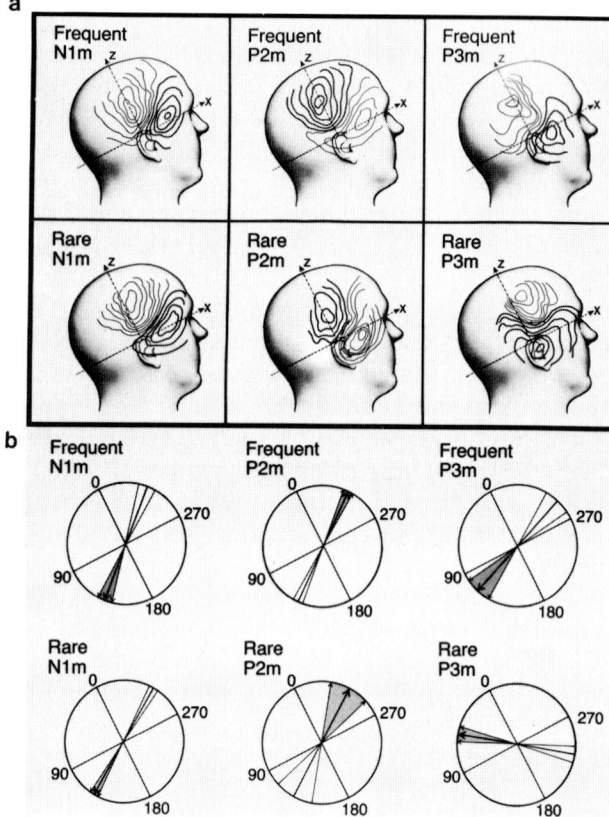

Figure 4 (a) Isocontour magnetic field maps for major peaks during frequent and rare stimulation. (b) Orientation of dipoles for magnetic fields for each peak.

Figure 3 Waveforms for the auditory evoked response, showing the appearance of P300 upon rare stimulation. (a) Electrical potentials at C_z. (b) Mean group average of 10 subjects, showing maximum and minimum magnetic fields. (c) Example of a single subject's magnetic waveforms.

N100, P200, and N2 waveforms can be identified, whereas rare stimuli produced N100, P200, and P300 peaks. Magnetic counterparts are in the next two rows of waveforms, maximum and minimum responses for the group average are in the middle, and a single subject's ER is on the bottom. Figure 4 shows the contour maps and orientation of the dipoles for all the peaks identified above for both frequent and rare stimulation. Note that the major difference during the P300 time period is a slight change in the orientation of the current flow so that the electrical potential at C_z changes from negative to positive.

Note that all the familiar peaks seen in the electrical waveforms have magnetic counterparts with clear extrema (maximum and minimum) that correspond temporally; however, this does not in and of itself establish that both have the same neural origins. One

obvious discrepancy between the electrical and the magnetic activity is the peak latency, with the magnetic peaks occurring at a later latency. This is illustrated in the left half of Fig. 5, which demonstrates that the late positive potential at C_z peaked at about 340 ms whereas the magnetic extrema peaked at approximately 465 ms, which raises the question of whether or not a common origin could produce both waveforms. The right portion of Fig. 5 illustrates the dipole strength calculated from the magnetic fields on the left. Note that the maximum point of dipole strength corresponds directly to the earlier peak seen on the electrical waveforms. The reason that the magnetic waveforms peak later is a time-dependent movement from medial to more lateral locations. Magnetic field strength is directly related to the distance from the sensors (placed laterally on the right hemisphere) according to the ratio $1/cm^2$. Thus, in this case the closer source, seen at a latency of 465 ms, half the distance of the deeper source at 340 ms, would be increased by a factor of 4 at the site of the sensors. Therefore, it does appear that both the electrical and

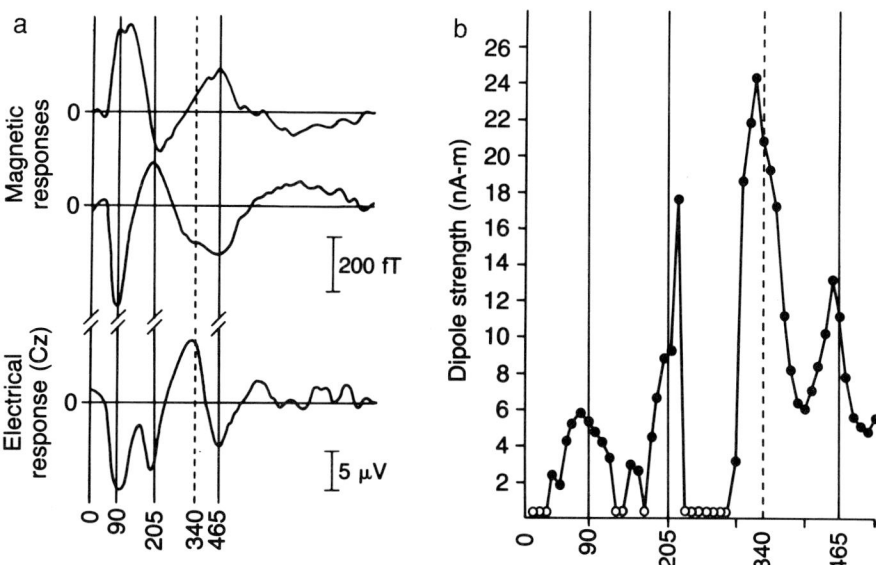

Figure 5 (a) Illustration of the difference in peaks for P300 between electrical and magnetic waveforms. (b) Plot of dipole strength, indicating that dipole strength is at its maximum at 340 ms, corresponding to the electrical peak.

the magnetic field activity were from the same generator.

Anatomically, the earlier peaks (e.g., N100 and P200) consistently localize to the primary sensory cortex for both auditory and visual stimulation. The localization of the late positive activity is more complicated. Depth electrode and lesion studies have indicated that P300-like activation occurs in the primary sensory areas, hippocampus, thalamus, frontal lobes, and parietal areas (Knight *et al.*, 1989; McCarthy *et al.*, 1989; Stapleton and Halgren, 1987). Auditory EP studies from our laboratory (Rogers *et al.*, 1991) using a rare (10%) oddball auditory signal indicated that P300 signals localized anywhere from deep structures

(hippocampus, thalamus, or both) to auditory cortex on the superior plane of the temporal lobe. Although the extreme values (most medial versus most lateral) suggested that the hippocampus and primary auditory cortex were involved, the overlap of the two sources temporally prevented us from forming a clear picture of these sources. However, two studies, oddball and omitted (Rogers *et al.*, 1992, 1993), using visual stimulation clearly indicated that there were two distinct sources, one on the primary visual cortex and the other in the vicinity of the hippocampus. Figure 6 demonstrates the hippocampal origin of a source from our visual missing stimulus experiment. Thus, we are now able to study both primary cortical and

Right hemisphere dipole

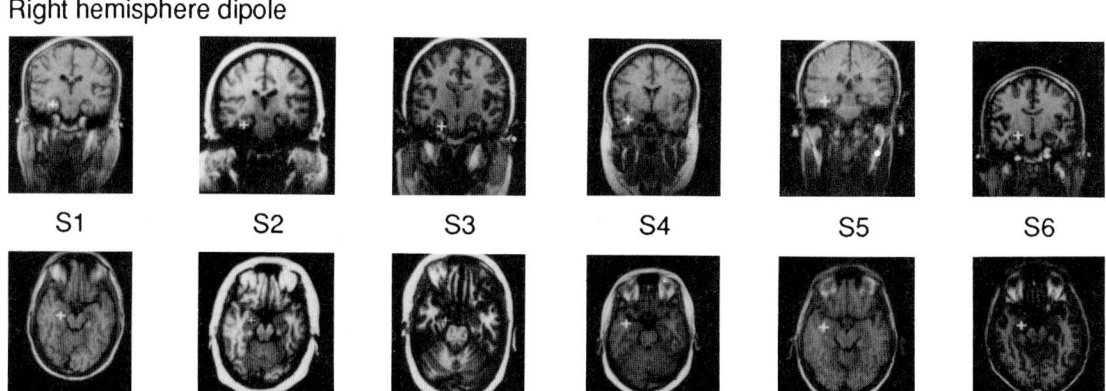

Figure 6 Location of the sources for 10 subjects (±SD) for the visual dipoles seen for P300, indicating multiple activation in the hippocampal region.

hippocampal activities during cognitive manipulations, which should provide new information on the contributions of these different neuronal systems.

IV. Visual Processing in the Middle Temporal Regions

Neuroscience studies using implanted electrodes in animals have demonstrated the involvement of inferior portions of the temporal lobe, including the superior temporal sulcus (STS) in polysensory processing with a predominance of vision (Baylis and Rolls, 1985). Neuroanatomical studies have revealed that inferior temporal (IT) regions of the brain receive afferents from all primary sensory modalities, including visual, auditory, and somatosensory (Underleider and Desimone, 1986). Individual neurons that respond to the shape, orientation, and color of visually presented stimuli have been identified in STS (Desimone *et al.*, 1985). However, STS appears to be primarily involved in motion detection and facial recognition (Bruce *et al.*, 1981). Reversible lesion and ablation studies have shown that these areas are implicated in visual attention, visual memory, and discrimination (Delacour, 1977). Recently, IT unit recordings have revealed cells that respond during heightened attention and memory (Fuster and Jervey, 1981). In humans, damage to the IT areas (including STS and the middle temporal gyrus) results in impaired visual discrimination and recognition of faces (Damasio *et al.*, 1982). To date, however, no externally recorded electromagnetic activity, corresponding to IT activity, in normal human subjects, has been reported.

In a recent study in our laboratory, 10 normal, right-handed subjects were tested using an oddball paradigm in which visual stimulation was delivered every 600 ms and lasted for 50 ms. In 10% of the trials, the stimulus was omitted on a random basis. Subjects were then instructed to count the number of missing flashes. In each run, responses from seven adjacent scalp locations were simultaneously recorded over the right hemisphere, with three to five successive runs being obtained.

The intracranial activity that gave rise to the observed magnetic field distribution was modeled as equivalent current dipoles. Dipole parameters (Cartesian coordinates, strength, and orientation) were estimated using a finite difference version of the Levenberg–Marquardt algorithm. Calculations were based on a model of a dipolar source within a sphere. The size and origin of the sphere were determined using a least-squares algorithm based on the digitized outer surface of the head, limited to the area in which

measurements were taken over the right hemisphere.

In all 10 subjects, two concurrent sets of activity, as defined by the presence of good dipolar source patterns, were easily discernible during two time periods: one occurring between 100 and 300 ms (mean, 180 ± 24.3 ms) and the other, between 300 and 600 ms (mean, 454.2 ± 22.1 ms). These periods of synchronized cortical activity correspond temporally to the early negative and later positive deflections of evoked potentials, which have been extensively studied in the past. Whether or not the dipolar sources identified by magnetic field measurements are the actual generator sites of the electrical potentials recorded along the midline has not been convincingly determined. However, some evidence has been offered to support this notion (Rogers *et al.*, 1991). Because previous studies, as described above, have characterized the magnetic field distributions during the late positive complex, we will now concentrate on the earlier magnetically recorded activity during the electrically negative deflection.

Localization of this early concurrent dipole, as indicated in Fig. 7, was in the vicinity of the superior temporal sulcus. This indicates that the source was generated in the STS, which results from a net dipole source perpendicular to the cortical surface within the

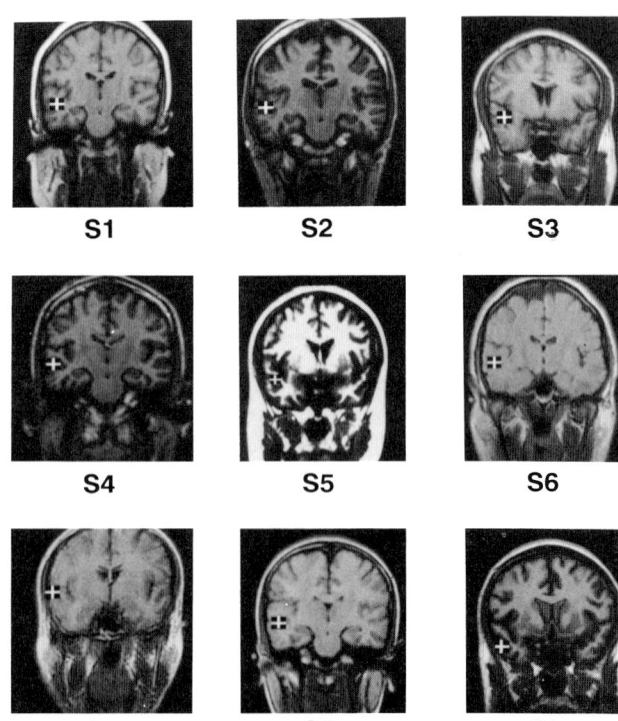

Figure 7   Locations of early negative components, indicating activation in the superior temporal sulcus.

sulcus and tangential to the outer surface of the head, which would produce a radial magnetic field pattern visible to external detectors. For comparison a recent study of the modality-specific functions of the major architectonic divisions of the inferior temporal area and superior temporal sulcus in a rhesus monkey indicated that a majority of individual cells responded to visual stimulation (Baylis and Rolls, 1985).

Because this magnetically detected activity, emanating from the region of the STS, occurred during the omission of stimulation, it apparently reflects internally initiated or endogenous neuronal activity. Animal studies have already suggested that different groups of cells in the STS area are activated either during different tasks, such as motion detection and complex visual discrimination, or by different aspects of an experimental procedure, such as the behavioral relevance of stimuli or demands on memory during delayed reaction tests. The ability to further study these processes noninvasively in intact humans could greatly enhance our ability to understand higher order visual processing. Additionally, because this area receives input from all sensory modalities, further studies could characterize how other sensory systems interact with and modify visual processing.

V. Prefrontal Contributions to Visual Attention

Since its discovery, the contingent negative variation (CNV) has been thought to originate in the vicinity of the frontal lobes (Walter and Crow, 1964). Although a significant amount of research has been devoted to clarifying the relations of CNV to stimulation/responding manipulations and to understanding prefrontal involvement in delay tasks using multiunit activity, lesion, and anatomic structure studies (Goldman-Rakic, 1987), much less has been done to combine this knowledge with data from cognitive neuroscience investigations in humans. Additionally, volume conduction of electrical potentials from remote simultaneous activity concomitant with these slow potentials makes precise localization technically difficult.

Nevertheless, recent cortical field potential studies accounting for depth–surface differences (Gemba *et al.*, 1990) confirm the prefrontal, premotor, and sensory-motor generation of earlier CNV components and motor potentials, even though some contributions from subcortical regions also occur, as shown for the readiness potential in the monkey (Bauer and Rebert, 1990). Interesting tomographic metabolic tracer studies have demonstrated that both prefrontal and ante-

rior cingulate regions participate in non-sensory-motor aspects of tasks (Roland and Friberg, 1985; Raichle, 1987), although temporal resolution limits and use of nonequivalent tasks remain problems for the desired theoretical integration.

Within the varied interpretations on the nature of prefrontal contributions to the organization of behavior, one area of study seems ubiquitous: regional specialization of function against widespread activation in a unified role (Luria, 1980; Goldman-Rakic, 1987). The first hypothesis, as old as the first clinical studies, is gaining support, although there is no consensus on the exact dimensions manifested in local differences. One possibility is a fundamental division between ventromedial and dorsolateral sectors, based on cortico–subcortical connections and manifesting itself as differing clinical conditions or deficits in the performance of specific neurocognitive tasks. Another possible specialization related to trends in cortico–cortical connectivity would be a dorsal versus ventral preferential activation corresponding to a spatial versus nonspatial attribute of tasks (Pandya and Yeterian, 1990).

In a recently initiated ongoing study in our laboratory, stimuli were presented in an array of LEDs composed of an exterior ring of 16 lights (approximately 30°) and a central rectangle of 5 × 3 lights. Two parallel computer programs controlled the interior or exterior lights, the first creating random patterns of 5 to 14 possible lights (the most central was continuously on as the eye fixation point) and the latter forming incomplete rings by keeping off 1, 2, or 3 lights in each of the four corners. Half of the trials started with a *p*, signaling the subject to attend to the peripherally presented stimuli, and half started with a *d* as the informative warning signal, which signaled the subject to attend to the internal pattern. A 1500-ms interval after the initial warning stimulus was followed by the presentation of the first stimulus (S_1); then another 1500-ms interval occurred before the presentation of the second pattern of lights (S_2). Subjects then had to determine if there was a match between the two sets on the designated task (central or foveal).

Preliminary inspections of the data to date suggest that, during the warning intervals in which differentiation of the task occurs, both produce a CNV pattern in the electrical potentials at F_z, but the MEG data indicate that differences in the distributions between foveal and central attention tasks are evident. More specifically, although both are located in prefrontal areas in close proximity, activation of foveal attention mechanisms demonstrated a more lateral–posterior localization than attention in the central visual field. This is in agreement with the architectonic and lesion studies mentioned above.

VI. Summary

Recent advances in electromagnetic mapping procedures appear to offer new promise in the understanding of neural mechanisms involved in high-order cognitive processing and should compliment exciting new findings being obtained using positron emission tomography, fast magnetic resonance imaging of local cerebral perfusion levels, and other recent functional imaging technologies. Within a few years, large arrays of more than 100 neuromagnetic sensors will allow three-dimensional studies of the functioning human brain, with high spatial resolution and temporal resolutions in the microsecond range. Recent studies have already demonstrated that MEG data can be used to construct tomographic images of local impressed currents (Ioannides *et al.*, 1993), which can subsequently be registered onto MRI scans to produce functional images that can be reconstructed to produce three-dimensional images.

Acknowledgments

This research was supported in part by Grants NS29540 and NS20806 from the National Institutes of Health, Bethesda, Maryland.

References

Barth, D. S., Sutherling, W., Broffman, J., and Beatty, J. (1986). Magnetic localization of a dipolar current source implanted in a sphere and a human cranium. *Electroencephalogr. Clin. Neurophysiol.* **63**, 260–273.

Bauer, H. H., and Rebert, C. S. (1990). Preliminary study on subcortical slow potentials related to the readiness potential in monkey. *Int. J. Psychophysiol.* **9**, 269–278.

Baumann, S. B., Rogers, R. L., Papanicolaou, A. C., and Saydjari, C. (1991). Intersession replicability of dipole parameters from three components of the auditory evoked magnetic field. *Brain Topogr.* **3**, 311–319.

Baylis, G. C., and Rolls, E. T. (1987). Subdivisions of the temporal lobe neocortex. *J. Neurosci.* **7**(2), 331–342.

Bruce, C., Desimone, R., and Gross, C. G. (1981). Visual properties of neurons in a polysensory area in superior temporal sulcus of the macaque. *J. Neurophysiol.* **46**(2), 369–384.

Cohen, D., Cuffin, B. N., Yunokuchi, K., Maniewski, R., Purcell, C., Cosgrove, G. R., Ives, J., Kennedy, J. G., and Schomer, D. L. (1990). MEG versus EEG localization test using implanted sources in the human brain. *Ann. Neurol.* **28**, 811–817.

Damasio, A. R., Damasio, H., and Van Hoesen, G. W. (1982). Prosopagnosia: Anatomical basis and behavioral mechanisms. *Neurology* **32**, 331–341.

Delacour, J. (1977). Inferotemporal cortex and visual memory. *Exp. Brain Res.* **28**, 301–310.

Desimone, R., Schein, S. J., Moran, J., and Ungerleider, L. G. (1985). Contour, color and shape analysis beyond the striate cortex. *Vis. Res.* **25**, 441–452.

Fuster, J. M., and Jervey, J. P. (1982). Neuronal firing in the inferotemporal cortex of the monkey in a visual memory task. *J. Neurosc.* **2**, 361–375.

Gemba, H., Sazaki, K., and Tsujimoto, T. (1990). Cortical field potentials associated with hand movements triggered by warning and imperative stimuli in the monkey. *Neurosc. Lett.* **113**, 275–280.

Goldman-Rakic, P. S. (1987). Circuitry of primate prefrontal cortex and regulation of behavior by representational memory. In "Handbook of Physiology—The Nervous System" (V. B. Mountcastle, Ed.), Vol. 5, Chap. 9. American Physiological Society.

Hari, R., and Makela, K. (1988). Modification of neuromagnetic responses of the human auditory cortex by masking sounds. *Exp. Brain Res.* **71**, 87–92.

Ioannides, A. A., Singh, K. D., Hasson, R., Baumann, S. B., Rogers, R. L., Guinto, F. C., and Papanicolaou, A. C. (1993). Comparison of single current dipole and magnetic field tomography analyses of the cortical response to auditory stimuli. *Brain Topogr.* **6**, 27–34.

Knight, R. T., Scabini, D., Woods, D. L., and Clayworth, C. C. (1989). Contribution of temporal parietal junction to the human auditory P3. *Brain Res.* **502**, 109–116.

Luria, A. R. (1980). "Higher Cortical Functions in Man." New York: Basic Books.

McCarthy, G., Wood, G. C., Williamson, P. D., and Spencer, D. D. (1989). Task dependent field potentials in human hippocampal formation. *J. Neurosc.* **9**, 4253–4268.

Pandya, D. N., and Yeterian, E. H. (1990). Prefrontal cortex in relation to other cortical areas in rhesus monkey: Architecture and connections. In "Progress in Brain Research" (H. Uylings, C. G. Van Eden, J. P. DeBruin, M. A. Corner, and M. G. Feenstra, Eds.), Vol. 85. London: Elsevier.

Papanicolaou, A. C., Baumann, B. S., Rogers, R. L., Saydjari, C., Amparo, E. G., and Eisenberg, H. M., (1990a). Localization of auditory response sources using MEG and MRI. *Arch. Neurol.* **47**, 33–37.

Papanicolaou, A. C., Rogers, R. L., Baumann, S. B., Saydjari, C., and Eisenberg, H. M. (1990b). Source localization of two evoked magnetic field components using two alternative procedures. *Exp. Brain Res.* **80**, 44–48.

Raichle, M. E. (1987). Circulatory and metabolic correlates of brain function in normal humans. In "Handbook of Physiology—The Nervous System" (V. B. Mountcastle, Ed.), Vol. 5, Chap. 16. American Physiological Society.

Reite, M., Zimmerman, J. F., and Zimmerman, J. E. (1981). Magnetic auditory evoked fields: Interhemispheric asymmetry. *Electroencephalogr. Clin. Neurophysiol.* **51**, 388–392.

Ritter, W., and Vaughan, H. G. (1969). Averaged evoked responses in vigilance and discrimination: A reassessment. *Science* **164**, 326–328.

Rogers, R. L., Papanicolaou, A. C., Baumann, S. B., Eisenberg, H. M., and Saydjari, C. (1990a). Spatially distributed cortical excitation patterns of auditory processing during contralateral and ipsilateral stimulation. *J. Cog. Neurosci.* **2**, 44–50.

Rogers, R. L., Papanicolaou, A. C., Baumann, S. B., Saydjari, C., and Eisenberg, H. M. (1990b). Neuromagnetic evidence of a dynamic excitation pattern generating the N100 auditory response. *Electroencephalogr. Clin. Neurophysiol.* **77**, 237–240.

Rogers, R. L., Baumann, S. B., Papanicolaou, A. C., Bourbon, T. W., Alagarsamy, S., and Eisenberg, H. M. (1991). Localization of the P3 sources using magnetoencephalography and magnetic resonance imaging. *Electroencephalogr. Clin. Neurophysiol.* **79**, 308–321.

Rogers, R. L., Papanicolaou, A. C., Baumann, S. B., and Eisenberg, H. M. (1992). Late magnetic fields and positive evoked potentials following infrequent and unpredictable omissions of visual stimuli. *Electroencephalogr. Clin. Neurophysiol.* **83,** 146–152.

Rogers, R. L., Papanicolaou, A. C., Basile, L. F., and Eisenberg, H. M. (1993). Magnetoencephalography reveals two distinct sources associated with late positive evoked potentials during visual oddball tasks. *Cereb. Cortex* **3,** 163–169.

Roland, P. E., and Friberg, L. (1985). Localization of cortical areas activated by thinking. *J. Neurophysiol.* **53,** 1219–1243.

Romani, G. L., Williamson, S., and Kaufman, L. (1982). Tonotopic organization of the human auditory cortex. *Science* **216,** 1339–1340.

Roth, W. T. (1973). Auditory evoked responses to unpredictable stimuli. *Psychophysiology* **36,** 219–225.

Squires, N. K., Squires, K. C., and Hillyard, S. A. (1975). Two varieties of long-latency positive waves evoked by unpredictable auditory stimuli in man. *Electroencephalogr. Clin. Neurophysiol.* **38,** 387–401.

Stapleton, J. M., and Halgren, E. (1987). Endogenous potentials evoked in simple cognitive tasks: Depth components and tasks correlates. *Electroencephalogr. Clin. Neurophysiol.* **76,** 73–85.

Underleider, L. G., and Desimone, R. (1986). Cortical connections of visual area MT in the macaque. *J. Comp. Neurol.* **248,** 190–222.

Walter, W. G., and Crow, H. J. (1964). Depth recording from the human brain. *Electroencephalogr. Clin. Neurophysiol.* **16,** 68–72.

Williamson, S., and Kaufman, L. (1987). Analysis of neuromagnetic signals. *In* "Handbook of Electroencephalography of Clinical Neurophysiology" (A. S. Gevins and A. Remond, Eds.), pp. 405–448. New York: Elsevier.

Index